全国高等中医药院校外国进修生教材

University Textbooks of Traditional Chinese Medicine
for Overseas Advanced Students

中医内科学
Traditional Chinese Internal Medicine

主编 彭 勃

Chief Editor Peng Bo

人民卫生出版社

People's Medical Publishing House

图书在版编目（CIP）数据

中医内科学/彭勃主编. —北京：
人民卫生出版社，2000
ISBN 7-117-03642-7

Ⅰ.中…　Ⅱ.彭…　Ⅲ.中医内科学
Ⅳ.R25

中国版本图书馆 CIP 数据核字（2000）第 10852 号

中 医 内 科 学

主　　编：	彭　勃
出版发行：	人民卫生出版社（中继线 67616688）
地　　址：	（100078）北京市丰台区方庄芳群园 3 区 3 号楼
网　　址：	http://www.pmph.com
E - mail：	pmph @ pmph.com
印　　刷：	北京人卫印刷厂
经　　销：	新华书店
开　　本：	787×1092　1/16　印张：34.5
字　　数：	791 千字
版　　次：	2000 年 5 月第 1 版　2002 年 4 月第 1 版第 2 次印刷
标准书号：	ISBN 7-117-03642-7/R·3643
定　　价：	58.00 元

著作权所有，请勿擅自用本书制作各类出版物，违者必究
（凡属质量问题请与本社发行部联系退换）

全国高等中医药院校外国进修生教材
总编辑委员会

顾　问　（按姓氏笔画排序）
　　　　　王延彬　韦贵康　皮持衡　刘忠德　杜　建
　　　　　李安邦　李任先　李明富　肖鲁伟　陈大舜
　　　　　范永升　尚炽昌　金志甲　郑守增　孟南华
　　　　　项　平　粟德林　高尔鑫　康锁彬　隋殿军
　　　　　谢建群　戴锡孟

主　任　吴秀芬

副主任　李道生　彭　勃

委　员　（按姓氏笔画排序）
　　　　　于铁成　冯照升　朱长仁　刘德贵　刘　毅
　　　　　齐　南　芦岳华　苏　华　李灿东　李明军
　　　　　杨公服　吴开建　张义胜　张天奉　张新仲
　　　　　张淑珍　图　娅　房家毅　赵树清　赵　毅
　　　　　饶　洪　施建明　姜敏杰　贺又舜　顾家柱
　　　　　柴可夫　黄庆娴　黄芩汉　崔洪江　曾福海

University Textbooks of Traditional Chinese Medicine for Overseas Advanced Students

Editorial Committee

Consultants (in the order of the strokes of Chinese surname)

Wang Yanbin	Wei Guikang	Pi Chiheng	Liu Zhongde
Du Jian	Li Anbang	Li Renxian	Li Mingfu
Xiao Luwei	Chen Dashun	Fan Yongsheng	Shang Chichang
Jin Zhijia	Zheng Shouzeng	Meng Nanhua	Xiang Ping
Li Delin	Gao Erxin	Kang Suobin	Sui Dianjun
Xie Jianqun	Dai Ximeng		

Director Wu Xiufen

Deputy Directors Li Daosheng Peng Bo

Committee Members (in the order of the strokes of Chinese surname)

Yu Tiecheng	Feng Zhaosheng	Zhu Changren	Liu Degui
Liu Yi	Qi Nan	Lu Yuehua	Su Hua
Li Candong	Li Mingjun	Yang Gongfu	Wu Kaijian
Zhang Yisheng	Zhang Tianfeng	Zhang Xinzhong	Zhang Shuzhen
Tu Ya	Fang Jiayi	Zhao Shuqing	Zhao Yi
Rao Hong	Shi Jianming	Jiang Minjie	He Youshun
Gu Jiazhu	Chai Kefu	Huang Qingxian	Huang Qinhan
Cui Hongjiang	Zeng Fuhai		

中医内科学

主　编　彭　勃（河南中医学院）

副主编　（按姓氏笔画排序）
　　　　　卢岳华（湖南中医学院）
　　　　　图　娅（北京中医药大学）
　　　　　柴可夫（浙江中医学院）
　　　　　谢建群（上海中医药大学）

编　委　（按姓氏笔画排序）
　　　　　于少民（黑龙江中医药大学）
　　　　　王思民（江西中医学院）
　　　　　卢岳华（湖南中医学院）
　　　　　朱长仁（南京中医药大学）
　　　　　刘　毅（天津中医学院）
　　　　　张　力（河南中医学院）
　　　　　张义胜（北京针灸骨伤学院）
　　　　　张淑珍（黑龙江中医药大学）
　　　　　张新仲（广州中医药大学）
　　　　　宋柏林（长春中医学院）
　　　　　图　娅（北京中医药大学）
　　　　　周　洁（天津中医学院）
　　　　　房家毅（河北医科大学中医学院）
　　　　　饶　洪（河南中医学院）
　　　　　赵会华（长春中医学院）
　　　　　赵清树（内蒙古医学院）
　　　　　施建明（新疆中医学院）
　　　　　柴可夫（浙江中医学院）
　　　　　黄庆娴（成都中医药大学）

　　　　谢建群（上海中医药大学）
　　　　彭　勃（河南中医学院）

主　译　朱忠宝（河南中医学院）

翻　译　朱忠宝（河南中医学院）
　　　　申　光（河南中医学院）
　　　　赵俊卿（河南中医学院）
　　　　张笑菲（河南中医学院）
　　　　石欲达（河南医科大学）
　　　　李震生（河南中医学院）
　　　　徐恒振（河南省教育委员会）
　　　　黄开传（郑州大学）
　　　　王洁华（河南中医学院）

Traditional Chinese Internal Medicine

Chief editor Peng Bo (Henan College of Traditional Chinese Medicine)
Vice-chief editors (in the order of the strokes of Chinese surname)
  Lu Yuehua (Hunan Traditional Chinese Medicine College)
  Tu Ya (Beijing University of Traditional Chinese Medicine)
  Chai Kefu (Zhejiang College of Traditional Chinese Medicine)
  Xie Jianqun (Shanghai University of Traditional Chinese Medicine)
Editors (in the order of the strokes of Chinese surname)
  Yu Shaomin (Heilongjiang University of Traditional Chinese Medicine)
  Wang Simin (Jiangxi College of Traditional Chinese Medicine)
  Lu Yuehua (Hunan College of Traditional Chinese Medicine)
  Zhu Changren (Nanjing University of Traditional Chinese Medicine)
  Liu Yi (Tianjin College of Traditional Chinese Medicine)
  Zhang Li (Henan College of Traditional Chinese Medicine)
  Zhang Yisheng (Beijing College of Acupuncture & Orthopaedics)
  Zhang Shuzhen (Heilongjiang University of Traditional Chinese Medicine)
  Zhang Xinzhong (Guangzhou University of Traditional Chinese Medicine)
  Song Bailin (Changchun College of Traditional Chinese Medicine)
  Tu Ya (Beijing University of Traditional Chinese Medicine)
  Zhou Jie (Tianjin College of Traditional Chinese Medicine)
  Fang Jiayi (Traditional Chinese Medicine College of Hebei Medical University)
  Rao Hong (Henan College of Traditional Chinese Medicine)
  Zhao Huihua (Changchun College of Traditional Chinese Medicine)
  Zhao Qingshu (Inner Mongolia College of Traditional Chinese Medicine)
  Shi Jianmin (Xinjiang College of Traditional Chinese Medicine)
  Chai Kefu (Zhejiang College of Traditional Chinese Medicine)
  Huang Qingxian (Chengdu University of Traditional Chinese Medicine)
  Xie Jianqun (Shanghai University of Traditional Chinese Medicine)
  Peng Bo (Henan College of Traditional Chinese Medicine)
Chief Translator Zhu Zhongbao (Henan College of Traditional Chinese Medicine)
Translators Zhu Zhongbao (Henan College of Traditional Chinese Medicine)
  Shen Guang (Henan College of Traditional Chinese Medicine)
  Zhao Junqing (Henan College of Traditional Chinese Medicine)
  Zhang Xiaofei (Henan College of Traditional Chinese Medicine)

Shi Yuda (Henan Medical University)
Li Zhensheng (Henan College of Traditional Chinese Medicine)
Xu Hengzhen (The Provincial Education Commission of Henan)
Huang Kaichuan (Zhengzhou University)
Wang Jiehua (Henan College of Traditional Chinese Medicine)

前 言

随着世界范围内中医药热潮的涌动，前来我国学习、研究中医药学的各国留学生（进修生）日益增多。已经形成了一支学习、继承、传播、发展中医药事业不可忽视的力量。为了适应中医药学高水平国际交流形势的迫切需要，在上级有关领导部门的支持下，1995 年在全国中医药高等教育国际交流与合作学会年会上，由北京中医药大学、广州中医药大学、河南中医学院、浙江中医学院等 21 所中医药高等院校发起协作编写这套"全国高等中医药院校外国进修生教材"，以期为促进中医药学科体系的弘扬传播，为进一步拓展高等中医药教育的国际交流与合作的事业做出应有的贡献。

本套系列教材采取英汉对照形式，包括《中医基础学》、《中医诊断学》、《中药学》、《方剂学》、《中医内科学》、《针灸学》六本。分别由浙江中医学院、北京中医药大学、福建中医学院、天津中医学院、河南中医学院和广州中医药大学担任主编单位。为确保本教材的编写质量，协编院校成立了教材编写委员会，由北京中医药大学国际学院院长吴秀芬教授任主任，广州中医药大学李道生教授、河南中医学院副院长彭勃教授任副主任，负责组织协调本套教材的中英文编写、翻译及审订、审校工作。

本套教材的编写原则是既坚持中医药学体系的系统性、科学性、独特性和实践性，又注意到阅读对象在学习时间、语言及民族文化心理等方面的特殊性，在确保教学内容的深度、广度的前提下，努力坚持文字简约、通顺易懂，篇幅精练、阐述明确、利于实用。

本套教材编写过程中基本按照教学大纲要求，并参照高等中医药院校五版（部分六版）教材和高等中医药院校外国进修生教材的主要内容，注重协调学术发展中的继承与创新、理论与实践的关系。各书主编及作者均为多年从事高等中医药对外教育第一线的教师，具有大量的实践经验和教学体会，善于针对留学生（进修生）特点进行教学。可以说是一套较为成熟的、结合中医药理论与对外教学实际的、实用性较强的系列教材。

在本套教材的英译工作中各校专家投入了大量精力，为尽可能统一规范英译中医名词术语问题，1996 年底在福州中医学院专门召开各书主要英译人员会议。各书在中文定稿时均专门召开主编、副主编审稿会，严格复审、终审，反复斟酌修改。充分注意到留学生语言及文化差异等特点。

中医药学走向世界，尤其是中医药学传统理论走向世界，面临着从实践技能的介绍到思维模式的沟通等等不同层面上的"跨文化传播"问题。因此，本系列教材经过全体编写人员和英译人员的不懈努力，也仅仅是为这一长期目标进行一些初步的探索。限于条件及水平，不足之处敬待使用者指出，以便不断促进高等中医药院校留学生教学工作的深入和提高。

全国中医药高等教育国际交流与合作学会
英汉对照全国高等中医药院校外国进修生教材编委会

PREFACE

Alongside the worldwide enormous upsurge of interest in traditional Chinese medicine more and more overseas (advanced) students come to China to pursue it, and they have become a force not to be ignored in study, inheritance, dissemination and development of traditional Chinese medicine. To meet the urgent high-leveled international exchange in this area, there arose an idea to compile a series of English-Chinese college textbooks of traditional Chinese medicine for overseas students on the 1995 annual meeting of the National Association of TCM Overseas Higher Education & Exahonge.

The motion was put forward by 21 universities and colleges of TCM headed by the Beijing University of TCM, Guangzhou University of TCM, Henan College of TCM, Zhejiang College of TCM, etc. with the support of the authority concerned. It is expected the series of textbooks will push dissemination of the scientific system of TCM and make due contribution to international exchange and cooperation in traditional Chinese medical education.

In bilingual form, the series includes six textbooks, namely: Basic Theory of Traditional Chinese Medicine, Traditional Chinese Diagnostics, Chinese Materia Medica, Chinese Medical Formulae, Traditional Chinese Internal Medicine and Acupuncture-Moxibustion.

The following six universities and colleges of TCM located in Zhejiang province, Beijing, Fujian province, Tianjin, Henan province and Guangzhou assume the responsibility for the chief editors. To ensure the quality an editorial committee has been established chaired by Prof. Wu Xiufen, Dean of the International School, Beijing University of TCM. The vice-chairmen are Prof. Li Daosheng, Guangzhou University of TCM and Prof. Peng Bo, Vice-président of the Henan College of TCM. They are in charge of coordination of the compilation, translation and editing.

The series adheres to the systematic scientific and practical nature and uniqueness of the traditional Chinese medical theory, and the specific characteristics of the readers' language, national, cultural psychology and their time spent on study. Predicated on the depth and breadth of the knowledge we advocate simple language easy to understand, limited space, clear exposition and practical usage.

In compilation the series is almost based on the requirement of the syllabus with reference to the mainstay of the Textbooks for Students of Colleges of TCM (6th edition) and the Textbooks for Foreign Advanced Students in association with inheritance and creation, theory and practice in academic progress. The chief editors and authors are faculty members of these universities and colleges engaged in education for foreign students for years. They have accumulated a wealth of experience in teaching of overseas students in accordance with their special characteristics. The series can be regarded as a well-thought-out, practical textbooks which combine the theory of TCM with experience in external teaching.

Great energies have been devoted to the English version. To standardize the Chinese medical terms a special meeting was called for the translators at the Fujian College of TCM at the end of 1996. Chief and deputy-chief editors have gone over the manuscripts and given their comments and suggestions. The series has gone through repeated revision and final revision and the characteristics of the foreign students' language and cultural difference are constantly stressed.

Introduction of traditional Chinese medical therapy, especially its theory to the world is actually a kind of cross-culture dissemination in different levels, from healing art to mode of thinking. With the efforts of the compiling staff and translators it is only a preliminary probe for the long-standing goal.

Because of the present condition and level, the editors hope that readers will comment on the shortcomings of the series to help promote the advance of TCM education for foreign students.

Editorial Committee,
University Textbooks of Traditional Chinese Medicine for
Overseas Advanced Students, National Association of
TCM Overseas Higher Education & Exchange

编写说明

本书是在全国高等中医药院校留学生教育协编教材编委会领导下，由全国16所高等中医药院校长期从事留学生教育的专家协作编写完成。主要供来华学习中医专业的留学生、进修生使用，也适用于世界各地的中医药爱好者。

本书以中国高等医药院校《中医内科学》教材为基础，针对留学生、进修生的需要和特点，结合留学生教育的实际，在体例和内容上做了一定的调整、提炼和补充。在总论中，主要增加了"中医内科学的特点"的介绍。在各论中，重点选择介绍40种病，每个病均按"概念"、"病因病机"、"诊断与鉴别"、"辨证论治"、"小结"、"思考题"等，分项论述。力求做到"概念"清晰准确、"病因病机"简明扼要、"诊断与鉴别"简练实用；"辨证论治"中，增加了"辨证要点"、"病机概要"、"调护要点"，以提纲挈领、突出重点、体现特色；"小结"主要以图表形式归纳，做到简明精练，便于总结和记忆；最后，以"思考题"的形式，列出该病的重点和难点，促进和帮助学生自学。书末附有"病名索引"和"方剂索引"。

由于不少留学生，特别是短期进修生都有一定的西医学基础，因此，本书在每个病的"概念"中归纳了常见的西医病名以资参照；在"辨证要点"中，也点出该证型常见的西医疾病；此外，还专编了"病名索引"，以便留学生在学习的过程中，中西互参，更好地理解和掌握中医学"同病异治、异病同治"的规律和特点。

中医专业留学生教育有着自身的规律和特点，由于我们水平有限，书中纰缪、粗浅之处在所难免，望同仁不吝指正，提出宝贵意见，以便进一步完善。

在本书翻译过程中，承蒙中国中医研究院蔡景峰教授审阅，在此表示衷心感谢！

全国高等中医药院校外国进修生教材

《中医内科学》编委会

FOREWORD

The purpose of this textbook is to satisfy the needs of overseas students who come to China to study traditional Chinese medicine, and those who are interested in TCM all over the world. Under the guidance of Editorial Committee of University Textbook of TCM for Overseas Advanced Students, the textbook is completed by the experts who have engaged for many years in teaching Internal Medicine of TCM to overseas students.

This textbook is based on the textbook of Internal Medicine of TCM adopted by Chinese TCM colleges with some adjustments, extraction and supplements in its style and contents in order to make it suitable for overseas students. In the "Introduction", the features of TCM are supplemented, while in the texts, forty diseases are discussed and each disease is discussed under the items of General, Etiology and Pathogenesis, Diagnosis and Discrimination, Selecting Treatment by Differentiating Syndromes, Summary and Discussions. In compiling the textbook, our efforts have been made to get General clear and accurate, Etiology and Pathogonesis concise, Diagnosis and Discrimination brief and practical, while in Selecting Treatment by Differentiating Syndromes, Main Points of Differentiation, Pathogenesis and Nursing Points are supplemented aiming to bring out the essentials, lay stress on the key points and reflect the features, Summary is in chart-form which makes the general idea of each text clear at a glance and easy to remember; Discussions are meant to lay out the key and difficult points to help the students to study independently; Recipe Index and Disease Index are attached at the end of the textbook.

Considering that many overseas students have some knowledge of Western Medicine, relative disease names by Western Medicine are included in General and Main Points of Differentiation for their reference. The Disease Index is aimed at helping the students to master the laws and features of "treating the same disease with different methods and vice versa" by means of making inter-references of TCM and Western Medicine.

The Compilers

目 录

总 论

1 绪论 ··· 1
  1.1 中医内科学的定义和范围 ·· 1
  1.2 中医内科学的特点 ··· 1
  1.3 学习中医内科学的要求和方法 ·· 4
2 中医内科学诊疗原则与方法 ··· 6
  2.1 五邪病机病证基本概念 ·· 6
  2.2 六经与卫气营血病机病证基本概念 ··· 14
  2.3 气血病机病证基本概念 ··· 16
  2.4 脏腑病机病证基本概念 ··· 18
  2.5 内科治疗 ··· 29

各 论

1 感冒 ··· 33
2 咳嗽 ··· 37
3 哮证 ··· 41
4 喘证 ··· 45
5 痰饮 ··· 50
6 自汗、盗汗 ··· 55
7 心悸 ··· 59
8 胸痹 ··· 63
9 厥证 ··· 67
10 中风 ··· 71
11 痉证 ··· 75
12 头痛 ··· 78
13 眩晕 ··· 82
14 不寐 ··· 85
15 郁证 ··· 88
16 癫狂 ··· 92
17 痫证 ··· 95

18	胃痛	97
19	呕吐	101
20	呃逆	104
21	泄泻	107
22	痢疾	111
23	便秘	115
24	虫证	118
25	腹痛	121
26	胁痛	124
27	黄疸	127
28	积聚	130
29	臌胀	133
30	血证	137
31	水肿	145
32	淋证	149
33	癃闭	153
34	腰痛	156
35	消渴	159
36	遗精	162
37	痹证	165
38	痿证	168
39	内伤发热	171
40	虚劳	175

附　录

| 1 | 方剂索引 | 181 |
| 2 | 西医病名索引 | 192 |

CONTENTS

General Programme

1 Introduction ··· 197

    1.1   The Definition and Scope of TCM Internal Medicine ············· 197
    1.2   The Characteristics of TCM Internal Medicine ····················· 197
    1.3   Requirements and Methods in Studying TCM Internal Medicine ············ 205

2 Therapeutic Principles and Methods of TCM Internal Medicine ········· 207

    2.1   Basic Concept of the Pathogenesis and Syndromes Caused by the Five Pathogenic Factors ··· 207
    2.2   Basic Concept of the Pathogenesis and Syndromes of the Six Meridians and *Wei*, *Qi*, *Ying* and *Xue* ····················· 221
    2.3   Basic Concept of the Pathogenesis and Syndromes of *Qi* and Blood ············ 226
    2.4   Basic Concept of the Pathogenesis and Syndromes of *Zang – Fu* Organs ········ 230
    2.5   Medical Treatment ··· 248

Each Exposition

1   **Cold** ·· 256
2   **Cough** (*Ke Sou*) ·· 262
3   **Asthma with Wheezing** ··· 270
4   **Dyspnea** ·· 277
5   **Fluid Retention** ·· 285
6   **Spontaneous Perspiration & Night Sweat** ·························· 294
7   **Palpitation** ·· 300
8   **Pectoral Pain with Stuffiness** ··· 306
9   **Syncope** (*Jue* **Syndrome**) ··· 314
10   **Apoplexy** ·· 321
11   **Convulsive Disease** ··· 329
12   **Headache** ·· 333
13   **Vertigo** (*Xuan Yun*) ·· 340
14   **Insomnia** ··· 345
15   **Melancholia** ··· 350

16	Mania – Depressive Psychosis	356
17	Epilepsy	361
18	Stomachache	365
19	Vomiting	371
20	Hiccup	377
21	Diarrhea	382
22	Dysentery	388
23	Constipation	394
24	Parasitic Syndrome (*Chong Zheng*)	400
25	Abdominal Pain	405
26	Hypochondriac Pain	411
27	Jaundice	416
28	The Syndrome of *Ji Ju* (Abdominal Mass)	422
29	Tympanites	428
30	Bleeding Syndrome	434
31	Edema	447
32	Stranguria	454
33	*Long Bi*	461
34	Lumbago	466
35	*Xiao Ke*	471
36	Spermatorrhea	476
37	*Bi* Syndrome	482
38	Flaccidity Syndrome (*Wei Zheng*)	487
39	Fever Due To Internal Injury	493
40	Consumptive Disease (*Xu Lao*)	500

Appendix

| 1 | Indexes of Recipes | 511 |
| 2 | Indexes of Diseases of Western Medicine | 531 |

总 论

1 绪论

1.1 中医内科学的定义和范围

中医内科学是用中医理论阐述内科所属病证的病因病机及其证治规律的一门临床学科。

中医内科学是突出体现中医学理论体系特色，突出代表中医实践体系优势，在中医学领域中占有重要位置的学科。

内科学有着广泛的治疗领域，按中医学理论可分为外感病、内伤病两大系列。外感病主要指《伤寒论》、《温病学》所说的伤寒、风温、暑温、湿温等热性病，它们主要是按六经、卫气营血和三焦的病理变化进行证候归类；内伤病包括《金匮要略》等书所说的脏腑经络诸病，它们主要是以脏腑、气血津液、经络的病理变化和病机学说指导辨证论治。外感病与内伤病既有区别又有联系。中医内科学就是在这一广阔的范围内，以中医理论阐述其发病原因、病变机制，探讨诊疗原则和方法。本书所讨论的内容以内伤病为主。

1.2 中医内科学的特点

中医内科学集中、突出体现了中医学理论与实践体系的特点。中医学作为研究生命现象、揭示疾病过程、探讨治疗机制和养生防病的医学学科，与其它各地域、民族的传统医学相比，与当代西医学相比，都显示出体系自身的特色。

中医学把人体看作是一个脏腑与体表之间相互协同的、精神思维活动与机体生理病理状态相互影响的有机整体。同时它还强调人的生命活动要适应外界自然环境和社会环境；并综合、宏观、动态地看待生命和疾病过程，这就是中医学的主要特色之一——整体观念。这种整体医学模式与当代西医学的生物-心理-社会医学模式同样科学先进，而它比后者的产生早了两千多年。中医学以中国古代哲学精华—阴阳学说、五行学说和天人相应论作为基本指导思想，使中医学辨证论治体系蕴涵着丰富的唯物辩证法精神。中医内科学将这种理论体系和指导思想具体地贯彻于临床领域，充分体现了中医学的特点和优势。

1.2.1 谨守病机 治病求本

病机，指疾病发生、发展与变化的机制和规律。中医理论认为：疾病过程中，病机的演变是反映病变本质、反映人体阴阳盛衰状况的关键所在。因此，在中医内科辨证论治过程中，极为重视"谨守病机"。

疾病种类繁多，临床症状复杂，个体差异显著，因而导致了病理状态下多种多样的临床表现。这些症状多表现为散在和局部，在疾病的某些阶段甚至会出现假象。因此，中医治病反对简单的头痛治头、脚痛医脚，而主张抓住证候类型、全面分析病机、追本溯源，即"治病求本"。

中医内科学，每一疾病都有不同的证候类型，每一证候都有其具体的病机，但从中医理论总体来看，可以概括为邪正盛衰、阴阳失调、气血失常三大规律。临证时无论患者病变表现多么复杂错综，多么异乎寻常，只要明辨证候，谨守病机，便能够达到治病求本之目的。

邪正盛衰　中医学发病理论认为：正气存内，邪不可干；邪之所凑，其气必虚。邪正的力量对比、交争是疾病发展和转归的根本原因。邪气亢盛则正气受损，疾病深入；正气强盛则驱邪外出，病势减退。所以，辨证论治过程中，首先要衡量某一具体疾病的某一具体阶段上正邪双方力量对比情况，以决定或攻邪，或扶正，或攻补兼施。

邪正盛衰直接导致疾病性质的虚实变化。邪气盛则实，即病变过程以邪气亢盛为矛盾的主导方面；精气夺则虚，指以正气（阴阳气血津液等）虚损为矛盾主导方面的病变反应。在内科学治疗领域内，实证和虚证以及虚实挟杂证极为常见。临床常见的痰涎壅盛、食滞不消、水湿内泛、瘀血内阻、热邪亢盛、腑气不通等，均以邪气亢盛为主；反之，气血生成不足或消耗过度、脏腑功能低下、津液化生不足、经络功能衰减等等，均以正气虚损为主。同时还必须注意，邪正力量对比在疾病状态中是贯穿始终的，又是在不同阶段表现各异的。另外，疾病本身就是邪正交争导致的结果。所以在临证中，纯虚无实与纯实无虚的状态是不存在的，应该强调的是"矛盾的主导方面。"

邪正盛衰在病变过程中会导致假象出现，即症状与疾病本质相反，如"大实有羸状，至虚有盛候"。真虚假实或真实假虚在疾病的许多关键阶段极易出现，所以临证时必须善于分析病机，把握本质，澄清真假，治病求本。

阴阳失调　中医学认为，阴平阳秘是机体健康状态总的概括。反之，各种致病因素导致人体的阴阳运动消长失去相对的动态平衡，形成阴阳偏盛偏衰或阴阳离绝，则表现为疾病发生或恶化。因此，阴阳是疾病发生发展的内在根据，阴阳失调是中医病机理论的重要组成部分。人生有形，不离阴阳。阴阳失调概括了机体脏腑、经络、气血、营卫失调等总体的病理关系，是对人体生命活动过程中出现的各种功能性、器质性病变的本质把握。

阴阳失调涵盖了人体病机变化，因而有着极为错综复杂的表现形式。总的可以概括为以下几大类别：

①阴阳偏盛。机能亢奋，热象显著者，称为阳盛，阳盛主要见于五志化火、六淫入内化热、气滞血瘀食积化热等一系列实热证；阴盛，则指机体在病变时表现出阴邪偏盛、机能障碍、寒象显著者，主要见于感受阴寒之邪或过食生冷导致寒邪直中脾胃、阴寒内盛等一系列实寒证。

从阴阳互根的观点来看，阴盛则阳病，实寒证时会有不同程度的阳气不足；同样，阳盛则阴病，邪热亢盛的实热证也会耗损阴津。但阴盛或阳盛是病机的主导方面。

②阴阳偏衰。包括阴虚、阳虚两方面。阳虚指人体功能减退、阳气虚损的病理变化，多由先天不足、后天失养及劳倦内伤、久病耗损导致。阳虚则阴相对偏胜，故阳虚则内寒，表现为畏寒肢冷、神疲倦息等虚寒证。阴虚指体内阴血、津液、精的亏耗，由此导致的滋养、濡润功能减退。阴虚则阳气失制，相对偏胜，阴虚则内热，故表现为五心烦

热、骨蒸潮热、盗汗咽干等虚热证。

阴阳互根理论还提示，阴损及阳、阳损及阴还能导致阴阳两虚的病理状态。这种情况下，必须把握病变本质，审因论治。此外，阴阳失调还有一类特殊病机，即阴阳格拒，包括阴盛格阳和阳盛格阴两方面。阴盛格阳在临床上表现为真寒假热；阳盛格阴表现为真热假寒。阴阳格拒的产生是由于阴邪（或阳邪）亢盛，内伏于里，迫阳（或阴）外出所致。

随着病机的变化，阴阳失调最危重的阶段是亡阴或亡阳导致的阴阳欲绝。亡阴由机体大量消耗阴血津液造成；亡阳为机体阳气耗竭或突然脱失，引起全身功能严重衰竭。此时如未能及时救治，便会发生"阴阳离决、精气乃绝"的严重后果。

气血失常 人体气血亦属一对阴阳关系。气属阳，主温煦，代表脏腑功能和机体正气；血属阴，主濡养，为生命活动的物质营养成分。气血之间又有相互促进，相互化生的生理联系。所以，气血失常的病机变化，既包括了气生化不足或耗散太过造成的气虚、气脱以及气的运行失常造成的气滞、气逆、气闭等气机失调，也包括了血液生成不足或消耗太过导致的血虚，还包括血液运行障碍出现的血瘀及血热出血等。此外，由于气血相互关联，临证还常常见到气滞血瘀、气虚血瘀、气不摄血、气随血脱、气血两虚等病机变化。

气血失常与脏腑功能活动有直接、密切的关系。因为肺主气，心主血；脾为气血生化之源，脾统血；肝藏血、主疏泄；肾主纳气，藏精，精血同源，所以，气血失常的病机变化总要落实到具体脏腑的功能低下或失调方面。关于气血病机与脏腑病机见2.3及2.4两节。

总之，千变万化的临床表现，反映出复杂多样的病机变化。临证时只要真正理解并善于把握邪正盛衰、阴阳失调、气血失常这些本质性的病机规律，便能够执简驭繁，治病求本。

1.2.2 辨病与辨证

中医学认识疾病和治疗疾病的基本原则是辨证论治，辨证论治也是中医内科学的显著特点之一。

中医内科学的治疗领域非常广阔，在进行辨证论治的过程中，辨证就是将四诊收集到的症状、体征及有关资料进行分析、综合，辨明病因、病性、病位、病势，得出证候判断的结论；论治则是以辨证为前提，在辨证的基础上针对病机确立相应的治疗原则和方法。辨证是决定治疗的前提和依据，论治是治疗的手段和方法。辨证论治的过程，就是认识疾病和解决疾病的过程。辨证和论治，是诊治疾病过程中相互联系、不可分割的两个方面，是理论和实践相结合的体现。

中医认识并治疗疾病，既辨病又辨证。"证"即"证候"，是机体在疾病发展过程中某一具体、特定阶段上的病理概括。一个证，涵盖了病位、病性、病因、邪正关系、气血阴阳盛衰变化等多种因素，能够全面、深刻、准确地揭示疾病发展过程中某一阶段病理变化的本质。而"病"则是疾病的名称，如痢疾、哮喘、中风、消渴等。"辨病"是鉴别区分不同的疾病；而"辨证"则是辨别同一疾病不同的证候类型，从而使论治更有针对性。如"感冒"是一种病，其中，包含多种证候类型，既有"风热表证"又有"风寒表证"，而这种"风寒表证"或"风热表证"就是对感冒病中某些具体病理变化的概括；

病位在表，病因属风寒或风热。而后才能确定用辛温解表或辛凉解表的方法，给以适当地治疗。由此可见，辨证论治既区别于头痛治头、脚痛医脚的局部对症疗法，又区别于不分主次，不分阶段，一方对一病的治疗方法。

综上所述，中医内科学的特点之一，就是辨病与辨证相结合，中医从汉唐时代始，多是在辨病的前提下辨证论治的。要学好中医内科学，就要深入学习和研究"病"与"证"的关系。由于中医内科学的病名常以疾病过程中最重要、最突出的症状来命名，有的能反映疾病的基本矛盾，有的则过于宏观和笼统；而证候则具体而详细地概括了该病发展过程中某一阶段的病理机制，对疾病的诊疗有着十分重要而现实的指导意义，因此，中医治病尤重"辨证"。

1.2.3 同病异治，异病同治

中医内科学的另一特点，是建立在辨证论治基础上，强调辨病与辨证相结合的"同病异治、异病同治。"

所谓同病，是指不同患者患有以相同主要症状为基本病变的疾病。然而由于患者体质的气血阴阳盛衰状况不同，发病时间、季节、地域不同，病理变化处于疾病过程的不同阶段，所反映出来的"证"势必有所差异。而这种表现在"证"方面的差异，就构成了同病异治的基础。因为，中医学辨证论治体系的特点与优势是集中地通过"证"体现出来的。中医内科学在诊疗疾病时，主要不是着眼于"病"，而是着眼于病机的区别，即重视"证"。在中医学里，"证"反映了具体的病机变化，证与病机是一致的。所患有同一种"病"的患者，可以有差异颇大的"证"，有了这种各自不同的"证"，必然要有治则治法完全不同的治疗手段。如"感冒"一病，由于发病季节不同，病因病机不同，人体正气强弱不同，就可分为风寒证、风热证、暑湿证、气虚、阴虚等不同证型，对这些不同的证型就应有针对性地采取辛温解表、辛凉解表、清暑祛湿解表、益气解表、滋阴解表等不同的治疗方法。这就是"同病异治。"

反之，不同疾病在其发展过程中的某一阶段，或不同疾病的患者机体在病变过程中某一阶段，可以出现相同的"证"——基本相同的病理机转，具有某种共性。这就是异病同治的前提。中医内科学的异病同治，就是不同的疾病在有共同的病机证候的前提下，可采取相同的治则治法。如：腹泻、脱肛、子宫脱垂、胃下垂等是完全不同的"病"，而其病变机制皆是由于脾气虚弱，不能升提统摄所致，那么，它们的"证"就相同。因此均可用补脾益气、升阳统摄的方法来治疗。这就是"异病同治"。

辨证论治作为指导临床诊治疾病的基本法则，要能辩证地看待病和证的关系，既可看到一种病可以包括几种不同的证，又能看到不同的病在其发展过程中可以出现同一种证。由此可见，中医学之所以强调"证"的概念，是因其蕴含着丰富的病机内容，是中医学独特的辨证论治体系的核心。"同病异治、异病同治"的前提与核心，就在于其"证"之异同——"证同治亦同，证异治亦异"。因此，同病异治、异病同治体现了中医内科学和整个中医学辨证论治理论体系的精神实质和特色优势。

1.3 学习中医内科学的要求和方法

中医内科学是运用中医基本理论阐述内科领域各种病证的病因病机及论治规律、探讨具体治法和疗效的临床学科，是中医学中极为重要的一门课程。

学习中医内科学的要求，是掌握本课程的基础理论、基本知识和基本技能，了解和掌握中医内科学的特点及常见病的治疗，提高临床和科学研究能力。

学习中医内科学的方法，包括系统的理论学习（课堂讲授）、课间教学见习和毕业前的临床实习三个阶段，而每一阶段的侧重点是不同的。理论学习要求比较深刻地理解中医基本理论的实质内涵，牢固掌握中医内科学的特点和辨证论治体系内容；课间教学见习则要求在教师带领下进行内科门诊诊断、辨证、拟方的见习和试诊，加强对理论教学的理解并接触临床，理论结合实践，增加感性认识；第三阶段则是直接在上级医师指导下进行内科临床实践，直接为患者服务，全面检验理论基础，锻炼提高临床基本技能以及分析病情、治疗疾病的综合能力——辨证论治的掌握和运用。

学习中医内科学，要对中医专业前期各基础学科经常复习，为中医内科学奠定坚实的基础。内科学里的某些病证，既有区别、又有联系，要前后互参。

学习中医内科学，要理论联系实际，善于综合、分析、判断，把握病变本质；要有扎实的诊断技能，只有准确地收集四诊资料，才有可能正确地辨证、有效地论治。

学习中医内科学，要牢固掌握中医内科学常用的辨证论治方法，掌握病机病证理论，通过"认识—实践—认识提高—指导实践"的反复强化过程，达到不断提高诊疗水平的目的。

学习中医内科学，要牢牢记住中医内科学的特点和优势：谨守病机、治病求本；辨病与辨证结合，重在辨证；同病异治与异病同治。充分发挥中医药学的独特优势，为全人类的健康做出贡献。

思考题

1. 为什么说"谨守病机、治病求本"是中医内科学的特点？
2. 你怎样理解"辨病与辨证结合"？哪一方面是中医学所侧重的？
3. 同病异治、异病同治的理论核心是什么？

2 中医内科学诊疗原则与方法

中医内科学的诊断治疗原则与方法集中体现了中医学辨证论治体系的特色和优势。诊疗原则，包括辨证与治则两大方面；治法则可按汗、清、下、和、温、补、消、涩、理气、理血、开窍、镇痉等归纳为十二法。

中医内科学常用的辨证方法，属《中医诊断学》中"辨证"部分。而运用于内科学临症治疗领域，则又有其一定的特殊性。因此，本书考虑到基础课程与临床运用之间的衔接问题，在这里按照中医内科杂病辨证论治常用的病机病证基本概念及分型方法，简要讲述五邪病机病证基本概念、六经与卫气营血病机病证基本概念、气血病机病证基本概念、脏腑病机病证基本概念等内容，以期在学习过程中做到温故知新，执简驭繁，不断提高中医内科辨证论治的水平。

2.1 五邪病机病证基本概念

概念：五邪是指由于脏腑功能失调而产生的类似于风、寒、湿、燥、火的五种病因病机变化。

风、寒、湿、燥、火病证，既可由外感六淫传变入里而致，又多见于脏腑病变过程中由内而生。凡因体内五邪病机变化产生的上述五种病证，均可称为"内风"、"内寒"、"内湿"、"内燥"、"内火"，以表示与六淫病因学说中相关概念的区别。

必须指出，五邪病机，既是脏腑病理变化的产物，又是继发影响脏腑功能活动的因素，因而必须明辨它与脏腑功能活动的密切关系，谨守病机，治病求本。

按照中医学基本理论，五脏、五邪在五行归属方面有着某种特定关系。在内科学临床的脏腑辨证论治全过程中起着重要的指导作用。这就是：风与肝同属"木"，风性主动，内风病变在于肝的功能活动失常；寒与肾同属"水"，水性寒滞，内寒病变责之于肾阳虚衰；湿与脾同属"土"，土性主长养万物而恶壅滞，内湿与脾脏阳气微弱密切相关；燥与肺同属"金"，内燥与肺宣发肃降、输布津液功能失常密切相关；火热之邪与心同属"火"，临床上常见的火邪亢盛与阴虚火旺多与心的功能失常有关。

同时，由于人体是一个复杂而有序、处于动态平衡状态中以五脏功能活动为中心的有机整体，脏腑气血之间的密切联系和协同作用，致使五脏在生理上息息相关，在病理上相互传变、影响。内风、内寒、内湿、内燥、内火的病机变化和病证表现，往往是以某脏为主，涉及其它相关脏腑，导致两脏或两脏以上功能异常而发生的。因此，探讨五邪病机病证，必须谨守病机、治病求本，明辨虚实、审别标本，分清脏腑病位、阴阳气血盛衰而治之。

2.1.1 风

内风与风邪有着共同的特性：轻扬上浮，善行数变，主动，一年四季均可发生。"风为百病之长"即概括了风证的多发性。

临床上以眩晕、震颤、抽搐、惊厥、颈项强直、四肢瘛疭、口眼㖞斜、角弓反张为见症者，属于"风证。"

风证包括外风、内风两大类。外风即伤风，风寒、风热、风湿、风水等；内风指肝阳化风，热极生风，血虚生风等。

本节重点讨论内风的病机病证。

中医学理论认为：头晕目眩、四肢抽搐、身体麻木、震颤、强直、甚者突然昏仆，不省人事，口眼歪斜，半身不遂或全身活动受限者，大多责之于肝与风。因为肝开窍于目，肝主筋，肝藏血，肝主疏泄，肝主怒，所以，由于脏腑功能失调产生的内风主要责之于肝的功能异常。

内风的病机特点是：

①易以侵犯人体头部为主要病变；

②易挟痰邪；

③易造成与内火结合的"风火相煽"病变。

导致内风的主要因素有：

（1）肝阳化风

【病机概要】 肝阴亏耗，肾阴受损，水不涵木，阴不潜阳，肝阳上亢，动风挟痰，上扰头部，蒙闭清窍。

【主症】 眩晕、欲仆、头痛剧烈，肢体麻木震颤，语言不利，手足蠕动，步履不稳。舌质红，脉弦细数或弦紧。病情严重则突然昏倒，舌强不语，口眼㖞斜，半身不遂（中风）。

【治法】 滋阴潜阳，平肝熄风。

【主方】 大定风珠[19]，镇肝熄风汤[291]等。

（2）热极生风

【病机概要】 邪热亢盛，伤及营血，燔灼肝经，内陷心包，热盛煽动肝风内起。

【主症】 高热烦渴，抽搐项强，两眼上翻，角弓反张，神志昏迷。舌质红绛，苔黄，脉弦数。

【治法】 清热凉肝，熄风醒神。

【主方】 羚羊钩藤汤[247]，安宫牛黄丸[111]，紫雪丹[267]等。

（3）阴（血）虚风动

【病机概要】 阴亏血少，不能濡养筋脉，虚风内动。

【主症】 肢体麻木，筋脉拘急，肌肉瞤动。舌质淡红、或舌红少津，脉细。

【治法】 滋阴养血，宁肝熄风。

【主方】 加减复脉汤[101]，补肝汤[142]，地黄饮子[104]等。

2.1.2 寒

内寒与寒邪在致病过程中有一致性：为阴邪，伤损阳气，在人体内易造成气血凝滞不通，气机闭塞的疼痛证候。外寒伤人多在冬季，而脏腑功能低下导致的内寒证，又称为阳虚、虚寒，在任何季节均可发生，但以冬季为甚。

临床上以筋脉拘挛，肢体不温，气血凝滞，出现疼痛及脏腑功能低下，阳气不足为主要见症者，属于"寒证。"

寒证包括内寒、外寒两大类。外寒为伤寒（寒邪伤于肌表）、中寒（寒邪直中脏腑）；内寒为机体阳气不足，阴寒之邪自内而生，主要责之于肾、脾、心功能低下。

中医学理论认为：畏寒肢冷，面色苍白，呕吐清涎，下利清谷，筋脉拘挛，局部冷痛，倦怠神疲，喜卧喜温，责之于阳虚内寒。因肾阳为一身阳气之根，脾阳为中阳之本，心阳鼓动血脉运行，同时心脾之阳全赖肾阳温煦扶助。肾阳虚衰，是导致虚寒病机的关键，诸多阳虚水泛，阳失温煦的病变，当从肾辨证论治。

内寒的病机特点是：

①伤人阳气；

②导致脏腑功能低下、紊乱；

③易造成疼痛，易聚饮停痰。

内寒常见以下证型：

(1) 阴寒内盛

【病机概要】 阳气衰微，失于温煦，阳衰则阴盛，阴盛则寒；阳微不能化气行水，寒水内聚，为饮为肿。

【主症】 形寒肢冷，重则四肢逆冷，呕吐清涎，下利清谷，面浮肢肿。舌苔白滑润，脉沉弦或沉细弱。

【治法】 温阳祛寒。

【主方】 四逆汤[80]，济生肾气丸[184]，真武汤[199]等。

(2) 脾肾阳虚

【病机概要】 多种原因耗损中阳，累及肾阳，或肾阳虚亏不能温养脾阳，导致脾肾阳虚。

【主症】 面色㿠白，腰膝或少腹冷痛，畏寒喜暖，五更泄泻，小便清长。舌淡胖，脉沉弱无力。

【治法】 温补脾肾。

【主方】 良附丸[139]，附子理中丸[146]等。

(3) 心阳不振

【病机概要】 久病或暴病伤损心阳，阳微不煦，阴寒内盛，闭阻胸阳。

【主症】 心悸胸闷，气短胸痛，受寒则痛势加剧，肢冷唇青，面色㿠白，形寒自汗。脉结代或涩。

【治法】 温阳益气，散寒通络。

【主方】 桂枝加附子汤[202]，栝楼薤白桂枝汤[210]，乌头桂枝汤[55]等。

2.1.3 湿（痰、饮）

湿为阴邪，易伤人体阳气，多先侵犯肢体下部，湿邪为患，病程迁延难愈。湿邪有内外之分，其中，外湿多由久居湿地，涉水淋雨，气候潮湿而侵入人体；内湿则责之于脾阳不足，不能正常运化水湿，导致人体内部水液代谢失常。必须注意：外湿伤人最易困顿脾阳，引动内湿；而脾阳虚衰，湿邪内生时，又极易招致外湿侵袭，故内外湿邪虽有不同，但又有密切的病机联系。所谓："同气相求"。凡临床表现出身体酸重肿痛，关节活动受限，食少纳呆，脘痞泄泻，头身重痛，苔白脉濡者，均属湿证。

外湿，包括寒湿、风湿、暑湿及湿热，多系外邪由体表肌腠而内侵，或流注关节，或损及脾胃。湿邪多兼挟其它邪气同时伤人。另外，湿邪内侵，可有从寒化、从热化的不同病理机转，而人体脏腑不同的功能，素质的差异，以及治疗失当则是形成上述转化的原因。

内湿既是病理产物，又是致病因素。内湿的形成，多因饮食失常，如恣食生冷酒醴肥甘，或饥饱失常。无论何种原因，均可损及脾肾功能，造成阳气虚弱，致脾失温运，水湿不化而凝痰聚饮。

本节重点讨论内湿。

内湿主要表现为：食欲不振，脘闷纳呆，便溏泄泻，肢体沉重浮肿。因内湿与痰饮一源而多歧，湿邪为患常兼挟痰饮，或停聚胸腹，或泛溢肌腠，或凝为痰邪，无所不至。同时，内湿责之于脾阳虚衰——本虚，而有形湿邪内聚又构成标实。所以湿邪为患，内外结合，病情缠绵难愈；而虚实并见，攻补均需慎重。临床辨证论治尤需分清主次，益脾温肾，化湿逐饮。

内湿的病机特点是：

①与脾阳虚有互为因果的关系，病情缠绵；

②既是病理产物，又是致病因素；

③易伤阳气，阻气停水，聚饮生痰，本虚标实。

内湿主要表现为以下几种类型：

(1) 寒湿困脾

【病机概要】 过食生冷，或起居不慎，外湿挟寒邪侵入机体；或内湿素盛，易感寒湿邪气，气机中阳被困，寒湿内生。

【主症】 脘腹闷胀，不思饮食，泛恶欲呕，腹痛溏泻，口淡不渴，头重如裹，肢体欠温，甚或身重浮肿。舌苔白滑或腻，脉濡缓。

【治法】 温中化湿。

【主方】 实脾饮[159]，胃苓汤[182]等。

(2) 湿热中阻

【病机概要】 感受湿热之邪或过食肥甘，酿成湿热，内蕴脾胃。

【主症】 脘痞呕恶，厌食口苦，口粘，渴不欲饮，小便短赤，或身热起伏，汗出热不解；或面目肌肤发黄，皮肤瘙痒。苔黄腻，脉濡数。

【治法】 清热化湿。

【主方】 连朴饮[133]，甘露消毒丹[74]等。

(3) 脾虚湿阻

【病机概要】 饮食不节，损伤脾胃，健运无权，升降失职，水湿内聚。

【主症】 面色萎黄，神疲乏力，四肢困重，脘腹不适，厌食油腻，纳呆，便溏泄泻。舌淡胖，苔薄而滑或腻，脉濡细。

【治法】 健脾化湿。

【主方】 香砂六君子汤[189]，实脾饮[159]等。

附1 痰

痰邪为患颇为广泛，故有"百病多由痰作祟"之说。痰的概念，既指排出体外的有形之痰，又指一类表现为痰的证候症状，如：胸闷脘痞，呕恶腹泻，眩晕心悸，皮肤麻木，关节肿胀，皮下肿块，癫狂等。由于痰的成因不同，又分为寒、热、燥、湿、风等多种痰，而各型之中又有虚实之分，脏腑病位之辨。

痰邪为患，证型颇多。概而言之，其病机总不越乎肺、脾、肾三脏功能失调所致。脾为生痰之源，因其主运化水湿；肺为贮痰之器，又为水之上源，肺失宣肃亦可凝津成痰；肾阳启动脾阳肺气，为一身元气之根，故又可因肾阳肾气虚弱导致水饮内聚，阻气生痰；此外，脏腑阴血不足，虚火内灼，也可炼液生痰。痰一旦形成，便随气升降，流布体内，或上蒙清窍，或注阻经络，变生诸多疾患。

证治类别：

(1) 痰阻于肺

【病机概要】 感受外邪、或咳喘日久，致肺不布津，聚而为痰。

【主症】 咳嗽气喘，或痰鸣有声，痰多色白，易于咯出，或伴见寒热表证。苔薄白腻，脉浮或滑。

【治法】 宣肺化痰。

【主方】 止嗽散[37]，杏苏散[130]等。

(2) 痰蒙心窍

【病机概要】 七情所伤，或感湿浊邪气，阻塞气机，气结痰凝，阻闭心窍。

【主症】 神昏癫狂，胸闷心痛，或昏倒于地，不省人事。苔白腻，脉滑。

【治法】 化痰开窍。

【主方】 导痰汤[121]，苏合香丸[128]等。

(3) 痰蕴脾胃

【病机概要】 饮食不节或思虑劳倦，脾胃受伤，脾失健运，生湿成痰。

【主症】 脘痞纳呆，恶心呕吐，倦怠乏力，身重嗜睡。苔白腻，舌体胖大，脉濡缓。

【治法】 健脾化痰。

【主方】 平胃散[70]，六君子汤[45]等。

(4) 痰郁于肝

【病机概要】 肝气郁结，气结痰凝，痰气互阻。

【主症】 咽中如有物梗塞，胸胁隐痛，嗳气，易怒善郁。苔薄白腻，脉弦滑。

【治法】 解郁化痰。

【主方】 四七汤[75]等。

(5) 痰动于肾

【病机概要】 久病及肾，肾阳亏虚，蒸化无权，水湿内停，上泛为痰；或肾阴亏耗，阴虚火旺，虚火灼津为痰。

【主症】 喘逆气促、舌淡脉沉细；或头晕耳鸣，腰膝酸软，舌红少苔，脉细数。

【治法】 温肾化痰，或滋肾化痰。

【主方】 济生肾气丸[184]，或金水六君煎[161]等。

(6) 痰留骨节经络

【病机概要】 痰浊留窜骨节经络，气血郁滞，络脉痹阻。

【主症】 骨节疼痛肿胀，肢体麻木不仁，或半身不遂，或口眼㖞斜，或见瘰疬、瘿气、结节、肿块。苔白腻，脉弦滑。

【治法】 软坚散结，通络化痰。

【主方】 四海舒郁丸[83]，指迷茯苓丸[179]等。

总之，痰与湿均由脾、肺、肾三脏功能低下所致，本于正虚。然痰停体内，常为实证，故临床多为本虚标实，需掌握急则治标、缓则治本及标本同治的原则。急则治其痰，缓则调理肺、脾、肾功能；同时，还需根据痰邪所兼挟邪气性质，采用针对性的措施治疗，如燥痰润而去之，湿痰燥而除之，顽痰软而逐之。

附2 饮

饮的成因与湿、痰有类似之处，为脾、肺、肾三脏功能失调，气化不利，水液代谢失常而导致。饮由停聚于体内的部位不同而分为四类：停于肠胃称为痰饮（狭义），停于胁下称为悬饮，泛溢肌肤称为溢饮，上犯胸肺称为支饮。饮停体内，总属本虚标实。

饮邪形成原因较多，但总的病机不外乎脾阳虚微，运化无权，水液停聚，蓄积为饮；肾阳不足，气化失职，不能温运脾阳，致使水饮内聚并流溢周身；肺为水之上源，肺气不能宣发输布津液，内蓄成饮。病机都属阳虚阴盛，水液代谢失常，水饮停积为患。

证治类别

（1）痰饮

【病机概要】 中阳不振，饮留胃肠。

【主症】 脘腹坚满而痛，胃中有振水声，呕吐痰涎，不欲饮水，头目眩晕，或肠间水声漉漉。苔白滑，脉滑。

【治法】 温阳化饮或攻逐水饮。

【主方】 苓桂术甘汤[150]，己椒苈黄丸[24]等。

（2）悬饮

【病机概要】 水流胁间，络脉被阻，气机升降不利。

【主症】 胸胁胀痛，咳唾、转侧、呼吸时加重，气短息促。苔白，脉沉弦。

【治法】 攻逐水饮。

【主方】 十枣汤[6]，葶苈大枣泻肺汤[261]等。

（3）溢饮

【病机概要】 肺脾之气输布失职，水饮泛溢。

【主症】 肢体痛重，甚或肢体浮肿，小便不利，或发热恶寒，无汗咳喘，痰多泡沫。苔白，脉弦紧。

【治法】 温化痰饮。

【主方】 小青龙汤[27]等。

（4）支饮

【病机概要】 饮犯胸肺，肺气上逆。

【主症】 咳喘胸满，甚则不能平卧，痰如白沫量多，久咳面目浮肿。苔白腻，脉弦紧。

【治法】 寒饮伏肺者，宜温肺化饮；脾肾阳虚者，宜温补脾肾。

【主方】 温肺化饮：小青龙汤[27]等；

温补脾肾：金匮肾气丸[163]，苓桂术甘汤[150]等。

2.1.4 燥

燥邪易伤津液，又易伤肺。使人出现口鼻干燥、咽干口渴，干咳少痰或痰中带血，皮肤干燥皲裂，毛发干枯不荣，肌肉消瘦干糙，大便干结等一系列"燥象"。燥邪致病，有外燥和内燥两类。外燥由感受外界燥邪而发病，邪从口鼻入，病由肺卫始，根据感受夏火之余气与近冬之寒气的不同，又有温燥与凉燥之分；内燥多见于高热、呕吐、腹泻、出汗出血过多之后。外燥多见于秋季，内燥则可见于四时。这里主要讨论内燥。

内燥病机，总括为津液耗伤，阴血亏损，病变主要涉及肺、胃、肾、肝。

内燥的病机特点是：

①易伤津耗液，损及阴血；

②易引动内风和内火（热）。

内燥常表现为以下类型：

（1）肺胃津伤

【病机概要】 热盛伤津或汗吐下诸法太过，伤津耗液。

【主症】 鼻咽干燥，口干口渴，干咳无痰，大便干结，小便短少，皮肤干燥无光泽。舌干少津。

【治法】 生津润燥。

【主方】 沙参麦冬汤[138]，增液汤[283]等。

（2）肝肾阴亏

【病机概要】 久病精血内夺，或大失血后难以骤生所致。

【主症】 咽干口燥，腰膝酸软，五心烦热，毛发干枯不荣，肌肉消瘦，遗精盗汗，妇女经闭。舌红少苔，脉细略数。

【治法】 滋阴养血。

【主方】 麦味地黄丸[125]，杞菊地黄丸[129]等。

2.1.5 火

中医学理论认为：热为火之渐，火为热之甚，所以临床常以"火热"并称。凡外感六淫，皆可入里化热化火；七情内郁，气机不畅，也可化热化火。中医理论常以"气有余便是火"来概括火邪为患的广泛性。

火为阳邪，具有易伤阴津，易上扰清窍，易动血耗血，易引动内风，兼挟痰浊的病机特点。

火邪为病，亦有内外之分。外火多系直接感受温热邪气所致；内火则由脏腑阴阳失调而成。其中，阳盛者属实火，病变涉及心、肝、肺胃，以心、肝为主，其症状为口舌糜烂，目赤口苦，咽喉干痛，牙龈肿痛，心烦躁怒等；阴虚者属虚火，病变涉及肺、肾、心、肝，而以肺、肾为主，症见五心烦热，低热盗汗，颧红、咽干目涩，头晕耳鸣等。故内火病有虚实之分，病位之别，其病机各异，治法不同，尤当详辨。

本节重点讨论内火。

火邪的主要病机特点是：

①病情变化迅速，易耗血、动风、挟痰；
②火邪伤人易上行，侵犯清窍、蒙蔽心神；
③火邪耗伤阴津，热象较著；
④内火多与情志因素、劳欲过度关系密切。

内火主要分为以下几种类型：

实火

（1）心火炽盛

【病机概要】 情志不调，郁而化火。

【主症】 心烦面赤，口渴欲饮，口舌生疮，失眠不宁。舌红脉数。

【治法】 清心泻火。

【主方】 泻心汤[153]等。

（2）肝火亢盛

【病机概要】 情志不遂，肝失疏泄，郁而化火，邪火上逆。

【主症】 头痛眩晕，耳鸣如潮，烦躁易怒，面红目赤，口苦咽干，胸胁灼痛。舌红苔黄，脉弦数。

【治法】 清泻肝火。

【主方】 龙胆泻肝汤[64]等。

虚火

（1）肾虚火动

【病机概要】 久病伤阴或亡血失精，肾阴亏耗，虚火内生。

【主症】 眩晕耳鸣，腰膝酸软，咽干口燥，健忘少寐，五心烦热，潮热盗汗，形体消瘦，遗精早泄。舌红而干，脉细数。

【治法】 滋肾降火。

【主方】 知柏地黄丸[160]等。

（2）肺虚火壅

【病机概要】 劳伤肺气或久咳耗阴，阴虚火旺。

【主症】 气短干咳，痰少粘稠或痰中带血丝，口干咽燥，颧红声嘶，骨蒸潮热，五心烦热。舌红少津，脉细数。

【治法】 滋阴润肺清火。

【主方】 百合固金汤[103]，秦艽鳖甲散[197]等。

小结

五邪病机直接与脏腑、阴阳、气血相关联，五邪致病是内科疾患中最常见、最普遍的病机变化。内生五邪既是由脏腑功能异常状态下的病机变化所产生，又是构成新的病理机转，进一步造成脏腑气血阴阳动态平衡的紊乱，使疾病复杂化的直接因素。所以，在中医内科学领域中，必须对五邪病机病证有本质的、准确的把握，才能指导临床辨证论治。

思考题

1. 五邪的概念与内生五邪概念的异同？

2. 内生五邪各自的病机特点是什么？

3. 内生五邪各有哪些证型？主要见症与治法各是什么？

2.2 六经与卫气营血病机病证基本概念

六经病机病证与卫气营血病机病证，是对外感热病进行证候归类辨证论治的两大类别，对内科学临床治疗都起着一定的指导作用，具有独特的意义和价值。而六经与卫气营血辨证方法，又需结合八纲、脏腑辨证理论，联系临证实际运用。

2.2.1 六经病机病证概要

概念：六经病机、六经病证以及六经辨证论治，来源于《伤寒论》确立的外感热病辨证体系。现分别简述如下：

(1) 太阳病

【病机概要】 太阳主六经之表，风寒邪气袭表，经气流行不畅。

【主症】 恶风寒，头痛，无汗或有汗，身痛项强。脉浮。

【治法】 表实无汗者，宜辛温解表；表虚有汗者，宜调和营卫。

【主方】 辛温解表，用麻黄汤[242]；调和营卫，用桂枝汤[200]。

(2) 阳明病

【病机概要】 邪入阳明气分，热盛灼伤胃津；邪入阳明腑，食积燥热内结。

【主症】 阳明经证：壮热、恶热、身大汗、口大渴、脉洪大；阳明腑实证：潮热汗出，腹部硬满拒按，便秘，甚则谵语。苔燥。

【治法】 阳明经证宜清热泻火；阳明腑证则攻泻实热。

【主方】 清热泻火用白虎汤[91]，攻泻实热选用大承气汤[21]，小承气汤[29]，调胃承气汤[218]。

(3) 少阳病

【病机概要】 少阳为六经枢机，主半表半里，病邪入侵，与正气分争于半表半里之间，气机升降疏泄不利。

【主症】 寒热往来，胸胁苦满，口苦咽干，默默不欲饮食。脉弦。

【治法】 和解少阳。

【主方】 小柴胡汤[30]。

(4) 太阴病

【病机概要】 太阴为三阴之首，太阴受邪，脾阳虚弱，寒湿中阻或寒邪直中、升降失常。

【主症】 腹满时痛，食欲不振，呕吐腹泻，口淡不渴。舌淡苔白，脉缓或迟。

【治法】 温中散寒。

【主方】 理中汤[229]等。

(5) 少阴病

【病机概要】 病入少阴，伤损心肾，根据机体阴阳盛衰状况又分两类：阴虚者从阳化热；阳虚者从阴化寒。

【主症】 少阴虚寒证以畏寒肢冷，嗜卧神疲，下利清谷，脉微细为主证；少阴虚热证以虚烦不眠，口干咽燥，脉细数为主证。

【治法】 寒化证宜回阳救逆；热化证则滋阴清热。

【主方】 寒化证用四逆汤[80]，热化证用黄连阿胶汤[231]。

(6) 厥阴病

【病机概要】 病入厥阴，厥热胜复，气机逆乱，寒热错杂。

【主症】 口渴不止，气上冲心，心中痛热，饥不欲食，厥逆下利，呕吐或吐蛔虫。

【治法】 温清并用。

【主方】 乌梅丸[56]。

2.2.2 卫气营血病机病证概要

卫气营血是中医温病学说创立的反映温病浅深轻重不同阶段的辨证论治体系，主要应用于外感发热性、传染性疾病的治疗领域。现简述如下：

(1) 卫分证

【病机概要】 温邪外袭，犯肺郁卫，气机不畅，邪正交争于卫分。

【主症】 发热口干，微恶风寒，可伴头痛咽痛，咳嗽。舌边尖红，脉浮数。

【治法】 辛凉解表。

【主方】 银翘散[255]，桑菊饮[227]等。

(2) 气分证

【病机概要】 风温之邪，侵犯肺胃，或湿热留恋三焦，邪正交争于气分。

【主症】 壮热恶热，口渴口苦，心烦懊恼，咳嗽，汗出热势不减，小便黄赤。脉洪大或沉实。

【治法】 清热透邪宣肺。

【主方】 栀子豉汤[237]，麻杏石甘汤[241]，白虎汤[91]。湿热留恋三焦者，用蒿芩清胆汤[276]，甘露消毒丹[74]等。

(3) 营分证

【病机概要】 温邪鸱张不解，内灼营阴，热陷心包，扰动心神。

【主症】 身热心烦，口干不寐，舌红绛，脉数，或斑疹隐隐，或神昏谵语，脉数。

【治法】 清营透热；或清心开窍。

【主方】 清营汤[252]或安宫牛黄丸[111]，紫雪丹[267]。

(4) 血分证

【病机概要】 温邪入于血分，病损心肝，煎耗真阴，累及于肾，动血、耗血，伤阴生风。

【主症】 高热，神昏或躁狂，斑疹显露，或吐血、衄血、便血、尿血，或手足搐动、痉厥。舌质深绛或光红如镜，脉虚数或促。

【治法】 凉血散血；或凉肝熄风；或滋阴熄风。

【主方】 犀角地黄汤[273]，凉肝熄风用羚羊钩藤汤[247]，滋阴熄风用大定风珠[19]。

小结

六经辨证是以经络命名，经络既有脏腑之隶属，又与六气和八纲相关，含义深远。所以六经辨证是将外感热病发生和发展过程，概括为六种不同的证候类型，以指导临床实践；而卫生营血辨证，是温病发生和发展全部过程的四个阶段，即温病由浅入深、由轻而重的四类证型。

六经辨证与卫气营血辨证有不少相似之处，如：都以辨治外感热病为主；都具有由表及里、由浅入深的发展、传变规律；温病学说的"卫分证"，"气分证"，其中一部分相当于《伤寒论》的"太阳病"、"阳明病"；发病初期多属表证，热盛时期多属里证、实证，后期多属虚证等。但六经辨证与卫气营血辨证又各有其不同的特点，如：伤寒治神昏谵语多用下法，温病增补了清心开窍法；伤寒偏重于回阳，处处顾其阳气，而温病偏重于救阴，处处顾护阴液。但综观二者辨证论治的基本内容，都是以八纲为总纲，以脏腑经络为基础的。我们要全面认识二者的异同和联系，从整体观点出发，将二者综合起来，灵活应用，才能达到正确辨证论治的目的。

思考题

1. 六经辨证的概念及适用范围是什么？
2. 卫气营血辨证的概念与辨证分型是什么？
3. 六经辨证与卫气营血辨证的关系？二者与八纲、脏腑辨证的关系怎样？

2.3 气血病机病证基本概念

中医学理论认为：气、血是人体生命活动最基本的动力和源泉。气为阳，血为阴，气与血有着阴阳相随、相互资生、相互促进、相互依存的关系。气对血，有温煦、化生、推动、统摄的作用；血对气，则有濡养、运载的功能。二者关系极为密切。

气和血既是人体脏腑功能活动所产生的物质，同时又作为脏腑功能活动必需的物质基础而在生命活动中不断的消耗，这种气血互化和消长的动态平衡维持着机体的健康状态。一旦某种因素影响了气血的相互关系、破坏了这种动态平衡，就会导致气血病变，产生气血亏虚、气不摄血、气随血脱、气滞血瘀等证。

气血之间在病变时互相影响，而气血的病变又必然影响到脏腑的功能活动。因此，讲气血病机病证，必须着眼于脏腑；讲脏腑辨证，也不能离开对气血病机的把握。只有这样，才能深刻体会和掌握中医内科学辨证思想的精华。

2.3.1 气病

气在中医理论体系中有两大含义：一指构成和维持人体生命活动的精微物质，如营气、宗气等；另一个含义是指机体各种功能活动及其表现，如脏气、经气等等。二者既有区别、又常常相互涵盖，这是中医基本理论的一大特点。

概括而言，气主温煦、推动、防御、固摄和气化作用。气属阳，所以，气虚时表现为一系列虚损不足及虚寒症状；而气有余便是火，气的运行障碍时可以郁而化火，热自内生。

气的运动称为气机，泛指机体生命活动过程中各组织器官（脏腑、经络）的功能表现。升降出入，构成了气机运动的基本形式。升降出入的正常与否直接依赖并反映出脏腑功能活动状况。

气的病变，可以概括为生成不足及运行异常两大类。常见类型有：

虚证

(1) 气虚

【病机概要】 久病体弱、饮食失调等多种因素导致元气生成不足或消耗过度，脏腑功能衰退。

【主症】 头晕目眩，倦怠乏力，少气懒言，自汗。舌淡脉虚。

【治法】 补气。

【主方】 四君子汤[77]。

(2) 气陷

【病机概要】 因气虚而导致气的升降失常，升举无力。

【主症】 头晕目花，少气倦怠，腹部有坠胀感，脱肛。舌淡苔白，脉弱。

【治法】 益气升提。

【主方】 补中益气汤[140]。

实证

(1) 气滞

【病机概要】 情志不舒、饮食失调、感受外邪等多种因素导致机体气机阻滞，运行不畅。

【主症】 胁腹胀痛，窜痛不定，时轻时重。苔薄，脉弦。

【治法】 行气导滞。

【主方】 金铃子散[162]，五磨饮子[43]等。

(2) 气逆

【病机概要】 气机升降失常，上逆不顺。多指肺、胃之气上逆及肝气升发太过所致的气火上逆。

【主症】 胃：呃逆、嗳气、呕吐；肝：头痛目眩昏厥、呕血；肺：咳嗽喘促。

【治法】 平冲降逆。

【主方】 苏子降气汤[127]，旋覆代赭汤[244]等。

2.3.2 血病

血是构成生命活动最重要的营养物质。血属阴，血主濡养。脾生血统血、肝藏血、心主血脉，血行脉中，由心阳鼓动运行，将营养成分输布周身。

血病一般表现为血虚、血瘀、出血。三者既有区别，又有联系。血虚可导致出血，而出血又可能是瘀血的病机；血瘀可使出血不止，瘀血不去则新血难生，又可导致血虚。

血病主要证型有：

(1) 血虚

【病机概要】 多种因素引起血液化生不足或消耗太过，均可血虚。

【主症】 面色无华，唇舌爪甲色淡，头晕眼花，心悸失眠，手足发麻。舌淡，脉细无力。

【治法】 补血。

【主方】 四物汤[79]。

（2）血瘀

【病机概要】 因气虚、气滞、寒凝、热结等导致血行障碍、瘀阻不畅。

【主症】 刺痛，痛处不移，拒按，局部紫癜、肿块、口唇爪甲色紫暗，肌肤甲错；瘀血阻于某一脏腑，便影响该脏腑功能而出现相应症状，如：胸痛咳血、呕血便血等。

【治法】 活血化瘀。

【主方】 血府逐瘀汤[119]。

（3）出血

【病机概要】 多由火热迫血妄行，或气虚不能摄血，或肾阴亏虚，阴虚火旺，虚火伤络，而致出血。

【主症】 咳血，吐血，便血，尿血，衄血。

【治法】 血热妄行者，宜泻热止血；气不摄血者，宜补气摄血；阴虚火旺者，宜滋阴降火。

【主方】 泻热止血，用犀角地黄汤[273]；补气摄血，用归脾汤[95]；滋阴降火，用茜根散[178]。

小结

气血病机病证的证治要点有：

1. 虚者补之、气虚宜补，主要是补肺、脾、肾之气；血虚当补血，因气血互生，故宜补血益气并施，以达补气生血之目的。

2. 瘀者散之、滞者行之。对气、血之实证，治宜理气、降气、行气、活血、行血、破瘀。

3. 出血需及时止血，要审因论治，用凉血止血，滋阴降火止血诸法；对气不摄血者，尤需牢记"有形之血难以速生，无形之气所当急固"这一治疗出血急重证的原则。

气血同病，主要表现为以下几种证型：

1. 气滞血瘀，由气滞导致血行障碍，治宜行气化瘀；
2. 气虚血瘀，气虚无力鼓动血行，治宜补气活血；
3. 气血两虚，气血生化不足或消耗过多，治宜气血双补；
4. 气虚失血，气虚失于统摄而出血、治宜补气摄血；
5. 气随血脱，出血导致气失所依而亡失，治宜止血固气。

思考题

1. 气、血的生理关系及在病理中的相互影响。
2. 血病病机病证的主要证型有哪些？

2.4 脏腑病机病证基本概念

脏腑功能失调的病理变化反映于临床的不同证候就是脏腑病证。而疾病过程中的脏腑功能失调及其产生的病理变化，则称之为脏腑病机。

中医内科学辨证论治的核心——脏腑辨证，就是基于对脏腑病证的把握和对脏腑病机的认识，是明确病变部位及性质的辨证方法。中医内科学诊疗方法中的五邪病机病证、六经、卫气营血、气血病机病证，都必须落实到脏腑，因为中医学理论的一条重要指导原则，即是以五脏为中心的有机整体观。

脏腑是构成人体的一个密切联系的整体。五脏之间有生克乘侮的关系，脏腑之间有表里的联系；经络将人体五脏六腑、四肢百骸、五官九窍、皮肉筋脉等联结为一个有机的统一体；气血津液由脏腑化生、输布，而脏腑又赖之进行生理活动。故脏腑病机病证既涉及气血津液，又与经络密切相关。虽然错综复杂，但归纳其证候性质，仍不出阴阳、表里、寒热、虚实八纲辨证的范围。因此，脏腑辨证还需以八纲辨证为基础。脏腑辨证和八纲辨证是中医内科学辨证论治的基础和核心。

2.4.1 肺（大肠）系病机病证概要

病机特点

（1）肺主气，司呼吸，故肺的病理表现，主要是气机出入升降失常；

（2）肺为娇脏，开窍于鼻，外合皮毛，故外邪内侵，首先犯肺；

（3）肺气宜宣肃，若肺气壅闭，则为咳喘；

（4）肺朝百脉，主治节，肺气失调，可致心血运行不利；

（5）肺主通调水道，下输膀胱，肺气不降，可致水液潴留；

（6）肺与大肠相表里，肺之肃降与大肠的传导功能互相影响。

肺系的病证，临床上常见有感冒、咳嗽、哮证、喘证、肺痈、肺痨、咳血、衄血等。

证治分类

实证

（1）寒邪犯肺

【病机概要】 外感寒邪、肺气不宣；寒饮内阻，肺失清肃。

【主症】 风寒外束者，症见恶寒发热，无汗，头痛身楚，鼻塞流清涕，咳痰稀薄，苔薄白，脉浮紧；寒饮内阻者，症见咳嗽频剧，气急身重，痰白如沫如涎，痰量多，苔白滑，脉浮或滑。

【治法】 宣肺散寒或温化痰饮。

【主方】 麻黄汤[242]，小青龙汤[27]。

（2）邪热乘肺

【病机概要】 风热上受或寒郁化热，痰热内蕴，肺失清肃。

【主症】 风热犯肺者，症见咳嗽痰黄，或流脓涕或恶风身热，咽痛，苔薄黄，脉浮数；痰热蕴肺者，症见咳吐大量黄稠痰，或有腥臭、或带脓血、或见喘逆痰鸣，咳则胸痛，烦渴引饮，溲赤便秘，舌红苔黄燥，脉滑数。

【治法】 疏风清热或清肺化痰。

【主方】 桑菊饮[227]，银翘散[255]，或清金化痰汤[248]等。

（3）痰浊阻肺

【病机概要】 感受外邪、或咳喘日久，以致肺不布津、聚为痰湿，或脾虚失运，湿聚成痰、上渍于肺。

【主症】 痰湿阻肺者，症见咳嗽痰多粘稠，色白或灰白，气息急促，苔白厚腻，脉濡滑；水饮伏肺者，症见咳喘痰鸣，胸胁支满疼痛，倚息不得卧，苔腻色黄，脉弦滑或数。

【治法】 燥湿化痰或泻肺逐饮。
【主方】 二陈汤[2]、平胃散[70]或葶苈大枣泻肺汤[261]、控涎丹[238]等。

虚证

(1) 阴虚肺燥

【病机概要】 外感燥邪，耗伤肺津；或风温诸邪伤津化燥；或痨虫袭肺、久咳伤肺、气血亏损，致肺阴不足，虚热内生，耗灼肺金。

【主症】 燥邪犯肺者，症见咳呛气逆，痰少而粘，或带血丝，口干咽痛，或伴微寒身热，苔薄质干，边尖红，脉细数；虚热内灼者，症见干咳少痰或痰中带血、声哑咽红、潮热盗汗，形体消瘦，舌红苔少，脉细数。

【治法】 清肺润燥，或滋阴润肺。

【主方】 桑杏汤[226]、清燥救肺汤[254]，或百合固金汤[103]、沙参麦冬汤[138]等。

(2) 肺气亏虚

【病机概要】 劳伤过度，或久咳伤肺，或气之化生不足。

【主症】 咳而短气，倦怠懒言，声音低怯，畏风自汗。舌淡苔薄白，脉虚弱。

【治法】 补益肺气。

【主方】 补肺汤[143]等。

兼证

(1) 脾虚及肺：兼见脾气虚、肺气虚病证。治宜培土生金，补益肺脾。方用六君子汤[45]等。

(2) 肺肾阴亏：兼见肺阴虚、肾阴虚病证。治宜滋肾养肺。方用六味地黄丸[46]、生脉散[84]等。

(3) 肝火犯肺：兼见肝郁、肺热病证。治宜清肝泻肺。方用黛蛤散[287]合泻白散[154]之类。

证治要点

①肺为娇脏，不耐寒热，用药宜清轻、辛平甘润，不宜重浊燥热。

②治肺之法，有直接与间接两种。直接治肺法是针对病因病机、采用宣肺、肃肺、清肺、泻肺、温肺、润肺、补肺、敛肺等法；间接治肺法是按五脏生克关系，采用诸如培土生金等多种方法来调节肺与它脏关系。

③肺系病证，可分为外感与内伤两大类，外感多属实证；内伤多为本虚标实。外感病在肺卫；内伤主要在肺，亦与心、肝、脾、肾相关，临证需全面考虑。

附 大肠病机病证概要

病机特点

肺与大肠互为表里，上下相应，肺气失宣则大肠腑气壅滞；大肠职司传导糟粕，受脾统摄，脾阳虚弱、传导失常；大肠又主津液的进一步吸收，脾阴不足，大肠津液亏乏导致排便不畅。

大肠病证，临床常见便秘、泄泻、痢疾、腹痛等。

证治分类

(1) 大肠实热证

【病机概要】 实热邪滞互结阳明之腑,闭塞不通。

【主症】 便秘不通,腹痛拒按,或发热呕逆,或纯利粪水、热结旁流,或烦躁谵语。舌苔黄燥或焦黄起芒刺,脉沉实有力。

【治法】 清热导滞。

【主方】 大承气汤[21]等。

(2) 大肠湿热证

【病机概要】 外感暑湿,或饮食不节、不洁,以致湿热蕴结大肠。

【主症】 腹泻或痢下赤白,里急后重,肛门灼热,腹痛,发热身重。苔黄腻,脉滑数。

【治法】 清化湿热。

【主方】 葛根芩连汤[260]或白头翁汤[88]等。

(3) 大肠虚寒证

【病机概要】 脾肾阳虚、或苦寒伤阳、或寒邪直中肠间所致。

【主症】 溏泻或久泻不止,腹满时痛,喜得温按,或肛门下脱、四肢欠温。脉细弱,舌淡苔薄白。

【治法】 温阳散寒。

【主方】 附子理中汤[146]等。

(4) 大肠津亏证

【病机概要】 大肠燥热伤津、或脾阴不足,不能下及大肠,致大肠津亏。

【主症】 大便秘结干燥,数日一行,或口臭咽燥,或头昏腹胀。舌红少津,苔黄燥,脉细。

【治法】 润肠通便。

【主方】麻子仁丸[240],增液承气汤[284]。

2.4.2 心(小肠)系病机病证概要

病机特点

(1) 心主血脉,又主神明,所以心的病理表现主要是血脉运行的障碍和情志思维活动的异常;

(2) 心包为心之外卫、故温邪逆传,多为心包所受;

(3) 心脏本身之病,多起自内伤。心阴虚的主要病机为心血亏耗,心阳虚的主要病机为心气不足;

(4) 心之热证和实证,多由情志抑郁,化火生痰、痰火上扰,或气滞血瘀、经脉瘀阻,或饮邪阻遏心阳。

证治分类

虚证

(1) 心阳(气)虚

【病机概要】 禀赋薄弱、久病体虚或暴病伤阳所致。

【主症】 心悸、气短、胸闷、心痛,或面色㿠白,形寒自汗。脉虚或结代。

【治法】 温心阳、益心气。

【主方】 桂枝加附子汤[202],养心汤[185]。

(2) 心阴（血）虚

【病机概要】 失血之后，或热病伤阴，或思虑过度，阴血暗耗；或由血之生化不足。

【主症】 心悸、心烦、惊惕不安，少寐多梦。舌红苔少，脉细数。

【治法】 滋阴养心安神。

【主方】 天王补心丹[32]，四物汤[79]等。

实证

(1) 痰火内扰

【病机概要】 情志不舒，气郁化火，煎熬津液成痰，痰火内扰，上蒙心包。

【主症】 心悸，癫狂，躁扰不寐。舌红赤或干裂，少苔，脉滑数。

【治法】 清心豁痰泻火。

【主方】 礞石滚痰丸[289]。

(2) 饮遏心阳

【病机概要】 停痰伏饮，阻遏心阳，气机不畅。

【主症】 心悸胸闷，眩晕阵作，呕吐痰涎。苔白腻，脉弦滑或沉紧。

【治法】 化饮除痰。

【主方】 茯苓甘草汤[174]，导痰汤[121]。

(3) 心血瘀阻

【病机概要】 心气或心阳亏虚，鼓动无力，气滞血瘀，络脉失和。

【主症】 心悸怔忡，心胸憋闷或刺痛，甚者心胸暴痛，口唇青紫，肢厥神昏。舌质暗或见瘀斑，脉细涩或结代。

【治法】 活血通络行瘀。

【主方】 血府逐瘀汤[119]等。

兼证

(1) 心脾两虚：兼见心气虚、脾气虚病证。治宜补益心脾，方用归脾汤[95]。

(2) 心肾不交：心阴不足，肾中虚火妄动，兼见心肾阴虚火旺病证。治宜交通心肾，方用黄连阿胶汤[231]、交泰丸[110]等。

(3) 心肺气虚：兼见心肺气阳亏虚病证。治宜补益心肺，方用保元汤[192]。

证治要点

①气属阳，血属阴，阴阳互根，心阳虚兼心气虚，心阴虚亦常兼心血虚。临证对此应注意相互关系，阴中求阳，阳中求阴，两者兼顾。

②临证治疗心系病证，须考虑心与脾、肺、肝、肾的关系。如心阳虚与饮遏心阳证，皆与脾阳不运有关；心阴虚与痰火内扰证，也与肝肾阴亏火旺有关，要整体把握和处理。

③心的病证有虚实之分，但虚实之间常兼夹互见，如心血瘀阻证常为因虚致实，表现为本虚标实，故临证需分清标本缓急。

④心主神明，心之气血阴阳失调均会扰及心神，临床治疗时须注意佐以宁心安神或重镇安神之品。

附 小肠病机病证概要

病机特点

心与小肠为表里，小肠受盛胃中水谷，主转输清浊。小肠之病，多由饮食失节，损伤脾胃下传而致。其病机为清浊不分、转输障碍。小肠的病证，虚寒多与脾胃损伤有关，而小肠实热多为心火下移所致。

小肠的病证，临床常见泄泻、腹痛、尿血等。

证治分类

（1）小肠虚寒

【病机概要】 饮食不节，损伤脾胃，小肠分清泌浊功能失常。

【主症】 肠鸣泄泻，小腹隐痛喜按。舌淡苔薄白，脉细缓。

【治法】 温通小肠。

【主方】 吴茱萸汤[135]。

（2）小肠实热

【病机概要】 多由心火下移小肠。

【主症】 心烦失眠，口舌生疮，溲赤涩痛，或见尿血。舌红苔黄，脉滑数。

【治法】 清心火，导热下行。

【主方】 导赤散[120]，凉膈散[213]。

2.4.3 脾（胃）系病机病证概要

病机特点

（1）脾与胃互为表里，脾升胃降，燥湿相济。若脾胃升降失常，则水谷的受纳、腐熟、转输等功能发生障碍，可见呕逆、泄泻等病证；

（2）脾主运化，胃主受纳腐熟，为气血生化之源。脾胃功能失常，则化源衰少，机体失养；

（3）脾主统血，脾气虚弱，气不摄血，血不归经，血证由生；

（4）脾主运化转输水湿，脾失健运，水津敷布失常，水湿停聚，为饮为肿。故脾病多与湿有关，而出现本虚标实之证。

脾胃系病证临床常见的病证有泄泻、胃痛、呃逆、呕吐、痰饮、吐血、便血等。

证治分类

虚证

（1）脾阳虚衰

【病机概要】 恣食生冷，或久病失养、或过施凉药，导致脾阳不振，运化无权。

【主症】 面黄脘冷，泛吐清水，纳少便溏，或见四肢不温。舌淡、苔白，脉濡弱。

【治法】 温运中阳。

【主方】 理中丸[229]。

（2）中气不足

【病机概要】 素体虚弱，或劳倦过度、久病耗伤；或由脾虚生化不足，升清无力。

【主症】 纳少腹胀，乏力懒言，肠鸣便溏，甚则脏器下垂、少腹下坠、脱肛。舌淡苔薄白，脉缓无力。

【治法】 补中益气。

【主方】 补中益气汤[140]。

实证

（1）寒湿困脾

【病机概要】 外感寒湿或湿邪内盛，中阳被遏，脾失运化。

【主症】 脘闷纳呆，头身困重，口粘不渴，大便不实或泄泻。苔白腻，脉濡。

【治法】 运脾化湿。

【主方】 胃苓汤[182]。

（2）湿热内蕴

【病机概要】 外感时邪，或素嗜酒甘，伤及脾胃、运化失常、湿热交阻、甚则薰蒸肝胆。

【主症】 胁胀脘闷，纳呆口苦，发热身重，溲赤便溏，甚则面目俱黄、皮肤发痒。苔黄腻，脉濡数。

【治法】 清热利湿。

【主方】 茵陈蒿汤[177]，五苓散[41]。

兼证

（1）脾胃不和：兼脾虚胃弱，升降失常的病证。治宜益气运中，调和脾胃。方用香砂六君子汤[189]等。

（2）脾肾阳虚：兼见脾肾两脏阳气虚弱病证。治宜健脾温肾。方用附子理中汤[146]、四神丸[82]等。

（3）脾湿犯肺：兼见脾虚失运，痰湿犯肺病证。治宜燥湿化痰。方用二陈汤[2]等。

（4）心脾两虚：见心病兼证。

证治要点

①脾病之病机病证多属本虚标实，临证应辨标本之缓急轻重而论治。

②脾喜燥恶湿，外湿易困脾，脾虚生内湿，故脾病与湿邪关系极为密切，不论寒热虚实诸证，均可兼见湿证。因而在治疗时需酌施燥湿、利湿、逐水、化湿之品。

③脾病多虚多寒，胃病多热多实，故古人概括为"实则阳明，虚则太阴"，所以，脾以升为健为补，胃以降为和为顺。

④脾胃位居中焦，为一身气机升降之枢，故脾胃与其它脏腑在病理上可互相影响，其中，尤与肝肾关系密切，因此在治疗上应从整体观念出发，综合考虑。

附 胃的病机病证概要

病机特点

胃主受纳腐熟，凡饮食不节、不洁，皆能影响于胃；胃为燥土，喜润恶燥，以降为顺，故胃病可见食积郁热等燥热证和呃逆、呕吐等胃失和降证。

胃的病证临床常见胃痛、嘈杂、呕吐、呃逆、便秘等。

证治分类

（1）胃寒

【病机概要】 胃阳素虚或过食生冷、寒邪内侵，寒凝于胃。

【主症】 胃脘冷痛，轻则绵绵不休，重则拘急剧痛，遇寒加剧，得温则减，呕吐清水。舌淡、苔白滑，脉迟。

【治法】 温胃散寒。
【主方】 良附丸[139]等。

(2) 胃热

【病机概要】 热邪犯胃、过食辛热或胃热素盛之体与情志郁火相并。

【主症】 胃脘灼痛，吞酸嘈杂，消谷善饥，喜冷饮或口臭，牙龈肿痛，出血。舌红少津，苔黄，脉滑数。

【治法】 清胃泄火。
【主方】 清胃散[250]。

(3) 胃虚

【病机概要】 火热之邪耗伤胃阴。

【主症】 口干唇燥，饥不欲食，或干呕呃逆，大便干燥。舌红少苔或光红，脉细数。

【治法】 养胃生津。
【主方】 益胃汤[217]等。

(4) 胃实

【病机概要】 饮食不节，食积不化。

【主症】 脘腹胀痛，厌食，嗳气，或呕吐酸腐食臭，大便不畅。苔垢腻，脉滑。

【治法】 消食导滞。
【主方】 保和丸[193]等。

2.4.4 肝（胆）系病机病证概要

病机特点

(1) 肝主疏泄，喜条达而恶抑郁，精神情志之调节功能与肝密切相关。若肝气郁结、可致肝脉阻滞；肝郁日久、气滞血瘀，可致癥瘕积聚；血瘀水停，可形成鼓胀；湿热内蕴，肝失疏泄，胆液外溢，可致黄疸；寒凝气滞，可形成疝气等证；

(2) 肝主藏血，有贮藏和调节血量的作用。肝病失藏，则可发生各种血证；肝血不足，筋脉失养，可致麻木、痿躄等证；

(3) 肝为风木之脏，体阴而用阳，主升主动。若肝阴耗伤，肝阳亢盛，化风内动、或肾水亏虚，肝失滋养，肝阳上亢，均可发生头痛、眩晕；若肝肾阴亏，肝阳暴张，血随气逆、挟痰挟火、蒙蔽清窍，则发为中风。

临床常见的肝系病证有：中风、眩晕、头痛、痉证、癫狂、厥证、积聚、鼓胀、吐血、衄血、耳鸣等。

证治分类

实证

(1) 肝气郁结

【病机概要】 郁怒伤肝、疏泄失常、气机阻滞、血行瘀阻。

【主症】 胁肋胀痛，呕逆嗳气、腹痛便泻、便后不爽，每因情志不遂而发作或加剧；或见癥瘕痞块、妇女月经不调。苔薄，脉弦。

【治法】 疏肝理气、破积散聚。

【主方】 柴胡疏肝散[211]，失笑散[86]。

(2) 肝火上炎

【病机概要】 肝胆疏泄无权,气郁化火,上扰巅顶。

【主症】 胁肋灼痛、呕吐苦水,头胀痛,眩晕,耳鸣如潮,目赤,烦怒,吐衄,溲赤便秘。舌红苔黄,脉弦数。

【治法】 清泻肝胆。

【主方】 龙胆泻肝汤[64]。

(3) 肝风内动

【病机概要】 肝气化火、阳气暴张,火随气窜、上冲巅顶。

【主症】 昏厥、痉挛、眩晕、麻木、头痛,并可见口眼㖞斜、语言不利、半身不遂等症。

【治法】 平肝熄风潜阳。

【主方】 天麻钩藤饮[33]等。

(4) 寒滞肝脉

【病机概要】 阴寒之邪侵袭肝经,肝气不畅、络脉痹阻。

【主症】 少腹胀痛,睾丸坠胀或阴囊收缩掣痛,形体虚怯,受寒则甚,得热则舒。舌润苔白,脉沉弦。

【治法】 温经暖肝。

【主方】 暖肝煎[277]等。

虚证

肝阴不足

【病机概要】 肾阴亏虚、水不涵木,或肝郁化火,火盛伤阴,阴不敛阳,虚风内动。

【主症】 眩晕头痛、耳鸣耳聋、鸣声低微,肢体麻木、肌肉瞤动、目干涩、少寐咽干。舌红少津,苔少,脉细数。

【治法】 宁肝滋肾,育阴潜阳。

【主方】 一贯煎[1]、杞菊地黄丸[129]。

兼证

肝气犯胃:兼见肝气郁结、胃失和降病证。治宜泄肝和胃。方用四逆散[81]合左金丸[67]。

肝脾不和:兼见肝郁、脾虚病证。治宜调理肝脾。方用逍遥散[222]。

肝胆不宁:兼见肝血不足,虚阳上扰,血不养心病证。治宜养肝清胆宁神。方用酸枣仁汤[280]。

肝肾阴虚:兼见肝肾阴精亏损、虚火内扰病证。治宜滋阴降火。方用大补阴丸[18]。

证治要点

①肝之病证,有虚实两类,而肝为刚脏,性喜升发,故肝病多见阳亢证候、以实证为多。但实证久延,易于耗伤肝阴,形成临床常见的本虚标实之证,辨证时尤当注意。

②肝病实证之中,肝气郁结、肝火上炎、肝风内动三者同出一源,属同一病理过程的不同阶段,不能截然分割,应做到见证知源、随证施治。

③肝病之虚证,常由肾阴不足,精不化血,而致肝阴不足、阳亢上扰,故治虚阳上亢、肝风内动时,要注意采用肝肾并治之法。

附　胆的病机病证

病机特点

（1）胆附于肝，与肝互为表里，关系密切，故肝气郁滞常影响胆汁的排泄，表现为肝胆同病；

（2）胆性刚直，故病理情况下多表现为火旺之证。

（3）因火热可煎熬津液为痰，故胆病又多兼痰。痰火常扰心神，因此在治疗时，既要注意泄胆化痰，又要清心安神。

胆的常见病证有：惊恐、不寐、耳鸣、眩晕等。

证治分类

（1）胆虚证　见"肝胆不宁"项。

（2）胆实证

【病机概要】　情志郁结，气郁痰生，痰热内扰，胆失疏泄，胃失和降。

【主症】　目眩耳聋，胸满胁痛，烦怒不寐，呕吐苦水，惊悸不宁。苔黄腻，脉弦滑。

【治法】　清化痰热，和胃降逆。

【主方】　黄连温胆汤[233]。

2.4.5　肾（膀胱）系病机病证概要

病机特点

（1）肾为先天之本，藏真阴而寓元阳，故只宜固藏，不宜泄露。禀赋薄弱、劳倦过度、久病失养等，皆可损伤精气，正所谓"五脏之伤，穷必及肾"，所以"肾无实证"，临证只须辨其阴虚抑或阳虚；

（2）肾主藏精，为人体生长、发育、生殖之源，若下元亏损，命门火衰，则为阳痿、五更泄泻；肾气亏耗，固摄失司，可致滑精、早泄；

（3）肾主水液，维持体内水液代谢平衡，若肾阳虚衰，关门不利，气不行水，水湿内聚或泛溢肌肤，则为饮为肿。

临床常见肾的病证有：消渴（下消）、水肿、癃闭、遗精、阳痿、腰痛、耳鸣、眩晕、泄泻等。

证治分类

（1）肾气不固

【病机概要】　劳损过度或久病失养，致肾气亏耗，失其封藏固摄之功。

【主症】　腰脊酸软，滑精早泄，听力减退，小便清频、尿后余沥、甚则不禁。舌淡苔薄白，脉弱。

【治法】　固摄肾气。

【主方】　大补元煎[17]、秘精丸[220]。

（2）肾不纳气

【病机概要】　劳伤肾气或久病气虚，气不归元，肾失摄纳。

【主症】　短气喘逆，动则尤甚，咳逆汗出、咳剧则小便失禁，面浮色白。舌淡苔薄，脉虚弱。

【治法】 纳气固肾。

【主方】 人参胡桃汤[10]、参蛤散[170]。

(3) 肾阳不振

【病机概要】 房劳伤肾或久病不愈，致下元亏损，命门火衰。

【主症】 腰酸腿软，形寒尿频、阳痿、头昏耳鸣。舌淡，脉沉弱。

【治法】 温补肾阳。

【主方】 右归丸[68]、金匮肾气丸[163]。

(4) 肾虚水泛

【病机概要】 肾阳亏耗，不能温化水液，水邪泛溢。

【主症】 水溢肌肤，则为周身浮肿，下肢尤甚，按之如泥，尿少；水泛为痰，则为咳逆痰多，动则喘息。舌淡苔白，脉沉滑。

【治法】 温阳化水。

【主方】 真武汤[199]、济生肾气丸[184]。

(5) 肾阴亏虚

【病机概要】 房劳过度或久病之后，真阴耗伤。

【主症】 头昏耳鸣、少寐健忘、腰酸腿软、遗精早泄，形体虚弱。舌红少苔，脉细。

【治法】 滋养肾阴。

【主方】 六味地黄丸[46]。

(6) 阴虚火旺

【病机概要】 肾阴亏耗，阴虚生内热。

【主症】 颧红唇赤，潮热盗汗，虚烦不寐，阳兴梦遗，口咽干痛。舌红苔少，脉细数。

【治法】 滋阴降火。

【主方】 知柏地黄丸[160]。

兼证

(1) 肾虚脾弱：兼见肾阳虚、脾气虚病证。治宜补火生土。方用附子理中汤[146]、四神丸[82]。

(2) 肾水凌心：兼见心肾阳虚、心阳被遏病证。治宜温化水气。方用真武汤[199]。

证治要点

①肾无表证与实证。肾之热证，属阴虚之变；肾之寒证，属阳虚之候。

②肾虚之证，分为阴虚、阳虚两大类。因此总的治疗原则是：只宜培养，不可攻伐。

③肾与其它脏腑关系密切。如：水不涵木，则肝阳上亢；子盗母气，可耗伤肺阴；水不上济，则心肾不交；火不生土，则脾阳不振。所以，临证辨治肾系病证，尤需注意脏腑间的相互影响。

附 膀胱病机病证概要

病机特点

膀胱与肾互为表里，肾主水液，膀胱贮存津液，化气行水，故二者联系紧密。肾的病变可直接影响于膀胱，其病理表现主要为气化无权。

常见的膀胱病证有：癃闭、遗尿、小便失禁等。

证治分类

（1）虚寒

【病机概要】 肾气亏虚、固摄无权，膀胱失约。

【主症】 小便频数、清长或失禁，尿有余沥。舌润苔白，脉沉细。

【治法】 固摄肾气。

【主方】 桑螵蛸散[228]。

（2）实（湿）热

【病机概要】 湿热之邪，下注膀胱。

【主症】 尿频、尿急、尿涩少而痛，尿黄赤混浊，或尿血、或尿有砂石，可伴发热，腰痛。舌红、苔黄腻，脉数。

【治法】 清利湿热。

【主方】 八正散[12]。

小结

脏腑病机病证，是中医内科学领域最重要，也最常用的诊疗原则和辨证方法，是中医学辨证论证体系的核心。脏腑辨证与脏腑病机，直接探讨和把握机体在疾病状况中五脏气血阴阳的虚实盛衰变化，所以能够明确病位，病性，能够了解脏腑之间相互关系在病理过程中的相互作用和影响。脏腑病机病证尽管错综复杂，千变万化，但仍是"万变不离其宗"——阴阳五行理论指导下的脏腑学说；仍然有明确简要的纲领可以把握——八纲：阴阳、表里、寒热、虚实。这是我们在学习中医内科学全过程中必须时刻注意的。

思考题

1. 脏腑病机病证概念是什么？它在中医内科学领域有什么样的作用？
2. 五脏辨证的病机病证分型及治则各有哪些？
3. 五脏的病机特点是什么？

2.5 内科治疗

2.5.1 治则

治则，是治疗原则的简称，是中医临床理论中的一个重要组成部分。治则的内容，是中医临床施治的指导思想，是制定治疗方法和处方用药的依据，是在对疾病整体病机病证深入分析的基础上，确立的论治原则。治则与治法不同，治则是宏观、整体、战略性的把握和指导；治法是微观、具体、战术性的施治措施与方法。因此，治则是中医学辨证论治体系中承上启下的重要一环。

这里主要介绍中医学的五大治疗原则：

1. 正治反治 正治法，又称逆治法，是临床最常用的治法。如寒者热之，热者寒之，虚者补之，实者泻之等。它适用于病机与症状表现一致，病情比较单纯的情况。选用药性，是逆证性而治。如风寒外束用辛温发表，温热犯肺用辛凉宣透等。

反治法，也称从治法，系特殊情况下，病情出现寒热虚实的假象时，抓住病机本质的一种治法。如寒因寒用（寒证用寒药），热因热用（热证用热药），塞因塞用（塞证用补药），通因通用（泻证用通药）等，它的特点，是采用方药的药性与症状表象相一致。如热深厥深用白虎汤，下利谵语用承气汤等。

2. **标本缓急** 标，是指疾病表现于临床的主要症状；本，是指疾病的病因病机。在病情变化过程中，一般是按照"急则治其标，缓则治其本"和"间者并行，甚者独行"的原则进行治疗。

急则治标，就是对紧急危重证，必须先行解决；缓则治本，就是对病情发展缓慢而平稳者，应主要从病的本质入手治疗。间者并行，是指在标本俱急的情况下，须标本同治；甚者独行，则指标急治标，本急治本的原则。

3. **扶正祛邪** 中医理论认为："正气存内、邪不可干"，"邪之所凑，其气必虚"。疾病的过程，在某种意义上可以说是正气与邪气交争的过程，邪胜于正则病进，正胜于邪则病退。扶正即是补益之法，用于正气虚；祛邪即是攻泻之法，用于邪气实。因此，扶正祛邪就是改变邪正双方的力量对比，使之向病愈转化。

扶正祛邪在临床往往是结合运用，既相辅相成，又有所侧重，总以扶正不留邪，祛邪不伤正为原则。

4. **脏腑补泻** 人体是一个有机的整体，脏腑之间生理上密切联系，病理上相互影响。基于此，临床上就应用脏腑间的生克表里关系，作为治疗上的补泻原则。这些原则可概括为以下三个方面：

（1）虚则补其母，实则泻其子

这是根据脏腑生克关系运用于临床的治疗原则。所谓"母"和"子"，是依五行相生的次序而言的。如：肾与肝是母子相生关系，肝血不足，就可以在补肝血的同时，通过间接地补益肾精，使精血互化，达到滋补肝血的作用，这就是"虚则补其母"；同样，如肝火偏盛，影响肾的封藏功能，致遗精梦泄，也可采用清泻肝火的办法，祛除实邪，使肾的病证痊愈，这也就是"实则泻其子"。

（2）壮水制阳和益火消阴

这是从脏腑病机入手的一种治本之法。壮水制阳，是指对于肾阴不足，虚阳上越之证，需用壮水——滋补肾阴的方药来根治；益火消阴，是指对肾阳亏虚、阴寒内盛之证，要用益火——温补肾阳的根治措施。

（3）泻表安里，开里通表和清里润表

这是根据脏腑的表里关系运用于治疗上的方法。适用于脏与腑之间表里俱病的情况。如，肺与大肠互为表里，当阳明实热，大便燥结而致肺气壅阻时，仅从肺治就很难收效，此时采用凉膈散泻表（大肠）以安里（肺），可收良效。

5. **三因制宜** 三因制宜，即因时、因地、因人制宜。是指治疗疾病应根据季节、地区以及人的体质、年龄、性别等不同情况而制定相应适宜的治疗方法。三因制宜的治疗原则，突出体现了中医学整体观念、辨证论治的特色优势，是提高临床疗效的重要保障。

2.5.2 治法

中医内科学在治疗原则的总体指导下，常用以下治疗方法。

解表法

治疗表证之法。发汗解肌驱邪，又称为汗法。包括辛凉解表、辛温解表、益气解表、辛凉透疹、辛散除湿、宣肺利水等。临床运用时需注意：吐泻亡血失精、疮疡、小便淋涩者禁用；发汗不可过度，以防伤阴耗阳；应考虑地域，体质差异；若有兼证可与它法配合应用。

清热法

治疗热证之法。清热泻火，凉血解毒，又称清法。包括清气分热，清营凉血，清热解毒、清脏腑热。运用清法需明辨寒热真假，寒热虚实，不可滥用；凡阴虚内热，需滋阴以清热，切忌苦寒直折；表邪未解者勿用；可用反治法治疗真热假寒证。

攻下法

泻有形实邪之法。通便泻浊，逐水涤痰，又称下法。包括寒下、热下、润下、逐水等。临证时需注意，邪在表或半表半里时不可妄用攻下，以免引邪入内；年高体弱、久病、妊娠时均宜慎用或不用；下法要中病而止，以免误伤正气而犯"虚虚"之戒。

和解法

和解少阳之法。治疗病入少阳半表半里，用以协调脏腑机能，达邪外出。又称和法。包括和解少阳、调和肝脾、调理胃肠等。和法惟病在少阳时常用之，临证尚需明辨少阳之表里，寒热之偏盛而变通用之。

温里法

治疗里寒之法。补益阳气、祛散寒邪。又称温法。包括温中祛寒，温经散寒，回阳救逆等。临证时必须明辨寒热真假，谨防为热深厥深的假寒证所迷惑。此外，回阳救逆时，必须防止温燥太过，反致耗血伤津散气。虚寒者则需甘温补虚。

补益法

治疗虚证之法。凡气血阴阳，脏腑虚弱诸证均宜补之。又称补法。包括补气、补血、补阴、补阳等。临证需注意防止被"至虚有盛候，大实有羸状"的假象所迷惑。补时要把握气血同源、阴阳互根的关系，注意于阴中求阳，阳中求阴，益气生血等。补法不可用于实证。

消法（消导、消散法）

治疗积聚实邪之法。包括消食导滞、消瘿化瘰、消水除肿、消结化石等。临床使用时必须注意：消法亦属祛邪之法，虚证不可滥用。临床常用消补兼施之法，消食滞、消水肿需与补脾并用；而消结石、消瘿瘰则宜与疏肝利胆诸法并用。

理气法

治疗气机失调之法。包括行气、降气。主要用于肝气郁结、肺气闭阻、胃失和降导致的气滞、气逆证。临床应分辨气之虚实，凡属实证者，均可用理气法治疗。由于理气药物辛燥苦温，运用时需防止过用伤阴耗液。

理血法

治疗血瘀及瘀血、出血之法。包括活血化瘀法、止血法。适用于血行不畅或瘀血内阻及咳血、吐血、衄血、便血、尿血等各种出血病证。临证时要注意气血关系，气滞可导致血瘀，气虚也可导致血瘀，使用理血法时需注意鉴别。理血可与温阳散寒、清热凉血、益气活血诸法并用，但孕妇尤当慎用。止血时还须防止留瘀，一般宜适当配伍一些活血化瘀药，使血止而瘀不留。

固涩法

治疗滑脱诸证之法。包括固表敛汗、涩肠止泻、涩精止遗等。用于肺气不固、自汗；肾气不固、遗精遗尿；脾气不固，下利脱肛等。涩法为补法之属，因此热证、实证、阴虚火亢均不宜使用。本法非治本之法，故需审证求因，临证应酌情与补气、温阳等法合用。

开窍法

开闭通窍以苏醒神志之法。包括凉开、温开法。凉开法用治热入心包的热闭诸证；温开法用治中风阴闭、痰厥、气厥诸证。开窍法以通窍醒神为治，但临证还需结合病机病证，酌用清热、通便、熄风、化痰等法。开窍药多含芳香挥发药物，不宜加热久煎。

镇痉法

治疗因各种原因引发的抽搐、惊厥、神昏诸证之法。包括清热熄风、镇肝熄风、养血熄风、祛风解痉等。临证时需明辨内风、外风以治之。内风需配合养阴柔肝、潜阳清热诸法；外风可祛而散之。祛风药多辛燥，用时谨防伤阴。

小结

中医内科治疗领域，在总的治疗原则指导下，常以上述十二法单独或配合运用，按疾病的发展过程的不同阶段适当选配，以充分体现中医学辨证论治思想的特色。

思考题

1. 中医内科五大治则是什么？
2. 内科学常用治法有哪几种？

各 论

1 感冒

概念

感冒是指感受触冒风邪或时令不正之气所致的常见外感疾病。

本病全年均可发生，尤以春、冬两季多见。临床表现以鼻塞流涕、咳嗽、喷嚏、恶风恶寒、发热、头身疼痛不适为主要特征。有轻重寒热之分。

西医的普通感冒、流行性感冒，可参考本病辨证论治。

病因病机

1. 外感风邪　风为百病之长，常兼挟寒邪、热邪、湿邪侵犯人体而致肺卫失调、营卫失和。

2. 卫阳不固　冬春气候多变，寒温失常，机体卫外之气不能及时调节适应，肌腠毛窍因卫阳不固而疏懈，更易感受外邪。

3. 平素体虚　正气不足、久病体虚，或素体阴阳偏盛偏衰，均易感受风邪。虚人外感在病变过程中有其特殊性。

4. 时邪致病　时令不正之气所致感冒，有不同程度的传染性，严重者可导致疫毒流行，病情严重并可变生它病。

外邪内侵，先犯上焦肺卫之气，口鼻皮毛等肺系部位首当其冲，所以感冒以鼻塞流涕、咳嗽身痛、恶风恶寒、发热等症状为特征。

病因病机要点：

外因 — 外感风寒、风热或时令不正之气 ┐
　　　　　　　　　　　　　　　　　　├ 外邪郁表，肺卫失和(有寒热虚实之别) — 感冒
内因 — 肺卫不固，正气相对不足 ┘

诊断与鉴别

感冒以恶风（恶寒）发热同时并见、肺系症状及全身不适感为症状特征，并以起病突然、病程短、病状轻浅为感冒与其它里证的鉴别要点。感冒尤其应与温疫初起相互鉴别：一般情况下，感冒发热不高或不发热；而温疫必有高热。感冒病程短，症状轻浅而且服解表药后脉静身凉，汗出症减；温疫则症状呈进行性加重，汗出而脉数，热不解，疫毒入里，传变复杂。尤其当冬春季节更需对患者密切观察，认真鉴别。

辨证论治

确诊为感冒后，应进一步辨证分型，以利于治疗。辨证要点如下：

感冒 ┬ 风寒:感受风寒邪气,恶风寒重,发热轻,无汗,身痛,脉浮紧;
　　 ├ 风热:感受风热邪气,恶风汗出发热,微渴,舌边尖红,咽痒,脉浮数;
　　 ├ 暑湿:季节性显著,身热汗少,头身沉重胀痛,苔薄黄而腻,脉濡或濡数;
　　 ├ 虚人外感:因平素阴阳气血不足,感受外邪时各有不同伴见症状,脉虚;
　　 └ 时行感冒:发病突然,恶寒高热,口渴,脉数有力,全身症状显著,传变快;

常见证型有:

1. 风寒感冒

【症状】 恶寒重,发热轻,无汗,头痛,肢体疼痛或不适,鼻塞声重,咳嗽,喷嚏,水样鼻涕,喉痒,痰稀薄白,口不渴或喜热饮。舌质如常,苔薄白,脉浮紧。

【辨证要点】 恶寒重,发热轻,无汗,流清涕,身痛。

本型常见于普通感冒。

【病机概要】 外感风寒,邪郁肺卫,肺系失于宣肃,正邪相搏于肌腠。

【治法】 辛温宣肺解表。

【主方】 荆防败毒散[173]。

如表寒重,身痛头痛者,可加麻黄、桂枝以宣肺散寒,温通表阳。

【调护要点】 适当休息,忌食生冷,慎避风寒。

2. 风热感冒

【症状】 身热较明显,微恶风寒,汗出,头胀痛,咳嗽痰粘黄量少,咽干或咽部红肿疼痛,鼻塞,涕黄浊,口渴欲饮。舌质如常或尖略红,苔薄黄而干,脉浮数。

【辨证要点】 身热明显,微恶风寒,汗出涕浊,咽痛。

【病机概要】 外感风热,犯肺伤津,热郁肌腠肺系,肺卫失宣。

【治法】 辛凉清肺解表。

【主方】 银翘散[255]。

如头痛甚者加桑叶、野菊花清利头目;咽红肿痛加山豆根、玄参、生甘草;咳痰黄粘稠者加黄芩、栝楼、知母以清宣肺热,化痰止咳。

【调护要点】 适当休息,多饮水,忌辛辣煎炸食物。

3. 暑湿感冒

【症状】 身热,微恶风,汗少,肢体酸重或疼痛,头昏闷胀痛,鼻流浊涕,咳嗽痰粘,口中粘腻,渴不多饮,心烦,胸闷泛呕,小便短赤。舌苔薄黄而腻,脉濡数。

【辨证要点】 夏季发病,身热,肢体酸重,头昏重胀,心烦泛呕。

【病机概要】 暑邪挟湿,伤人阳气,湿邪重浊,故易伤表阳、阻清窍、伤肺气、遏中阳。

【治法】 清暑祛湿解表。

【主方】 新加香薷饮[278]。

如热重于湿,热象明显,可加黄连、青蒿、荷叶、芦根清暑泄热;湿重于热,湿邪困表者,可加藿香、佩兰化湿宣表;里湿偏重者,可加苍术、半夏、陈皮和中化湿;小便短赤不利者,可加六一散[44]、黄柏、赤茯苓,清热利湿。

【调护要点】 宜清淡饮食,少食生冷瓜果,忌肥甘厚味。

4. 气虚感冒

【症状】 恶寒较著，发热不明显，无汗或自汗不止，全身倦怠酸楚，咳嗽声低，咳痰无力，微喘，诸症动则加剧。舌淡胖苔薄白，脉无力。

【辨证要点】 素体虚弱，恶寒重，发热轻，咳痰无力，倦怠，脉虚。

【病机概要】 阳气虚弱，卫表不固，正虚邪恋，反复难愈。

【治法】 扶正达邪。

【主方】 参苏饮[168]或玉屏风散[61]。

【调护要点】 慎起居，避风寒；忌食生冷，饮食以富含营养、易于消化为原则。

5. 阴虚感冒

【症状】 身热，微恶风寒，少汗，头昏，口干心烦，干咳少痰。舌红少苔，脉细数。

【辨证要点】 身热少汗，心烦干咳，舌红少苔。

【病机概要】 阴津素亏，复感表邪，无以作汗达邪。

【治法】 滋阴解表。

【主方】 加减葳蕤汤[102]。

口渴咽干症状明显者，可加沙参、麦冬等养阴生津。

【调护要点】 宜清淡易消化饮食，忌食辛辣煎炸油腻之品。

6. 时行感冒

【症状】 突然恶寒，甚则寒战，高热，周身酸痛，剧烈头痛，面色潮红，目赤，倦怠乏力，咽部充血或伴纳呆，恶心，便秘，不咳或微咳，少见鼻塞流涕等症。脉数。

【辨证要点】 流行性发病。起病急骤，恶寒高热，头身剧痛，乏力，呼吸道症状轻而全身症状重。

本型可见于流行性感冒。

【病机概要】 感受时行毒气，犯卫郁肺，热邪伤津，毒气伤阳。

【治法】 清热解毒。

【主方】 清瘟败毒饮[253]。

若热毒症状明显，加大青叶、板蓝根、虎杖、蒲公英等；邪热壅肺而咳喘，加石膏、黄芩以清泻肺热，伴有正气虚损症状者，可酌加益气固脱，生津养阴诸药。本证病情多变，须严密观察，谨防邪毒内陷。

【调护要点】 预防为主。流行季节减少社交活动，口服板蓝根冲剂等，室内可用熏醋法消毒。患者应注意休息，减少活动，按时服药并随时与医护配合，观察病情，防止病邪传变。

小结

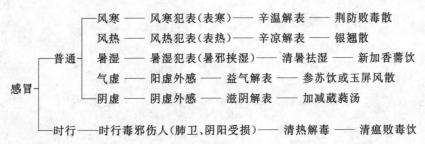

思考题

1. 试述普通感冒与时行感冒的区别。
2. 感冒分为几种证型？各型的辨证要点和治法、主方是什么？

2 咳嗽

概念

咳嗽是肺系疾病的主要证候。咳为有声无痰,嗽为有痰无声,但临床难以截然区别。咳嗽不仅是一种具有独立性的证候,又是肺系疾病的一个常见症状。

以咳嗽为主要表现的病证较多,主要分为外感、内伤两大类别。西医学的多种呼吸系统病患,如上呼吸道感染、支气管炎、肺炎、肺结核、支气管扩张、慢性咽喉炎、肺癌等均可参考本篇辨证治疗。

病因病机

1. 外邪侵袭　肺主气、司呼吸,自然界的"天气"直通于肺,故外邪可由口鼻或皮毛入内,壅遏肺气、伤损肺阴、阻塞肺气出入而引起咳嗽。外邪中最易引发咳嗽者为风、寒、燥、热(火)。

2. 脏腑功能失常　五脏六腑功能失常,均可阻塞气机升降而累及肺主气功能,引发咳嗽,临床称之为"内邪干肺"。临床以脾湿生痰犯肺,肝郁化火伤肺,肾失摄纳累肺致咳为多见。

3. 肺脏自病　肺系外感,迁延不愈伤损肺气,或肺阴久耗,失于清润,均可引发肺主气功能失常,宣发清肃失权,导致咳嗽。

总之,无论外邪侵袭或脏腑失常,都必须损及肺脏,才能引发咳嗽一证出现。所以,咳嗽的病因病机,不止于肺,也不离于肺。

病因病机要点:

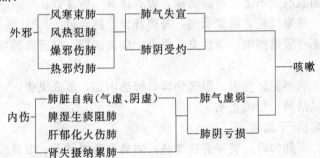

诊断与鉴别

临床以咳嗽为主要见症者,可诊断为本证。咳为有声无痰,嗽为有痰无声的传统说法,因临证难于截然分开,且实际指导意义不大,故可不必过于拘泥。咳嗽既是一个相对独立的证候,又是肺系多种疾患的症状。因此,临床治疗中要在诊断明确的前提下审证求因,分型论治。

辨证论治

咳嗽一证,明确诊断较易,而分型论治最为关键。外感内伤皆可导致咳嗽,五脏六腑内伤皆可令人咳嗽，病因繁多，病机复杂，辨证论治尤当慎重准确。首先需根据咳嗽时间久暂、节律、性质、诱因及伴见症状以区别外感或内伤，并分清寒热虚实，辨证审因，以期指导治疗。

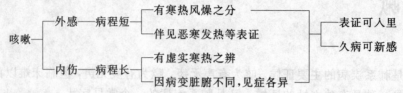

常见证型如下：

外感咳嗽

1. 风寒束肺

【症状】 咳嗽声重，咳痰稀白，气急咽痒。伴见头痛，鼻塞流清涕，肢体酸楚，恶寒发热，无汗。舌淡苔薄白，脉浮或浮紧。

【辨证要点】 咳痰稀白，伴见风寒表证。

本型常见于上呼吸道感染及急性支气管炎初起。

【病机概要】 风寒束肺，阻遏肺气，壅闭腠理。

【治法】 疏风散寒，宣肺止咳。

【主方】 杏苏散[130]，止嗽散[37]。

若风寒重，加麻黄宣肺散寒；若痰湿重，加半夏、厚朴、茯苓化痰燥湿；若外寒内热，气急身热者，加石膏、黄芩、桑白皮以解表清热。

【调护要点】 避风寒，忌食生冷及辛辣等刺激性食物。

2. 风热犯肺

【症状】 咳嗽频作，气粗声嘶，咽喉干燥疼痛，痰黄粘不爽，口微渴。伴见头痛，身热，恶风汗出，四肢酸楚不适，鼻流黄涕。舌苔薄黄，脉浮数。

【辨证要点】 咳嗽气粗，痰黄咽痛，身热汗出。脉浮数。

本型多见于上呼吸道感染、急性支气管炎、肺炎初期、流行性感冒、慢性支气管炎合并感染。

【病机概要】 风热犯肺伤表，阻气伤津，肺热内郁，蒸液成痰。

【治法】 疏风清肺，化痰止咳。

【主方】 桑菊饮[227]加减。

如热邪郁肺，可加知母、黄芩清宣肺热；咽痛重者加射干、山豆根清热利咽；气急似喘加前胡、牛蒡宣肺利气；伤阴重者加沙参、天花粉生津清热。

【调护要点】 忌食煎炸辛辣、油腻食物，节饮食，戒烟酒。

3. 风燥伤肺

【症状】 干咳呛咳，喉痒咽干，痰少而粘难以咯出，或有血丝。伴见鼻干唇燥，甚则咳后胸痛，鼻塞头痛，微有寒热。舌尖红，苔薄黄而干，脉细而略数。

【辨证要点】 干咳喉痒，痰少而粘，难咯出，或带血丝。

本型可见于肺结核、慢性支气管炎、慢性咽炎、肺癌等。

【病机概要】 燥邪伤肺，灼肺伤津，气机不利，表卫不和。

【治法】 疏风清肺，润燥止咳。

【主方】 桑杏汤[226]。

若伤津较重，可加玉竹、麦冬等滋养肺阴；热重可加石膏、知母清肺泄热；燥邪偏凉者，可以温润药物治之，如杏苏散[130]加款冬花、百部、紫菀等清宣温润止咳。

【调护要点】 忌食辛辣煎炸食物，戒烟酒。

内伤咳嗽

1. 痰湿蕴肺

【症状】 咳嗽反复发作，咳声重浊，痰多色白或粘腻成块，脘闷纳呆，神疲乏力，呕恶便溏。苔白腻，脉濡滑。

【辨证要点】 咳声重浊，痰多脘闷，呕恶纳呆，苔白腻。

本型可见于慢性支气管炎、肺气肿等。

【病机概要】 脾湿生痰，上阻于肺，壅遏肺气，累损宣肃功能。

【治法】 健脾燥湿，化痰止咳。

【主方】 二陈汤[2]或三子养亲汤[14]加减。

若中阳重虚，寒痰阻肺，可加细辛、干姜温肺化痰；若脾虚神倦严重，加党参、白术、炙甘草温阳益脾。缓解期可服六君子汤[45]。

【调护要点】 宜食易消化的温性食品，忌劳伤耗气，忌生冷油腻，戒烟酒。

2. 痰热壅肺

【症状】 咳嗽气喘息粗，或喉中有痰声，痰多质粘稠或色黄，咳吐不爽，有腥味，甚者咳唾血痰，胸胁胀满，咳时痛甚，面赤身热，口干欲饮。舌质红、苔黄腻，脉滑数。

【辨证要点】 咳喘息粗，胸满痰黄，面赤身热，舌红苔黄，脉滑数。

本型可见于肺脓疡、支气管扩张合并感染、大叶性肺炎、肺癌。

【病机概要】 邪热壅遏肺气，灼液成痰，伤损脉络，阻滞气机。

【治法】 清热化痰，肃肺止咳。

【主方】 清金化痰汤[248]加减。

若痰黄腥臭如脓，可加鱼腥草、薏苡仁、冬瓜子；胸满喘逆，可加葶苈子；痰火伤津者，可加天冬、麦冬、花粉、沙参等养阴生津。

【调护要点】 戒烟酒，勿食辛辣油腻助火生痰类食物。

3. 肝火犯肺

【症状】 咳逆阵作，咳时面赤咽干，自觉痰滞喉咽不易咯出，量少质粘；咳时痛引胸胁，口苦，症状随情绪变化而增减。舌苔薄黄少津，脉弦数。

【辨证要点】 气逆咳嗽随情绪变化而增减，咳时痛引胸胁，脉弦数。

本型见于结核性胸膜炎、慢性咽喉炎、气管炎。

【病机概要】 肝气郁而化火，上炎侮肺，肺失清肃，木火刑金，灼液成痰。

【治法】 平肝降火，清肺止咳。

【主方】 黛蛤散[287]合泻白散[154]。

若肝火偏盛，可加丹皮、山栀子；若气逆痰促，可加苏子、竹茹、枇杷叶、枳壳、旋覆花；若痰粘咽燥，可加贝母、海浮石、天花粉、麦冬等化痰生津敛肺止咳。

【调护要点】 调情志，戒烟酒，忌食辛辣助火耗气食品。

4. 肺气虚弱

【症状】 咳声低微,喘促气短,动则加剧,痰少质稀,形神疲惫,畏风寒,肢冷自汗,面色无华。舌苔淡白,脉沉细弱。

【辨证要点】 咳喘气短,动则加剧,肢冷自汗,脉沉细弱。

本型可见于肺气肿、肺心病、慢性支气管炎、肺癌。

【病机概要】 肺虚气耗,摄纳无权,气机升降失司而咳喘频作。

【治法】 补肺益气,止咳定喘。

【主方】 补肺汤[143]加减。

若寒痰较重,可加苏子、细辛、桂枝;若兼肾虚失摄作喘,可加蛤蚧、磁石、沉香。肺气虚之咳嗽多兼喘,治疗应权衡主次,调理肺肾阴阳以治之。

【调护要点】 慎起居,避风寒;戒烟酒及刺激性食品,忌食生冷伤阳食物,宜食补而不腻之品。

5. 肺阴亏虚

【症状】 干咳声促,少痰或痰中带血丝,甚则咳血,口燥咽干声嘶,午后潮热,心烦颧红,盗汗失眠,体瘦神疲。舌红少苔,脉细数。

【辨证要点】 干咳咽干,咳血或痰中带血,潮热盗汗,舌红苔少。

本型常见于肺结核、慢性支气管炎、结核性胸膜炎、肺癌。

【病机概要】 肺阴亏虚,虚热内灼,肺失清润,阴津虚耗而致咳,虚火伤络而咯血。

【治法】 滋阴润肺,止咳化痰。

【主方】 沙参麦冬汤[138]加减。

咳而气促者,可加五味子、诃子收敛肺气;潮热、阴虚重者,可加青蒿、鳖甲、地骨皮、银柴胡、胡黄连以清虚热;咯痰咯血可加藕节、丹皮、山栀清热止血;咳久不愈者,可加熟地、五味子、山萸肉滋阴益肾。

【调护要点】 戒烟酒,忌食辛辣助火伤阴食物。

小结

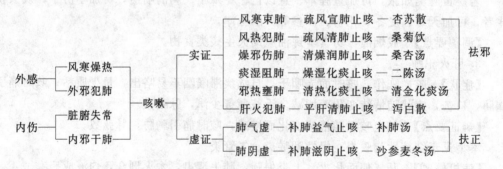

思考题

1. 咳嗽分为哪几大类?如何辨识外感咳嗽与内伤咳嗽的不同?

2. 外感咳嗽各型的症状、诊断要点和治法、主方各是什么?

3. 咳嗽主要涉及哪些脏腑?其病机是什么?

3 哮证

概念

哮证是一种发作性的痰鸣气喘疾患，以呼吸急促困难，喉间哮鸣有声，甚则不能平卧为特征。

由于哮必兼喘，本病又名哮喘，专指发作性呼吸气促、喉中痰鸣者。肺系疾病其他气喘疾患，不属本论范围，但亦可与本论辨证论治内容联系互参。

西医学的支气管哮喘（内源性、外源性、混合性）、慢性喘息性支气管炎，肺气肿等可参考本篇辨证论治。

病因病机

哮证属发作性疾患，病因分为内因、外因两类。

1. 内因　内因又称为夙根，多由宿痰内伏于肺而致。宿痰的成因，可大致分为寒、热二种。

（1）寒痰：屡感风寒，失于表散，邪客肺腧；或久食生冷，伤损肺气，不能布津而成痰；或久病阳气虚弱，形寒饮冷伤肺气而导致寒痰内生。

（2）热痰：过食辛辣甘肥，酿痰生热，上干于肺；或因寒痰郁久化热而成热痰；久病伤阴及素体阳盛者，亦多见热痰内蕴。

2. 外因　外因又称为诱因，是导致哮证发作的直接因素。诱因可大致分为外邪侵袭、饮食失当、情志变化、劳倦过度几类。

外邪侵袭　由于气候突变，机体未能及时适应，风寒暑湿皆可引发哮证；吸入花粉、烟尘、刺激性气味等，也可致哮证发作。

饮食失当　饮食偏嗜，过食肥甘辛辣，或进食海腥膻味，都可成为诱发哮证的因素。

情志变化　七情剧烈变化波动，阻滞气机升降，肺气不利而引动内因，也可诱发哮证。

劳倦过度　劳倦太过，伤损脾肾肺气，引动内郁之伏邪，导致哮证发作。

病因病机要点：

内因：素有寒热痰邪，蕴伏于肺，或久病、禀弱体虚、肺气虚亏　　　　　　　　　　　　　　引发伏痰，痰随气升 — 邪实正虚 — 哮证
诱因：外邪侵袭，饮食失当，情志变化，劳倦过度，触发内邪

诊断与鉴别

本证在发作期因症状特征显著而易于与他病鉴别。临床以发作性呼吸急促，喉间哮鸣有声为诊断及鉴别要点。询问病史，有明显诱因，多数患者有发作史。哮证发作多有先兆，如喉痒，鼻痒，胸闷等。

哮与喘的区别可从病史及症状两方面着眼：喘证无反复发作史，为气息急促或低弱不足导致的呼吸困难，喉中无哮鸣音；哮必兼有喘息，而喘证不必兼哮鸣。

哮与咳的区别也可由病史询问而明确。哮证发作突然，缓解迅速，间歇期形同常人；而咳嗽虽有时兼见痰鸣气喘，却与发作性哮证显著不同，临床较易区别。

哮证，从西医学角度来讲，是由某种过敏源引起的机体（肺部）变态反应，故呈发作性。从中医学理论来看，总属邪实正虚。发作期以邪实为主，间歇期以正虚为主。

哮证与喘证、咳嗽的鉴别要点

鉴别 \ 病名	哮 证	喘 证	咳 嗽
病 史	反复性、间歇性发作	进行性加重、持续	进行性加重、持续
症 状	喉中哮鸣、气急	呼吸困难、气促、喘	咳嗽、可兼见喘、哮
诱 因	明显	不明显	不明显

辨证论治

明确诊断后，应根据发作期、间歇期不同情况，区别寒热虚实，进行辨证论治。

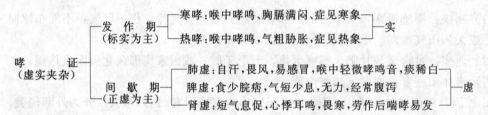

常见证型

发作期

1. 寒哮

【症状】 呼吸急促，喉中哮鸣有声，痰白，胸膈满闷如塞，咳不甚，面色晦暗有青色，口不渴或喜热饮；每因感寒遇冷而诱发，形寒肢冷，或见头痛发热。舌苔白滑，脉弦紧或浮紧。

【辨证要点】 喉中哮鸣气急，感寒遇冷而发，常有鼻喉作痒等先兆。苔白滑。

【病机概要】 寒痰伏肺，感邪诱发，气道阻塞，痰气相搏，胸阳被遏。

【治法】 温肺散寒，化痰止哮。

【主方】 射干麻黄汤[221]，小青龙汤[27]。

两方均可治疗寒哮。若痰多咽喉不利者，可首选射干麻黄汤；若寒邪较重者，可用小青龙汤温散表里之寒。治疗后哮喘渐平，则可按扶正补虚诸法巩固疗效。若诸症未见缓解而神疲汗出，呼吸艰难，累损心阳，欲成脱证者，加补肾纳气固脱类方药，并中西医结合救治。

【调护要点】 慎起居，避风寒，戒劳作，忌食生冷。

2. 热哮

【症状】 呼吸气急声粗,喉间痰鸣如吼,呛咳阵作,胸满胁胀,烦闷不宁,痰黄或白,粘浊质稠,咯吐不利;汗出,口渴喜冷饮,面赤口苦,不恶寒,或兼头痛,发热。舌红苔黄腻,脉滑数或弦滑。

【辨证要点】 气急声粗,痰鸣如吼,痰稠烦满,舌红苔黄腻。

【病机概要】 痰热内蕴,外邪引动,痰火相搏,气道阻塞,邪热壅盛。

【治法】 宣肺清热,豁痰止哮。

【主方】 定喘汤[158],越婢加半夏汤[263]。

两方均为寒温并用。因热哮多由寒郁化火而成,治疗亦不可一味寒凉直折。若表寒内热,可加桂枝、石膏、知母;若邪热伤阴,形瘦咽干,盗汗虚烦,可酌加麦冬、沙参、虫草,以清热养阴,化痰止哮;若诸症加剧,欲成脱证,急宜中西医结合救治。

【调护要点】 忌食辛辣甘肥,慎起居。

间歇期

1. 肺虚

【症状】 自汗畏风,易患感冒,每因气候变化而诱发哮证;鼻塞流清涕,气短声低,喉中常有轻微哮鸣音,咳痰清稀色白,面色㿠白。舌质淡,苔薄白,脉细弱或虚大。

【辨证要点】 自汗畏风,易感冒,喉中轻微哮鸣音。哮喘每因气候变化而复发。

【病机概要】 肺卫气虚,卫外不固,痰饮蕴肺。

【治法】 补肺益气,固表实卫。

【主方】 玉屏风散[61]。

若表虚明显,畏寒畏风者,可加桂枝、白芍、生姜、大枣调和营卫以固表;若气阴两亏,口干咽红少痰者,可合用生脉散[84]以益气养阴。

【调护要点】 避免过敏原刺激,忌生冷,慎起居。

2. 脾虚

【症状】 食少脘痞,大便不实,每因食油腻食物而腹泻,常由饮食失当诱发哮喘,痰多气短,体倦乏力。舌质淡,苔白滑或腻,脉细弱。

【辨证要点】 食少脘闷,便溏体倦。哮喘常由饮食失当而发。

【病机概要】 脾气虚弱,健运无权,中气不足,痰湿内蕴。

【治法】 健脾化痰。

【主方】 六君子汤加减[45]。

若脾阳不振、寒象明显者,可加干姜、肉豆蔻温运脾阳。

【调护要点】 慎起居,避寒邪;忌食肥甘生冷,忌暴饮暴食。

3. 肾虚

【症状】 平素气短息促,动则加剧,吸气不利,心悸头晕耳鸣,腰膝酸软,神疲乏力,每因过劳后哮证发作;畏寒肢冷自汗,面色苍白。舌质淡而胖嫩,脉沉细。肾阴虚者可见烦热颧红,汗出而粘,舌红少津,脉细数。

【辨证要点】 短气息促,动则加剧,腰酸神疲;或烦热颧红。常因过劳诱发哮喘。

【病机概要】 肾中阴阳偏虚,摄纳失权,气不归根。

【治法】 补肾摄纳。

【主方】 金匮肾气丸[163]或七味都气丸[8]。

金匮肾气丸适用于肾气肾阳偏虚者；七味都气丸重在益肾纳气。阴虚明显者去温补药加麦冬、当归、龟板胶。

【调护要点】 戒劳作，节房事；宜食富含营养且易消化食物。

小结

哮证作为一种发作性肺系疾患，诱因在发病过程中非常重要，要重视预防，减少或杜绝诱因。在间歇期注意固养肺、脾、肾之正气。但由于本病正虚邪伏之内因仍为主要矛盾，因此，应依标本缓急的治则调治。

本证颇为顽固，反复发作，迁延难愈。部分青少年患者待成年肾气充盛后自行缓解。若哮证大发作，症状危重，呈喘脱危象时，需及时中西医结合救治。

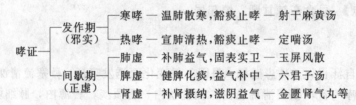

思考题

1. 如何区别寒哮与热哮？
2. 哮证间歇期应从哪几型辨证论治？
3. 哮证发作期分几型？其辨证要点、治法、主方是什么？

4 喘证

概念

喘证是以呼吸困难为特征的肺系疾患。患者因呼吸困难而呈张口抬肩、鼻翼煽动、不能平卧状,严重者每致喘脱。

喘证涉及多种急、慢性疾病,是肺系疾病的主要证候,也可由全身其它脏腑病变而影响于肺所致。临床治疗需辨病与辨证相结合进行。

西医学的慢性喘息性支气管炎、急性支气管炎、肺气肿、肺心病、肺结核、肺不张、癔病性喘息、肺癌、纵隔肿瘤等以喘为主症者,均可参考本病辨证论治。

病因病机

喘证形成的原因可分为外感、内伤两大类。无论外感或内伤首先累及何脏何腑,都要影响肺的主气司呼吸功能,进而导致喘证发生。

1. 外邪侵袭 重感风寒或风热犯肺,内壅肺气,外郁皮肤腠理,或蕴邪伤肺,或炼液成痰,均可导致清肃失司,气逆作喘。

2. 饮食失当 嗜食甘肥生冷或辛辣之品、饮酒过度,脾运失健,痰浊内生,上干于肺,壅阻肺气,气机升降不利,发为喘促;若痰湿郁久化热,痰火交阻,肺气上逆,亦可导致喘促。

3. 情志失调 情志抑郁,忧思气结,肝气上逆,肺失肃降,气逆而喘。

4. 劳欲久病 久病过劳,耗伤肺气肺阴,气失所主而喘促;或久病损脾,或纵欲伤肾,脾为生痰之源,肾为纳气之本,两脏受损,影响及肺而致喘。

喘证病机主要在于肺肾二脏。因肺为气之主,肾为气之根。喘证主要分为虚实两大类,实喘当责之肺,虚喘当责之肾。总而言之,喘证由气机升降出入失常引起。

病因病机要点:

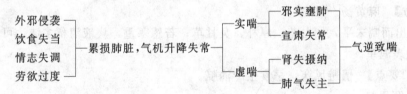

诊断与鉴别

喘证是以呼吸困难、甚则张口抬肩、鼻翼煽动为特征的肺系疾患。临床上应与咳嗽、哮证、气短相互鉴别。与哮、咳的鉴别见"哮证"。

喘证与气短鉴别要点

鉴别\病名	喘 证	气 短
症状	呼吸困难,张口抬肩,鼻翼煽动	少气,呼吸微弱浅促,似喘而无声

(续表)

病名\鉴别	喘 证	气 短
体位	不能平卧	喜卧,能平卧
病性	有虚实之分	一般皆为虚证

辨证论治

明确诊断为喘证后,应首先辨明虚实。

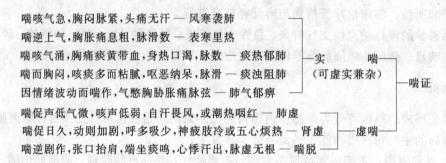

常见证型如下:

实喘

1. 风寒袭肺

【症状】 喘促气急,胸闷咳嗽,痰多色白质稀;兼见恶寒头痛,无汗,口不渴,或见发热。舌苔薄白,脉浮紧。

【辨证要点】 喘促气急,痰多色白质稀,兼见风寒表实证。

本型常见于喘息性支气管炎、急性支气管炎之喘息、肺气肿。

【病机概要】 风寒郁表袭肺,邪气壅实,肺气失宣,寒邪凝液成痰而致喘。

【治法】 宣肺散寒平喘。

【主方】 麻黄汤[242]加减。

若汗出而喘未平,加白芍、厚朴、炙甘草;若感寒重,痰液清稀多沫,可用小青龙汤[27],发表温里。

【调护要点】 慎避风寒,忌食生冷油腻。

2. 表寒里热

【症状】 喘逆气急声粗,胸部胀痛,鼻翼煽动,痰粘稠、咳吐不爽,伴见形寒身热,烦闷身痛,有汗或无汗,口渴。舌红苔薄白或黄,脉浮数或滑数。

【辨证要点】 喘逆气粗声高,形寒身热,脉浮数或滑数。

本证常见于肺炎、支气管扩张合并感染、肺气肿、肺心病合并感染。

【病机概要】 寒邪束表未解,入里化热,郁遏肺气,气逆而喘。

【治法】 宣肺泻热平喘。

【主方】 麻杏石甘汤[241]。

热甚可加黄芩、桑白皮、全栝楼;痰多可加葶苈子、射干。

【调护要点】 忌食辛辣肥甘，忌烟酒，饮食宜清淡。

3. 痰热郁肺

【症状】 喘咳气涌，胸胀痛，痰多色黄质稠，或夹血色，伴见心胸烦热，身热汗出，口渴喜冷饮，咽干，面红，尿赤，大便秘结。苔黄腻，脉滑数。

【辨证要点】 喘咳气涌，胸中烦热胀痛，痰黄稠，苔黄腻。

本证常见于肺炎、支气管扩张合并感染、肺气肿及肺心病合并感染、肺癌、纵隔肿瘤等。

【病机概要】 邪热壅肺，灼津成痰，闭阻气机，肃降无权。

【治法】 清热涤痰平喘。

【主方】 桑白皮汤[225]。

若热邪偏重，身热较甚，加石膏、知母清气泻热；口渴咽干，加天花粉生津清热；喘促气涌，不能平卧者，加葶苈子、大黄、芒硝通腑泻浊降气；痰味腥重者，加鱼腥草、薏苡仁。

【调护要点】 忌食辛辣油腻，忌烟酒。

4. 痰浊阻肺

【症状】 喘咳胸满闷窒，甚则仰息，痰多粘腻色白，咯吐不爽，口粘无味，纳呆恶心。舌苔厚腻色白，脉滑。

【辨证要点】 喘咳胸闷仰息，痰多粘腻色白，恶心纳呆，苔厚白腻。

本证常见于肺不张、肺气肿、肺心病、慢性喘息性支气管炎、矽肺。

【病机概要】 中阳失运，酿痰壅肺，肺气不降，窒满致喘。

【治法】 化痰降气平喘。

【主方】 二陈汤[2]合三子养亲汤[14]。

若脾运呆滞较重者，加苍术、厚朴燥湿理脾；气逆喘咳重者，加贝母、麻黄宣肺平喘。

【调护要点】 宜食清淡易消化之品，忌食甘肥煎炸之物。

5. 肺气郁闭

【症状】 每因情绪刺激而致喘，突然呼吸急促，但喉中痰声不著，气憋胸闷而痛，咽中如物窒塞，或见失眠、胁痛、心悸、脉弦。

【辨证要点】 喘促发作与情绪郁怒有关，气憋胸闷，咽中窒塞感明显，脉弦。

本证可见于癔病性喘息。

【病机概要】 肝郁气逆，犯肺致喘。

【治法】 开郁降气平喘。

【主方】 五磨饮子[43]加减。

若心悸失眠重者，加酸枣仁、远志。

【调护要点】 调情志、忌郁怒；忌食辛辣厚味。

虚喘

1. 肺虚

【症状】 喘促气怯，喉有鼾声，咳声低微，语言无力，痰液稀薄，自汗畏风；或呛咳痰少，咽喉不利，烦热面红。舌质淡红或舌红苔剥，脉象软弱或细数。

【辨证要点】 喘促短气，气怯声低，脉弱。

本证常见于慢性喘息性支气管炎、肺不张、肺气肿、肺心病。

【病机概要】 肺虚致喘可分为肺气虚和肺阴虚两类。肺气虚，则卫外不固；肺阴虚，则虚火上炎。

【治法】 补肺益气，养阴平喘。

【主方】 生脉散[84]合补肺汤[143]。

若气虚阳亏，寒痰内盛，可加干姜、甘草、钟乳石温肺化痰定喘；若阴虚较甚者，可加玉竹、沙参、百合养阴定喘；若兼见食少便溏，腹部有气坠感，则为肺脾两虚，治宜升提益气定喘，可酌加补中益气汤[140]之类药物。

【调护要点】 避风寒，慎劳作，忌辛辣。

2. 肾虚

【症状】 喘促日久，呼多吸少，动则喘甚，气不得续，形神疲惫，肢冷跗肿，汗出，面青唇紫或淡白，舌淡，苔白或黑而湿润，脉微细或沉弱；或喘咳咽干，面红烦躁，足冷，汗出如油，舌红少津，脉细数。

【辨证要点】 喘促日久，呼多吸少，肢冷跗肿，脉微细沉弱；或喘咳咽干，面赤足冷，舌红少津。

本证可见于肺心病、肺气肿、肺不张、肺结核。

【病机概要】 肾虚致喘亦分为肾气虚和肾阴虚两大类。肾气亏虚，失于固纳，气不归根而致喘；若肾中真阴亏耗，孤阳上越，则气失摄纳而致喘。

【治法】 补肾纳气，滋阴定喘。

【主方】 金匮肾气丸[163]，参蛤散[170]或七味都气丸[8]。

若肾气虚者，可用金匮肾气丸温补肾中阳气；气喘冲逆，脐下筑动者，可用参蛤散纳气定喘；肾阴亏耗致喘，可用七味都气丸加减以滋阴纳气；若见颧红额汗之戴阳症者，可加龙骨、牡蛎以潜阳平喘。

肾虚致喘多为久病，一般以阳损及阴为多见，在善后调理期应常服紫河车粉、胡桃肉等扶正固本。

【调护要点】 避风寒，戒劳作，节房事。

3. 喘脱

【症状】 喘逆剧作，张口抬肩，鼻翼煽动，端坐不能平卧，或见痰鸣，心慌动悸，烦躁，面青唇紫，汗出如珠，肢冷神疲，脉浮大无根或见歇止，或脉来模糊不清，或见躁烦内热，咽干颧红，汗出粘手。脉细数无根。

【辨证要点】 喘逆严重，不能平卧，大汗肢冷，脉散乱无根；或躁扰颧红，汗出粘手，脉细数无根。

本证可见于肺心病、心衰、肺癌、纵隔肿瘤等。

【病机概要】 肺气欲竭，心肾阳衰，阴阳欲绝，元气耗散；或真阴耗竭，孤阳失于维系，冲气上逆。

【治法】 扶阳益阴，固脱平喘。

【主方】 参附汤[167]送服黑锡丹[268]。

亦可用独参汤[194]加龙骨、牡蛎、西洋参、五味子等。

【调护要点】 喘证发展到喘脱，为最危重阶段，除中医药扶正固脱治疗外，有必要中西医结合抢救。加强护理，严密观察。

小结

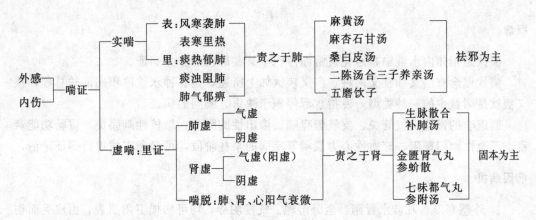

思考题

1. 哮与喘有何联系与区别？
2. 实喘、虚喘如何鉴别？各有哪几种证型？
3. 各型喘证的辨证要点、治法、主方是什么？

5 痰饮

概念

痰饮是指体内水液输布运化失常而停积于某些部位的一类病证。

痰饮概念有广义和狭义两种。广义痰饮如上所述,是各种水饮停积病证的总称;狭义痰饮是诸饮中的一种类型,专指水邪停积于脾胃、肠间的病证。

西医学的慢性支气管炎、支气管哮喘、渗出性胸膜炎、结核性胸膜炎、胃肠功能紊乱、不全性幽门梗阻、充血性心力衰竭等疾病的某些阶段,可参考本病进行辨证论治。

病因病机

1. 外感寒湿　凡涉水冒雨、坐卧湿地、气候阴冷,均可伤损卫阳肌表,由皮毛而伤及肺气。肺失宣发,寒湿之邪由表入里,浸渍肌肉,内困脾胃,以致外湿引动内湿,水津停滞,积而成饮。

2. 饮食不当　大量饮冷水、茶水、生冷食品,冷热相搏,中阳暴遏,脾失运化,水湿之邪自内而生,津液不能正常代谢而化生成饮。

3. 劳欲所伤　凡劳倦过度伤脾,或纵欲过度伤肾,阳气虚耗,运化功能失常,均可导致水湿内停而成痰饮。

中医学理论认为,三焦是气化的场所,上焦(肺)有宣发津液,肃降水湿作用;中焦(脾)有运化水谷和水液作用;下焦(肾)有蒸化水液,分清泌浊作用。所以,如果三焦某一部分脏腑失职、气机闭塞,必将影响机体水液吸收、运行、排泄的正常过程,导致水饮停积,发生痰饮病证。

病因病机要点:

外感寒湿 — 伤卫阳、伤肺气 ┐
饮食不当 — 伤脾阳　　　　├ 阳虚阴盛,三焦输化失调,水饮停积 — 痰饮
劳倦纵欲 — 伤肾阳、伤脾阳 ┘

诊断与鉴别

痰、饮、水、湿的鉴别

病名	病机	特　点
痰	津液不归正化,停积而成	多厚浊,无处不到,病变多端,多因热煎熬而成,为阳邪
饮		呈稀涎,多停于体内局部,多由寒积聚而生,为阴邪
水		为清液,每泛溢体表、全身,属阴类,但有阴阳之分
湿		粘而滞,发病缓慢,缠绵难解,属阴邪,每与它邪相兼为患

痰饮还须与其它病证如哮证、喘证、水肿相互区别。痰饮中各型(痰饮、悬饮、溢

饮、支饮）是依水邪停聚部位从病理角度命名，而哮证、喘证、水肿是以病证特点命名。痰饮与水肿同属津液病变，但前者饮邪停积于局部，后者水液泛滥于全身。因而有区别，也有某些内在的联系。

辨证论治

痰饮的辨证，应首先依水液停积的不同部位而分为四类证型，即痰饮、悬饮、溢饮、支饮。

四类证型的鉴别如下：

鉴别 病名	病位	病机	主 要 症 状
痰饮	停留胃肠	脾阳虚弱	心下痞闷、胃肠中沥沥水声、呕痰沫
悬饮	水流胁下	肺气失宣	胸胁刺痛、心下痞硬、干呕
溢饮	泛溢肢体	肺脾失职	肢体浮肿疼痛、无汗、喘咳
支饮	支撑胸肺	肺气虚弱	咳喘不能平卧、痰白量多

痰饮的治疗，当以温化为原则。因其病机主要是阳虚阴盛，本虚标实，故健脾温肾为其正治；发汗、利水、攻逐，乃为治标权宜之法。

痰饮

1. 脾阳虚弱

【症状】 胸胁支满、心下痞闷，胃中有振水音，脘腹喜温畏寒，背微恶寒，呕吐清水痰涎，口渴不欲饮，饮水易呕，心悸气短，食少便溏，形体渐瘦。舌苔白滑，脉弦细而滑。

【辨证要点】 心下痞闷，胃中有振水声，畏寒喜温，食少便溏。

本证常见于胃肠功能紊乱、不完全性幽门梗阻、充血性心力衰竭等。

【病机概要】 饮停中焦，脾阳不振，寒湿内聚，清阳不升。

【治法】 温运脾阳，化饮降逆。

【主方】 苓桂术甘汤[150]或小半夏加茯苓汤[25]。

若脾阳虚水饮严重，可用苓桂术甘汤；若水停心下，胃失和降者，可用小半夏加茯苓汤；若小便不利，心悸眩冒，可加泽泻、猪苓；若胃脘冷痛，涎沫频吐者，可加肉桂、干姜、吴茱萸温中降逆；心下痞闷严重者，可加枳实行气消痞。

【调护要点】 避风寒，忌生冷油腻食物。

2. 饮留胃肠

【症状】 脘腹坚满或痛，自利，利后症减，继而又加重；水走肠间漉漉有声，或便秘腹满，口舌干燥、不欲饮水。苔或黄或白而腻，脉沉弦或伏，重取乃得。

【辨证要点】 腹满自利或便秘，口干不欲饮，肠间有水声，脉沉弦。

本证常见于胃肠神经官能症。

【病机概要】 水饮留滞肠胃，饮邪难尽新饮又积，阳气被遏。

【治法】 攻下逐饮。

【主方】 己椒苈黄丸[24]或甘遂半夏汤[73]。

若饮在肠间，郁而化热者，可用己椒苈黄丸前后分消；若水饮在胃肠间，可用甘遂半夏汤攻守兼施。若饮邪上逆，胸满严重者，可加枳实、厚朴利气行水。但攻逐水饮时必须注意顾护正气，不可攻伐太过，更伤中阳。

【调护要点】 忌食生冷肥甘之品。

悬饮

1. 邪犯胸肺

【症状】 胸胁刺痛，呼吸或活动时加剧，心下痞硬，寒热往来或发热不恶寒，汗少或有汗而热不解，咳嗽气急，痰少干呕，口苦咽干。苔薄或白或黄，脉弦数。

【辨证要点】 胸胁刺痛因呼吸、活动而加剧，心下痞硬，干呕口苦。脉弦数。

本证常见于胸膜炎、肺炎、支气管炎、支气管哮喘等。

【病机概要】 时邪外袭，热郁胸肺，肺气失宣，邪蕴少阳。

【治法】 和解宣利。

【主方】 柴枳半夏汤[212]。

若见咳嗽气粗，胁痛较剧，可用本方加桑白皮、白芥子；若心下痞硬，口苦干呕较重，可加半夏、栝楼；热象明显，汗出较多者，可加麻杏石甘汤[241]合用。

【调护要点】 忌肥甘、辛辣；慎起居，避外邪。

2. 饮停胸胁

【症状】 咳唾引痛，呼吸困难，咳逆喘促不得平卧，或仅能偏卧于饮停一侧，患侧肋间胀满，甚则胸廓隆起。舌苔薄白腻，脉沉弦或弦滑。

【辨证要点】 咳喘气逆不能平卧，胸胁引痛，脉弦滑。

本证常见于渗出性胸膜炎、肺炎、支气管哮喘。

【病机概要】 饮停气滞，脉络不通，肺气痹窒，饮邪上迫。

【治法】 逐水祛饮。

【主方】 十枣汤[6]。

本方主治水饮结胸，体壮邪实，水邪结多者。若邪实体虚，可用控涎丹[238]宣肺理气祛饮，药力较缓。十枣汤、控涎丹服后见呕吐、腹泻剧烈，可暂停服二、三日，改用椒目栝楼汤[265]导水除饮；若痰涎偏盛，可加薤白、杏仁；若体虚食少，饮停日久，可加桂枝、白术、甘草通阳化饮。凡病久或体虚者，不宜峻攻。

【调护要点】 忌食生冷油腻之品；加强护理，慎避外邪。

3. 络气不和

【症状】 胸胁闷痛不舒，有刺痛或灼痛感，呼吸不畅或有闷咳；甚则迁延不已，遇阴雨时加重。舌质暗，苔薄，脉弦。

【辨证要点】 胸胁疼痛，如灼如刺，闷咳胸满，舌暗脉弦。

本证常见于陈旧性胸膜炎等。

【病机概要】 饮邪久郁，气滞络痹。

【治法】 理气和络。

【主方】 香附旋覆花汤[188]加减。

若胸闷苔腻，痰气郁阻较重者，可加栝楼、枳壳；若久病入络，疼痛明显者，加当归、桃仁、红花、没药等；若咳痰量多而稀者，为水饮不净，可加冬瓜皮、桑白皮、通草等。

【调护要点】 忌食辛辣煎炸油腻之品；调情志，忌忧思郁怒。

4. 阴虚内热

【症状】 呛咳阵作，口干咽燥，咯痰量少质粘，或见午后潮热，颧红盗汗，心烦失眠，伴胸胁闷痛，病程较长，形体消瘦。舌红少苔，脉细小而数。

【辨证要点】 呛咳咽干，痰少质粘，颧红盗汗，舌红少苔。

本证常见于结核性胸膜炎等。

【病机概要】 饮阻气郁，化热伤阴，阴虚肺燥，络脉失和。

【治法】 滋阴清热，通络祛饮。

【主方】 沙参麦冬汤[138]合泻白散[154]。

若干咳痰少咽干，胸痛舌红者，用沙参麦冬汤；若呛咳气逆，肌肤蒸热者，用泻白散。若潮热甚者，为阴伤较重，可加鳖甲、白薇、玄参；若咳呛剧作可加川贝、百部；胸胁闷痛严重，加丝瓜络、栝楼皮、郁金、枳壳；兼见久病正虚，神疲气短者，可酌加黄芪、五味子、白术、太子参等。

【调护要点】 忌辛辣醇酒，戒房事。

溢饮

【症状】 身体疼痛沉重，肢体浮肿，恶寒，无汗；或见喘咳，痰多而色白有沫，胸闷干呕，不欲饮水。苔白，脉弦紧。

【辨证要点】 身重疼痛，肢体浮肿，恶寒无汗，喘咳，痰白而多。

本证常见于支气管炎。

【病机概要】 外感风寒，肌腠郁闭，肺脾失职，水饮流溢四肢体表。

【治法】 发表化饮。

【主方】 小青龙汤[27]。

若肢体浮肿较重而尿少者，可加茯苓、猪苓、泽泻；若饮邪化热，烦躁，苔白黄相兼者，可加石膏；若寒象不明显者，可去干姜、细辛。

【调护要点】 慎避风寒，忌食生冷肥甘。

支饮

1. 寒饮伏肺

【症状】 咳逆喘满不得平卧，痰白量多有沫，病程迁延，天寒受凉则加剧，甚则面浮跗肿；或平素伏而不作，遇寒即发，发作时腰疼背痛，身体振振瞤动，发热恶寒。舌苔白滑或白腻，脉弦紧。

【辨证要点】 咳逆喘满不得卧，痰白量多，感寒即发。

本证可见于慢性支气管炎、肺气肿、肺心病、充血性心力衰、肾功能衰竭等。

【病机概要】 饮邪迫肺，痰阻气壅，寒饮内盛，水饮泛溢。

【治法】 温肺化饮。

【主方】 小青龙汤[27]。

若饮多寒少，表证不显者，可用葶苈大枣泻肺汤[261]；若体虚，表证不显者，用苓甘五味姜辛汤[149]；若胸满气逆苔浊者，用小青龙汤加白芥子、莱菔子；若饮邪壅实，胸痛烦闷者，可用小青龙汤配甘遂、大戟。邪实下虚，郁饮化热，症见心下痞硬，面色黧黑，烦渴咳逆者，用木防己汤[35]行水散结、补虚清热；寒饮郁久化热，症见痰稠咽燥，舌红少津者，可用麦门冬汤[124]加栝楼、木防己、川贝生津化饮清热。

【调护要点】 避风寒，调饮食，忌生冷肥甘。

2. 脾肾阳虚

【症状】 喘促气短，动则加剧，或咳而气怯，痰多食少，胸闷神疲，畏寒肢冷，小腹拘急，脐下悸动，足跗浮肿，小便不利，或口吐涎沫，头目昏眩。舌苔白润或灰暗而腻，舌质胖大，脉沉细。

【辨证要点】 喘促气短，畏寒肢冷，足跗浮肿，食少痰多，头目昏眩。舌体胖大，脉沉细。

本证常见于肺气肿、支气管哮喘、充血性心力衰竭等。

【病机概要】 饮邪日久，伤及脾肾，温运无权，水饮泛逆。

【治法】 温补脾肾，蠲化水饮。

【主方】 金匮肾气丸[163]、苓桂术甘汤[150]。

若脾虚严重者，首选苓桂术甘汤健脾化饮；肾虚严重者，选用金匮肾气丸温肾化饮。食少痰多者，可加半夏、陈皮、砂仁、白蔻；脐下悸动、头目昏眩者，可用五苓散[41]或真武汤[199]降逆化气平饮。

【调护要点】 慎避风寒，忌食生冷；戒劳作，节房事。

小结

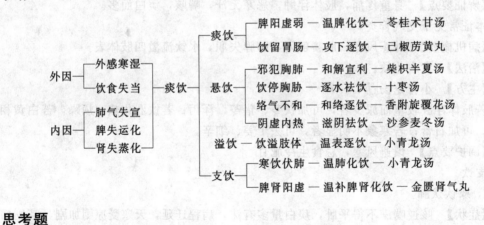

思考题

1. 广义痰饮分几大类？如何鉴别？
2. 痰、饮、水、湿有何异同？
3. 临床上对支饮怎样辨证论治？

6 自汗、盗汗

概念

　　自汗、盗汗是由于阴阳失调、腠理不固，致汗液外泄失常的一类病证。自汗为非睡眠状态中时汗出，动则加剧；盗汗为睡眠中汗出，而醒后自止。自汗、盗汗既是一种相对独立的病证，又是某些疾病过程中的症状，因此，临床较为常见。

　　西医学的植物神经功能紊乱、结核病、风湿热、甲状腺功能亢进、低血糖症、更年期综合征、休克等疾病的某些阶段以自汗、盗汗为主症者，可参考本病进行辨证论治。

病因病机

　　1. 肺气不足　肺主皮毛、司卫气。肺气不足则卫气失于固护，腠理开合失司而自汗。

　　2. 营卫不和　营卫同源而营行脉中，卫行肌腠。营卫失和，卫外失司，汗泄失常而自汗。

　　3. 阳气虚弱　阳气虚耗，不能收敛阴液，阴液外泄而致自汗不止，可导致汗多亡阳。

　　4. 阴虚火旺　亡血失精，热病伤阴，阴津亏耗，虚火内生，迫劫阴津作汗而泄，形成盗汗。

　　5. 邪热郁蒸　肝火湿热内蕴，蒸迫津液外泄，导致自汗。

　　病因病机要点：

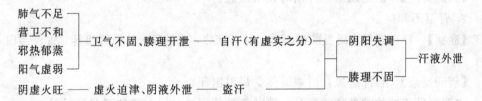

诊断与鉴别

　　自汗以非睡眠时汗出为特征；盗汗以睡眠汗出、醒后汗止为特征，临床易于诊断与鉴别。

　　自汗、盗汗应与脱汗、战汗相鉴别。

　　其主要鉴别如下：

鉴别\病名	自　汗	脱　汗	战　汗	盗　汗
病因病机	肺气不足，营卫不和，阳气虚弱，邪热郁蒸	正气欲脱，阳不敛阴。常见于危重病人	外感热病，正邪交争。常见于急性热病	阴精亏耗，虚火内生，阴津被扰，不能自藏

(续表)

病名鉴别	自汗	脱汗	战汗	盗汗
临床表现	醒时汗出,常兼表证,全身症状较轻	醒时或昏睡汗出,大汗淋漓,四肢厥冷,病情危重	发热烦渴,突然恶寒战栗,继而汗出	睡眠汗出,醒后即止

辨证论治

自汗、盗汗临床较易诊断及鉴别。在辨证论治时,应着重辨别阴阳虚实。自汗多属虚证,而其中邪热郁蒸为实证;盗汗为虚证,有心、肺、肾阴亏之别。

常见证型如下:

自汗

1. 肺气不固

【症状】 汗出,恶风寒,动则尤甚,易于感冒,面色㿠白,体倦乏力。苔薄白,脉细弱。

【辨证要点】 汗出,恶风寒。易患感冒。

本型常见于植物神经功能紊乱、低血糖症等。

【病机概要】 体虚肺气不足,皮毛肌腠不固。

【治法】 益气固表止汗。

【主方】 玉屏风散[61]。

汗出过多者可加入麻黄根、浮小麦、煅牡蛎敛阴止汗。

【调护要点】 慎避风寒,汗出时尤须注意。

2. 营卫不和

【症状】 汗出恶风,周身酸楚不适,时有寒热,或半身、某局部出汗。舌苔薄白,脉缓。

【辨证要点】 自汗恶风,时寒时热,局部出汗。

本型可见于植物神经功能紊乱、甲状腺功能亢进、风湿热的某些阶段等。

【病机概要】 体弱正虚,阴阳失调,营卫失和,腠理不固。

【治法】 调和营卫。

【主方】 桂枝汤[200]加减。

汗出过多者,可加煅龙骨、煅牡蛎固摄敛汗;气虚者加黄芪益气固表;阳虚畏寒者加附子温阳;失眠或半身汗出者,可用甘麦大枣汤[71]。

【调护要点】 慎避风寒,忌肥甘。

3. 阳气虚弱

【症状】 久病阳虚或重病患者,突然汗出不止,语声低微,神疲体倦,呼吸短促,四肢不温,脉弱。

【辨证要点】 久病重病中,突然汗出不止。

本型常见于低血糖症、休克。

【病机概要】 久病重病阳气虚微,阳不敛阴。

【治法】 益气温阳敛汗。

【主方】 生脉散[84]加减。

本型须及时止汗并对症治疗全身虚弱诸症状,以防病变加剧,转为亡阴或亡阳脱汗。

若汗出不止,四肢不温明显,可加黄芪、人参益气扶阳,或加煅龙骨、牡蛎敛汗固摄;病情转剧者,用参附汤[167]回阳救逆,敛汗固脱。

【调护要点】 静卧休息,密切观察病情。注意补充水分,忌食生冷,慎避风寒。必要时,采取综合治疗措施。

4. 邪热郁蒸

【症状】 汗出蒸蒸不止,面赤烘热,躁扰不宁,肢节烦痛,汗出身热不退,口苦,溲黄,便干。舌红苔黄,脉数而有力。

【辨证要点】 汗出蒸蒸,身热不退,口苦,溲黄,舌红苔黄,脉数。

本型可见于风湿热、更年期综合征、甲状腺功能亢进等。

【病机概要】 肝火亢盛或湿热内蕴,蒸腾津液外泄。

【治法】 清肝泄热,化湿和营。

【主方】 龙胆泻肝汤[64]。

若汗多伤津,口渴引饮者,可加天花粉、鲜芦根、石斛;热结便闭者,可加生大黄、芒硝通腑泻浊;热势不盛,湿热之象明显者,可用四妙丸[76];酌加竹叶、山栀子、黄连清心除烦。

【调护要点】 适量饮水,补充阴液;忌食辛辣肥甘;调情志,忌郁怒。

盗汗

1. 心血不足

【症状】 睡眠汗出,醒后即止,心悸少寐,多梦神疲,气短乏力,面色无华。舌质淡,苔薄,脉虚。

【辨证要点】 盗汗,心悸,多梦,舌淡。

本型可见于结核病、植物神经功能紊乱、更年期综合征等。

【病机概要】 心血亏耗,虚火内扰,阴津外泄。

【治法】 补血养心敛汗。

【主方】 归脾汤[95]。

汗多者加煅龙骨、煅牡蛎、五味子、浮小麦等;阴伤有热象者加青蒿、知母、地骨皮等。

【调护要点】 忌食辛辣耗气伤阴食品。慎起居,避风寒,调情志。

2. 肺肾阴虚

【症状】 盗汗潮热,虚烦少寐,干咳日久,腰膝酸软,五心烦热,形体消瘦;女子月经量少色红,经期不调,梦交;男子遗精。舌红少苔,脉细数。

【辨证要点】 盗汗潮热,干咳消瘦,腰酸遗精,舌红苔少。

本型可见于结核病、甲状腺功能亢进、更年期综合征等疾病的某些阶段。

【病机概要】 亡血失精,肺肾阴亏,虚火内炽,迫汗外泄。

【治法】 滋阴降火敛汗。

【主方】 当归六黄汤[113]。

若潮热烘作，加知母、地骨皮、龟板等；若盗汗较重，可加煅龙骨、煅牡蛎、麻黄根等；虚热甚者，除方中重用黄柏外，可加青蒿、鳖甲、银柴胡等。

【调护要点】 调起居，戒房劳；忌食辛辣之品，宜清淡养阴饮食。

小结

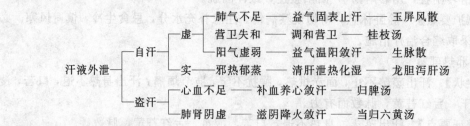

思考题

1. 自汗与盗汗、脱汗、战汗如何鉴别？
2. 自汗分哪几种证候类型？为什么虚证和实证都可以引起自汗？
3. 盗汗各型的辨证要点，病机概要，治法和主方是什么？

7 心悸

概念

心悸包括惊悸和怔忡，是指病人自觉心中悸动、惊惕不安，甚则不能自主的一种病证。

西医学中的各种器质性和功能性心脏病，如病毒性心肌炎、心律失常，以及心脏神经官能症、充血性心力衰竭、甲状腺功能亢进、贫血、低血糖症等疾病，表现以心悸为主症者，均可参照本病辨证论治。

病因病机

1. 心虚胆怯　平素心虚胆怯，由于突然惊恐，使心惊神慌不能自主；或因大怒伤肝，大恐伤肾，阴虚于下，火逆于上，动撼心神，而发惊悸。

2. 心血不足　久病体虚，失血过多，或思虑过度，劳伤心脾，脾胃生化无源，气血两亏，阴血亏损，心失所养，不能藏神，致神不安而志不宁，出现心慌心悸。

3. 阴虚火旺　久病体虚，伤及肾阴；或肾水素亏，虚火妄动，上扰心神，遂成本病。

4. 心阳不振　大病久病之后，阳气衰弱，不能温养心脉，导致心悸不安。

5. 水饮凌心　脾肾阳虚，不能蒸化水液，停聚而为饮，饮邪上犯，心阳被抑，因而引起心悸。

6. 瘀血阻络　心阳不振，血液运行不畅，或风寒湿邪搏于血脉，内犯于心，以致心脉痹阻，营血运行不畅，引起心中悸动不安。

病因病机要点：

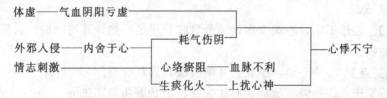

诊断与鉴别

心悸是以病人自觉心中悸动，惊惕不安为特征。惊悸和怔忡二者均有心慌心跳，但在病因和病情上有区别：

鉴别 \ 病名	惊　悸	怔　忡
病　因	常因外因而成；或因惊恐，或因恼怒	多因内因引起；或阴血亏损，或心阳不足
病　情	发作心悸，时作时止，属阵发性，病来虽速，但病势浅而短暂	稍劳即发，持续不已，发病虽渐，但病较重

辨证论治

在明确心悸的诊断后，要进一步辨证。首先，要看病人是否有"心跳"、"心慌"不能自主的自觉症状；其次，要区别其性质，是属实证还是虚证，是心阳虚还是心阴虚，是挟痰还是挟瘀；第三，从病因和病情上区别是惊悸还是怔忡。

常见证型：

1. 心虚胆怯

【症状】 心悸，善惊易恐，坐卧不安，少寐多梦。舌苔薄白或如常，脉象动数或虚弦。

【辨证要点】 心中悸动，善恐易惊。

本型常见于心脏神经官能症。

【病机概要】 惊则气乱，心不藏神，气血逆乱。

【治法】 镇惊定志，养心安神。

【主方】 安神定志丸[112]。

惊悸严重者，可加琥珀、磁石镇惊安神；若心胆虚怯者，可加炙甘草以补益心气；若心阴不足，加柏子仁、五味子、酸枣仁以养心安神，收敛心气。

【调护要点】 怡养性情，保持精神乐观。

2. 心血不足

【症状】 心悸头晕，面色无华，倦怠无力。舌质淡红，脉象细弱。

【辨证要点】 心悸伴头晕，面色无华，脉细。

本型常见于贫血、低血糖症、病毒性心肌炎、心律失常。

【病机概要】 心血虚损，外不华面，内不养心充脑振脉。

【治法】 补血养心，益气安神。

【主方】 归脾汤[95]。

若见心动悸而脉结代者，宜用炙甘草汤[165]益气养血，滋阴复脉；若热病后期，损及心阴而心悸者，则用生脉散[84]以益气养阴。

【调护要点】 加强营养，戒劳作。

3. 阴虚火旺

【症状】 心悸不宁，心烦少寐，头晕目眩，手足心热，耳鸣腰酸。舌质红，少苔或无苔，脉细数。

【辨证要点】 心悸心烦，少寐，耳鸣腰酸，舌红少苔。

本证可见于心脏神经官能症、心律失常、甲状腺功能亢进等。

【病机概要】 肾阴不足，水不济火，心火内动，扰动心神。

【治法】 滋阴清火，养心安神。

【主方】 天王补心丹[32]。

若伴腰酸梦遗者，可用知柏地黄丸[160]。

【调护要点】 忌辛辣，戒烟酒，节房事。

4. 心阳不振

【症状】 心悸不安，胸闷气短，面色苍白，形寒肢冷。舌质淡，脉象虚弱或沉细。

【辨证要点】 心悸气短，形寒肢冷，脉沉弱。

本证可见于病毒性心肌炎、充血性心力衰竭、心律失常、心脏神经官能症、贫血、低血糖症。

【病机概要】 久病体虚，心失温养，心阳不振，鼓动无力。

【治法】 温补心阳,安神定悸。
【主方】 桂枝甘草龙骨牡蛎汤[201]。
若病情较重,汗出肢冷,可加人参、附子回阳救逆。
【调护要点】 戒劳作,忌生冷,避风寒。

5. 水饮凌心

【症状】 心悸眩晕,胸脘痞闷,形寒肢冷,小便短少,或下肢浮肿,渴不欲饮,恶心吐涎。舌苔白滑,脉弦滑。

【辨证要点】 心悸眩晕,脘痞肢冷,恶心吐涎,苔白滑。

本型可见于充血性心力衰竭、病毒性心肌炎、贫血等。

【病机概要】 阳虚不能化水,水邪内停,上凌于心;饮阻于中,清阳不布。

【治法】 振奋心阳,化气行水。
【主方】 苓桂术甘汤[150]。
若水饮上逆,呕恶吐涎者,加半夏、陈皮、生姜以和胃降逆;如属肾阳虚衰不能制水,水气凌心者,宜真武汤[199]。
【调护要点】 忌生冷肥甘。水肿较甚者,低盐饮食。

6. 心血瘀阻

【症状】 心悸不安,胸闷不舒,心痛时作,或见唇色青紫。舌质紫暗或有瘀斑,脉涩或结代。

【辨证要点】 心悸伴胸闷心痛,舌质紫暗或有瘀斑。

本型常见于冠心病、心脏神经官能症等。

【病机概要】 心脉瘀阻,心失所养,心阳遏滞,脉络瘀阻。

【治法】 活血化瘀,理气通络。
【主方】 桃仁红花煎[206]。
若心悸较重者,可酌加生龙骨、生牡蛎以镇心安神。
【调护要点】 避免剧烈运动,忌忧思恼怒。

小结

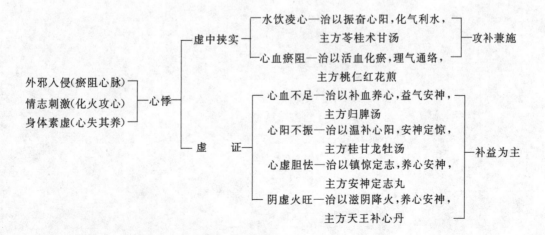

思考题

1. 心悸的发病机制是什么？
2. 心悸虚证常见哪些证型？其辨证要点、治法、主方各是什么？
3. 惊悸与怔忡如何鉴别？

8 胸痹

概念

　　胸痹是指胸部闷痛，甚则胸痛彻背、短气、喘息不得卧为主症的一种疾病。

　　西医学的冠状动脉粥样硬化性心脏病、风湿性心脏病、病毒性心肌炎、心肌病及心脏神经官能症、胸膜炎等具有胸痹表现者，均可参照本病辨证论治。

病因病机

　　1. 寒邪内侵　素体阳衰，胸阳不足，阴寒之邪乘虚侵袭，寒凝气滞，痹阻胸阳而成胸痹。

　　2. 饮食不当　饮食不节，如过食肥甘生冷，或嗜酒成癖，以致脾胃损伤，运化失健，聚湿成痰。痰阻脉络，则气滞血瘀、胸阳失展而成胸痹。

　　3. 情志失调　忧思伤脾，脾虚气结，气结则津液不得输布，遂聚而为痰；郁怒伤肝，肝失疏泄，肝郁气滞，甚则气郁化火，灼津成痰。气滞痰阻，血行失畅，脉络不利，胸阳不运，心脉痹阻不通则发为胸痹。

　　4. 年迈体虚　年迈之人，肾气渐衰，如肾阳虚衰，则不能鼓舞五脏之阳，导致心气不足或心阳不振；肾阴亏虚，则不能滋养五脏之阴，可引起心阴内耗。本虚标实，导致气滞、血瘀，而使胸阳失运，心脉阻滞，发生胸痹。

　　以上病因病机，可二者或三者并存，或交互为患。一般来讲，总属本虚标实。

　　病因病机要点：

```
寒邪内侵┐
饮食不当│
情志失调├──胸阳不振，气滞血瘀──胸痹
年迈体虚┘
```

诊断与鉴别

　　胸痹是以胸部闷痛，甚则胸痛彻背为特征。真心痛是胸痹发展的危重阶段，而胃脘痛与悬饮也均伴有胸痛，应予鉴别。

鉴别＼病名	胸　痹	悬　饮	真心痛	胃脘痛
疼痛部位	胸部	胸胁部	胸部（偶见胃脘、肩背部）	胃脘部
疼痛性质	憋闷窒痛，历时短暂，休息或用药后可缓解	胀痛，持续不解，呼吸时疼痛加重	疼痛剧烈，持续不解	多为胀痛、隐痛
伴见症状	可引及左侧肩背疼痛。常于劳累、情绪激动后突然发作	多伴咳嗽、咯痰、肋间饱满等症	伴汗出肢冷、唇紫、手足青至节、脉结代等	嗳气、呕恶、泛酸

辨证论治

在对胸痹明确诊断后,辨证首当掌握虚实、分清标本:

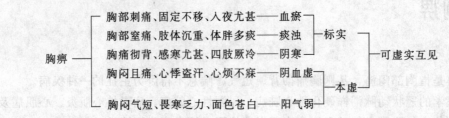

常见证型如下:

1. 心血瘀阻

【症状】 胸部刺痛,固定不移,入夜尤甚,时或心悸不宁。舌质紫暗,脉象沉涩。

【辨证要点】 胸部刺痛,固定不移,舌质紫暗。

本型常见于急性心肌梗死、心绞痛等。

【病机概要】 气郁日久,瘀血内停,络脉不通。

【治法】 活血化瘀,通络止痛。

【主方】 血府逐瘀汤[119]。

若胸痹甚者,可加五灵脂、郁金、延胡索;若血瘀轻者,可改用丹参饮[51]。

【调护要点】 调情志,戒郁怒;慎起居,避风寒;忌生冷肥甘,忌烟酒。

2. 痰浊壅塞

【症状】 胸闷如窒而痛,或痛引肩背,气短喘促,肢体沉重,形体肥胖,痰多。苔浊腻,脉滑。

【辨证要点】 胸闷窒痛,痰多,苔腻,脉滑。

本型可见于冠心病心绞痛、心肌梗死。

【病机概要】 痰浊盘踞,胸阳失展,脉络阻滞。

【治法】 通阳泄浊,豁痰开结。

【主方】 栝楼薤白半夏汤[208]。

若痰浊较甚者,可加入干姜、陈皮、白蔻仁等,以通阳豁痰,温中理气。

【调护要点】 忌烟酒及肥甘厚味。

3. 阴寒凝滞

【症状】 胸痛彻背,感寒痛甚,胸闷气短,心悸,重则喘息不能平卧,面色苍白,四肢厥冷。舌苔白,脉沉细。

【辨证要点】 胸痛彻背,感寒尤甚,面白肢冷,脉沉细。

本型常见于冠心病心绞痛、胸膜炎、心肌病等。

【病机概要】 寒邪内侵,阳气不足,气机阻痹。

【治法】 辛温通阳,开痹散寒。

【主方】 栝楼薤白白酒汤[209]。

可加枳实、桂枝、附子、丹参、檀香等加强通阳开痹、散寒通络之效。若痰湿内盛,胸痛伴有咳唾痰涎,可加生姜、陈皮、茯苓、杏仁等,以行气化痰;若症见心痛彻背、背痛彻心，痛剧而无休止，身寒肢冷，喘息不得卧，脉沉紧者，此为阴寒极盛，胸痹之重证，宜用乌头赤石脂丸[54]合苏合香丸[128]以芳香温通而止痛。

【调护要点】 适当休息，注意保暖，忌食生冷。

4.心肾阴虚

【症状】 胸闷且痛，心悸盗汗，心烦不寐，腰酸膝软，耳鸣，头晕。舌红或有紫斑，苔少，脉细数或见细涩。

【辨证要点】 胸闷痛，心悸盗汗，腰酸耳鸣，舌红苔少。

本证常见于冠心病、心脏神经官能症。

【病机概要】 病久体虚，心肾阴伤，脉络失充，气血不畅。

【治法】 滋阴益肾，养心安神。

【主方】 左归饮[66]。

若心阴亏虚，心烦不寐较甚者，可加麦冬、五味子、柏子仁、酸枣仁等以养心安神；若闷痛较甚者，可加当归、丹参、川芎、郁金等，以养血通络；若阴虚阳亢而见头晕目眩、舌体麻木者，可加制首乌、女贞子、钩藤、生石决明、生牡蛎、鳖甲等，以滋阴潜阳。

【调护要点】 慎房事，戒劳伤；调情志，忌辛辣。

5.气阴两虚

【症状】 胸闷隐痛，时作时止，心悸气短，倦怠懒言，面色少华，头晕目眩，遇劳则甚。舌偏红，或有齿印，脉细弱无力或结代。

【辨证要点】 胸闷隐痛，心悸气短，遇劳则甚，脉细弱无力。

本证可见于心肌病、心脏神经官能症、隐性冠心病、陈旧性心肌梗塞等。

【病机概要】 胸痹日久，气阴两虚，气虚则无以行血，阴虚则脉络不利。

【治法】 益气养阴，活血通络。

【主方】 生脉散[84]合人参养营汤[11]。

若胸痛较甚，可加丹参、参三七、益母草、郁金、五灵脂等以活血通络；若脉结代，为气虚血少，血不养心所致，可合炙甘草汤[165]以益气养血，滋阴复脉。

【调护要点】 勿过劳，忌辛辣。

6.阳气虚衰

【症状】 胸闷气短，甚则胸痛彻背，心悸，汗出，畏寒肢冷，腰酸乏力，面色苍白，唇甲淡白或青紫。舌淡白或紫暗，脉沉细或沉微欲绝。

【辨证要点】 胸闷气短，畏寒肢冷，自汗乏力，脉沉细。

本证常见于冠心病心绞痛、心肌病、病毒性心肌炎等。

【病机概要】 阳气虚衰，胸阳不运，气机痹阻，血行瘀滞。

【治法】 益气温阳，活血通络。

【主方】 参附汤[167]合右归饮[69]。

若见面色唇甲青紫，大汗出，四肢厥冷，脉微欲绝者，为心阳欲脱，可重用红参、附子，并加煅龙骨、煅牡蛎，以回阳救逆固脱；若阳损及阴，阴阳两虚者，可加麦冬、五味子以温阳滋阴并用。

【调护要点】 注意保暖，勿使过劳；忌食生冷。

小结

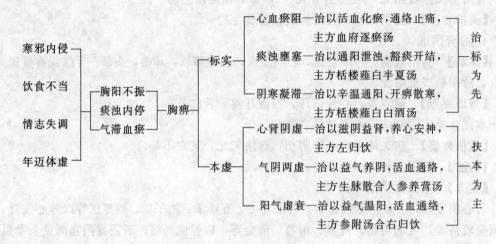

本虚标实、虚实挟杂者,当分虚实主次,兼顾同治。

思考题

1. 胸痹临床上常见有哪几种证型?
2. 试述胸痹阴寒凝滞、痰浊壅塞、心血瘀阻各证的辨证要点及治疗方法。

9 厥证

概念

厥证是以突然昏倒，不省人事，四肢厥冷为主要表现的一种病证。

西医学的癔病性昏厥、血管抑制性晕厥、高血压脑病、脑血管痉挛、低血糖症、出血性及心源性休克、肺性脑病等引起的昏厥，可参考本篇辨证论治。

病因病机

1. 气厥　恼怒惊骇、情志过极，以致气机逆乱，上壅心胸，蒙闭窍隧，引起昏倒；或由于元气素弱，又遇惊恐，或因疲劳过度，以致阳气消乏，气虚下陷，清阳不升，造成昏厥。

2. 血厥　肝阳素旺，又加暴怒，以致血随气逆，气血上壅，清窍不利，突然昏倒；或因久病血虚及产后或其它原因致失血过多，气随血脱，发生昏厥。

3. 痰厥　形盛气弱之人，恣食酒酪肥甘之品，脾胃受伤，运化失常，聚湿生痰，痰浊内阻，气机不利，偶因恼怒气逆，痰随气升，上蒙清窍，以致突然眩仆而厥。

4. 食厥　饮食不节，积滞内停，转输失常，气机受阻，以致窒闷而厥。

病因病机要点：气机突然逆乱，升降乖戾—气血运行失常—厥证。

诊断与鉴别

厥证以突然昏倒、不省人事、四肢厥冷为特征。随时随地均可发生。

本病与中风、痫证均有突然昏迷这一症状，与蛔厥同有四肢厥冷等症状，应予鉴别：

病名 鉴别	厥　证	中　风 （中脏腑）	痫　证	蛔　厥
神志	不清	昏迷	不清	一般神志清楚
伴见症状	突然昏倒，四肢厥冷	可见口眼㖞斜，半身不遂	口吐涎沫，两目上视，四肢抽搐或喉中作猪羊叫声	脘腹剧痛，按之有块，四肢厥冷或呕吐蛔虫
清醒后状态	无口眼㖞斜及半身不遂	多有后遗症	一如常人	驱蛔安脏后一如常人

辨证论治

厥证发生，各有明显诱因：

厥证
- 气厥
  - 虚证—平素体弱，厥前有过度疲劳、饥饿受寒等
  - 实证—多因郁怒忧思等精神刺激而发
- 血厥
  - 虚证—失血过多，常发生于大出血、月经过多或分娩之后
  - 实证—多因暴怒所致
- 痰厥——好发于恣食肥甘、体胖湿盛之人
- 食厥——暴饮暴食之后

常见证型如下：

气厥

1. 实证

【症状】 突然昏倒,不省人事,口噤拳握,呼吸气粗,或四肢厥冷,苔薄白,脉伏或沉弦。

【辨证要点】 多发于精神刺激后,突然昏倒,口噤肢厥,息粗脉弦。

本型常见于癔病性昏厥、血管抑制性晕厥(迷走神经晕厥)。

【病机概要】 肝气不舒,气机逆乱,上壅心胸,阻塞清窍。

【治法】 顺气开郁。

【主方】 五磨饮子[43]。

可酌加入白豆蔻、檀香、丁香、藿香之类,以理气宽胸;若肝阳偏亢,症见头晕而痛,面赤者,可加入钩藤、石决明、磁石等药,以平肝潜阳;若醒后时时啼笑无常,睡眠不宁者,可加茯神、远志、酸枣仁等,以安神宁志。

因精神刺激常可导致本证反复发作,故平时可常服逍遥散[222]以理气达郁。

【调护要点】 注意情志调摄,避免恼怒诱发。

2. 虚证

【症状】 眩晕昏仆,面色苍白,呼吸微弱,汗出肢冷。舌质淡,脉沉微。

【辨证要点】 眩晕昏仆,汗出肢冷,息微脉弱。

本型常见于低血糖休克、心源性休克、血管抑制性晕厥等。

【病机概要】 元气虚弱,气机不相顺接,中气下陷,清阳不升。

【治法】 补气回阳。

【主方】 四味回阳饮[78]。

若表虚自汗者,可加黄芪、白术等以益气固表;若汗出不止者,可加煅龙骨、煅牡蛎等以固涩止汗;若纳食不香,咳嗽痰多者,可加白术、茯苓、陈皮、半夏等以健脾化痰;若心悸不宁者,可加远志、酸枣仁等以养心安神。

【调护要点】 戒劳作,避风寒,调情志,忌生冷。

血厥

1. 实证

【症状】 突然昏倒,不省人事,牙关紧闭,面赤唇紫。舌红,脉多沉弦。

【辨证要点】 多发于暴怒之后,突然昏倒,牙关紧闭,面赤唇紫。

本型多见于脑血管痉挛、高血压脑病、心源性休克等。

【病机概要】 由于暴怒肝气上逆,血随气升,上蔽神明,闭塞清窍。

【治法】 活血顺气。

【主方】 通瘀煎[224]。

若急躁易怒、眩晕头痛者,可加钩藤、石决明、龙胆草、菊花、珍珠母、远志、石菖蒲等以平肝宁神。

【调护要点】 调情志,戒恼怒;忌辛辣烟酒。密切观察病情。

2. 虚证

【症状】 突然昏厥,面色苍白,口唇无华,四肢震颤,目陷口张,自汗肤冷,呼吸微弱。舌淡,脉芤或细数无力。

【辨证要点】 多发于失血过多后,突然昏厥,面唇无华,震颤肤冷,口张舌淡。本型常见于失血性及心源性休克、低血糖休克等。

【病机概要】 失血过多,血不上承。

【治法】 补益气血。

【主方】 独参汤[194]、人参养营汤[11]。

急用独参汤灌服,以益气回阳;继服人参养营汤。若出血不止者,可加仙鹤草、藕节、侧柏叶以止血;若自汗肤冷,呼吸微弱者,可加附子、干姜等以温阳;若心悸寐少者,可加龙眼肉、远志、酸枣仁等以养心宁神。

【调护要点】 密切观察病情。注意休息,加强营养。

痰厥

【症状】 突然昏厥,喉有痰声,或呕吐涎沫,呼吸气粗。苔白腻,脉沉滑。

【辨证要点】 突然昏厥,喉有痰声,苔白腻。

本型可见于肺性脑病、高血压脑病等。

【病机概要】 素多痰湿,恼怒气逆,痰壅气机,上闭清窍。

【治法】 行气豁痰。

【主方】 导痰汤[121]。

若痰气壅盛者,可加苡仁、白芥子以化痰降气;若痰湿化热,症见口干便秘、苔黄腻、脉滑数者,可加黄芩、栀子、竹茹、栝楼仁等,以清热降火。

【调护要点】 忌食肥甘油腻之品。

食厥

【症状】 暴饮过食之后,突发昏厥,气息窒塞,脘腹胀满。苔厚腻,脉滑实。

【辨证要点】 昏厥多发于暴饮暴食之后,苔厚腻,脉滑实。

【病机概要】 暴饮多食,食滞中脘,气逆于上,清窍闭塞。

【治法】 和中消导。

【主方】 神术散[186]合保和丸[193]。

若食后不久,首用盐汤探吐以去实邪;继用神术散合保和丸。若腹胀而大便不通者,可用小承气汤[29]导滞下行。

【调护要点】 节制饮食,宜少食、素食,忌暴饮暴食。

小结

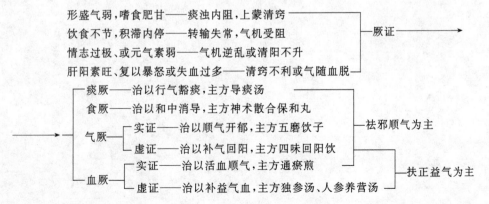

思考题

1. 厥证的临床特征是什么？与中风、痫证有何区别？
2. 气厥、血厥、痰厥的病机和治法各有何不同？

10 中风

概念

中风又名卒中，是以卒然昏仆、不省人事，伴口眼㖞斜、半身不遂、语言不利，或不经昏仆而仅以㖞僻不遂为主症的一种疾病。

西医学的高血压性脑溢血、脑血栓形成、脑栓塞、蛛网膜下隙出血、腔隙性脑梗死、一过性脑缺血，以及周围性面神经麻痹等出现上述症状者，可参考本病辨证论治。

病因病机

1. 积损正衰　年老体衰，肝肾阴虚，肝阳偏亢；或思念过度，气血亏损，阴亏于下，阳亢风动，气血上逆，上蒙元神，突发中风。

2. 饮食不节　嗜酒肥甘，或形盛气弱，脾失健运，聚湿成痰，痰郁化热，以致肝风夹杂痰火，横窜经络，蒙蔽清窍，突然昏仆，㖞僻不遂。

3. 情志所伤　五志过极，心火暴盛，或素体阴虚，复因情志所伤，肝阳暴动，气血上逆，心神昏冒，因而卒倒无知。

4. 气虚邪中　气血不足，脉络空虚，风邪乘虚入中经络，气血痹阻，或痰湿素盛，外风引动痰湿，闭阻经络，而致㖞僻不遂。

病因病机要点：

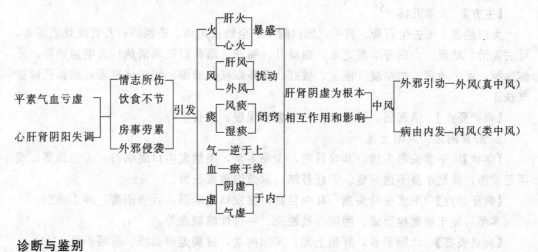

诊断与鉴别

本病以起病急骤、证见多端、变化迅速为发病特点，以卒然昏仆，伴以口眼㖞斜、半身不遂、语言不利或不经昏仆，而仅以㖞斜不遂为临床特征。临床上以内因引发者居多，但也有因外邪侵袭而引发者。因本病起病急骤、证见多端、变化迅速，与风性善行数变的特征相似，故以"中风"名之。与《伤寒论》中，风寒之邪侵犯太阳经出现的"中风"证，名同实异。

厥证、痫证，均有突然昏仆的症状，应予鉴别，请参考厥证节。本病也与痉证症状有相似之处，鉴别如下：

病　名 鉴　别	中　风	痉证
口眼㖞斜、半身不遂	有	无
四肢抽搐、甚则角弓反张	无	有

辨证论治

本病的发生，有轻重缓急的差别：

轻者—局限于血脉经络，而无脏腑病变及神志症状—中经络；

重者—累及脏腑，伴神志改变—中脏腑。

中经络

1. 络脉空虚，风邪入中

【症状】 肌肤不仁，手足麻木，突然口眼㖞斜，语言不利，口角流涎，甚则半身不遂，或兼见恶寒，发热，肢体拘急，关节酸痛等症。苔薄白，脉浮数。

【辨证要点】 肌肤不仁，手足麻木，突发口眼㖞斜语言不利，或兼见外邪袭表症状。神志清醒。

本型常见于面神经麻痹、一过性脑缺血、腔隙性脑梗死。

【病机概要】 正气不足，络脉空虚，卫外不固，风邪乘虚入中经络，痹阻气血。

【治法】 祛风、养血、通络。

【主方】 大秦艽汤[22]。

无内热者，可去生石膏、黄芩，加白附子、全蝎祛风痰、通经络；若有风热表证者，可去羌活、防风、当归等辛温之品，加桑叶、菊花、薄荷以疏风清热；若呕逆痰盛，苔腻脉滑，可去地黄，加半夏、南星、橘红、茯苓以祛痰燥湿；年老体衰者，加黄芪以益气扶正。

【调护要点】 慎起居，避风邪；注意患侧保暖；忌食生冷。

2. 肝肾阴虚，风阳上扰

【症状】 平素头晕头痛，耳鸣目眩，少寐多梦，突然发生口眼㖞斜，舌强语蹇，或手足重滞，甚则半身不遂等症。舌红苔腻，脉弦细数或弦滑。

【辨证要点】 平素头晕头痛，耳鸣目眩，突发口眼㖞斜，舌强语蹇。神志清醒。

本型可见于脑血栓形成、腔隙性脑梗死、一过性脑缺血等。

【病机概要】 肾阴素亏，肝阳上亢，风阳内动，挟痰走窜经络，脉络不畅。

【治法】 滋阴潜阳，熄风通络。

【主方】 镇肝熄风汤[291]。

可加天麻、钩藤、菊花以增强平肝熄风之力。痰热较重者，加胆星、竹沥、川贝母以化痰清热；头痛较重者，加羚羊角、石决明、夏枯草以清熄风阳。

【调护要点】 注意患侧保暖；宜清淡、低脂饮食；调情志，忌恼怒激动；戒房劳。

中脏腑

中脏腑的主要表现是突然昏倒，不省人事。临床上有闭证和脱证的区别。

闭证——邪实内闭为主——实证——急宜祛邪；

脱证——阳气欲脱为主——虚证——急宜扶正。

1. 闭证　闭证的主要症状是：突然昏仆，不省人事，牙关紧闭，两手握固，二便不通，肢体强痉。在辨证时注意有阳闭和阴闭之别。

（1）阳闭

【症状】　除上述闭证的症状外，还有面赤身热，气粗口臭，躁扰不宁。苔黄腻，脉弦滑而数。

【辨证要点】　突然昏仆，面赤身热，牙关紧闭，大小便闭。苔黄腻，脉弦滑数。

本型常见于脑栓塞、高血压性脑溢血、蛛网膜下腔出血等。

【病机概要】　肝阳暴张，阳升风动，气血上逆，挟痰挟火，蒙蔽清窍。

【治法】　清肝熄风，辛凉开窍。

【主方】　至宝丹[109]或安宫牛黄丸[111]。

先灌服上药，继用羚羊角汤[246]以清肝熄风、育阴潜阳。如有抽搐，可加全蝎、蜈蚣、僵蚕；痰多者，可加竹沥、天竺黄、胆南星；如痰多昏睡者，可加郁金、菖蒲以增强豁痰透窍之力。

【调护要点】　减少搬动，避免刺激，严密观察。

（2）阴闭

【症状】　除上述闭证的症状外，还有面白唇暗，静卧不烦，四肢不温，痰涎壅盛。苔白腻，脉沉滑缓。

【辨证要点】　突然昏仆，牙关紧闭，面白唇暗，四肢不温。苔白腻，脉沉滑缓。

本型可见于高血压性脑溢血、蛛网膜下腔出血。

【病机概要】　痰湿偏盛，风挟痰湿，上蒙清窍，内闭经络。

【治法】　豁痰熄风，辛温开窍。

【主方】　苏合香丸[128]。

继用涤痰汤[215]豁痰熄风，可加天麻、钩藤以平肝熄风。

【调护要点】　昏迷期间，注意清除痰涎、预防感染，保持大便通畅。

2. 脱证

【症状】　突然昏仆，不省人事，目合口张，鼻鼾息微，手撒肢冷，汗多，大小便失禁，肢体软瘫。舌痿，脉细弱或脉微欲绝。

【辨证要点】　突然昏仆，目合口张，手撒肢冷，汗多肢软，二便失禁，脉弱。

本型常见于高血压性脑溢血、蛛网膜下隙出血。

【病机概要】　阳浮于上，阴竭于下，正气虚脱，心神颓败。

【治法】　益气回阳，救阴固脱。

【主方】　参附汤[167]合生脉散[84]。

如汗多不止者，可加黄芪、煅龙骨、煅牡蛎、山萸肉，以敛汗固脱。

【调护要点】　注意保暖，避免刺激，严密观察。

3. 后遗证　中风经过救治，神志清醒后，多留有不同程度的后遗证，如半身不遂，言语不利，口眼㖞斜等。要抓紧时机，积极治疗。同时配合针灸、推拿、按摩等综合疗法，并适当活动锻炼,以提高疗效。

(1) 半身不遂　半身不遂,肢体无力,并伴患侧手足浮肿、口眼㖞斜、面色萎黄、舌淡、脉细弱无力,属气虚血滞、脉络瘀阻。治宜补气活血、通经活络。主方为补阳还五汤[141]。

(2) 语言不利　舌强语蹇,肢体麻木,脉弦滑者,属风痰阻络,方用解语丹[279],以宣窍行气通络。

若语言不利,心悸气短,及腰膝酸软,属肾虚精亏,用地黄饮子[104],去肉桂、附子,加杏仁、桔梗、木蝴蝶,以开音利窍。

(3) 口眼㖞斜　多由风痰阻于络道所致。治宜祛风、除痰、通络,方用牵正散[181]。

小结

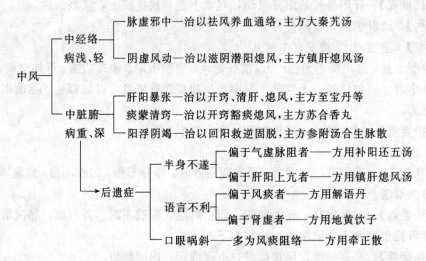

思考题

1. 中经络和中脏腑在病机和症状上有何异同?
2. 什么叫闭证和脱证?两者有何区别?
3. 中风恢复期如何进行治疗?

11 痉证

概念

痉证是以项背强急,四肢抽搐,甚至角弓反张为主要表现的病证。

西医学中的流行性脑脊髓膜炎、流行性乙型脑炎、结核性脑膜炎,以及高热惊厥、手足搐搦症、脑肿瘤等,凡以项背强急、四肢抽搐等为主症者,均可参照本病辨证论治。

病因病机

1. 邪壅经络　风寒湿邪,壅滞脉络,气血运行不利,筋脉失养,拘急而成痉。
2. 热甚发痉　热甚于里,消灼津液,阴液被伤,筋脉失于濡养,引起痉证。
3. 阴血亏损　素体阴虚血虚,或因亡血,或因汗下太过,致使阴血损伤,难以濡养筋脉,因而成痉。

病因病机要点:

```
外因——邪壅脉络,气血不畅 ┐
                          ├筋脉拘急——痉证
内因——阴血亏竭,失其濡养 ┘
```

诊断与鉴别

痉证以项背强急,四肢抽搐,甚至角弓反张为特征。发病无明显季节性。

中风与痫证均有筋脉拘急的抽搐症状,应予鉴别。与中风的鉴别见中风篇,与痫证鉴别如下:

病名 鉴别	痉　　证	痫　　证
筋脉症状	项背强急、四肢抽搐,甚至角弓反张	昏迷时,筋脉拘急,四肢抽搐
伴见症状	见于多种疾病过程中,可伴见其它疾病的症状	发作时多吐涎沫,或发出异常叫声,醒后如常人

辨证论治

临证宜详辨外感、内伤及虚实。

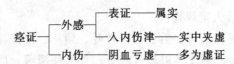

常见证型如下:

1. 邪壅经络

【症状】 头痛、项背强直，恶寒发热，肢体酸重。苔白腻，脉浮紧。

【辨证要点】 项背强直，头痛，恶寒发热，苔白腻。

本型可见于流行性脑脊髓膜炎、流行性乙型脑炎、结核性脑膜炎初期等。

【病机概要】 风寒湿邪，阻滞经络，体表营卫不利。

【治法】 祛风散寒，和营燥湿。

【主方】 羌活胜湿汤[155]。

如寒邪较甚，病属刚痉，方选葛根汤[259]；如风邪偏盛，头痛汗出，脉沉细，病属柔痉，方用栝楼桂枝汤[207]；若筋脉拘急，渴不欲饮，小便短赤，苔黄腻，脉滑数，为湿热入络，方用三仁汤[15]，以清热化湿，疏通经络。

【调护要点】 慎避寒湿，忌食生冷。

2. 热甚发痉

【症状】 发热胸闷，口噤龂齿，项背强直，甚至角弓反张，手足挛急；腹胀便秘，咽干口渴，心烦急躁，甚则神昏谵语。苔黄腻，脉弦数。

【辨证要点】 项背强直，口噤龂齿，发热烦躁，甚至角弓反张。苔黄腻，脉弦数。

本型多见于流行性脑脊髓膜炎、流行性乙型脑炎、结核性脑膜炎以及其它高热惊厥病证。

【病机概要】 邪热薰蒸阳明气分，宿滞中焦，腑气不通；热盛伤津，筋脉失养，邪热上扰神明。

【治法】 泄热存津，养阴增液。

【主方】 增液承气汤[284]。

如热盛伤津，并无腑实证，可用白虎加人参汤[89]，以清热救津；如抽搐较甚者，可酌加地龙、全蝎、菊花、钩藤等熄风通络之品；如烦躁甚者，可加淡竹叶，栀子等清心除烦。

【调护要点】 注意观察神志、出汗、大小便的变化，以便及时随证施治；抽搐时宜加强护理，防止窒息、骨折等并发症的产生。

3. 阴血亏虚

【症状】 素体阴血亏虚，或在失血、汗、下太过之后，项背强急，四肢抽搐，头目昏眩，自汗、神疲、气短。舌淡红，脉弦细。

【辨证要点】 项背强急，四肢抽搐，头目昏眩，舌淡苔少，脉细。

本型可见于各型脑炎、脑膜炎及手足抽搦症、脑肿瘤等。

【病机概要】 阴血两虚，不能营养筋脉，血虚不能上奉于脑，元气耗伤，卫外不固。

【治法】 滋阴养血。

【主方】 四物汤[79]合大定风珠[19]。

若头晕、虚烦、失眠者，可加栀子、淡竹叶、菊花、夜交藤以清热宁神；如纳呆腹满者，可加砂仁、鸡内金、陈皮等以理气和胃；如大便溏薄，面色㿠白，可加党参、白术等益气健脾。

【调护要点】 宜多食新鲜瓜果和润养食品，忌食辛辣。

小结

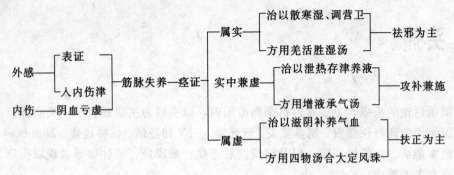

思考题

1. 痉证的主要病机是什么？
2. 邪壅经络证、热甚发痉证、阴血亏虚证的治疗方法和代表方剂各是什么？

12 头痛

概念

本篇所讨论的头痛,主要是内科杂病范围内,以头痛为主要症状的一类病证。

西医学中的流行性感冒、副鼻窦炎、青光眼、三叉神经痛、枕神经痛、高血压病、贫血、神经官能症、血管性头痛、以及脑震荡后遗症、脑膜炎、脑肿瘤等表现以头痛为主者,均可参考本篇辨证论治。

病因病机

1. 外感头痛　起居不慎,坐卧当风,感受风寒湿热等外邪。外邪自表侵袭于经络,上犯巅顶,清阳之气受阻,气血不畅,阻遏络道,而致头痛。

2. 内伤头痛　脑赖脾胃水谷精微及肝肾精血濡养,输布气血上充于脑。肝因情志所伤,失于疏泄,郁而化火,上扰清空,可为头痛;或因肾水不足,水不涵木,导致肝肾阴亏,肝阳上亢,上扰清空而致头痛;或因脾胃虚弱,生化不足,营血亏虚,不能上充于脑髓而致头痛。

病因病机要点:

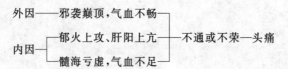

诊断与鉴别

中医内科学所述的头痛,是以头痛为主要症状特征的一类病证,一年四季均可发生。头痛和眩晕可单独发生,亦可同时互见,二者比较如下:

病名 鉴别	头　　痛	眩　　晕
从发病看	外感、内伤	内伤多见
从辨证上看	虚实夹杂居多	虚证为主

辨证论治

头痛的辨证,应该注意辨别致病原因,还应注意头痛之性质、时间之久暂、特点及部位等。

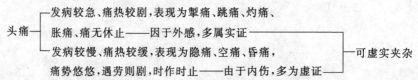

常见证型如下：

外感

1. 风寒头痛

【症状】　头痛时作，痛连项背，恶风畏寒，遇风尤剧，口不渴。苔薄白，脉浮。

【辨证要点】　头痛，恶风寒，苔薄白。

本型常见于流行性感冒。

【病机概要】　风寒外袭肌表，清阳之气被遏，不得宣达。

【治法】　疏散风寒。

【主方】　川芎茶调散[23]。

若寒邪侵犯厥阴经，引起巅顶头痛，干呕，吐涎沫，甚则四肢厥冷者，治用吴茱萸汤[135]，去人参、大枣加半夏、藁本、川芎等，以温散降逆。

【调护要点】　慎避风寒、忌食生冷。

2. 风热头痛

【症状】　头痛而胀，甚则头痛如裂，发热恶风，面红目赤，口渴欲饮，便秘溲黄。舌红苔黄，脉浮数。

【辨证要点】　头痛而胀，发热、溲黄便秘。苔黄，脉浮数。

本型可见于流行性感冒、脑膜炎、血管性头痛等。

【病机概要】　风热之邪，上扰清窍，热盛耗津。

【治法】　疏风清热。

【主方】　芎芷石膏汤[106]。

方中羌活、藁本偏于辛温，可改用黄芩、薄荷、山栀子以辛凉清解。若热盛伤津严重，可酌加知母、石斛、天花粉等生津止渴。

【调护要点】　忌食辛辣。

3. 风湿头痛

【症状】　头痛如裹，肢体困重，纳呆胸闷，小便不利，大便或溏。苔白腻，脉濡。

【辨证要点】　头痛如裹，肢体困重，胸闷纳呆，苔白腻。

本型可见于神经官能症、副鼻窦炎、流行性感冒等。

【病机概要】　风湿外感，上犯巅顶，阻遏清窍；湿浊中阻，清阳不布。

【治法】　祛风胜湿。

【主方】　羌活胜湿汤[155]。

若湿浊中阻，症见胸闷纳呆、便溏，可加苍术、厚朴、陈皮、枳壳等以燥湿宽中。

【调护要点】　宜食清淡，忌肥甘。

内伤

1. 肝阳头痛

【症状】　头痛而眩，心烦易怒，夜眠不宁或兼胁痛，面赤口苦。苔薄黄，脉弦有力。

【辨证要点】　头痛而眩，心烦易怒，胁痛口苦，脉弦。

本型多见于高血压病、更年期高血压等病症。

【病机概要】　肝阳偏亢，上扰清窍；肝火偏亢，扰乱心神。

【治法】　平肝潜阳。

【主方】 天麻钩藤饮[33]。

可在方中加入牡蛎、龙骨加强重镇潜阳之功。若头痛甚剧，伴胁痛口苦，便秘溲赤，肝火偏旺者，可加郁金、龙胆草、夏枯草以清肝泄火；若肝肾阴虚，症见头痛朝轻暮重，或遇劳加剧，脉弦细者，可加生地、何首乌、女贞子、枸杞子等滋养肝肾。

【调护要点】 注意情志调摄；忌食辛辣动火之品。

2. 肾虚头痛

【症状】 头痛且空，每兼眩晕，遇劳加重，腰膝酸软，神疲乏力，遗精带下，耳鸣少寐。舌红少苔，脉细无力。

【辨证要点】 头痛伴眩晕，腰膝痠软，耳鸣少寐，脉弱。

本型常见于神经衰弱性头痛等。

【病机概要】 肾虚髓不上荣于脑，脑海空虚；腰为肾府，肾虚腰骨失养。

【治法】 养阴补肾。

【主方】 大补元煎[17]。

如病情好转，可常服杞菊地黄丸[129]，补肾阴以巩固疗效；若头痛而畏寒，四肢不温，舌淡、脉沉细而缓，可用右归丸[68]，温补肾阳，填补精血。

【调护要点】 加强调养，宜食血肉有情之品；慎起居，戒房劳。

3. 血虚头痛

【症状】 头痛而晕，心悸不宁，神疲乏力，面色㿠白。舌淡，苔薄白，脉细弱。

【辨证要点】 头痛而晕，面白心悸，舌淡脉弱。

本型常见于各种贫血引起的头痛。

【病机概要】 血虚气弱，不能上荣于脑；气血不足，心神失养。

【治法】 补养气血。

【主方】 加味四物汤[98]。

若气虚明显，神疲乏力严重，遇劳加剧，汗出气短，可加黄芪、人参。

【调护要点】 加强营养，注意休息。

4. 痰浊头痛

【症状】 头痛昏蒙，胸脘满闷，呕恶痰涎。苔白腻，脉滑。

【辨证要点】 头痛昏蒙，呕恶痰涎，苔白腻，脉滑。

本型常见于高血压病、血管性头痛、神经官能症等。

【病机概要】 脾失健运，痰浊中阻，上蒙清窍，清阳不展。

【治法】 化痰降逆。

【主方】 半夏白术天麻汤[92]。

可加入厚朴、白蒺藜等协助其化痰降逆。若痰浊郁久化热，症见口苦，大便不畅，苔黄腻，脉滑数，可加黄芩、竹茹、枳实以行气、清热、燥湿。

【调护要点】 忌肥甘厚味。

5. 瘀血头痛

【症状】 头痛经久不愈，痛处固定不移，痛如锥刺，或有头部外伤史。舌紫，苔薄白，脉细弱。

【辨证要点】 头痛经久不愈，痛如锥刺，固定不移。舌紫或有瘀斑。

本型常见于脑震荡后遗症、脑肿瘤等。

【病机概要】 瘀血内停，脉络不畅。

【治法】 活血化瘀。

【主方】 通窍活血汤[223]。

可酌加郁金、菖蒲、细辛、白芷以理气宣窍止痛。头痛甚者，可加虫类搜逐之品，如全蝎、蜈蚣、地鳖虫等；如头痛久而不愈伴气血不足者，酌加黄芪、当归补益气血。

【调护要点】 起居有时，劳逸结合，避风寒，忌肥甘。

小结

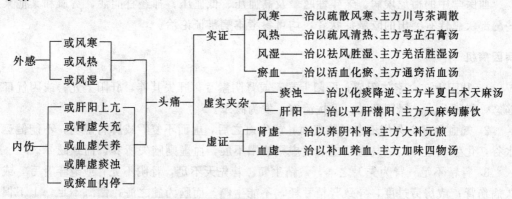

思考题

1. 外感头痛与内伤头痛的症状特点有何不同？
2. 分别说明肝阳、血虚、痰浊、血瘀头痛的症状特点及治法、主方。

13 眩晕

概念

眩是眼花，晕指头晕。眩晕是指头晕眼花，重者如坐车船，旋转不定，不能久立，甚或伴有恶心、呕吐、汗出等症的一种病证。

西医学中的梅尼埃病、老年性眩晕及高血压、低血压、神经官能症、贫血和其他某些脑部疾患伴有突出的眩晕症状者，均可参考本病辨证论治。

病因病机

1. 肝阳上亢　素体阳盛，肝阳上亢；或肾阴素亏，肝失其养，肝阳上亢；或因忧郁恼怒，气郁化火，风阳升动，上扰清空，发为眩晕。

2. 气血亏虚　久病不愈耗伤气血；或失血之后，虚而不复；或脾胃虚弱，不能健运水谷，化生气血，以致气血两虚，气虚则清阳不展，血虚则脑失所养，而致眩晕。

3. 肾精不足　肾为先天之本，藏精生髓。若先天不足，肾阴不充；或老年肾亏，或久病伤肾；或房劳过度，导致肾精亏耗，不能生髓。而脑为髓之海，髓海不足，上下俱虚，发生眩晕。

4. 痰浊中阻　嗜酒肥甘，饥饱劳倦，伤于脾胃，健运失司，聚湿生痰，痰湿中阻，则清阳不升，浊阴不降，引起眩晕。

病因病机要点：

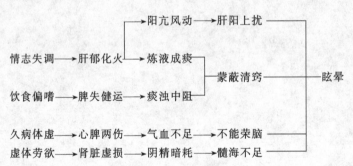

诊断与鉴别

眩晕以头晕目眩为主要特征。发病无明显季节性。

眩晕有时兼有头痛，头痛也可伴有眩晕。详细鉴别，参见头痛篇。

辨证论治

在对眩晕明确诊断后，应进行辨证。临床上眩晕以虚证或虚中挟实为多，但其中又以肝阳上亢及气血亏虚较为常见。

1. 肝阳上亢

【症状】 眩晕耳鸣,头痛且胀,每因烦恼而头晕、头痛加剧,面时潮红,急躁易怒,少寐多梦,口苦。舌红,苔黄,脉弦。

【辨证要点】 眩晕耳鸣,头痛且胀,多因恼怒而加剧。

本型常见于高血压病。

【病机概要】 肝阳上亢,上冒清空。

【治法】 平肝潜阳,滋养肝肾。

【主方】 天麻钩藤饮[33]。

如肝火过盛,可加龙胆草、菊花、丹皮等以增强清肝泄热之力;如大便秘结可加用当归龙荟丸[114],以泄肝通腑;如眩晕急剧,手足麻木,甚则震颤,筋惕肉瞤,有阳动化风之势者,可加龙骨、牡蛎、珍珠母等,以镇肝熄风。

【调护要点】 戒躁怒,忌辛辣。

2. 气血亏虚

【症状】 眩晕,动则加剧,劳累即发,面色㿠白,唇甲不华,发色不泽,心悸少寐,神疲懒言,饮食减少。舌淡,脉细弱。

【辨证要点】 眩晕,动则加剧,劳累即发,面色㿠白,舌淡脉弱。

本型常见于贫血性眩晕。

【病机概要】 气虚清阳不展,血虚脑失所养。

【治法】 补益气血,健运脾胃。

【主方】 归脾汤[95]。

若食少便溏,脾胃较弱者,当归宜炒,木香宜煨,并酌加茯苓、苡仁、泽泻、砂仁、神曲等,以增强健脾和胃之力;如血虚甚者,可加熟地、阿胶,并重用黄芪以补气生血;若兼见形寒肢冷,腹中隐痛,可加桂枝、干姜以温中助阳。

【调护要点】 宜进富有营养之品,不宜过劳。

3. 肾精不足

【症状】 眩晕而见精神萎靡,少寐多梦健忘,腰膝痠软,遗精耳鸣。偏于阴虚者,五心烦热,舌红,脉弦细数;偏于阳虚者,四肢不温,形寒肢冷。舌淡,脉沉细无力。

【辨证要点】 眩晕,腰膝痠软,遗精,耳鸣。偏阴虚者,有虚热征象;偏于阳虚者,有畏寒表现。

本型可见于老年性眩晕和贫血性眩晕及梅尼埃病。

【病机概要】 肾精不足,不能上充于脑,下健其腰;肾虚精关失约。偏阴虚者生内热;偏阳虚者生外寒。

【治法】 偏阴虚者,治以补肾滋阴;偏阳虚者,治以补肾助阳。

【主方】 偏阴虚者用左归丸[65]。若内热明显者,可加炙鳖甲、知母、黄柏、地骨皮等以滋阴清热;偏阳虚者用右归丸[68]。若眩晕较甚,阴虚阳浮者,二方均可加龙骨、牡蛎、珍珠母等以潜浮阳。

【调护要点】 平素可多食血肉有情之品。戒房劳。

4. 痰浊中阻

【症状】 眩晕而见头重如蒙,胸闷呕恶,食少多寐。苔白腻,脉濡滑。

【辨证要点】 眩晕、头重如蒙,胸闷恶心,苔白腻,脉濡滑。

本型多见于高血压病、梅尼埃病、老年性眩晕等。

【病机概要】 痰浊中阻，蒙蔽清阳，浊阴不降，气机不利。

【治法】 燥湿祛痰，健脾和胃。

【主方】 半夏白术天麻汤[92]。

若眩晕较甚，呕吐频作者，加代赭石、竹茹、生姜以镇逆止呕；若脘闷不食，加白蔻仁，砂仁等芳香和胃；若耳鸣重听，加葱白、郁金、菖蒲以通阳开窍；若痰阻气机，郁而化火，症见头目胀痛，心烦口苦，渴不多饮，苔黄腻，脉弦滑者，宜温胆汤[270]，加黄连、黄芩等苦寒燥湿之品，以化痰泄热。

【调护要点】 宜食清淡，忌肥甘油腻之品。

小结

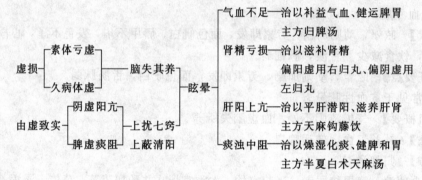

思考题

1. 眩晕的主要病机有哪些？
2. 试述肝阳上亢、气血不足、肾精亏损、痰浊中阻四证的主症、治法和方药。

14 不寐

概念

不寐是指经常不能获得正常睡眠为特征的一种病证。

西医学中的神经官能症、以及一部分以失眠为主要表现的慢性疾病（如高血压性失眠，消化不良性失眠，贫血性失眠），均可参照本病辨证论治。

病因病机

1. 思虑劳倦太过，伤及心脾 心伤则阴血暗耗，神不守舍；脾伤则食少纳呆，生化之源不足，营血亏虚，不能上奉于心，以致心神不安。

2. 阳不交阴、心肾不交 素体虚弱，或久病之人，肾阴暗耗，不能上奉于心，水不济火，则心阳独亢；或五志过极，心火内炽，不能下交于肾，心肾失交；心火亢盛，热扰神明，神志不宁，因而不寐。

3. 阴虚火旺，肝阳扰动 情志所伤，肝失条达，气郁不舒，郁而化火，火性上炎；或阴虚阳亢扰动心神，神不安宁以致不寐。

4. 心虚胆怯，心神不安 心虚胆怯，决断无权，遇事易惊，心神不安，也能导致不寐。

5. 胃气不和，夜卧不安 饮食不节，肠胃受伤，宿食停滞，酿为痰热，壅遏于中，痰热上扰，胃气不和，以致不得安寐。

病因病机要点：

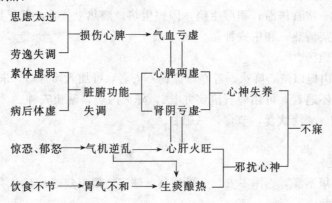

诊断与鉴别

不寐是以经常不能获得正常睡眠为特征，一般多伴有食纳乏味、精神萎靡等症。如睡眠时间较少，但精神不减，无其他不适感觉者，不应视作病态。老年人夜醒后不能再睡，多属正常现象。因一时情志影响，或生活环境改变，引起偶尔失眠者，也不属病态。

辨证论治

临床辨证，要明确本病主要特征为入寐艰难，或寐而不酣。其次要分清虚实。

虚证——多属阴血不足，责在心脾肝肾。

实证——多因肝郁化火、食滞、痰浊、胃腑不和。

常见证型如下：

实证

1. 肝郁化火

【症状】 不寐，性情急躁易怒，不思饮食，口渴喜饮，目赤口苦，小便黄赤，大便秘结。舌红，苔黄，脉弦而数。

【辨证要点】 不寐，急躁易怒，目赤口苦。脉弦数。

本型多见于神经衰弱性失眠。

【病机概要】 多因恼怒伤肝，肝失条达，气郁化火，上扰心神致不寐。

【治法】 疏肝泻热，佐以安神。

【主方】 龙胆泻肝汤[64]。

可加茯神、龙骨、牡蛎，以镇心宁神。如胸闷胁胀，善太息者，加郁金、香附之类以疏肝开郁。

【调护要点】 调情志，忌恼怒扰思，忌食辛辣。

2. 痰热内扰

【症状】 不寐，头重，痰多胸闷，恶食嗳气，吞酸恶心，心烦口苦，目眩。苔腻而黄，脉滑数。

【辨证要点】 不寐，痰多胸闷，恶食吞酸，苔黄腻，脉滑数。

本型多见于消化不良性失眠。

【病机概要】 宿食停滞，积湿生痰，因痰生热，痰热上扰，心烦不寐。

【治法】 化痰清热，和中安神。

【主方】 温胆汤[270]。

可加黄连、山栀以清心降火。若心悸惊惕不安者，可加入珍珠母、朱砂以镇惊定志；若痰热重而大便不通者，可用礞石滚痰丸[289]，降火泻热，逐痰安神。

【调护要点】 清淡饮食，节食，忌肥甘。

虚证

1. 阴虚火旺

【症状】 心烦不寐，心悸不安，头晕耳鸣，健忘，腰痠梦遗，五心烦热，口干津少。舌红苔少，脉细数。

【辨证要点】 心烦不寐，腰痠梦遗，五心烦热。舌红苔少。

本型常见于高血压性失眠。

【病机概要】 肾阴不足，不能上交于心，心肝火旺，虚热扰神。

【治法】 滋阴降火，养心安神。

【主方】 黄连阿胶汤[231]。

若阳升面热，眩晕耳鸣重者，可加牡蛎、龟板、磁石等重镇潜阳。

【调护要点】 忌食辛辣，慎房事，戒劳伤。

2. 心脾两虚

【症状】 多梦易醒，心悸健忘，头晕目眩，肢倦神疲，饮食无味，面色少华。舌淡，苔薄，脉细弱。

【辨证要点】 多梦易醒，心悸健忘，纳少肢倦。舌淡，脉弱。

本型可见于贫血性失眠。

【病机概要】 心脾亏虚，血不养心，神不守舍。

【治法】 补养心脾，以生气血。

【主方】 归脾汤[95]。

如心血不足较甚者，可加熟地、白芍、阿胶以养心血；如不寐较重者，酌加五味子、柏子仁以养心安神，或加合欢花、夜交藤、龙骨、牡蛎，以镇静安神；如兼见脘闷纳呆，苔滑腻者，加半夏、陈皮、茯苓、厚朴等，以健脾理气化痰。

【调护要点】 适当休息，进食富有营养之品。

3. 心胆气虚

【症状】 不寐或多梦，易于惊醒，胆怯心悸，遇事善惊，气短倦怠，小便清长。舌淡，脉弦细。

【辨证要点】 不寐或多梦，易于惊醒，胆怯心悸，遇事善惊。

本型多见于神经衰弱性失眠。

【病机概要】 心虚则心神不安，胆虚则善惊易恐。

【治法】 益气镇惊，安神定志。

【主方】 安神定志丸[112]。

若血虚阳浮，虚烦不寐者，宜用酸枣仁汤[280]。

【调护要点】 加强体魄锻炼；调节情志；睡前忌喝浓茶、咖啡，少吸烟。

小结

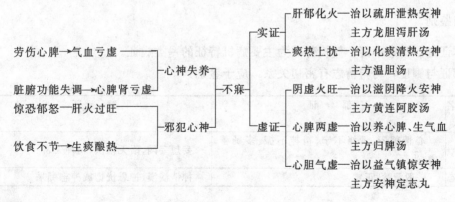

思考题

1. 不寐的主要病因有哪些？
2. 试述肝郁化火、心脾两虚二证的辨证要点和治法及主方。

15 郁证

概念

郁证是指由于情志不舒、气机郁滞所引起的以心情抑郁，情绪不宁，胁肋胀痛，或易怒善哭，以及咽中如有异物梗阻、失眠等多种复杂症状为表现的一类病证。

西医学中的神经官能症、更年期综合征等表现此类症状者，可参考本病辨证论治。

病因病机

1. 郁怒不畅，肝失条达，气失疏泄，而致肝气郁结。气郁日久可化火，气滞又可导致血瘀不行。若肝郁及脾，或思虑不解，劳倦伤脾，均能使脾失健运，蕴湿生痰，导致气滞痰郁。

2. 情志不遂，肝郁抑脾，耗伤心气，营血渐耗，心失所养，神失所藏，即所谓忧郁伤神，可致心神不安。若久郁伤脾，饮食减少，生化乏源，则气血不足，心脾两虚；郁久化火，易伤阴血，累及于肾，阴虚火旺，由此发展成种种虚损之象。

病因病机要点：

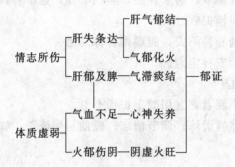

诊断与鉴别

本证是以情志不舒、气机郁滞为主要病机特征的一类病证。

郁证与癫证，均与情志有密切关系，应予鉴别：

病名 鉴别	郁 证	癫 证
症状特点	心情郁闷、情绪不宁、精神不振、多疑善虑、失眠	妄想妄闻、语无伦次、精神失常
神志状态	一般清楚、正常	神情淡漠、神思恍惚或神志痴呆

辨证论治

在对郁证明确诊断后，应进行辨证。首先要区别虚实，然后依证治之。实证以舒肝理气为主；虚证以益气血、扶正为法。

实证

1. 肝气郁结

【症状】 精神抑郁，情绪不宁，善太息，胸胁胀痛，痛无定处，脘闷嗳气，腹胀纳呆，或呕吐，女子月经不行。苔薄腻，脉弦。

【辨证要点】 精神抑郁，善太息，胸胁胀痛。脉弦。

本型常见于神经官能症、更年期综合征。

【病机概要】 情志所伤，肝失条达，肝气郁滞，气机不畅。

【治法】 疏肝理气解郁。

【主方】 柴胡疏肝散[211]。

可加郁金、青皮以助解郁之功。在服药的同时，可常服越鞠丸[264]以行气解郁。如嗳气频作，胸脘不舒，酌加旋覆花、代赭石、陈皮，以平肝降逆；兼有食滞腹胀者，可加山楂、神曲、鸡内金，以消食化滞。

【调护要点】 保持情绪乐观，减轻精神负担。医护人员和患者家属要对患者体贴关心。

2. 气郁化火

【症状】 性情急躁易怒，胸闷胁胀，嘈杂吞酸，口干而苦，大便秘结，或头痛，目赤，耳鸣。舌红，苔黄，脉弦数。

【辨证要点】 急躁易怒，口干而苦。舌红，苔黄，脉弦数。

本型多见于神经官能症。

【病机概要】 气郁化火，火性炎上，肝火犯胃伤津。

【治法】 清肝泻火，解郁和胃。

【主方】 丹栀逍遥散[52]合左金丸[67]。

若大便秘结较甚者，可加龙胆草、大黄以泻火通便。

【调护要点】 同肝气郁结证，并注意少食辛辣动火之品。

3. 气滞痰郁

【症状】 咽中不适，如有物梗阻，咯之不出，咽之不下，胸中窒闷，或兼胁痛。苔白腻，脉弦滑。

【辨证要点】 咽中不适，如有物梗阻，胸中窒闷。

本型多见于神经官能症。

【病机概要】 肝郁乘脾，脾运不健，生湿聚痰，气失舒展。

【治法】 化痰利气解郁。

【主方】 半夏厚朴汤[93]。

可加制香附、枳实、佛手、旋覆花、代赭石等，以增强理气开郁、化痰降逆之效。如兼见呕恶、口苦、苔黄而腻，证属痰热，可用温胆汤[270]加黄芩、贝母、栝楼之类，以化痰清热，而利气机。

【调护要点】 保持心情舒畅，宜清淡饮食。

虚证

1. 忧郁伤神

【症状】 精神恍惚，心神不宁，悲忧善哭，时时欠伸。舌淡，苔薄白，脉弦细。

【辨证要点】 精神恍惚，悲忧善哭，时时欠伸。

本型多见于癔病。

【病机概要】 忧郁不解，心气耗伤，营血暗耗，心神失养。
【治法】 养心安神。
【主方】 甘麦大枣汤[71]。
可加柏子仁、枣仁、茯神、合欢花等，以加强养心安神之功。
【调护要点】 医护人员应态度和蔼，应用心理疗法调治。

2. 心脾两虚

【症状】 多思善虑，心悸胆怯，少寐健忘，面色少华，头晕神疲，食欲不振。舌淡，脉细弱。
【辨证要点】 多思善虑，心悸，少寐，面色不华，神疲纳差。
本型常见于神经官能症。
【病机概要】 劳心思虑，脾不健运，心失所养，心脾两虚。
【治法】 健脾养心，益气补血。
【主方】 归脾汤[95]。
可酌加郁金、合欢花之类以开郁安神。
【调护要点】 怡养性情，保持乐观，调摄饮食。

3. 阴虚火旺

【症状】 心烦易怒，心悸，少寐，眩晕，或遗精腰痠。妇女则月经不调。舌红，脉弦细而数。
【辨证要点】 少寐心烦，眩晕，心悸。舌红少苔，脉弦细而数。
本型多见于更年期综合征。
【病机概要】 肝肾阴虚，营血暗耗，心神失养，虚热上扰。
【治法】 滋阴清热，镇心安神。
【主方】 滋水清肝饮[271]。
可加入珍珠母、磁石、生铁落等重镇安神。腰痠遗精乏力者，加龟板、知母、杜仲、牡蛎等，以益肾固精；月经不调者，加香附、益母草以理气开郁调经。
【调护要点】 怡养性情，保持乐观。忌食辛辣醇酒。

小结

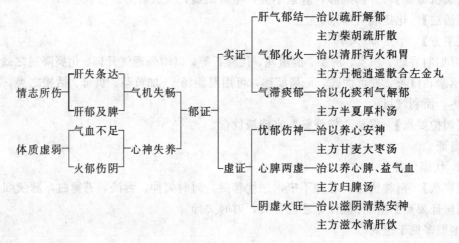

思考题

1. 郁证的基本概念是什么？
2. 肝气郁结和心脾两虚证的病因病机、症状、治法、主方各是什么？

16 癫狂

概念

癫狂是指精神错乱、神志失常的一类疾患。癫证以沉默痴呆，语无伦次，静而多喜为特征；狂证以喧扰不宁，躁妄打骂，动而多怒为特征。

西医学中的精神分裂症、躁狂抑郁症、更年期精神病、心因性反应及部分神经官能症等可参照本病辨证论治。

病因病机

1. 阴阳失调　机体阴阳平衡失调，不能相互维系，以致阴虚于下，阳亢于上，心神被扰，神明逆乱而发癫狂。

2. 情志抑郁　恼怒惊恐，损伤肝肾，或喜怒无常，心阴亏耗，肝肾阴液不足，木失濡润，屈而不伸，则默默寡言痴呆，语无伦次；或心阴不足，心火暴张，肝胆气逆，则狂言狂语，骂詈不休。如此等等，均能发为癫狂。

3. 痰气上扰　痰气上扰清窍，蒙蔽心神，神志逆乱，狂躁不宁，歌笑骂詈，逾垣上屋而为癫狂。

4. 气血凝滞　气滞血凝，经络不畅，脑气与脏腑之气不相连接而发狂。

病因病机要点：

```
阴阳失调 ┐ ┌思虑抑郁——心脾气结┐       ┌痰气郁结——癫
         ├─┤                    ├痰蒙心神─┤
情志所伤 ┘ └惊恐恼怒——肝胆气逆┘       └痰火上扰——狂
```

诊断与鉴别

癫狂属精神失常的一类病证。癫证以静而多喜为特征；狂证以动而多怒为特征。癫狂与痫证均有神志失常，但痫证平素一如常人，发则眩仆倒地，昏不知人，而癫狂则平常均伴有不同程度的神志失常。痫证有发病前突发"羊叫声"且吐涎沫，而癫狂则少见，是为其区别。

辨证论治

癫狂证的主要病因病机为气郁痰火，阴阳失调，其病变在肝胆心脾。临床上应首先区别癫证与狂证之不同。

```
       ┌癫证——精神抑郁、沉默痴呆、喃喃自语——治当疏肝理气,化痰开窍
癫狂 ──┤
       └狂证——喧扰打骂、狂躁不宁——治当镇心祛痰,清肝泻火
```

常见证型如下：

癫

1. 痰气郁结

【症状】 精神抑郁，表情淡漠，神志痴呆，语无伦次，或喃喃独语，喜怒无常，不思饮食。舌苔腻，脉弦滑。

【辨证要点】 精神抑郁，神志痴呆，语无伦次，苔腻，脉滑。

本型常见于抑郁症、更年期忧郁症、神经官能症。

【病机概要】 思虑太过，脾气不升，肝气被郁，气郁痰结，阻蔽神明。

【治法】 理气解郁，化痰开窍。

【主方】 顺气导痰汤[191]。

甚者可用控涎丹[238]，以除胸膈之痰浊。如神思迷惘，表情呆钝，言语错乱，目瞪不瞬，舌苔白腻，为痰迷心窍，治宜豁痰宣窍，理气散结。先用苏合香丸[128]芳香开窍，继用四七汤[75]加陈胆星、郁金、菖蒲、远志之类以化痰行气。

【调护要点】 注意精神治疗，少食肥甘生痰之品。

2. 心脾两虚

【症状】 神思恍惚，魂梦颠倒，心悸易惊，善悲欲哭，肢体困乏，饮食减少。舌淡，脉细无力。

【辨证要点】 神思恍惚，心悸易惊，纳少倦怠，舌淡，脉细。

本型可见于更年期精神病、神经官能症。

【病机概要】 心血内亏，心神失养，血少气衰，脾失健运。

【治法】 健脾养心，益气安神。

【主方】 养心汤[185]。

临床上与甘麦大枣汤[71]合用以养心润燥，为治疗癫狂悲伤欲哭、精神恍惚之常用良方。

【调护要点】 加强精神治疗，注意饮食营养。

狂

1. 痰火上扰

【症状】 病起急骤，先有性情急躁，头痛失眠，两目怒视，面红目赤，突然狂乱无知，逾垣上屋，骂詈叫号，不避亲疏，或毁物伤人，气力逾常，不食不眠。舌红绛，苔黄腻，脉弦大滑数。

【辨证要点】 病起急骤，面红目赤，狂乱无知，不食不眠，舌绛，苔黄腻，脉弦大滑数。

本型常见于躁狂症、精神分裂症。

【病机概要】 暴怒伤肝，肝火暴张，鼓动痰热，上扰神明。

【治法】 镇心涤痰，泻肝清火。

【主方】 生铁落饮[85]。

如痰火壅盛而苔黄腻者，同时用礞石滚痰丸[289]泻火逐痰；再用安宫牛黄丸[111]清心开窍；如属阳明热盛、大便秘结，苔黄糙，脉实大者，可用加减承气汤[100]，以荡涤秽浊，清泻胃肠实火。

【调护要点】 发作时宜加强安全防范，以防意外。忌食辛辣肥甘。

2. 火盛伤阴

【症状】 狂病日久，其势渐减，且有疲惫之象，多言善惊，时而烦躁，形瘦面红。舌红苔少,脉细数。

【辨证要点】 狂病日久,疲惫,烦躁,舌红苔少。

本型多于躁狂症后期。

【病机概要】 狂久不已,耗气伤阴,气不足则狂势渐减;阴不足则心火上炎。

【治法】 滋阴降火,安神定志。

【主方】 二阴煎[3]。

可合用定志丸[156]以资调理。

【调护要点】 注意生活调摄,忌烟酒辛辣。

小结

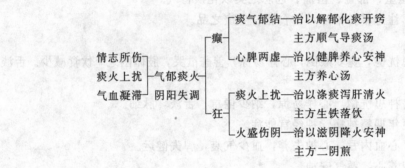

思考题

1. 癫与狂在病机和临床表现上的区别是什么?
2. 痰气郁结的癫证和痰火上扰的狂证,各自的症状、治则、主方是什么?

17 痫证

概念

痫证是一种发作性神志异常的疾病。其特征为发作性精神恍惚，甚则突然仆倒，昏不知人，口吐涎沫，两目上视，四肢抽搐，或作猪羊叫声，移时苏醒。

西医学中的癫痫，可参考本病辨证论治。

病因病机

1. 七情失调　突发惊厥，造成气机逆乱，进而损伤脏腑，肝肾受损，致阴不敛阳而生热生风。

2. 先天因素　病始于幼年者，与先天因素有关。若母体突受惊恐，或导致气机逆乱，或导致精伤而肾亏。母体精气耗伤，可使胎儿发育异常，出生后，遂易发生痫证。

3. 脑部外伤　因跌扑撞击，或出生时难产，均能致颅脑受伤，气血瘀阻，络脉不和，发为癫痫。

病因病机要点：

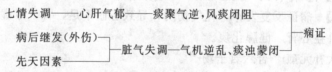

诊断与鉴别

痫证是以发作性神志恍惚，或突然仆倒，昏不知人，口吐涎沫，喉中如作猪羊叫声为特征。该病随时随地均可发作。

痫证与中风、厥证均有突然仆倒、昏不知人的主症，应予鉴别。详见中风与厥证节。

辨证论治

临床辨证时，应分标本虚实，进而论治。频繁发作者，以治标为主，着重豁痰顺气、熄风开窍定痫；平时以治本为重，宜健脾化痰，补益肝肾，养心安神。

常见证型如下：

1. 风痰闭阻

【症状】　发作前，常有眩晕、胸闷、乏力等先兆，发则突然跌倒，神志不清，抽搐吐涎，或伴尖叫与二便失禁。也有短暂神志不清，或精神恍惚而无抽搐者。苔白腻，脉弦滑。

【辨证要点】　平时神清，发则突然昏仆，抽搐吐涎，口中尖叫，或仅有短暂精神恍惚。

【病机概要】　肝风内动，痰随风动，风痰闭阻，心神被蒙；痰浊内生，风痰上涌。

【治法】　涤痰熄风，开窍定痫。

【主方】　定痫丸[157]。

【调护要点】 平时生活要有规律,饮食宜清淡,忌酒、羊肉等动火诱发之品。避免到危险地带从事危险性工作,以免发生意外。

2. 痰火内盛

【症状】 发作时昏仆,抽搐吐涎,或有吼叫。平时情绪急躁,心烦失眠,咯痰不爽,口苦而干,便秘。舌红,苔黄腻,脉弦滑数。

【辨证要点】 发作时昏仆,叫声如吼;平素有烦躁、口苦便秘等痰热证。舌红,苔黄腻,脉滑数。

【病机概要】 肝火偏旺,火动生风,煎熬津液,结而为痰,风动痰升,阻塞心窍。

【治法】 清肝泻火,化痰开窍。

【主方】 龙胆泻肝汤[64]合涤痰汤[215]。

可加入石决明、钩藤、竹沥、地龙等加强平肝熄风、化痰定痫之力。若痰火壅实,大便秘结,可用竹沥达痰丸[117],以祛痰泻火。

【调护要点】 少食辛辣肥甘油腻,以免动火生痰;防止患者独自到危险境地,或做危险工作;发作时要解开衣扣,头偏向一侧,防止痰涎吸入气管。

3. 心肾亏虚

【症状】 癫痫发作日久,健忘,心悸,头晕目眩,腰膝酸软,神疲乏力。苔薄腻,脉细弱。

【辨证要点】 发作日久,健忘心悸,腰酸神疲。

【病机概要】 痫证反复发作,耗气伤阴,导致心血不足,肾气亏虚。

【治法】 补益心肾,健脾化痰。

【主方】 大补元煎[17]合六君子汤[45]。

偏于肾虚为主者,可用河车大造丸[152]调治。若痫证日久不愈,而见神志恍惚、恐惧、抑郁、焦虑,可合甘麦大枣汤[71]养心润燥。

【调护要点】 进行适当体育锻炼,避免过度精神刺激。慎房事。

小结

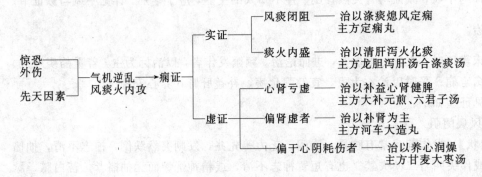

思考题

1. 痫证的发病机制是什么?
2. 风痰闭阻与痰火内盛的证治方药各是什么?

18 胃痛

概念

胃痛是指以胃脘部近心窝处经常发生疼痛为主症的疾患。

西医学中的胃及十二指肠溃疡、急慢性胃炎、胃下垂、胃神经官能症、胃粘膜脱垂症及胃癌等病表现上述症状时，可参考本病辨证论治。

病因病机

1. 病邪犯胃　外感寒邪，恣食生冷，以致寒积于中，胃阳被遏，气失舒展，而致胃痛。

2. 肝气郁结　忧思恼怒伤肝，肝气不能疏泄，横逆犯胃，气机阻塞，胃失和降，因而发生胃痛。

3. 脾胃虚寒　劳倦过度，饥饱失常，均可损伤脾胃，使中气虚寒而痛。

病因病机要点：

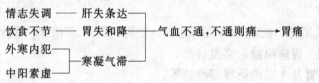

诊断与鉴别

胃痛以心窝以下、脐以上部位发生的经常性或突发性疼痛为主要症状，其疼痛有胀痛、刺痛、隐痛、剧痛等不同。在疼痛的同时，常伴见脘腹胀满、嗳腐吞酸、恶心呕吐、不思饮食、大便或干或溏等脾胃症状以及神疲乏力、面黄、消瘦、浮肿等全身症状。

胃痛应与真心痛、腹痛、胁痛进行鉴别。真心痛为胸痹之重证，其疼痛偏于左侧胸膺部，每突然发作，疼痛剧烈，或如锥刺，或心胸闷痛窒塞，难以忍受。症状及预后与胃痛截然不同。腹痛则以胃脘以下耻骨毛际以上整个部位的疼痛为主症，与胃痛的部位有所不同，但胃处腹中，与肠相连，因而在个别特殊病证中，胃痛可以影响及腹，而腹痛亦可牵连及胃，应注意辨别。胁痛是以一侧或双侧胁部胀痛为主症，可资鉴别。

辨证论治

胃痛临床辨证，当分虚实两类。

虚证——发病缓，病程长，痛势缓，喜按。

实证——发病急，病程短，痛势剧，拒按。

常见证型如下：

1. 寒邪客胃

【症状】　胃痛暴作，畏寒喜暖，局部热敷痛减，口不渴或喜热饮。苔薄白，脉弦紧。

【辨证要点】 胃痛暴作，恶寒喜温。

本型可见于急慢性胃炎、胃溃疡、十二指肠球部溃疡等。

【病机概要】 寒邪客胃，阳气被阻，不通则痛。

【治法】 散寒止痛。

【主方】 轻症可用局部温熨，或服生姜红糖汤。较重者可用良附丸[139]加味。如不效，可用半夏厚朴汤[93]。兼挟食滞者可加枳实、神曲、鸡内金等以消食导滞。

【调护要点】 忌食生冷，宜食生姜、红糖等暖胃之品。

2. 饮食停滞

【症状】 胃脘胀闷，甚则疼痛，嗳腐吞酸，呕吐不消化食物，吐后痛减，或大便不爽。苔厚腻，脉滑。

【辨证要点】 胃脘胀满恶食，嗳腐吞酸。

本型常见于急性胃炎、胃及十二指肠球部溃疡。

【病机概要】 饮停食滞，阻滞胃肠，气机不利，传导受阻。

【治法】 消食导滞。

【主方】 保和丸[193]加枳实、槟榔等。如不效，可用小承气汤[29]加木香、香附等。如受寒停食，郁而化热，胃痛较急，兼苔黄、便秘，或见发热者，再加芒硝以下之。

【调护要点】 宜清淡饮食，少食。

3. 脾胃虚寒

【症状】 胃痛隐隐，泛吐清水，喜暖喜按，手足不温，大便溏薄。舌淡苔白，脉弱或沉细。

【辨证要点】 胃痛隐隐，喜温喜按。

本型可见于胃及十二指肠球部溃疡等。

【病机概要】 脾胃虚寒，阳气不运，水饮停聚。

【治法】 温中散寒。

【主方】 黄芪建中汤[235]。

若泛酸者，可加吴茱萸暖肝温胃以制酸，亦可酌加瓦楞子；泛吐清水较多者，可加干姜、陈皮、半夏、茯苓等以温胃化饮；如寒胜而痛甚，肢冷呕吐，可用大建中汤[20]温运中气，或理中丸[229]温中散寒。中阳得运，则寒邪自散，诸证悉除。

【调护要点】 忌食生冷，慎避寒湿。

4. 肝气犯胃

【症状】 胃脘胀闷，攻撑作痛，脘痛连胁，嗳气频繁，大便不畅，每因情志郁怒而痛作或加重。苔薄白，脉沉弦。

【辨证要点】 胃痛胀闷，攻撑连胁。病情与情志因素有关。

本型常见于胃神经官能症、慢性胃炎。

【病机概要】 情志不舒，肝气郁结，横逆犯胃。

【治法】 疏肝理气。

【主方】 柴胡疏肝散[211]。

可选加郁金、青皮、木香等以加强理气解郁之效。若疼痛较甚者，可加川楝子、延胡索以加强理气止痛；嗳气较频者，可加沉香、旋覆花以顺气降逆，也可用沉香降气散[136]。

【调护要点】 调节情志，避免不良刺激。

5. 肝胃郁热

【症状】 胃脘灼痛，痛势急迫，烦躁易怒，泛酸嘈杂，口干口苦。舌红苔黄，脉弦或数。

【辨证要点】 胃灼痛，嘈杂烦怒，口干苦。

本型多见于急性胃炎、胃及十二指肠溃疡，胃粘膜脱垂症。

【病机概要】 肝气郁结，日久化热，邪热犯胃，逆而上冲。

【治法】 清肝泄热，和胃止痛。

【主方】 化肝煎[49]。

可加左金丸[67]辛开苦降。内热最易伤阴，故可选加香橼、佛手、绿萼梅等理气而不伤阴的解郁止痛药。

【调护要点】 忌食辛辣、油腻之品。

6. 瘀血停滞

【症状】 胃脘疼痛，痛有定处而拒按，或痛如针刺，食后痛甚，或见吐血便黑。舌质紫暗，脉涩。

【辨证要点】 痛有定处，或痛有针刺感。

本型可见于胃癌、胃溃疡、胃粘膜脱垂症。

【病机概要】 气滞日久，瘀血停滞，胃络内损，不通则痛。

【治法】 化瘀通络，理气和胃。

【主方】 失笑散[86]合丹参饮[51]。

若见呕血及黑便等出血现象者，宜去檀香、砂仁，加茜草炭、三七、降香等化瘀止血。

【调护要点】 宜食易消化饮食，忌生冷，勿过食。

7. 胃阴亏虚

【症状】 胃痛隐隐，口燥咽干，大便干结。舌红少津，脉细数。

【辨证要点】 胃痛隐隐，口燥咽干，舌红少津。

本型可见于慢性萎缩性胃炎等。

【病机概要】 胃痛日久，阴虚气滞，胃络失养，虚热内扰。

【治法】 养阴益胃。

【主方】 一贯煎[1]合芍药甘草汤[108]。

可酌选加香橼、佛手、绿萼梅等药调气止痛，若胃中嘈杂，或有吞酸者，可加左金丸[67]以制酸和胃；胃酸明显减少者，当酌加乌梅、诃子肉等，以增强酸甘化阴之力；若便秘，可酌加麻仁、栝楼仁以润肠通便。

【调护要点】 宜进食易消化之品，忌食辛辣油腻、生冷、粗硬之食物。并以少吃多餐为宜。

小结

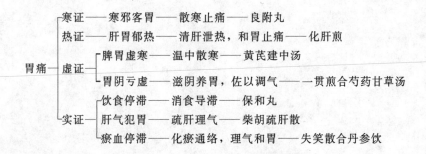

思考题

1. 胃痛和真心痛有何不同？
2. 胃痛的病因病机主要有哪些？
3. 如何对肝气犯胃、脾胃虚寒证进行辨证治疗？

19 呕吐

概念

呕吐是指胃气上逆，迫使胃内容物从口而出的病证。

呕吐可以单独出现，亦可伴见于多种急、慢性疾病中。西医学中的急、慢性胃炎，消化性溃疡、食源性呕吐、神经源性呕吐、耳源性呕吐、精神性呕吐以及其他疾病以呕吐为主症者，均可参照本病辨证论治。

病因病机

1. 外邪侵袭　感受风、寒、暑、湿之邪以及秽浊之气，侵犯胃腑，致胃失和降，水谷随气逆而上，发生呕吐。
2. 饮食不节　饮食过多，或生冷油腻之物停滞不化，以致胃气不能下行，上逆而呕吐；或脾胃运化失常，导致水谷不能化为精微，停痰留饮，积于中脘，痰饮上逆，亦可发生呕吐。
3. 情志失调　忧思恼怒，以致肝失条达，横逆犯胃，胃气不降，食随气逆，导致呕吐。
4. 脾胃虚弱　病后脾胃虚弱，中阳不振，寒浊中阻；或胃阴不足，失其润降，而致呕吐。

病因病机要点：

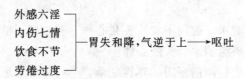

诊断与鉴别

凡以呕吐为主要临床表现者，皆可按本病辨证论治。

呕吐、反胃、呃逆三者，都是胃气上逆的病变，应注意鉴别：呕吐是有声有物；反胃是朝食暮吐，暮食朝吐，食良久复吐，宿食不化；呃逆为喉间呃呃连声、声短而频、令人不能自制，不难辨识。

辨证论治

呕吐当辨别虚实，实证多为外邪、饮食所伤，发病较急，病程较短；虚证多为脾胃运化功能减弱，发病缓慢，病程较长。现分述如下：

实证

1. 外邪犯胃

【症状】突然呕吐，来势较急，可伴恶寒发热头身疼痛，或胸闷懊恼，胃脘疼痛，腹泻，口粘腻。苔白腻，脉濡缓。

【辨证要点】 突然呕吐，头身疼痛或有寒热。

本型常见于胃肠型流行性感冒、急性胃炎、胆囊炎、胰腺炎等。

【病机概要】 外邪犯胃，动扰胃腑，气机不利，浊气上逆。

【治法】 祛邪解表，芳香化浊。

【主方】 藿香正气散[288]。

若兼有宿滞、胸闷腹胀者，去白术、甘草、大枣，加鸡内金、神曲消导积滞；如表邪偏重，寒热无汗，可加防风、荆芥之类以祛风解表；夏令感受暑湿，呕吐而兼心烦口渴者，本方去甘温之药，加入黄连、佩兰、荷叶之属，以清暑解热；如感受秽浊之气，可先服玉枢丹[60]以辟秽止呕。

【调护要点】 忌食生冷肥甘，避风寒。

2. 饮食停滞

【症状】 呕吐酸腐，脘腹胀满，疼痛拒按，嗳气厌食，得食愈甚，吐后反感舒畅，大便或溏或秘。舌苔厚腻，脉滑实。

【辨证要点】 呕吐酸腐，嗳气厌食。

本型常见于急性胃炎，幽门梗阻。

【病机概要】 饮食停滞，运化失常，气机受阻，浊气上逆。

【治法】 消食化滞，和胃降逆。

【主方】 保和丸[193]。

如积滞较多，腹满便秘，可加枳实、大黄导滞通腑，使浊气下行，则呕吐可止；若由胃中积热上冲，食已即吐，口臭而渴，苔黄脉数者，宜用竹茹汤[118]以清胃降逆。

【调护要点】 宜少食、素食。

3. 痰饮内阻

【症状】 呕吐痰涎清水，脘闷不食，头眩心悸。苔白腻，脉滑。

【辨证要点】 呕吐痰涎清水，头眩心悸。

本型常见于慢性胃炎、幽门梗阻、耳性眩晕。

【病机概要】 脾失运化，痰饮内停，胃失和降，浊饮上逆。

【治法】 健脾温中，化饮降逆。

【主方】 小半夏汤[26]。

如吐清水痰涎多者，可加用牵牛子，白芥子各2克，研末装胶囊，每日分三次吞服，可增强化痰蠲饮的作用。如痰郁化热，壅阻于胃，胃失和降，出现眩晕、心烦、少寐、恶心呕吐等证，可用温胆汤[270]以清胆和胃，除痰止呕。

【调护要点】 饮食宜清淡，忌肥甘、生冷；戒烟酒；并保持劳逸适度，以防诱发。

4. 肝气犯胃

【症状】 呕吐吞酸，嗳气频繁，胸胁闷痛，每因情绪郁怒而加重。舌边红，苔薄腻，脉弦。

【辨证要点】 呕吐吞酸，嗳气胁痛，发作常与情志波动有关。

本型可见于急慢性胃炎、胃及十二指肠球部溃疡、精神性呕吐等。

【病机概要】 肝气不舒，横逆犯胃，胃失和降。

【治法】 舒肝和胃，降逆止呕。

【主方】 半夏厚朴汤[93]合左金丸[67]加减。

若并见口苦嘈杂，大便秘结者，酌加大黄、枳实以通腑降浊；如热象较甚，可加竹茹、山栀以清肝降火。

【调护要点】 保持心情舒畅，避免精神刺激。

虚证

1. 脾胃虚寒

【症状】 饮食稍多即脘胀不舒，甚则恶心呕吐，倦怠乏力，口干不欲饮，喜暖恶寒，面色㿠白，甚则四肢不温，大便溏薄。舌质淡，苔白腻，脉象濡弱。

【辨证要点】 饮食稍有不慎即吐，肢冷便溏。

本型常见于慢性胃炎、消化性溃疡。

【病机概要】 脾胃虚弱，中阳不振，运化失常。

【治法】 温中健脾，和胃降逆。

【主方】 理中丸[229]。

可加砂仁、半夏、陈皮之类以理气降逆。呕吐不止者，加吴茱萸以温中降逆止呕。

【调护要点】 宜少食多餐，忌食生冷。

2. 胃阴不足

【症状】 呕吐反复发作，时作干呕，口燥咽干，似饥而不欲食。舌红少津，脉细数。

【辨证要点】 干呕，口燥咽干，舌红少津。

本型可见于慢性萎缩性胃炎、幽门梗阻、精神性呕吐等。

【病机概要】 胃热不清，耗伤胃阴，胃失濡养、气失和降。

【治法】 滋养胃阴，降逆止呕。

【主方】 麦门冬汤[124]。

如津伤过甚，则半夏宜少用，人参改沙参，再加石斛、天花粉、竹茹、知母之类以生津养胃；若大便干结者，加火麻仁、栝楼仁之类润肠通便。

【调护要点】 忌食肥甘厚味、辛辣、香燥。忌烟酒。

小结

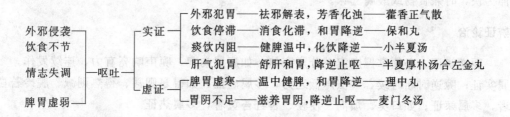

思考题

1. 试述呕吐发生的病因病机。
2. 呕吐的常见证型有哪些？并试述其主症、治法和方药。

20 呃逆

概念

呃逆是指以气逆上冲，喉间呃呃连声，声短而频，令人不能自制为特征的病证。

本证常见于西医学中的胃肠神经官能症。某些食管、胃、肠、腹膜、纵隔和脑部疾患引起的呃逆，亦可参考本篇辨证论治。

病因病机

1. 饮食不节　如过食生冷或寒凉药物，寒气蕴蓄于中，胃阳被遏；或过食辛热之品，过服温燥药物，燥热内盛，均可引起呃逆。

2. 情志不和　精神刺激，情志不和，气郁化火，肝火犯胃，或痰滞内阻，郁久化热，以致胃气不降，上逆而为呃逆。

3. 正气亏虚　重病久病之后，或误用吐、下之剂，耗伤中气，或损及胃阴，均可使胃失和降而发生呃逆。如病深及肾，则呃逆多由肾气失于摄纳，引起冲气上乘，挟胃气动膈所致。

病因病机要点：

```
饮食不节 ┐
情志抑郁 ┼─ 邪犯于胃 ┐
正气亏虚 ── 虚气上逆 ┴─ 胃气上逆 ── 呃逆
```

诊断与鉴别

因气逆于上而喉间呃呃连声，令人不能自制者，均可诊断为呃逆。呃逆、干呕、嗳气三者，同属胃气上逆之病变，但特征各异：干呕以有声无物、呕吐涎沫为特征，其声重浊而长，与呃逆声短而频，不能自制有别；嗳气则指气郁中焦，胸膈胀满，须嗳而得伸为快，时兼食物或酸腐气味。

辨证论治

呃逆辨证，必须掌握虚实，分辨寒热。如病属初起，呃声响亮有力，连续发作，多属实证；呃逆时断时续，气怯声低乏力，多属虚证。如得寒则甚、得热则减、脘冷苔白者，多属寒证；如口臭、烦渴、便秘、舌红苔黄者，多属热证。

常见证型如下：

实证

1. 胃中寒冷

【症状】　呃声沉缓有力，膈间及胃脘不舒，得热则减，得寒则甚，饮食减少，口不渴。舌苔白润，脉迟缓。

【辨证要点】　呃声沉缓有力，得热则减，得寒则甚。

本型常见于胃肠神经官能症、食管炎、胃炎。

【病机概要】 寒邪阻遏，胃失通降，气逆于上。

【治法】 温中祛寒，降逆止呃。

【主方】 丁香散[7]。

如寒重者，可加肉桂、吴茱萸以温阳散寒降逆；如挟痰滞不化，脘闷嗳腐，可加厚朴、枳实、陈皮行气化痰消滞。

【调护要点】 勿食生冷或饮冷，避风寒。

2. 胃火上逆

【症状】 呃声洪亮，连续有力，冲逆而出，口臭烦渴，溲赤便秘。舌苔黄，脉滑数。

【辨证要点】 呃声洪亮，口臭烦渴，溲赤便秘。

本型常见于胃炎、胃扩张。

【病机概要】 宿食痰浊，久蕴胃中，郁而化火，胃火上冲。

【治法】 清胃降逆，泄热止呃。

【主方】 竹叶石膏汤[116]加柿蒂、竹茹。

如大便秘结，脘腹痞满，可合用小承气汤[29]以通腑泄热，腑气通则胃气降，而呃逆自止。

【调护要点】 忌食辛辣煎炒之品。

3. 气机郁滞

【症状】 呃逆连声，常因情志不畅而诱发或加重，伴有胸闷，纳减，脘胁胀闷，肠鸣矢气。舌苔薄白，脉弦。

【辨证要点】 呃逆连声，常因情志不畅而诱发或加重。

本型常见于癔病、胃炎。

【病机概要】 情志抑郁，肝气横逆，胃气上冲。

【治法】 顺气降逆，和胃止呃。

【主方】 五磨饮子[43]。

可加丁香、代赭石降逆止呃，川楝子、郁金舒肝解郁。如气郁化火，心烦、便秘、口苦、舌质红、脉弦数者，可加山栀、黄连等泄肝和胃；若气逆痰阻，则可有头目昏眩，或时有恶心，舌苔薄腻，脉弦滑，可合旋覆代赭汤[244]，二陈汤[2]化裁，以顺气降逆，化痰和胃。

【调护要点】 避免精神刺激，保持心情舒畅。

虚证

1. 脾胃阳虚

【症状】 呃声低弱，气不接续，面色苍白，手足不温，食少脘胀，困倦无力。舌淡苔白，脉沉细弱。

【辨证要点】 呃声低弱，手足不温，食少脘胀。

本型可见于尿毒症、晚期胃癌等。

【病机概要】 脾胃虚弱，升降不利，虚气上逆。

【治法】 温补脾胃，和中降逆。

【主方】 理中汤[229]加吴茱萸、丁香。

若呃逆不止，心下痞硬，可合用旋覆代赭汤[244]以重镇和中降逆；如肾阳亦虚，见形寒肢冷，腰膝酸软，舌体胖嫩，脉沉迟者，可加附子、肉桂以温肾助阳；如兼有食滞，可稍佐陈皮、麦芽之类以理气化滞；若中气大亏，呃声低弱难续，食少便溏，体倦乏力，脉虚者，宜用补中益气汤[140]。

【调护要点】 忌食生冷、油腻之品，可常服生姜红糖水，或口含姜片，并注意保暖。

2. 胃阴不足

【症状】 呃声急促而不连续，口干舌燥，烦躁不安。舌质红而干或有裂纹，脉细数。

【辨证要点】 呃声急促，口干舌燥，舌红而干。

本型可见于脑部炎症、脑瘤、脑溢血、胃肠神经官能症、尿毒症、肠梗阻等。

【病机概要】 热病耗津，或汗、吐太过，阴液亏损，胃失濡润，气失和降。

【治法】 养胃生津，和胃止呃。

【主方】 益胃汤[217]。

可加枇杷叶、石斛、柿蒂等，以降逆止呃。如胃气大虚，不思饮食，则合用橘皮竹茹汤[286]以益气和中。

【调护要点】 宜食清淡甘凉食物，如绿豆汤、藕粉、梨汁等；忌烟、酒、葱、蒜、辣椒等辛温之品。

小结

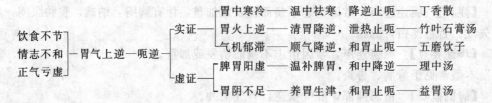

思考题

1. 呃逆的虚、实、寒、热有哪些特征？
2. 呃逆的病机有几大类？
3. 呃逆的实证有哪些常见证型？如何辨证治疗？

21 泄泻

概念

泄泻是指排便次数增多,粪便稀薄,甚至泻如水样的一种病证。

西医的急、慢性肠炎、非特异性溃疡性结肠炎、胃肠神经官能症等引起的腹泻,可参考本病辨证论治。

病因病机

1. 感受外邪　外邪引起的泄泻,以寒、湿、暑、热为常见,其中尤以湿邪居多。由于脾喜燥恶湿,而外感湿邪又最易困伤脾阳,使脾失健运,清浊不分,发生泄泻。

2. 饮食所伤　暴食暴饮或过食肥甘、或贪食生冷、误食不洁,损伤脾胃、传导失职、升降失调,而致泄泻。

3. 情志失调　脾胃素虚,或有宿食停滞,复因忧思恼怒、惊恐不安,以致肝气郁结,横逆乘脾,运化失常,遂成泄泻。

4. 脾胃虚弱　饮食不节、劳倦内伤、久病缠绵,均可导致脾胃虚弱。胃不受纳,脾失健运,水谷停滞、清浊不分,混杂而下,而成泄泻。

5. 肾阳虚衰　久病之后、损伤肾阳,或年迈体衰、阳气不足、脾失温煦,运化失常,而致泄泻。

病因病机要点：外因——湿胜致脾伤 ┐
　　　　　　　内因——脾虚致湿阻 ┘ 运化失常——泄泻

诊断与鉴别

泄泻是以排便次数增多,粪便清稀为特征。一年四季均可发病,但以夏秋两季为多见。

本病与痢疾的病变部位都在肠间,都有腹痛和排便异常,应予鉴别：

鉴别 \ 病名	泄　泻	痢　疾
大　便	粪便稀溏,甚至泻下如水样,泻下较爽利	痢下赤白脓血,泻下不爽
腹　痛	或有或无,伴肠鸣脘胀,呈阵发性,泻后痛止	必有腹痛,伴里急后重,呈持续性,便后仍痛或痛减而不能止
粪　检	一般无明显异常,或可见少量红、白、脓细胞	可见大量红细胞、脓细胞

辨证论治

在对泄泻病明确诊断后,应进行辨证。首先,要区别寒、热、虚、实。

泄泻
- 大便清稀，完谷不化，畏寒腹冷，腹痛喜温—寒证
- 便色黄褐而臭，泻下急迫，肛门灼热　　　—热证
- 发病急、泻下腹痛，痛势急，拒按，泻后痛减—实证
- 病程较长，泄泻次数较少，腹隐痛，喜揉按—虚证

可兼夹互见

常见证型如下：

感受外邪

1. 寒湿困脾

【症状】　泄泻清稀，甚至如水样，腹痛肠鸣，脘闷食少。或兼恶寒发热，鼻塞头痛，肢体酸痛。舌淡苔薄白或白腻，脉濡缓。

【辨证要点】　泄泻清稀，腹痛肠鸣。

本型常见于急性肠炎。

【病机概要】　寒湿郁表，内侵肠胃，脾失健运，升降失调。

【治法】　芳香化湿，散寒解表。

【主方】　藿香正气散[288]。

若寒湿表证较重，可加荆芥、防风、羌活、独活、蔓荆子；湿邪偏重，证见胸闷腹胀、体倦、苔白腻者，重用苍术、厚朴、云苓或用胃苓汤[182]。若大便如水样，可在上述基础上加用车前子、泽泻以分利水湿。

【调护要点】　忌食生冷，避风寒。

2. 湿热壅遏

【症状】　泄泻腹痛，泻下急迫，或泻而欠爽，粪色黄褐而臭味较大，肛门灼热，烦热口渴，溲少色黄。舌红苔黄腻，脉濡数或滑数。

【辨证要点】　泻下急迫，粪色黄褐、便臭灼肛。苔黄腻，脉数。

本型亦常见于急性肠炎。

【病机概要】　湿热或暑湿之邪壅遏，内迫肠胃，传化失常。

【治法】　清热利湿。

【主方】　葛根芩连汤[260]。

若湿邪偏重，见胸腹满闷，渴不欲饮，可加平胃散[70]燥湿宽中；发于盛夏，偏暑湿，证见泄泻如水，自汗面垢，可加藿香、香薷、扁豆衣、荷叶等，以清暑化湿；若挟食滞，见纳呆厌食，加神曲、麦芽、山楂以消积化滞。

【调护要点】　忌食荤腥油腻及甜食。

3. 食滞肠胃

【症状】　泻下粪便臭如败卵，腹痛肠鸣，泻后痛减，伴有不消化之物，脘腹痞满，嗳腐酸臭，不思饮食。舌苔垢浊或厚腻，脉滑。

【辨证要点】　粪便臭如败卵，嗳腐酸臭，厌食。苔厚腻，脉滑。

本型常见于急性肠炎。

【病机概要】　宿食不化，阻滞胃肠，气机不利，传导失常。

【治法】　消食导滞。

【主方】　保和丸[193]。

若食滞较重，泻而不畅者，或可采用"通因通用"之法，用枳实导滞丸[172]消积导滞、

清利湿热。此型病人,小儿多见,临床宜用消食药配以生大黄、枳实等通导之品,祛邪以安正,万不可畏攻留寇,延误病情。

【调护要点】 宜少食、素食。

4. 肝气乘脾

【症状】 每因抑郁恼怒或情绪紧张之时,发生腹痛泄泻,平素常胸胁胀闷、嗳气食少。舌淡红,脉弦。

【辨证要点】 泄泻与情志郁怒变化有关,胁胀、脉弦。

此型多见于肠神经官能症,亦可见于慢性非特异性结肠炎。

【病机概要】 肝气郁结,横逆犯脾,气机失调,运化失常。

【治法】 抑肝扶脾。

【主方】 痛泻要方[269]。

若肝郁明显,证见胁胀满、太息口苦者,酌加柴胡、香附、郁金、青皮等,以增疏肝解郁之功;若兼嗳腐、脘胀等食滞证时,加鸡内金、麦芽、山楂等消食去积。

【调护要点】 忌忧思郁怒。

5. 脾胃虚弱

【症状】 大便时溏时泻,水谷不化,稍进油腻食物,则大便次数增多、饮食减少,脘腹胀闷不舒,面色萎黄,体倦乏力。舌淡苔白,脉细弱。

【辨证要点】 大便时溏时泻,面黄体倦,病程较长。

本型可见于慢性肠炎、慢性非特异性溃疡性结肠炎等。

【病机概要】 脾胃亏虚,运化无力,水谷不化,清浊不分。

【治法】 健脾益胃。

【主方】 参苓白术散[169]。

若脾阳不振,阴寒内盛,表现腹中冷痛,手足不温者,宜予理中汤[229]加吴茱萸、肉桂以温中散寒;若久泻不止,中气下陷而出现脱肛者,可用补中益气汤[140]益气升提。

【调护要点】 宜少食多餐;忌食生冷、油腻,忌过食。

6. 肾阳虚衰

【症状】 泄泻多在黎明前发生,腹部作痛,肠鸣即泻,泻后即安,形寒肢冷,腰膝酸软。舌淡苔白,脉沉细。

【辨证要点】 五更泻(鸡鸣泻),畏寒腰酸,脉沉细。

本型可见于慢性肠炎、慢性非特异性结肠炎等。

【病机概要】 肾阳亏虚,脾失温养,运化失常。

【治法】 温肾健脾,固涩止泻。

【主方】 四神丸[82]。

肾阳虚多兼脾阳虚,故常以四神丸合理中丸[229]施治;若见年老体衰,久泻不止,中气下陷,宜加黄芪、党参、白术、山药益气健脾,合桃花汤[205]以固涩止泻。

【调护要点】 宜食炒面、小米汤等温性食品;忌食生冷。

小结

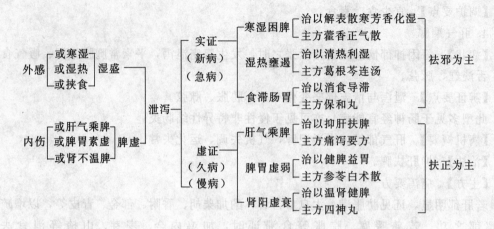

思考题

1. 临床应如何区分泄泻的寒热虚实证？
2. 泄泻分为哪几个证候类型，其辨证要点、治法和主方各是什么？
3. 泄泻和痢疾如何鉴别？

22 痢疾

概念

痢疾是以大便次数增多,腹痛,里急后重,下痢赤白脓血为主症的疾病。是夏秋季常见的肠道传染病。

与本病相关的西医疾病有:急、慢性细菌性痢疾和急、慢性阿米巴痢疾。此外,慢性非特异性溃疡性结肠炎、血吸虫病、结肠过敏、结肠直肠恶性肿瘤等,以下痢为主症者,均可参考本病辨证论治。

病因病机

1. 外感时邪　暑湿、疫毒之邪侵及肠胃,湿热郁蒸,或疫毒弥漫,气血阻滞,与暑湿、疫毒相搏结,化为脓血而成为湿热痢或疫毒痢。

2. 内伤饮食　素好肥甘酒炙之品,或食入腐垢不洁之物,酿生湿热,蕴结肠中,传导失司,气血凝滞,化为脓血,则生湿热痢;亦有恣食生冷瓜果,脾胃受损,脾虚不运,水湿内停,中阳受阻,湿从寒化,寒湿蕴滞,气机不行,气滞血瘀,与肠中腐浊之气相搏结,化为脓血而成寒湿痢。

病因病机要点:

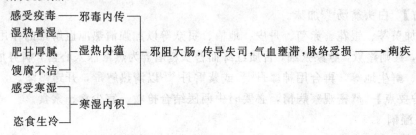

诊断与鉴别

凡具大便次数增多而量少,痢下赤白粘冻,腹痛,里急后重者,均可诊断为痢疾。急性痢疾多发生于夏秋季节,而慢性痢疾则四季可见。

痢疾与泄泻临床症状相似,两者病位同在胃肠,病因亦不易分辨,皆多发于夏秋之季,因此,需将二者予以鉴别(详见"泄泻"一节)。

辨证论治

在对痢疾明确诊断后,应进行辨证。首先,要注意区别寒、热、虚、实。

若下痢赤白而清稀,无热臭,面白形寒,或腹痛隐隐、喜温喜按,为寒证;里急后重明显,舌质红、苔黄腻、脉滑数或濡数,或见发热,甚至高热不退,则为热证;若里急后重、便后不减,腹痛喜按、痛势绵绵,多为虚证;若里急后重、便后得减,腹痛胀满、痛而拒按,痛时窘迫欲便,便后痛暂减轻者,多为实证。

常见证型如下：

1. 湿热痢

【症状】 腹痛，里急后重，下痢赤白相杂，肛门灼热，小便短赤。舌苔黄腻，脉滑数。

【辨证要点】 肛门灼热，小便短赤。

本型多见于急性细菌性痢疾。

【病机概要】 湿热之邪壅滞肠中，脉络受伤，气血瘀滞，传导失司。

【治法】 清热导滞，调气行血。

【主方】 芍药汤[107]。

兼有恶寒发热，头痛等表证者，加葛根、连翘、荆芥等；挟食滞者，加六曲、山楂；如热重下痢，赤多白少，或纯赤痢，发热较重，口渴引饮，舌红苔黄，脉滑数者，可用白头翁汤[88]清热解毒，酌加银花、芍药、枳实、甘草。

【调护要点】 注意休息，宜进清淡易消化的流质或半流质饮食，忌辛辣肥甘。

2. 疫毒痢

【症状】 发病急骤，头痛烦躁，壮热口渴，腹痛剧烈，甚则神昏痉厥。痢下鲜紫脓血，便次频繁，里急后重甚于湿热痢。舌质红绛，苔黄燥，脉滑数。

【辨证要点】 发病急骤，壮热烦躁，甚至有神志症状，腹痛、里急后重较剧。

本型多见于中毒性痢疾、急性血吸虫病。

【病机概要】 疫毒之邪，熏灼肠道，耗伤气血，蒙蔽清窍。

【治法】 清热凉血，解毒化积。

【主方】 白头翁汤[88]加味。

可酌加黄芩、银花、赤芍、丹皮、地榆、贯众等以加强清热凉血解毒的作用。如见神昏谵语，甚则痉厥，脉象弦细，舌质红绛而苔黄糙者，为热毒深入心营，病势危急，可加羚羊角、鲜生地等，再合用神犀丹[187]或紫雪丹[267]以清热解毒，开窍镇痉。

【调护要点】 严密观察病情，必要时中西医结合抢救。宜少食、素食。

3. 寒湿痢

【症状】 痢下赤白粘冻，白多赤少，或纯为白冻，伴有腹痛，里急后重，饮食乏味，胃脘饱闷，头身重困。舌质淡，苔白腻，脉濡缓。

【辨证要点】 痢下赤少白多或纯为白冻，脘闷，头身重困。

本型多见于慢性细菌性痢疾、慢性非特异性溃疡性结肠炎、结肠过敏。

【病机概要】 寒湿滞留肠道，气机阻滞，传导失常。

【治法】 温中散寒，化湿导滞。

【主方】 胃苓汤[182]加减。

因痢疾不宜过利小便，故泽泻、猪苓不宜选用。若寒邪较著者，可于原方中加用炮姜、肉桂之类以散寒调气。

【调护要点】 忌食生冷瓜果，以免助寒，重伤脾胃之阳。饮食宜清淡素洁，如小米粥等。

4. 阴虚痢

【症状】 痢下赤白脓血，或下鲜血粘稠，脐腹灼痛，虚坐努责，食少，心烦口干。舌质红绛少苔，或舌光红乏津，脉细数。

【辨证要点】 痢下赤白，或下鲜血粘稠，虚坐努责。舌红绛或光红。

本型常见于慢性细菌性痢疾、慢性非特异性溃疡性结肠炎、结肠癌、直肠癌等。

【病机概要】 久痢缠绵，湿热未尽，阴液伤耗，邪滞肠间。

【治法】 养阴和营，清肠止痢。

【主方】 驻车丸[166]加减。

可加白芍、甘草以酸甘化阴，和营止痛；加栝楼以滑利气机。如虚热灼津而见口渴、尿少、舌干者，可加沙参、石斛养阴生津；若见痢下血多者，可加丹皮、赤芍、旱莲草、地榆炭以凉血止血；若湿热未清，而见口苦、肛门灼热者，可加黄柏、秦皮以清解湿热。

【调护要点】 忌食辛辣煎炸之品；戒劳作。

5. 虚寒痢

【症状】 下痢稀薄，带有白冻，甚则滑脱不禁，或腹部隐痛，食少神疲，四肢不温，腰酸怕冷。舌淡苔薄白，脉沉细而弱。

【辨证要点】 下痢稀薄或白冻，或滑脱不禁，肢冷腰酸。

本型多见于慢性细菌性痢疾、慢性非特异性溃疡性结肠炎、结肠过敏。

【病机概要】 痢久，寒湿留滞肠中，脾肾阳虚，中气下陷，固摄无权。

【治法】 温补脾肾，收涩固脱。

【主方】 真人养脏汤[198]加减。

若虚寒较甚者，可配合附子理中汤[146]温中散寒；若积滞未尽者，应少佐消导积滞之品，如枳壳、山楂、神曲等，或加入莱菔子；若久痢而脾虚气陷，脱肛少气者，可改用补中益气汤[140]，益气补中、升清举陷。

【调护要点】 宜进食营养丰富但不油腻之品。戒劳作，避风寒。

6. 休息痢

【症状】 下痢时发时止，日久难愈，饮食减少，倦怠怯冷，嗜卧，临厕腹痛里急，大便夹有粘液或见赤色。舌质淡苔腻，脉濡或虚数。

【辨证要点】 下痢时发时止，经年不愈。

本型常见于慢性细菌性痢疾、慢性阿米巴痢疾、慢性非特异性溃疡性结肠炎、慢性血吸虫病。

【病机概要】 下痢日久，正虚邪恋，寒热错杂，肠胃传导失司。

【治法】 温中清肠，调气化滞。

【主方】 连理汤[134]加味。

可加槟榔、木香、枳实等以调气化滞。

【调护要点】 以清淡易消化的饮食为主，夏秋季节可经常食用生大蒜或马齿苋作菜肴以资预防。注意锻炼身体，劳逸结合，增强体质。

小结

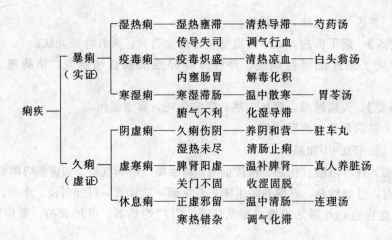

思考题

1. 何谓痢疾？分几个证型？
2. 湿热痢和休息痢怎样进行辨证论治？
3. 试述疫毒痢的病理特点、临床表现及治疗措施。

23 便秘

概念

便秘是指大便秘结不通，排便时间延长，或欲大便而艰涩不畅的一种病证。

老年性便秘、饮食性便秘、习惯性便秘、精神神经性便秘，均可参考本篇辨证论治。

病因病机

1. 胃肠燥热 阳盛之体，或饮酒过度，嗜食辛热厚味，以致胃肠积热；或热病之后，余热留恋，耗伤津液，导致肠道燥热。津液失于输布而不能下润，于是大便干结，难以排出。

2. 气机郁滞 忧愁思虑，或久坐少动，往往引起气机郁滞，使肠胃消化、通降、传导功能失常，因之糟粕内停，不能下行，造成大便秘结。

3. 气血两亏 劳倦内伤，或病后、产后以及老年人，气血两亏。气虚则大肠传送无力，血虚、津少则不能滋润大肠，都能造成大便排出困难。

4. 阴寒凝结 身体虚弱，或年高体衰，真阳亏损，温煦无权，以致阴邪凝结而大便艰难。

病因病机要点：

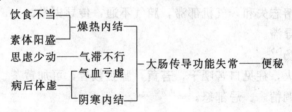

诊断与鉴别

便秘的诊断，问诊时要了解患者平时的生活、饮食、排便习惯，以辨明便秘的原因。

便秘的一般表现，为大便燥结，排出困难，经常三、五日或七、八日才一次，有时甚至更久。便秘日久，常可引发其他症状。部分患者由于便秘，腑气阻滞，往往引起腹中胀满，甚则疼痛以及食欲减退、头晕脑胀、睡眠不安等症。长期便秘，会引起痔疮、便血、肛裂等。便秘日久，在左下腹部可触及到索条状，或大小不等包块，此为粪便所致，需与癥瘕、积聚鉴别。若是便秘之包块，通下之后即消失或减少；癥积则推之不移、按之不动，通下之后不消；瘕聚则推之能移、按之能动、时聚时散。

辨证论治

便秘的辨证可分热秘、气秘、虚秘、冷秘，也可分为虚实两大类。实秘包括热秘与气秘；虚秘包括气虚、血虚、阳虚（冷秘）。

便秘的治疗应以通下为主，但不可单纯用泻下药，应结合病机加以配伍。实秘治以清热润肠，顺气行滞；虚秘治以益气养血，温通开秘。

常见证型如下：

1. 热秘

【症状】 大便干结，小便短赤，面红身热，或兼有腹胀腹痛，口干口臭。舌红苔黄或黄燥，脉滑数。

【辨证要点】 大便干结，身热溲赤，腹胀痛。

本型可见于饮食性便秘或热病之后引起的便秘。

【病机概要】 肠胃积热，津液耗伤，燥屎内停，腑气不通。

【治法】 清热润肠。

【主方】 麻子仁丸[240]。

燥结较盛，大便多日不通，加玄明粉软坚散结、清热通便；若兼肝经郁火，见目赤、易怒、舌红、脉弦者，加龙胆草、黄芩、山栀清热泻火，或配服更衣丸[131]凉肝通便。素有痔疮，属肠胃燥热，大便秘结，引起便血量多者，加槐花、地榆凉血止血；燥热不甚，无明显其他症状者，可服青麟丸[148]以清腑缓下，以免再秘。

【调护要点】 忌食煎炒、肥甘、酒类、辛辣；宜食清淡。

2. 气秘

【症状】 大便秘结，欲便不得，嗳气频作，胸胁痞满，甚则腹中胀痛，纳食减少。舌苔薄腻，脉弦。

【辨证要点】 大便秘结，欲便不得，嗳气频作，胸胁痞满。

本型常见于胃肠神经官能症。

【病机概要】 情志失和，气机郁滞，腑气不通，传导失常。

【治法】 顺气导滞。

【主方】 六磨汤[47]。

若气郁日久化火，症见口苦咽干，苔黄，脉弦数者，可加黄芩、山栀以清热泻火。

【调护要点】 调情志、忌郁怒。

3. 虚秘

(1) 气虚

【症状】 虽有便意，但临厕努挣乏力，挣则汗出气短，大便多不干硬，便后疲乏，面色㿠白，神疲气怯。舌质淡，苔薄白，脉虚。

【辨证要点】 临厕努挣乏力，汗出气短，神疲气怯。脉虚。

本型可见于老年性便秘，习惯性便秘，饮食性便秘等。

【病机概要】 肺脾气虚，大肠传送无力。

【治法】 益气润肠。

【主方】 黄芪汤[234]。

若气虚明显者，可加党参、白术以增强补气之功；若气虚下陷，肛门坠胀，可合用补中益气汤[140]以益气举陷，使脾肺之气得以内充，则传送有力，大便通畅。

【调护要点】 忌食辛辣，宜多食蔬菜瓜果，蜂蜜等；戒过劳；并养成定时大便的习惯。

(2) 血虚

【症状】 大便干结，面色淡白无华，心悸，头晕目眩，唇舌淡白，脉细。

【辨证要点】 大便秘结，面无华，唇舌淡，脉细。

本型可见于老人、产妇及疾病恢复期体质羸弱者。

【病机概要】 血虚津少，不能滑利肠道。

【治法】 养血润燥。

【主方】 润肠丸[214]。

若因阴血虚少而生内热，出现烦热、口干、舌红少津，可加玄参、生首乌、知母以清热生津；若津液已复，便仍干燥，可用五仁丸[39]以润肠通便。

【调护要点】 调起居，戒劳作。可配合以药膳食疗，如黑芝麻、胡桃肉、松子仁等，研细，加蜜冲服。

4. 冷秘

【症状】 大便艰涩，排出困难，小便清长，面色㿠白，四肢不温，喜热怕冷，腹中冷痛，或腰脊酸冷。舌淡苔白，脉沉迟。

【辨证要点】 大便艰难，腹中冷痛，四肢不温。

【病机概要】 阳气虚衰，寒自内生，气机阻滞，肠道传送无力。

【治法】 温阳通便。

【主方】 济川煎[183]。

若为阴寒内盛，可用半硫丸[94]。

【调护要点】 忌食生冷、慎避风寒。

此外，保持精神舒畅，进行身体锻炼以及注意饮食，定时大便等，均有利于便秘的治疗。至于热病之后，或其他久病患者，由于水谷不进而不大便者，不必急于通便，只须扶养胃气，待饮食渐增，则大便自能正常排出。

小结

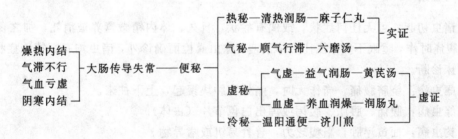

思考题

1. 试述便秘的病因病机。
2. 治疗便秘应如何正确使用通下法？
3. 便秘常分几种证型，其辨证要点、治法、主方各是什么？

24 虫证

概念

虫证是指寄生在人体肠道的虫类所引起的病证。

蛔虫病、绦虫病、钩虫病、蛲虫病、姜片虫病等引起的症状，可参考本病辨证论治。

病因病机

1. 饮食所致　饮食因素为虫证产生的主要根源，其中包括饮食失节和饮食不洁两方面。饮食失节如：恣食厚味生冷，过食甘甜之物等。饮食不洁如：食品未洗净，沾有虫卵；食用未熟之鱼、肉类；手指爪甲、衣被附有虫卵，随饮食入口成病。

2. 由肤而入　如钩虫病的发生，除饮食不洁外，往往由于人们在耕作之时，皮肤接触泥土，钩蚴钻入皮肤，进入人体。

3. 湿热内蕴　湿热有利于虫邪寄生，而虫邪作乱，又可扰乱气机，使脏腑失和，湿热内生。

4. 正虚虫动　若脏腑气虚，功能失调，尤其是脾胃虚弱之时，虫类乘虚而动，诸病乃生。

病因病机要点：

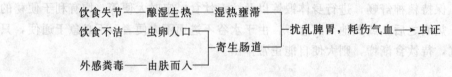

诊断与鉴别

诸虫初起，可无任何症状，或偶有症状，日久，体内精微营养被消耗，加之食欲减退，腹痛时作，睡眠不安，往往形体消瘦。除由粪检而确诊外，诸虫均有其特殊症状，可资临床诊断。

蛔虫病：绕脐腹痛，痛作无时，痛处有肿块聚起，上下往来。

绦虫病：腹痛、腹胀、腹泻或泻出白色节片（虫体）。

钩虫病：面黄浮肿，羸瘦乏力，善食易饥或嗜异物。

蛲虫病：夜间肛痒、肛门周围可见蠕动白色小虫，睡眠不安。

姜片虫病：一般无明显症状，后期始有轻度的腹痛、腹泻。

临床上，钩虫病的黄浮需与黄疸病相鉴别，黄疸病的黄呈全身皮肤、巩膜黄染，无浮肿，伴胁痛、小便黄赤如茶、纳差等症状，病属湿热内盛；钩虫病则面部呈黄色，有浮肿，而巩膜无黄染，伴神疲乏力等症。

辨证论治

虫证的辨证必须辨明病之新久、虚实，而后治疗。一般先予驱虫，虫去后再予调理脾胃。

1. 蛔虫病

【症状】 脐周腹痛,时作时止,胃脘嘈杂,甚或吐虫、便虫、腹中虫瘕,较严重者表现为不思饮食,面黄肌瘦,鼻孔作痒,睡中龄齿流涎。

【辨证要点】 脐周作痛,时作时止,鼻孔作痒,睡中龄齿流涎。

【病机概要】 蛔虫内扰,气机紊乱,湿热内生。

【治法】 驱虫安蛔,健脾和胃。

【主方】 化虫丸[48],乌梅丸[56]。

化虫丸适用于蛔虫证腹痛不剧或腹不痛时,以驱除蛔虫,消除病因。乌梅丸适用于腹中疼痛较剧,及有恶心呕吐者,以安蛔定痛。

【调护要点】 注意饮食卫生。

2. 绦虫病

【症状】 腹部隐痛或胀满,或有腹泻,肛门作痒,久则消瘦乏力,大便中或衬裤上有时发现白色节片。

【辨证要点】 腹痛或胀、便出白色节片。

【病机概要】 虫居肠中,阻滞气机,扰乱脾胃,运化失健,精微被耗。

【治法】 祛除绦虫,调理脾胃。

【主方】 可服用下列简易方:

①槟榔合南瓜子,服药2小时后,用玄明粉9～18克,溶化于温开水中顿服,约2～3小时后,即有虫体排出。

②雷丸研粉,每次20克,1日1次,连服3天。

③石榴根皮25克,水煎服。但胃病患者不宜此药。

【调护要点】 驱虫需连头节同时排出,方能彻底治愈。驱虫后宜服健运脾胃中药。注意饮食卫生,不吃不熟的猪、牛肉。

3. 钩虫病

(1) 脾虚湿滞

【症状】 面色萎黄或面黄而虚浮,善食易饥,食后腹胀,或异嗜生米、茶叶、木炭之类,神疲肢软。舌淡苔薄,脉濡。

【辨证要点】 面黄浮肿,善食易饥或嗜异物。

【病机概要】 钩虫扰乱气机,脾胃失于健运,生化乏源,气血亏虚,水湿积滞。

【治法】 健脾燥湿,和中补血。

【主方】 黄病绛矾丸[236]。

(2) 气血两虚

【症状】 颜面、肌肤萎黄或苍白,面足、甚至全身浮肿,脘闷不舒,倦怠乏力,精神不振,眩晕耳鸣,心悸气短。舌质淡胖,脉弱。

【辨证要点】 肤色萎黄或苍白,面足浮肿,心悸气短。

【病机概要】 虫居肠中,吸食水谷精微,损耗人体气血,气血亏虚。

【治法】 补益气血。

【主方】 八珍汤[13]。

脘闷纳差者,加木香、砂仁理气调胃。

钩虫病均需要进行驱虫治疗。可酌情采用榧子、雷丸、槟榔、百部、鹤虱、贯众等药。

【调护要点】 注意局部皮肤防护,勿赤脚及赤身着地。宜进食富于营养而又易于消化的食物。重症病人应注意休息。

4. 蛲虫病

【症状】 肛门奇痒,夜间尤甚,睡眠不安,作痒时可在肛门周围发现蠕动的白色小虫,甚者可见精神烦躁,夜寐不安,头昏纳少,面黄肌瘦,或恶心呕吐,腹痛腹泻。

【辨证要点】 夜间肛痒,肛门周围可见白色小虫蠕动。

【病机概要】 虫行肛门,蠕动作痒,虫居肠间,脾失健运,气机郁滞。

【治法】 驱虫止痒。

【主方】 追虫丸[196]。

亦可选用使君子、鹤虱、榧子、槟榔等驱虫药。

除内服药物外,尚可外用百部煎汤灌肠。

【调护要点】 注意个人卫生,勤换衣裤,勤洗被褥。

5. 姜片虫病

【症状】 一般可无临床症状,有的患者可见轻度腹痛、腹泻或恶心呕吐,病久则见精神倦怠,或腹胀浮肿。

【辨证要点】 轻度腹痛、腹泻或倦怠,浮肿。

【病机概要】 虫积于肠,纳运失司,气机阻滞;病久脾胃虚弱,气血亏损,水湿不化。

【治法】 驱虫为主,佐以健脾。

【主方】 驱虫可用槟榔50克,碎后加清水先浸一夜,再浓煎1小时,空腹顿服,连服2~3日。

健脾和胃则用香砂六君子汤[189]。若见腹胀水肿,加用车前草、五加皮、陈葫芦以渗湿利水。

【调护要点】 注意饮食卫生,蔬菜洗净,食品煮熟,生菱、荸荠应沸水烫洗后吃。

小结

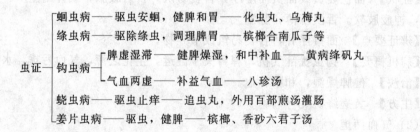

思考题

1. 虫证是如何发生的?
2. 蛔居肠中有哪些临床表现?如何治疗?
3. 治疗绦虫病的有效方药有哪些?

25 腹痛

概念

腹痛是指胃脘以下，耻骨毛际以上部位疼痛为主要表现的一种病证。

腹痛病证所涉及的范围较广。西医学中的肠痉挛、急性胰腺炎、胃肠神经官能症、部分肠炎和结肠炎、粘连性肠梗阻、肠系膜及腹膜病等，凡以腹痛为主症者，均可参考本病辨证论治。

病因病机

1. 感受外邪　寒热暑湿之邪侵入腹中，使脾胃运化失常，留滞于中，以致气机阻滞，发生腹痛。

2. 饮食不节　暴饮暴食，或恣食不洁之品；或过食膏粱厚味辛辣之物，致食物停滞不化，酿成湿热；或热结肠胃而腑气不通，均能导致腹痛。

3. 情志失调　情志怫郁，恼怒伤肝，木失条达，气血郁滞；或肝气横逆，乘犯脾胃，以致脾胃不和，气机不畅，均可导致腹痛。

4. 阳气素虚　脾阳不振，健运无权；或寒湿停滞，渐致脾阳衰惫，气血不足，不能温养脏腑，遂致腹痛。

此外，腹部手术后或跌仆损伤亦可导致气滞血瘀、脉络阻塞而引起腹痛。

病因病机要点：

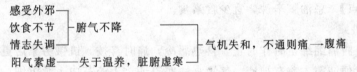

诊断与鉴别

临床上，凡以胃脘以下、耻骨毛际以上部位疼痛为主要表现者，即属腹痛。

内科腹痛，当与肠痈、疝气、霍乱、痢疾、积聚等腹痛相鉴别。肠痈腹痛，多在右下腹，痛重拒按，右足喜屈而畏伸；疝气腹痛，多伴有少腹拘急，痛引阴股；霍乱腹痛，多伴有上吐下泻，绞痛不已，厥冷转筋等；痢疾腹痛，多伴有后重急迫，便下脓血等；积聚之痛，多见腹中包块，有形可征。其他诸如妇科腹痛，多伴有经带胎产之异常。

辨证论治

腹痛的辨证，应注意分别疼痛的性质。凡痛势急剧，痛时拒按者，多属实证；若痛势隐隐，痛时喜按者，多为虚证；凡疼痛急迫，腹胀便秘，得热痛势不减者，多为热证；如疼痛遇冷加剧，得热敷或进热食后减轻者，多为寒证；凡腹部胀闷，走窜不定，多由气滞所致；腹部刺痛，固定不移者，属血瘀为病。

常见证型如下：

1. 寒邪内阻

【症状】 腹痛急暴，得温痛减，遇冷更甚，口和不渴，小便清利，大便自可或溏薄。舌苔白腻，脉沉紧。

【辨证要点】 遇寒痛甚，得温痛减。

本型可见于肠痉挛及肠炎性腹痛等。

【病机概要】 寒邪入侵，阳气不运，气血被阻。

【治法】 温中散寒。

【主方】 良附丸[139]合正气天香散[62]。

若寒重，痛势剧烈，手足逆冷，脉沉细者，可加入附子、肉桂辛热通阳，散寒止痛；若少腹拘急冷痛，属肝经寒凝气滞者，可加吴茱萸、小茴香、沉香以暖肝散寒；腹中冷痛，兼见便秘，可加附子，大黄以温通腑气。

【调护要点】 勿食生冷及油腻之品，避风寒。

2. 湿热壅滞

【症状】 腹痛拒按，胸闷不舒，大便秘结或溏滞不爽，烦渴引饮，自汗，小便短赤。舌苔黄腻，脉滑数。

【辨证要点】 腹痛拒按，胸闷不舒，便秘溲赤，苔黄腻，脉数。

本型可见于急性肠炎、急性胰腺炎、肠梗阻等疾病。

【病机概要】 湿热内结，气机壅滞，腑气不通。

【治法】 泄热通腑。

【主方】 大承气汤[21]。

如燥结不甚而湿热重者，可去芒硝加黄芩、山栀等；如痛引两胁者，可加柴胡、郁金。

【调护要点】 忌油腻辛辣，宜少食素食。

3. 中虚脏寒

【症状】 腹痛绵绵，时作时止，喜热恶冷，痛时喜按，饥饿劳累后更甚，得食或休息后稍减，大便溏薄，兼有神疲、气短、怯寒等证。舌淡苔白，脉沉细。

【辨证要点】 腹痛喜按，便溏，怯寒，得食痛减。

本型可见于慢性肠炎及肠系膜、腹膜方面的慢性炎症。

【病机概要】 脾阳不振，寒从内生，脉络失养。

【治法】 温中补虚，缓急止痛。

【主方】 小建中汤[28]。

如见神倦少气，或大便虽软而艰难者，为气虚无力，可加黄芪以补气；若虚寒腹痛见证较重，呕吐肢冷脉微者，用大建中汤[20]以温中散寒；若腹痛自利、肢冷、脉沉迟者，则属脾肾阳虚，用附子理中汤[146]以温补脾肾。

【调护要点】 宜进易于消化的温热食物，勿食生冷油腻之品。

4. 饮食积滞

【症状】 脘腹胀满疼痛，拒按，恶食，嗳腐吞酸，或痛而欲泻，泻后痛减，或大便秘结。舌苔腻，脉滑实。

【辨证要点】 腹胀痛，拒按，恶食，嗳腐。

本型多见于急性胃肠炎，不完全性肠梗阻等。

【病机概要】 宿食不化，停滞肠胃，升降失司，运化无权，腑气不行，浊气上逆。

【治法】 消食导滞。

【主方】 保和丸[193]或枳实导滞丸[172]。

【调护要点】 节饮食，勿过饱，少食多餐，或适当禁食。

5. 气滞血瘀

【症状】 以气滞为主者，证见脘腹胀闷或痛，攻窜不定，痛引少腹，得嗳气或矢气则胀痛酌减，遇恼怒则加剧，苔薄，脉弦；以血瘀为主者，则痛势较剧，痛处不移，舌质青紫，脉弦或涩。

【辨证要点】 气滞以胀痛为主，攻窜不定；血瘀以刺痛为主，痛处不移。

本型可见于急性胰腺炎、肠粘连、慢性非特异性溃疡性结肠炎、胃肠神经官能症等。

【病机概要】 肝气不舒，气机郁滞，不通则痛；久痛入络，瘀血阻滞。

【治法】 调气活血。以气滞为主者，宜疏肝理气；以血瘀为主者，宜活血化瘀。

【主方】 柴胡疏肝散[211]、少腹逐瘀汤[57]。

气滞与血瘀，气滞病浅，血瘀病深；先气滞而后血瘀，血瘀又常兼气滞。因此，治疗血瘀常加用理气药物，使气行则血行；治疗气滞亦可加入活血药物，如郁金、延胡索等，使血行气亦行。

【调护要点】 慎饮食，忌暴饮暴食；调情志，戒忧思郁怒。

小结

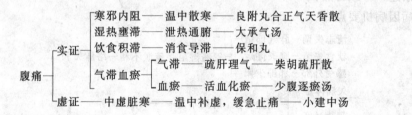

思考题

1. 如何理解腹痛的病因病机？
2. 试述腹痛的辨证要点及类证鉴别。
3. 寒邪内阻、气滞血瘀及中虚脏寒之腹痛的症状、治法及方药是什么？

26 胁痛

概念

胁痛是以一侧或两侧胁肋部疼痛为主要表现的病证，也是临床上常见的一种自觉症状。

胁痛可见于西医学中多种疾病，如急性肝炎、慢性肝炎、肝寄生虫病、肝脓疡、肝硬化、肝癌，以及急性胆囊炎、慢性胆囊炎、胆石症、胆道蛔虫病、肋间神经炎等。凡以胁痛为主要症状表现者，均可参考本病辨证论治。

病因病机

1. 肝气郁结　情志抑郁，或暴怒伤肝，肝失条达，疏泄不利，气阻络痹而致胁痛。
2. 瘀血停着　气郁日久，血流不畅，瘀血停积，胁络痹阻，出现胁痛；或强力负重，胁络受伤，瘀血停留，阻塞胁络，致使胁痛。
3. 肝阴不足　久病或劳欲过度，精血亏损，肝阴不足，血虚不能养肝，使脉络失养，导致胁痛。
4. 肝胆湿热　外邪内侵，或饮食所伤，脾失健运，痰湿中阻，气郁化热，肝胆失其疏泄条达，导致胁痛。

病因病机要点：

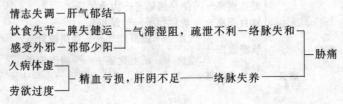

诊断与鉴别

凡以一侧或两侧胁肋疼痛为主要临床表现者，即可诊断为胁痛。

胁痛在临床上应与胸痛、胃痛相鉴别。因为胁痛、胸痛、胃痛均有肝郁气滞证型，由于其病机基本相同，所以，临床表现上有相同之处，诊断时易于混淆，须认真鉴别之。

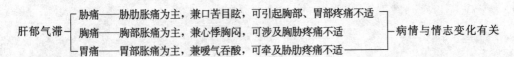

辨证论治

胁痛的辨证，当以气血为主。一般胀痛多属气郁，且疼痛呈游走无定；刺痛多属血瘀，而痛有定所；隐痛多属阴虚，其痛绵绵。至于湿热之胁痛，多表现为疼痛剧烈，且伴有口苦苔黄。

常见证型如下:

1. 肝气郁结

【症状】 胁肋胀痛,或左或右,或两胁均痛,走窜不定,疼痛每因情志变化而增减,胸闷气短;饮食减少,嗳气频作。舌苔薄白,脉弦或弦细。

【辨证要点】 胁肋胀痛,走窜不定,发病与情志因素有关。

本型多见于急、慢性肝炎和急、慢性胆囊炎。

【病机概要】 肝郁气滞,疏泄不利,气阻胁络。

【治法】 疏肝理气。

【主方】 柴胡疏肝散[211]。

可配以制香附、青陈皮、郁金、延胡索、川楝子理气解郁止痛。若气郁较甚,胁痛经久不止,可酌加绿萼梅、丝瓜络、佛手片、白蒺藜、玫瑰花、合欢花等理气解郁;若气郁化火,胁痛如灼,口干而苦,心烦易怒,二便不畅,舌红苔黄,脉弦数,可选用丹栀逍遥散[52]加黄连、郁金清肝解郁。

【调护要点】 调情志,忌郁怒,忌辛辣、油腻。

2. 瘀血停着

【症状】 胁痛经久不已,其痛如刺,部位固定,入夜尤甚,或胁下可扪及癥块。舌质紫暗、苔薄白,脉沉涩。

【辨证要点】 胁肋刺痛,痛有定处,入夜尤甚。

本型可见于慢性肝炎、肝硬化、肝癌。

【病机概要】 气滞血瘀,瘀血停着,痹阻胁络。

【治法】 理气通络,活血化瘀。

【主方】 旋覆花汤[245]。

方中亦可酌加郁金、桃仁、延胡索、当归以增强理气活血之力。若瘀较重者,可用复元活血汤[190]以活血祛瘀,通经活络;若胁肋下有癥块,而正气未衰者,可加三棱、莪术、地鳖虫等以增强破瘀消坚之力。

【调护要点】 注意生活规律,作到起居有节,清心寡欲。饮食以清淡之品为宜。

3. 肝阴不足

【症状】 胁肋隐痛,悠悠不休,遇劳加重,口干咽燥,心中烦热,头晕目眩,精神倦怠。舌红少苔,脉细弦或细数。

【辨证要点】 胁肋隐痛,咽燥心烦,舌红少苔。

本型常见于慢性肝炎、肝硬化。

【病机概要】 精血亏损,肝阴不足,胁络失养。

【治法】 滋阴养血,柔肝和络。

【主方】 一贯煎[1]。

心中烦热可加炒栀子、酸枣仁以清热安神;头晕目眩可加黄精、女贞子、菊花以益肾清肝。

【调护要点】 饮食以新鲜蔬菜水果、豆制品及动物蛋白为主;忌食辛辣厚味及油腻食物。慎房事,戒劳伤。

4. 肝胆湿热

【症状】 胁痛口苦，胸闷纳呆，恶心呕吐，目赤或目黄、身黄、小便黄赤。舌苔黄腻，脉弦滑数。

【辨证要点】 胁痛口苦，目黄、身黄、小便黄赤。苔黄腻，脉滑数。

本型常见于黄疸型病毒性肝炎、急性胆囊炎、胆道蛔虫病等。

【病机概要】 肝胆湿热，疏泄失常，胁络不和。

【治法】 清热利湿。

【主方】 龙胆泻肝汤[64]。

若发热、黄疸者，可加茵陈、黄柏以清热利湿除黄；若胁肋剧痛，呕吐蛔虫者，先以乌梅丸[56]安蛔，继则除蛔；若湿热煎熬，结成砂石，阻滞胆道，症见胁肋剧痛，连及肩背，可加金钱草、海金砂、郁金等，以利胆排石；若热盛伤津，大便秘结，腹部胀满者，可加大黄、芒硝以泄热通便。

【调护要点】 戒劳伤。忌食肥甘辛辣滋腻之品；宜食蔬菜、水果、豆制品等清淡食物。

小结

```
          ┌实证┬─肝气郁结──疏肝理气──柴胡疏肝散
          │    ├─瘀血停着──理气通络，活血化瘀──旋覆花汤
胁痛─┤    └─肝胆湿热──清热利湿──龙胆泻肝汤
          └虚证───肝阴不足──滋阴养血，柔肝和络──一贯煎
```

思考题

1. 试述胁痛的病因病机。
2. 胁痛常见的证候类型有哪些？其辨证要点是什么？
3. 肝气郁结胁痛的临床表现有哪些特点？如何治疗？

27 黄疸

概念

黄疸是以目黄、身黄、小便黄为主要症状的病证。其中以目黄为本病的重要特征。

本病与西医论述的黄疸含义相同,大致涉及西医学中的肝细胞性黄疸、阻塞性黄疸和溶血性黄疸。临床常见的黄疸型病毒性肝炎、黄疸型传染性单核细胞增多症、瘀胆型肝炎、胆囊炎、胆石症、钩端螺旋体病、药物中毒性肝损伤等,凡出现黄疸者,均可参照本病辨证论治。

病因病机

1. 感受外邪　时邪、湿热外袭,郁而不达,内阻中焦,脾胃运化失常,湿热交蒸,不得泄越,熏蒸肝胆,以致肝失疏泄,胆汁外溢,浸渍肌肤,下流膀胱,而使身目小便俱黄。

2. 饮食所伤　饮食不洁,饥饱失常,或嗜酒过度,皆能损伤脾胃,以致运化功能失常,湿浊内生,郁而化热,熏蒸于肝胆,胆汁不循常道,熏染肌肤而发病。

3. 脾胃虚寒　素体脾胃阳虚,或病后脾阳受伤,湿浊内阻,湿从寒化,寒湿郁滞中焦,胆液被阻,溢于肌肤而发黄疸。

4. 积聚转化　积聚日久不消,瘀血阻滞胆道,胆汁外溢而产生黄疸;或黄疸缠绵不愈,湿邪阻滞气机,气滞血瘀,亦可出现多种瘀血症状。

前两种因素,皆因湿从热化,发为阳黄;后两种因素则因湿从寒化,发为阴黄。

病因病机要点:

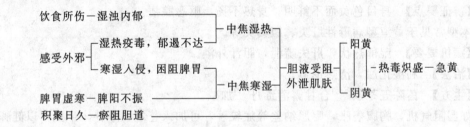

诊断与鉴别

黄疸的诊断依据是:目黄、身黄、小便黄赤。其中以目黄最有诊断价值,因目黄是最早出现而最晚消失的指征。

临床上应注意将黄疸与虚黄进行鉴别。黄疸病机为湿蕴肝脾,胆汁外溢,其主症为目黄、身黄、小便黄;虚黄病机为气血不足,肌肤失养,其主症为面及全身萎黄,双目不黄。

辨证论治

黄疸的辨证,主要是分清阳黄和阴黄。阳黄病程较短,黄色鲜明,属于热证、实证;阴黄病程较长,黄色晦暗,属于寒证、虚证。阳黄和阴黄在一定条件下可相互转化。阳黄失于治疗，迁延日久，脾阳不振，湿从寒化，可转为阴黄；阴黄由于重感外邪，湿热内蒸，胆汁外泄，熏于肌肤，可变为阳黄。而后者的阳黄与前者不同，是虚中挟实，病情比较复杂。

常见证型如下：

阳黄

1. 热重于湿

【症状】 身目俱黄，黄色鲜明，发热口渴。或见心中懊侬，腹部胀满，口干而苦，恶心呕吐，大便秘结，小便短少黄赤。舌苔黄腻，脉弦数。

【辨证要点】 身目俱黄，黄色鲜明，发热口渴。

本型常见于急性黄疸型病毒性肝炎、传染性单核细胞增多症、胆囊炎等。

【病机概要】 湿热蕴蒸，胆汁外溢。

【治法】 清热利湿，解毒散结。

【主方】 茵陈蒿汤[177]。

本方可加茯苓、猪苓、滑石等渗湿之品，以助湿热从小便而去；若腹部胀满，可加郁金、川楝子、青皮疏肝理气；若恶心、呕吐，加橘皮、竹茹以降逆止呕；如心烦懊侬，可加黄连、龙胆草；若兼心烦失眠、衄血者，可酌加赤芍、丹皮凉血止血；若便通热减，舌苔渐化，可加用健脾化湿之品，如白术、茯苓等，并酌减苦寒清热之品，以防脾阳损伤而转为阴黄。

【调护要点】 宜进富有营养的软食或半流质食品；禁食辛热、醇酒及油腻之品。注意卧床休息，保持心情舒畅。

2. 湿重于热

【症状】 身目俱黄，但不鲜明，身热不扬，头重身困，胸脘痞满，食欲减退，渴不多饮，恶心呕吐，腹胀，便稀不爽，小便短黄。舌苔厚腻微黄，脉弦滑或濡缓。

【辨证要点】 身目色黄而不鲜明，身热不扬，呕恶脘痞。

本型常见于黄疸型病毒性肝炎、胆囊炎等。

【病机概要】 湿郁热伏，肝失疏泄，胆汁外溢。

【治法】 利湿化浊，清热退黄。

【主方】 茵陈五苓散[175]合甘露消毒丹[74]加减。

如湿阻气机，胸腹痞胀，呕恶纳差等症较著，可加入苍术、厚朴、半夏，以健脾燥湿，行气和胃。

【调护要点】 节饮食，禁酒类，忌辛热肥甘。

急黄

【症状】 发病急骤，黄疸迅速加深，其色如金，高热烦渴，胁痛腹满，神昏谵语，或见衄血、便血，或肌肤出现瘀斑。舌质红绛，苔黄而燥，脉弦滑数或细数。

【辨证要点】 发病急，进展快，黄疸其色如金，高热烦渴，神昏谵语，可见血证。

本型可见于急性或亚急性重症肝炎。

【病机概要】 热毒入侵，毒性猛烈，熏灼肝胆，胆汁泛溢。

【治法】 清热解毒，凉营开窍。

【主方】 犀角散[274]。

可加生地、丹皮、玄参、石斛等以增强清热凉血之力。如神昏谵语可配服安宫牛黄丸[111]或至宝丹[109]以凉开透窍；如衄血、便血或肌肤瘀斑重者，可加地榆炭、柏叶炭等凉血止血之品；如小便短少不利，或出现腹水者，可加木通、白茅根、车前草、大腹皮等，以清热利尿。

【调护要点】 卧床休息，严密观察病情。宜进流质食物；禁食辛辣、肥腻、油炸之品。

阴黄

【症状】 身目俱黄，黄色晦暗，或如烟熏，纳少脘闷，或见腹胀，大便不实，神疲畏寒，口淡不渴。舌质淡，苔腻，脉濡缓或沉迟。

【辨证要点】 黄色晦暗，脘闷便溏，神疲脉缓。

本型可见于瘀胆型肝炎、慢性黄疸型病毒性肝炎等。

【病机概要】 寒湿内阻，阳气不宣，土壅木郁，胆汁泛溢。

【治法】 健脾和胃，温化寒湿。

【主方】 茵陈术附汤[176]。

可加郁金、厚朴、茯苓、泽泻等行气利湿之品。若兼木郁脾虚，肝脾失调，症见脘腹胀满，胁肋隐痛，不思饮食，肢体困倦，大便时干时溏，脉弦细者，治宜疏肝扶脾，配服逍遥散[222]；若兼胁下癥积胀痛，固定不移，肤色暗黄，舌质暗红，脉弦细，属气血两虚，浊邪瘀阻脉络，可用硝石矾石散[266]，以化浊祛痰软坚；若黄疸日久，气滞血瘀，兼见癥块，胸胁刺痛，拒按，宜服鳖甲煎丸[290]，以活血化瘀；若脾胃虚寒，腹胀纳呆，倦怠乏力者，可配服香砂六君子汤[189]以健脾和胃。

【调护要点】 宜进食富于营养而易于消化的饮食，禁食生冷油腻之品。戒劳伤，忌房事。

小结

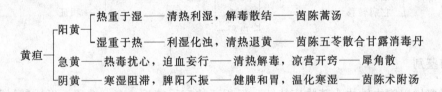

思考题

1. 何谓黄疸？试述其病因病机。
2. 试述阳黄、阴黄、急黄的鉴别。
3. 试述阳黄的主证、治法及代表方剂。

28 积聚

概念

积聚是指腹内结块，或痛或胀的病证。积属有形，结块固定不移，痛有定处，病在血分，是为脏病；聚属无形，包块聚散无常，痛无定处，病在气分，是为腑病。

西医学中的胃神经官能症、肠梗阻、幽门梗阻、肠扭转、肠套叠、肝脾肿大、肝硬化、腹腔肿瘤等病，均可参考本病进行辨证论治。

病因病机

1. 情志失调　情志抑郁，肝气不舒，脏腑失和，气机阻滞，脉络受阻，血行不畅，气滞血瘀，日积月累而成积聚。

2. 饮食内伤　酒食不节，脾失健运，湿浊凝聚成痰；痰与气阻，血行不畅，脉络壅塞。

3. 感受寒湿　寒湿侵袭，脾阳不运，湿痰内聚，气血瘀滞，积块乃成。

4. 它病转移　黄疸病后，或黄疸经久不退，湿邪留恋，气血阻滞；或久疟不愈，湿痰凝滞，脉络痹阻；或感染血吸虫，肝脾不和，气血凝滞；或久泻、久痢之后，脾气虚弱，营血运行涩滞，均可导致积聚的形成。

病因病机要点：

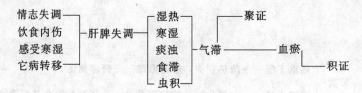

诊断与鉴别

积聚均以腹内结块为其临床特征，但积证的病程较长，有一个逐渐形成的过程，以腹内可扪及大小不同、质地较硬的包块，固定不移，痛有定处为特点，其病较重，较难治；聚证的病程较短，其发作有时、休止不定，以腹中气聚有形，攻窜胀痛，痛无定处，气散则胀痛包块消失为特点，其病较轻，较易治。

积聚应与痞满相鉴别。痞满是脘腹部痞塞胀满，是一种自觉症状，而无块状物可扪及；积聚则是腹内结块，或痛或胀，不仅有自觉症状，而且有结块可扪及。

辨证论治

临床所见积聚之证，虽有积证与聚证之别，但每有先因气滞成聚，久聚血瘀为积者，故临床上多以积聚并称。

常见证型如下：

聚证

1. 肝气郁滞

【症状】 腹中气聚,攻窜胀痛,时聚时散,脘胁胀闷不适。苔薄,脉弦。

【辨证要点】 腹中气聚窜痛,时聚时散。

本型可见于胃神经官能症。

【病机概要】 肝失疏泄,气结成形,或气机逆乱。

【治法】 疏肝解郁,行气消聚。

【主方】 逍遥散[222]。

如气滞较甚者,可加香附、青皮、广木香等疏肝理气之品;如兼瘀象,加延胡索、莪术等;如年老或体虚者,可加党参以顾其本;如寒湿中阻,症见脘腹痞满,食少纳呆,舌苔白腻,脉弦缓者,可用木香顺气散[36]以温中散寒,行气化湿。

【调护要点】 调情志,忌郁怒。

2. 食滞痰阻

【症状】 腹胀或痛,便秘,纳呆,时有如条状物聚起在腹部,重按则胀痛更甚。舌苔腻,脉弦滑。

【辨证要点】 腹部时有条状物聚起,拒按,便秘,纳呆。

本型可见于不完全肠梗阻、肠套叠等。

【病机概要】 食滞肠道,脾运失司,湿痰内生,痰食互阻,气机不畅。

【治法】 导滞通便,理气化痰。

【主方】 六磨汤[47]。

痰湿盛者,可加陈皮、半夏、茯苓以增强化痰和中之力。若痰湿较重,兼有食滞,腑气虽通,苔腻不化者,可用平胃散[70]加山楂、六曲等,以健脾消导,燥湿化痰。聚证虽实证多见,但反复发作,易损伤脾气,可常服香砂六君子汤[189],健脾和中,以扶正气。

【调护要点】 忌食肥甘厚腻及辛辣刺激之品,宜少食、素食。

积证

1. 气滞血阻

【症状】 积块软而不坚,固着不移,胀痛并见,舌苔薄,脉弦。

【辨证要点】 积块软而不移,胀痛并见。

本型可见于肝脾肿大、肠梗阻、肠套叠。

【病机概要】 气滞血阻,脉络不和,积而成块。

【治法】 理气活血,通络消积。

【主方】 金铃子散[162]合失笑散[86]。

若气滞血瘀较甚,兼有寒象者,可用大七气汤[16];若见寒热身痛,舌苔白腻,脉浮弦大者,是兼外感风寒之表证,宜宣表理气,通滞去积,可用五积散[42]。

【调护要点】 调情志,慎起居,避风寒。

2. 瘀血内结

【症状】 腹部积块明显,硬痛不移,面黯消瘦;纳减乏力,时有寒热,女子或见月经不下。舌质紫或有瘀斑瘀点,脉细涩。

【辨证要点】 积块硬痛不移,舌紫暗。

本型常见于肝脾肿大、肝硬化、腹腔肿瘤等。

【病机概要】 积块日久,气血凝结,脉络阻塞。

【治法】 祛瘀软坚,兼调脾胃。

【主方】 膈下逐瘀汤[282]。

可加川楝子、三棱、莪术等以增强祛瘀软坚之力。如积块大而坚硬作痛,可合用鳖甲煎丸[290]以化瘀软坚。

【调护要点】 忌郁怒、戒劳作。

3. 正虚瘀结

【症状】 久病体弱,积块坚硬,疼痛逐渐加剧,面色萎黄或黧黑,消瘦脱形,饮食大减。舌质淡紫无苔,脉细数或弦细。

【辨证要点】 积块坚硬,消瘦脱形,面色萎黄或黧黑。

本型可见于肝硬化、肝癌、胃癌等。

【治法】 大补气血,活血化瘀。

【主方】 八珍汤[13]合化积丸[50]。

若阴伤较甚,头晕目眩,舌光无苔,脉细数者,可加生地、北沙参、枸杞子、石斛等养阴生津;若见牙龈出血、鼻衄,酌加山栀、丹皮、白茅根、茜草、三七等凉血化瘀止血;若阳气虚弱,畏寒肢冷,舌淡白,脉沉细者,加黄芪、附子、肉桂、泽泻等,以温阳益气,利水消肿。

【调护要点】 慎起居,节饮食,调情志,戒劳作。

小结

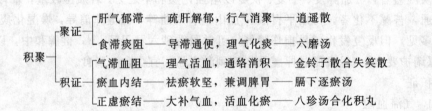

思考题

1. 试述积聚的病因病机要点。
2. 积与聚有什么区别与联系?
3. 试述聚证中肝气郁滞证的主症、病机、治法及方药。

29 臌胀

概念

臌胀是指腹部胀大,绷急如鼓,皮色苍黄,脉络显露为特征的病证。

本病主要见于西医学中的肝硬化腹水。另外,结核性腹膜炎、腹腔肿瘤、慢性缩窄性心包炎、肾病综合征等发生腹水而出现类似臌胀的证候时,亦可参考本病辨证论治。

病因病机

1. 酒食不节 嗜酒过度,或恣食甘肥厚腻,酿湿生热,蕴聚中焦,清浊相混,水谷精微失于输布,湿浊内聚,遂成臌胀。

2. 情志所伤 忧思郁怒,伤及肝脾,肝失疏泄,气机滞涩,日久由气及血,络脉瘀阻。肝失疏泄,克伐脾胃,脾失健运,则水湿内停,气血水壅结而成臌胀。

3. 虫毒感染 虫(血吸虫)毒感染后,未及时治疗,内伤肝脾,脉络瘀塞,气机不畅,升降失常,清浊相混,积渐而成臌胀。

4. 病后续发 凡因它病损伤肝脾,导致肝失疏泄,脾失健运者,均有续发臌胀的可能。如黄疸病久,肝脾俱伤,气血凝滞,脉络瘀阻,渐成臌胀。积聚日久,积块增大,气机壅滞更甚,可引起水湿停聚。

病因病机概要:

酒食不节
情志失调 } 肝脾肾三脏受损
虫毒感染 } 气滞、血瘀、水停 → 臌胀
病后续发

诊断与鉴别

臌胀病以患者腹部臌起胀大为临床主要特征。臌胀初起,以气胀为主,患者虽感腹胀,但按之尚柔软,叩之如鼓,仅在转侧时有振水声。臌胀后期,则腹水显著增多,腹部胀大绷急,按之坚满,并可出现脐心突出,青筋暴露,脉络瘀阻等症状。另外,患者面色多属萎黄,巩膜或见黄染,体表肌肤有红纹赤缕等,可作为诊断的参考。

臌胀应与水肿相鉴别。臌胀以腹胀大为主,四肢肿不甚明显,晚期方伴肢体浮肿,每兼见面色青晦,面颈部有血痣赤缕,胁下癥积坚硬,腹皮青筋暴露;水肿之浮肿多从眼睑开始,继则延及头面及肢体,或下肢先肿,后及全身,每见面色㿠白,腰酸倦怠等,亦可伴见腹水。

辨证论治

臌胀辨证,首当辨别病性虚实。一般来说,热者多实,寒者多虚;脉滑有力者多实,脉浮微细者多虚;气息粗壮者多实,形色憔悴,声音短促者多虚;年青少壮,气血壅滞者多实,中衰积劳,神倦气怯者多虚。

常见证型如下：

1. 气滞湿阻

【症状】 腹胀按之不坚，胁下胀满或疼痛，饮食减少，食后作胀，嗳气不适，小便短少。舌苔白腻，脉弦。

【辨证要点】 腹胀，按之不坚，胁下胀痛，食后胀甚。

本型常见于肝硬化腹水。

【病机概要】 肝郁脾虚，湿阻中焦，浊气充塞。

【治法】 疏肝理气，行湿散满。

【主方】 柴胡疏肝散[211]或胃苓汤[182]。

如胸脘痞闷，腹胀，嗳气为快，偏于气滞者，可酌加佛手、沉香、木香调畅气机；如湿阻中焦，尿少，腹胀，苔腻者，加砂仁、大腹皮、泽泻、车前子以加强健脾利湿作用；若脾阳不振，神倦便溏，舌质淡者，当酌加党参、附片、干姜、川椒以温阳益气，健脾化湿；如兼胁下刺痛，舌紫，脉涩，气滞血瘀者，可加延胡索、莪术、丹参等活血化瘀药。

【调护要点】 保持心情舒畅，尽量减少不良精神刺激。生活起居有节，饮食以清淡为主。

2. 寒湿困脾

【症状】 腹大胀满，按之如囊裹水，甚则颜面微浮，下肢浮肿，脘腹痞胀，得热稍舒，精神困倦，怯寒懒动，尿少便溏。舌苔白腻，脉缓。

【辨证要点】 腹大，按之如囊裹水，怯寒困倦，浮肿，便溏。

本型常见于肝硬化腹水、肾病综合征。

【病机概要】 脾阳不振，寒湿停聚，水蓄不行。

【治法】 温中健脾，行气利水。

【主方】 实脾饮[159]。

如水湿过重，可加肉桂、猪苓、泽泻以助膀胱之气化而利小便；如气虚息短者，可酌加黄芪、党参以补肺脾之气；如胁腹痛胀，可加郁金、青皮、砂仁等以理气宽中。

【调护要点】 忌食生冷肥甘，避寒湿。

3. 湿热蕴结

【症状】 腹大坚满，脘腹撑急，烦热口苦，渴不欲饮，或有面目皮肤发黄，小便赤涩，大便秘结或溏垢。舌边尖红，苔黄腻或兼灰黑，脉弦数。

【辨证要点】 腹大坚满，烦热口苦，面黄溲赤。

本型可见于肝硬化腹水、腹腔肿瘤。

【病机概要】 湿热互结，浊水停聚，气机不利。

【治法】 清热利湿，攻下逐水。

【主方】 中满分消丸[38]合茵陈蒿汤[177]。

如热势较重，常加连翘、龙胆草、半边莲清热解毒；小便赤涩不利者，加陈葫芦、蟋蟀粉（另吞服）行水开窍。若病势突变，骤然大量吐血、下血，病情危急者，可用犀角地黄汤[273]加参三七、仙鹤草、地榆等清热凉血止血。如湿热偏重，蒙蔽心包，神识昏迷，烦躁不安，甚则怒目狂叫，四肢抽搐颤动，便秘尿赤，苔黄，脉数，用安宫牛黄丸[111]或至宝丹[109]清热凉开透窍；如痰浊偏重，静卧嗜睡，语无伦次，昏迷逐渐加深，舌苔厚腻，脉濡细，可用苏合香丸[128]芳香温通开窍。

【调护要点】 卧床休息，宜清淡饮食为主，忌食煎炸、辛辣、坚硬食物。

4．肝脾血瘀

【症状】 腹大坚满，脉络怒张，胁腹刺痛，面色黧黑，面颈胸臂有血痣，呈丝纹状，手掌赤痕，唇色紫褐，口渴，饮水不能下，大便色黑。舌质紫红或有紫斑，脉细涩或芤。

【辨证要点】 腹大坚满，脉络怒张，胁腹刺痛，舌质紫暗。

本型常见于肝硬化腹水，腹腔内肿瘤。

【病机概要】 水湿内停，血脉滞涩，隧道不通。

【治法】 活血化瘀，行气利水。

【主方】 调营饮[219]。

若胁下癥积明显肿大，可选加穿山甲、地鳖虫、水蛭、虻虫、牡蛎等，或配合鳖甲煎丸[290]内服，以化瘀消癥。如病久体虚，气血不足，或攻逐之后，正气受损，宜用八珍汤[13]补养气血；若大便色黑，可加参三七、茜草、侧柏叶等化瘀止血。

【调护要点】 饮食宜清淡，忌食煎炸、辛辣、坚硬食物。

5．脾肾阳虚

【症状】 腹大胀满不舒，早宽暮急，面色苍黄，或呈㿠白，脘闷纳呆，心悸，神疲畏寒，肢冷或下肢浮肿，小便短少不利。舌质胖淡紫，脉沉弦无力。

【辨证要点】 腹大胀满，入暮尤甚，神疲畏寒，腿肿，舌淡。

本型多见于肾病综合征、肝硬化腹水、慢性缩窄性心包炎。

【治法】 温补脾肾，化气行水。

【主方】 附子理中汤[146]合五苓散[41]。

如下肢浮肿，小便短少者，可加入济生肾气丸[184]以滋阴助阳，化气行水。伴腹壁青筋暴露等血瘀兼证者，可稍加赤芍、桃仁、三棱、莪术之类以活血化瘀。

【调护要点】 卧床休息，多应取半卧位。饮食宜清淡，忌肥甘油腻之品。

6．肝肾阴虚

【症状】 腹大坚满，甚则青筋暴露，形体消瘦，面色黧黑，唇紫，口燥，心烦，齿鼻时有衄血，小便短赤。舌质红绛少津，脉弦细数。

【辨证要点】 腹大坚满，青筋暴露，口燥心烦，齿鼻衄血，舌绛少津。

本型常见于肝硬化腹水，结核性腹膜炎腹水，腹腔肿瘤。

【病机概要】 肝肾阴虚，气机郁滞，水湿内停，血行不畅。

【治法】 滋养肝肾，凉血化瘀。

【主方】 一贯煎[1]合膈下逐瘀汤[282]。

若内热口干，舌绛少津，可加玄参、石斛；若兼有潮热，加银柴胡、地骨皮；小便少者，加猪苓、滑石；齿鼻衄血，加仙鹤草、茅根之类；若见神志昏迷，急用紫雪丹[267]或安宫牛黄丸[111]以凉营清热开窍。

【调护要点】 宜进清淡、富有营养且易于消化之食物；调畅情志，戒房劳，避外感之邪。

小结

$$\left.\begin{array}{l}\text{酒食不节}\\\text{情志失调}\\\text{虫毒感染}\\\text{病后续发}\end{array}\right\}臌胀\begin{cases}\text{气滞湿阻——疏肝理气，行湿散满——柴胡疏肝散、胃苓汤}\\\text{寒湿困脾——温中健脾，行气利水——实脾饮}\\\text{湿热蕴结——清热利湿，攻下逐水——中满分消丸，茵陈蒿汤}\\\text{肝脾血瘀——活血化瘀，化气利水——调营饮}\\\text{脾肾阳虚——温补脾肾，化气行水——附子理中汤、五苓散}\\\text{肝肾阴虚——滋养肝肾，凉血化瘀——一贯煎、膈下逐瘀汤}\end{cases}$$

思考题

1. 什么叫臌胀？
2. 试述臌胀发病的主要病机和主要证型。
3. 试述臌胀寒湿困脾、湿热蕴结、肝肾阴虚型的主症、治法和常用方剂。

30 血证

概念

　　血证是指血不循经或自九窍排出体外，或渗溢于肌肤的一类出血性病证。在内科范围内，常见的有鼻衄、齿衄、咳血、吐血、便血、尿血、紫斑等血证。

　　西医学中多种急、慢性疾病所引起的出血，如再生障碍性贫血、急性白血病、血小板减少性紫癜、肺结核、支气管扩张、肺炎、支气管肺癌、消化性溃疡、胃癌、门脉性肝硬化、肾小球肾炎、肾结核、肾肿瘤、慢性非特异性溃疡性结肠炎等所引起的出血性疾病，均可参考本病进行辨证论治。

病因病机

　　1. 感受外邪　外感风邪，肺有燥热，风热相搏，肺失清肃，肺络受伤，以致咳血、衄血。
　　2. 饮食失节　饮酒过多或过食辛燥之品，以致燥热蕴积于胃肠，化火灼伤血络而外溢，形成吐血、衄血、便血。
　　3. 情志过极　情志过极则火动于内，气逆于上，迫血妄行而成血证。如郁怒伤肝，肝气横逆犯胃，胃络损伤而引起吐血；肝气郁结，肝火犯肺，血随火升则导致衄血、咳血。
　　4. 劳倦过度　劳倦过度导致心、脾、肾的损伤，若伤气则致气不摄血，伤精则致阴虚火旺，进而引起出血。
　　5. 热病或久病之后　热病或久病使阴津伤耗，以致阴虚火旺；或使正气亏耗，气虚不摄；或为血络瘀阻，血不循经而导致出血。

诊断与鉴别

　　血证是以血液不循常道，或上溢于口鼻诸窍（如鼻衄、咳血、吐血），或下泄于前后二阴（如尿血，便血），或渗出于肌肤（如紫斑）为特征。

　　临床上，应注意咳血、咯血与吐血的鉴别。血随咳嗽而出为咳血，血自肺来；一咯就出为咯血；血随呕吐而出为吐血，血由胃出。若咳血量多，亦可咯而即出，而咳嗽症状不显著。但咳血多混有痰液，血色鲜红，呈泡沫状；咯血多为小血块或盈口，可随痰咯出。吐血可混有食物残渣，血色紫暗或暗红，或成块，几乎均伴便血。

　　血便须注意远血与近血的鉴别。远血其位在胃、小肠，血与粪便相混，血色如黑漆色或黯紫色。近血来自乙状结肠、直肠、肛门，血便分开，或便外裹血，色多鲜红。

　　尿中有血，分为尿血与血淋两种。排尿不痛者为尿血；尿血兼小便滴沥涩痛者为血淋。本节仅讨论尿血，血淋在淋证中论述。

辨证论治

　　血证辨证，首先应辨清出血的部位及脏腑病位，其次应辨清证候的虚实，分清实热、阴虚和气虚的不同。一般来说，实热证病势急，病程短，血色鲜紫深红，质浓稠，血涌量多，体质多壮实，兼见一般实热症状；阴虚证病势缓，病程长，血色鲜红或淡红，时作时止,血量一般不多,形体偏瘦,兼见一般阴虚内热症状;气虚证病多久延不愈,血色暗淡,质稀,出血量少,亦可暴急量多,体质虚弱,伴一般阳气亏虚症状。

对血证的治疗,可归纳为治火、治气、治血三原则。治火,即实火当清热泻火,虚火当滋阴降火;治气,即实证当清气降气,虚证当补气益气;治血,即凉血止血,收敛止血,活血止血之法。

下面分述各种血证的辨证治疗:

鼻衄

1. 热邪犯肺

【症状】 鼻燥衄血,口干咽痛,或兼有身热,咳嗽痰少。舌质红苔薄,脉数。

【辨证要点】 鼻衄,口干鼻燥,身热。

本型常见于感染性、发作性疾病的鼻出血。

【病机概要】 肺内积热,耗伤肺阴,血热妄行。

【治法】 清泄肺热,凉血止血。

【主方】 桑菊饮[227]。

可加丹皮、茅根、旱莲草、侧柏叶凉血止血。肺热盛而无表证者,去薄荷、桔梗,加黄芩、栀子清泄肺热;阴伤较甚,口、鼻、咽干燥显著者,加玄参、麦冬、生地养阴润肺。

【调护要点】 注意气候变化,避免感受外邪。忌食辛辣煎炸之品。

2. 胃热炽盛

【症状】 鼻衄,或兼齿衄,血色鲜红,口渴欲饮,鼻燥,口干臭秽,烦躁,便秘。舌红苔黄,脉数。

【辨证要点】 鼻衄,色红量多,口渴,便秘。舌红苔黄,脉数。

本型常见于发热性疾病的鼻出血、原发性血小板减少性紫癜。

【病机概要】 胃火上炎,迫血妄行。

【治法】 清胃泻火,凉血止血。

【主方】 玉女煎[59]。

可加茅根、大蓟、小蓟、藕节之类凉血止血。热势甚者,加山栀、丹皮、黄芩清热泻火;大便秘结加生大黄通腑泻热;阴伤较甚,口渴,舌红苔少,脉细数者,加天花粉、石斛、玉竹养胃生津。

【调护要点】 忌烟、酒及辛辣动火之物。

3. 肝火上炎

【症状】 鼻衄,头痛,目眩,耳鸣,烦躁易怒,两目红赤,口苦。舌红,脉弦数。

【辨证要点】 鼻衄,头痛,目赤,口苦。

本型可见于高血压病、发热性疾病。

【病机概要】 气郁化火,肝火上炎,迫血妄行。

【治法】 清肝泻火,凉血止血。

【主方】 龙胆泻肝汤[64]。

可加白茅根、蒲黄、大蓟、小蓟、藕节等凉血止血。若阴液亏耗,口鼻干燥,舌红少津,脉细数者,可去车前草、泽泻、当归,酌加玄参、麦冬、女贞子、旱莲草养阴清热。

【调护要点】 调情志,忌恼怒,忌食辛燥之品。

4. 气血亏损

【症状】 鼻衄,或兼齿衄,肌衄,神疲乏力,面色㿠白,头晕,耳鸣,心悸,夜寐不宁。舌质淡，脉细无力。

【辨证要点】 鼻衄，面色㿠白，头晕，心悸，神疲。

本型常见于再生障碍性贫血、白血病。

【病机概要】 气血亏虚，气虚不能摄血，血溢脉外。

【治法】 补气摄血。

【主方】 归脾汤[95]。

可加仙鹤草、阿胶、茜草等加强其止血作用。

【调护要点】 宜进食富含营养之食品，戒劳伤。

齿衄

1. 胃火炽盛

【症状】 齿衄血色鲜红，齿龈红肿疼痛，头痛，口臭，便秘，舌红苔黄，脉洪数。

【辨证要点】 齿衄血色鲜红，齿龈疼痛，口臭，便秘。

本型多见于血小板减少性紫癜、再生障碍性贫血。

【病机概要】 胃火上熏，灼伤脉络。

【治法】 清胃泻火，凉血止血。

【主方】 加味清胃散[99]合泻心汤[153]。

可酌加白茅根、大蓟、藕节以凉血止血。

【调护要点】 忌烟、酒及辛辣香燥之品。

2. 阴虚火旺

【症状】 齿衄，血色淡红，常因受热及烦劳而诱发，齿摇不坚。舌红苔少，脉细数。

【辨证要点】 齿衄，齿摇不坚，舌红苔少。

本型常见于血小板减少性紫癜、再生障碍性贫血。

【病机概要】 肝肾阴虚，相火上浮，热迫血行。

【治法】 滋阴降火，凉血止血。

【主方】 滋水清肝饮[271]合茜根散[178]。

虚火较甚而见低热，手足心热者，加地骨皮、白薇、知母清退虚热。

【调护要点】 忌烟、酒及辛辣动火之物。

咳血

1. 燥热伤肺

【症状】 喉痒咳嗽，痰中带血，口干鼻燥，或有身热。舌红少津，苔薄黄，脉数。

【辨证要点】 喉痒咳嗽，痰中带血。

本型可见于急性气管——支气管炎、细菌性肺炎等。

【病机概要】 风热燥邪，损伤于肺，肺失清肃，肺络受损。

【治法】 清热润肺，宁络止血。

【主方】 桑杏汤[226]。

可加白茅根、茜草根等凉血止血；津伤较甚者，可酌加玄参、麦冬等养阴润燥。

【调护要点】 避免劳倦过度。饮食应营养丰富，易于消化。忌食辛燥之品。

2. 肝火犯肺

【症状】 咳嗽阵作，痰中带血或纯血鲜红，胸胁胀痛，烦躁易怒，口苦。舌质红，苔薄黄，脉弦数。

【辨证要点】 咳嗽，痰中带血，胸胁胀痛。

本型多见于支气管扩张、肺结核。

【病机概要】 肝火上炎，肺失清肃，肺络受损。

【治法】 清肝泻肺，凉血止血。

【主方】 泻白散[154]合黛蛤散[287]。

可酌加生地、旱莲草、茅根、大小蓟等凉血止血。肝火较甚，头晕目赤，心烦易怒者，加丹皮、栀子、黄芩清肝泻火；若咳血量较多，纯血鲜红，可用犀角地黄汤[273]加三七粉冲服，以清热泻火，凉血止血。

【调护要点】 调情志，忌恼怒，忌烟、酒及辛辣动火之物。

3. 阴虚肺热

【症状】 咳嗽痰少，痰中带血或反复咳血，血色鲜红，口干咽燥，颧红，潮热盗汗。舌红苔少，脉细数。

【辨证要点】 咳嗽咽干，痰中带血，潮热盗汗。

本型常见于肺结核、肺癌。

【病机概要】 阴虚肺热，肺失清肃，火热灼肺，损伤肺络。

【治法】 滋阴润肺，宁络止血。

【主方】 百合固金丸[103]。

可加白及、藕节、白茅根、茜草等止血，反复咳血及咳血量多者，加阿胶、三七养血止血；潮热、颧红者，加青蒿、鳖甲、地骨皮、白薇等清退虚热；盗汗加糯稻根、浮小麦、五味子、牡蛎等收敛固涩。

【调护要点】 忌食辛辣，忌烟酒。

吐血

1. 胃热壅盛

【症状】 脘腹胀闷，甚则作痛，吐血色红或紫黯，常夹有食物残渣，口臭，便秘或大便色黑。舌红苔黄腻，脉滑数。

【辨证要点】 吐血色红，脘腹胀闷，口臭，便秘。脉滑数。

本型常见于急慢性胃炎、消化性溃疡。

【病机概要】 胃中积热，热伤胃络，胃失和降。

【治法】 清胃泻火，化瘀止血。

【主方】 泻心汤[153]合十灰散[5]。

胃气上逆而致恶心呕吐者，加代赭石、竹茹、旋覆花和胃降逆。

【调护要点】 忌暴饮暴食，忌食辛辣及烟酒。

2. 肝火犯胃

【症状】 吐血色红或紫黯，口苦胁痛，心烦易怒，寐少梦多。舌质红绛，脉弦数。

【辨证要点】 吐血色红，口苦，胁痛。

本型常见于急慢性胃炎、消化性溃疡。

【病机概要】 肝火上炎，横逆犯胃，胃络损伤。

【治法】 泻肝清胃，凉血止血。

【主方】 龙胆泻肝汤[64]。

可酌加白茅根、藕节、旱莲草,茜草凉血止血。

【调护要点】 保持精神愉快,忌食难于消化以及辛辣动火的食品。

3. 气虚血溢

【症状】 吐血缠绵不止,时轻时重,血色暗淡,神疲乏力,心悸气短,面色苍白。舌质淡,脉细弱。

【辨证要点】 吐血缠绵不止,心悸气短,神疲,脉虚。

本型常见于胃、十二指肠球部溃疡出血。

【病机概要】 中气亏虚,统血无能,血液外溢。

【治法】 健脾养心,益气摄血。

【主方】 归脾汤[95]。

可酌加仙鹤草、白及、乌贼骨、炮姜炭等温经固涩止血。

【调护要点】 忌食烟酒及辛辣动火之品,并重视精神和生活起居的调养,宜食富含营养又不油腻的食品。

便血

1. 肠道湿热

【症状】 便血鲜红,大便不畅或稀溏,或有腹痛,口苦。苔黄腻,脉濡数。

【辨证要点】 便血鲜红,口苦,苔黄腻。

本型常见于慢性非特异性溃疡性结肠炎。

【病机概要】 湿热蕴结,肠道脉络受损,传化失常,气机阻滞。

【治法】 清化湿热,凉血止血。

【主方】 地榆散[105]。

【调护要点】 忌烟、酒,忌食辛辣肥甘。

2. 脾胃虚寒

【症状】 便血紫黯或呈黑便,神疲,便溏,舌淡。

本型常见于慢性非特异性溃疡性结肠炎、胃、十二指肠球部溃疡。

【病机概要】 脾胃虚寒,中气不足,统血无力,血溢肠胃。

【治法】 健脾温中,养血止血。

【主方】 黄土汤[230]。

可加白及、乌贼骨收敛止血,三七、花蕊石活血止血。阳虚较甚,畏寒肢冷者,加鹿角霜、炮姜、艾叶等温阳止血。

【调护要点】 调起居,避风寒,忌食生冷,戒过劳。

尿血

1. 下焦热盛

【症状】 小便黄赤灼热,尿血鲜红,心烦口渴,面赤口疮,夜寐不安。舌红,脉数。

【辨证要点】 小便黄赤灼热带血,血色鲜红。

本型可见于急性肾小球肾炎、肾结核、肾肿瘤。

【病机概要】 热迫下焦,脉络受损,血渗膀胱。

【治法】 清热,泻火,凉血止血。

【主方】 小蓟饮子[31]。

【调护要点】 忌食辛辣厚味。

2. 肾虚火旺

【症状】 小便短赤带血，头晕耳鸣，颧红潮热，腰膝酸软。舌红，脉细数。

【辨证要点】 小便短赤带血，耳鸣潮热，腰膝酸软。

本型常见于肾结核、肾肿瘤。

【病机概要】 肾阴亏虚，虚火内炽，灼伤脉络。

【治法】 滋阴降火，凉血止血。

【主方】 知柏地黄丸[160]。

可加旱莲草、大小蓟、藕节、蒲黄凉血止血。

【调护要点】 调起居，戒房劳，忌烟酒及辛辣之品。

3. 脾不统血

【症状】 久病尿血，面色不华，体倦乏力，气短声低，或兼齿衄、肌衄。舌质淡，脉细弱。

【辨证要点】 久病尿血，面色不华，气短乏力，舌淡，脉弱。

本型可见于血液病等所出现的血尿。

【病机概要】 脾气亏损，统血无力，血不循经。

【治法】 补脾摄血。

【主方】 归脾汤[95]。

【调护要点】 宜食富含营养食品，但忌油腻和过食，以免腻胃、伤胃。

4. 肾气不固

【症状】 久病尿血，色淡红，头晕耳鸣，精神困惫，腰脊酸痛。舌质淡，脉沉弱。

【辨证要点】 久病尿血，血色淡红，耳鸣，腰酸。

本型可见于肾肿瘤、肾结核等。

【病机概要】 肾气不固，封藏失职，血随尿出。

【治法】 补益肾气，固摄止血。

【主方】 无比山药丸[34]。

【调护要点】 节制房事。忌食烟酒及辛辣刺激之品。

紫斑

1. 血热妄行

【症状】 皮肤出现青紫斑点或斑块，或伴有鼻衄，齿衄，便血，尿血，或有发热，口渴，便秘。舌红，苔黄，脉弦数。

【辨证要点】 皮肤见青紫斑点或斑块，发热，口渴，便秘。舌红苔黄，脉数。

本型常见于血小板减少性紫癜、再生障碍性贫血、急性白血病等。

【病机概要】 热壅脉络，迫血妄行。

【治法】 清热解毒，凉血止血。

【主方】 犀角地黄汤[273]。

热毒炽盛，发热，出血广泛者，加生石膏、龙胆草、紫草，冲服紫雪丹[267]。

【调护要点】 避免劳累，注意冷暖变化，预防感受外邪。饮食应富于营养，易于消化。忌食辛辣，忌烟酒。

2. 阴虚火旺

【症状】 皮肤青紫斑点或斑块时发时止，常伴鼻衄、齿衄或月经过多，颧红，心烦，口渴，手足心热，或有潮热、盗汗。舌质红、苔少，脉细数。

【辨证要点】 皮肤瘀斑、瘀点，色红或紫红，潮热，盗汗。舌红苔少。

本型常见于血小板减少性紫癜、过敏性紫癜、再生障碍性贫血。

【病机概要】 阴虚火旺，虚火伤络，血溢肌腠。

【治法】 滋阴降火，宁络止血。

【主方】 茜根散[178]。

阴虚较甚者，可酌加玄参、龟板、旱莲草等养阴清热。

【调护要点】 饮食应富于营养，易于消化，避免辛辣动火之物以及鱼、虾、蟹、牛乳等腥味之品。

3. 气不摄血

【症状】 久病不愈，反复发生肌衄，神疲乏力，头晕目眩，面色苍白或萎黄，食欲不振。舌质淡，脉细弱。

【辨证要点】 皮肤紫斑色暗淡，反复发作，过劳则甚。

本型常见于血小板减少性紫癜、慢性再生障碍性贫血。

【病机概要】 气血亏耗，气不摄血，血溢肌腠。

【治法】 补气摄血。

【主方】 归脾汤[95]。

可酌情选加仙鹤草、棕榈炭、地榆、蒲黄、茜草根、紫草，以增强止血及化瘀消斑的作用。若兼肾气不足而见腰膝酸软者，可加山茱萸、菟丝子、续断补肾益气。

【调护要点】 增强身体素质，避免感受外邪，忌食烟酒及辛辣动火之品。宜食富含营养，易于消化之品。忌过劳。

小结

- 血证
  - 鼻衄
    - 热邪犯肺—清泄肺热，凉血止血—桑菊饮
    - 胃热炽盛—清胃泻火，凉血止血—玉女煎
    - 肝火上炎—清肝泻火，凉血止血—龙胆泻肝汤
    - 气血亏损—补气摄血—归脾汤
  - 齿衄
    - 胃火炽盛—清胃泻火，凉血止血—加味清胃散合泻心汤
    - 阴虚火旺—滋阴降火，凉血止血—滋水清肝饮合茜根散
  - 咳血
    - 燥热伤肺—清热润肺，宁络止血—桑杏汤
    - 肝火犯肺—清肝泻肺，凉血止血—泻白散合黛蛤散
    - 阴虚肺热—滋阴润肺，宁络止血—百合固金汤
  - 吐血
    - 胃热壅盛—清胃泻火，化瘀止血—泻心汤合十灰散
    - 肝火犯胃—泻肝清胃，凉血止血—龙胆泻肝汤
    - 气虚血溢—健脾养心，益气摄血—归脾汤
  - 便血
    - 肠道湿热—清化湿热，凉血止血—地榆散
    - 脾胃虚寒—健脾温中，养血止血—黄土汤
  - 尿血
    - 下焦热盛—清热泻火，凉血止血—小蓟饮子
    - 肾虚火旺—滋阴降火，凉血止血—知柏地黄丸
    - 脾不统血—补脾摄血—归脾汤
    - 肾气不固—补益肾气，固摄止血—无比山药丸
  - 紫斑
    - 血热妄行—清热解毒，凉血止血—犀角地黄汤
    - 阴虚火旺—滋阴降火，宁络止血—茜根散
    - 气不摄血—补气摄血—归脾汤

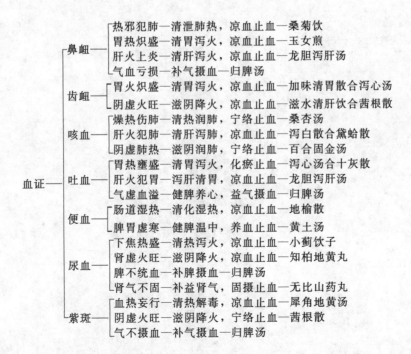

思考题

1. 什么叫血证？临床常见的血证有哪些？
2. 治疗血证的基本治则有哪些？
3. 咳血和吐血如何区别？各自有哪些常见证型？其辨证要点及治法、主方各是什么？

31 水肿

概念

水肿是指体内水液潴留、泛溢肌肤，引起眼睑、头面、四肢甚至全身浮肿的一类病证。水肿重证可伴见胸水、腹水。

西医学中的急、慢性肾炎和肾病综合征、心源性水肿、特发性水肿、经前期紧张综合征、粘液性水肿及营养障碍所致的水肿，均可参考本病辨证论治。

病因病机

水肿是全身脏腑功能低下或紊乱、气化失常的一种临床表现。当主要责之于肺、脾、肾及三焦气化不利，病本在肾。

1. 风邪外袭，肺失通调　肺为水之上源，主宣发肃降，肺为邪舍则宣降不利，水道不通，风水相搏，泛溢肌腠。

2. 湿毒浸渍，脾气受困　疮痈肿毒或湿邪内合于脾，脾之运化功能不利，水液代谢失常，水邪泛溢肌肤。

3. 湿热内蕴，三焦壅滞　湿热久郁化热，弥漫三焦，壅遏气机，水邪不化，水道不通，泛溢周身，发为水肿。

4. 肾气虚损，阳微水泛　多种原因导致肾精亏耗，肾气内伐，阳气衰微，不能启动脾肺化气行水，膀胱开合失司，水邪内停，泛为水肿。

病因病机概要：

风邪外袭——肺失宣降，水道不通　┐
湿毒内侵——脾气受困，运化失职　├—水邪内聚，泛溢肌肤→水肿
湿热壅盛——三焦气化失司，气滞水停　│
劳伤虚损——肾元虚耗，阳微水泛　┘

诊断与鉴别

水肿病证，以肌肤水肿为诊断依据。水肿病须与饮证、臌胀鉴别。

病名 鉴别	水 肿	臌 胀	饮 证
病因病机	肺、脾、肾水液代谢障碍	肝、脾、肾三脏功能失调	肺、脾、肾气化功能失调
病证特点	多有肾病史，面色㿠白。以头面、四肢肌肤松弛处水肿明显。仅在病重时方出现胸水或腹水。腹皮无青筋暴露	一般有肝病史，面色青晦，以腹水为主，水多在腹腔，四肢一般不肿，严重时，下肢呈轻度水肿。腹皮青筋暴露	水饮多停于体内局部

辨证论治

水肿辨证，需以阴阳为纲，辨明表里、寒热、虚实；同时尤需注意病机的转化，标本缓急。常见证型如下：

阳水

1. 风水泛滥

【症状】 眼睑浮肿为首见，继之四肢及周身悉肿，来势迅速，伴见发热恶寒，肢节酸楚，小便不利，或见咳喘咽痛。舌质偏红或偏白，脉浮滑或沉紧。

【辨证要点】 眼睑浮肿，迅即全身皆肿，伴有风寒或风热表证。

本型常见于急性肾炎初期。

【病机概要】 风邪袭肺，肺失宣肃，水道不通，水邪泛溢。

【治法】 散风清热，宣肺行水。

【主方】 越婢加术汤[262]。

偏于风热者，可酌加宣肺清热之茅根、连翘、板蓝根等；偏于风寒者，加苏叶、防风、桂枝，酌减石膏；若汗出恶风，属卫阳虚，可用防己黄芪汤[122]补肺卫利水湿。

【调护要点】 饮食宜清淡，避风寒，戒劳作。

2. 湿毒侵淫

【症状】 眼睑浮肿，延及周身，小便不利，肌肤疮痍、甚则溃烂，伴见恶风发热。舌红苔薄黄，脉浮滑数。

【辨证要点】 眼睑先肿，延及周身，风热表证，身发疮痍，脉浮滑数。

本证可见于急性肾炎。

【病机概要】 湿毒郁滞肺卫，内传脏腑，脾肺气机不利，湿毒化热，水湿泛溢。

【治法】 宣肺解毒，利湿消肿。

【主方】 麻黄连翘赤小豆汤[243]。

湿毒内蕴热盛者，可酌加银花、公英、板蓝根、紫花地丁；若脓溃糜烂者，加苦参、土茯苓，若血热红肿甚者，加丹皮、赤芍药、大黄。

【调护要点】 忌辛辣煎炙。慎起居。

3. 水湿浸渍

【症状】 周身水肿，按之没指，身体困重，小便短少，胸闷泛恶，食欲不振。苔白腻，脉沉缓。起病缓慢，病势迁延。

【辨证要点】 周身水肿，按之没指，病程长，身困重，泛恶胸闷。

本型可见于慢性肾炎、肾病综合征、右心功能衰竭、营养不良性水肿。

【病机概要】 水湿内聚，脾阳被困，脾失健运，水湿不化，溢于肌肤。

【治法】 健脾化湿，通阳利水。

【主方】 胃苓汤[182]合五皮饮[40]。

肿甚而喘者，加麻黄、葶苈子、杏仁宣肺利水以平喘。

【调护要点】 宜食易消化、高营养、低盐食物。

4. 湿热壅盛

【症状】 遍身浮肿，皮肤绷紧光亮，脘痞烦渴，溲赤便秘。苔黄腻，脉滑数或沉数。

【辨证要点】 周身浮肿,皮肤绷紧而光亮,脘闷烦热,溲赤便秘,苔黄腻。

本型可见于急性肾炎。

【治法】 分利湿热。

【主方】 疏凿饮子[275]。

肿势较重者,可用五苓散[41];兼见喘逆者,酌用葶苈大枣泻肺汤[261];湿热久郁伤及阴津,热象较重者,可选用猪苓汤[257];腹满便秘严重者,可用己椒苈黄丸[24]。

【调护要点】 清淡低盐饮食,忌烟酒辛辣。

阴水

1. 脾阳虚衰

【症状】 身肿,腰以下为甚,按之凹陷难复,脘闷腹胀,食少便溏,面色萎黄,神疲肢冷,尿少。舌淡,苔白腻,脉沉缓。

【辨证要点】 指凹性水肿,腰以下为甚,神疲肢冷,食少便溏,脉沉缓。

本型常见于慢性肾炎、肾病综合征、心源性水肿、营养不良性水肿、粘液性水肿后期。

【病机概要】 脾阳虚衰,运化失司,阳不化气,水邪泛溢。

【治法】 温运脾阳,利水除湿。

【主方】 实脾饮[159]。

若气虚症状明显者,酌加人参、黄芪温中益脾;尿少肿甚者,酌加桂枝、泽泻,以助膀胱化气行水。

【调护要点】 慎避风寒,宜低盐高营养饮食。

2. 肾气衰微

【症状】 头面全身浮肿,腰下尤甚,按之凹陷不起,心悸气促,腰酸重冷痛,少尿或多尿,神疲肢冷,面色㿠白或灰滞。舌淡胖,苔白,脉沉迟细弱。

【辨证要点】 全身指凹性水肿,腰以下为甚,腰酸重冷痛,神疲肢冷,脉沉迟细弱。

本型常见于慢性肾炎及肾病、心源性水肿、营养不良性水肿、粘液性水肿后期。

【治法】 温肾助阳,化气行水。

【主方】 济生肾气丸[184]合真武汤[199]。

若尿清长量多,去泽泻、车前子加桑螵蛸、补骨脂;若心悸、口唇紫绀,重用附子,加桂枝、丹参、干姜温阳化瘀;若气喘气促,酌加蛤蚧、五味子或黑锡丹[268]吞服;若神倦、泛恶、口中有尿味,加附子、黄连、大黄。

【调护要点】 低盐饮食;慎避风寒,加强调护。

小结

水肿为临床常见病证。水肿辨证须紧密结合脏腑(肾、脾、肺)功能的变化,明辨阴阳,分清标本,注意虚实寒热转化;水肿一证的治疗大法,常用宣肺发汗、健脾温肾、化瘀降浊、利尿逐水等多种,临证须准确辨证,严谨论治。

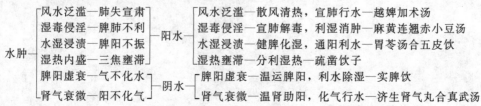

思考题

1. 简述水肿病因病机。
2. 怎样鉴别水肿与臌胀？
3. 简述阳水各型的症状、辨证要点及治法、主方。

32 淋证

概念

淋证是指小便频数短涩，滴沥刺痛，欲出未尽，小腹拘急，或痛引腰腹的病证。

西医学中的泌尿系感染、泌尿系结石、泌尿系结核、前列腺炎、乳糜尿、泌尿系肿瘤见上述症状者，可参考本病辨证论治。

病因病机

1. **膀胱湿热**　多食辛辣肥甘之品，或嗜酒太过，酿成湿热，下注膀胱，发而为淋。若小便灼热刺痛者，为热淋；若湿热蕴积，尿液受其煎熬，日积月累，尿中杂质结为砂石，则为石淋；若湿热蕴结于下，以致气化不利，无以分清泌浊，脂液随小便而去，小便如脂如膏，则为膏淋；若热盛伤络，迫血妄行，小便涩痛有血，则为血淋。

2. **脾肾两虚**　久淋不愈，湿热耗伤正气，或年老久病体弱，劳累过度，房室不节，均可导致脾肾亏虚。脾虚则中气下陷，肾虚则下元不固，因而小便淋漓不已。如遇劳即发者，则为劳淋；中气不足，气虚下陷者，则为气淋；肾气亏虚，下元不固，不能制约而脂液下泄，尿液浑浊，则为膏淋；肾阴亏虚，虚火灼络，尿中夹血，则为血淋。

3. **肝郁气滞**　大怒伤肝，气滞不畅，气郁化火，郁于下焦，影响膀胱气化，则少腹作胀，小便艰涩而痛，余沥不尽，而发为气淋。此属气淋的实证，中气下陷所致气淋，是为气淋的虚证。

诊断与鉴别

淋证与其他病证的鉴别：

1. **癃闭**　癃闭以排尿困难、小便量少，甚则点滴全无为特征。排尿困难与淋证相似，但淋证尿频而痛，癃闭无尿痛。

2. **尿血**　血淋和尿血都以小便出血、尿色红赤、甚至溺出纯血为共有症状，其鉴别要点是有无尿痛。一般以痛者为血淋，不痛者为尿血。

3. **尿浊**　淋证的小便浑浊需与尿浊相鉴别，尿浊排尿时无疼痛滞涩感，与淋证不同。

辨证论治

1. **热淋**

【症状】　小便短数，灼热刺痛，溺色黄赤，少腹拘急胀痛，或有寒热、口苦、呕恶，或腰痛拒按，或大便秘结。苔黄腻，脉濡数。

【辨证要点】　小便短数，灼热刺痛，溲赤便秘，苔黄腻。

本证常见于尿道炎、膀胱炎、肾盂肾炎等泌尿系感染，以及膀胱结核、肾结核。

【病机概要】　湿热蕴结，壅于下焦，膀胱气化失司。

【治法】　清热利湿通淋。

【主方】 八正散[12]。

若大便秘结腹胀者，可重用生大黄，并加用枳实，以通腑泄热；若伴见寒热、口苦、呕恶者，可合小柴胡汤[30]以和解少阳；若湿热伤阴者，可去大黄，加生地、知母、白茅根以养阴清热。

【调护要点】 忌食辛辣肥甘，宜清淡饮食，多饮水。

2. 石淋

【症状】 尿中时夹砂石，小便艰涩，或排尿时突然中断，尿道窘迫疼痛，少腹拘急，或腰腹绞痛难忍，尿中带血，舌红，苔薄黄，脉弦或带数。若病久砂石不去，可伴见面色不华，精神萎靡，少气乏力，舌淡有齿痕，脉细而弱；或腰腹隐痛，手足心热，舌红少苔，脉细数。

【辨证要点】 排尿时突然中断，尿道疼痛，少腹拘急，或尿中带血。

本证常见于泌尿系结石。

【病机概要】 嗜食肥甘辛辣之品，致湿热壅于下焦，煎熬尿液，结为砂石，阻塞尿路，损伤脉络。

【治法】 清热利湿，通淋排石。

【主方】 石韦散[63]。

腰腹绞痛者，可加芍药、甘草以缓急止痛；如尿中带血，可加小蓟、生地、藕节以凉血止血；如兼发热，可加蒲公英、黄柏、大黄，以清热泻火；如石淋日久，证见虚实夹杂，当标本兼顾；气血亏虚者，宜二神散[4]合八珍汤[13]；阴液耗伤者，宜六味地黄丸[46]合石韦散[63]。

【调护要点】 宜食清素，忌食辛辣肥甘之品。

3. 气淋

【症状】

实证 小便涩滞，淋沥不爽，少腹满痛。苔薄白，脉沉弦。

虚证 少腹坠胀，尿有余沥，面色㿠白。舌质淡，脉虚细无力。

【辨证要点】 实证为小便涩滞，少腹满痛，脉弦；虚证为少腹坠胀，尿有余沥，脉虚。

本证常见于泌尿系结核、膀胱肿瘤、前列腺炎等。

【治法】 实证宜利气疏导；虚证宜补中益气。

【主方】 实证用沉香散[137]加味。

胸闷胁胀者，可加青皮、乌药、小茴香以疏通肝气；日久气滞血瘀者，可加红花、赤芍、牛膝以活血行瘀。

虚证用补中益气汤[140]。

兼血虚肾亏者，可用八珍汤[13]倍茯苓加杜仲、枸杞子、怀牛膝，以益气养血，脾肾双补。

【调护要点】 调情志，忌郁怒，慎起居，戒劳作。

4. 血淋

【症状】

实证 小便热涩刺痛，尿色深红，或挟有血块，疼痛满急加剧，或见心烦。苔黄，脉滑数。

虚证　尿色淡红，尿痛涩滞不显著，腰酸膝软，神疲乏力。舌淡红，脉细数。

【辨证要点】　实证尿血红紫，虚证淡红；实证刺痛满急，虚证则不明显。

本证常见于急性肾盂肾炎、膀胱炎、尿路感染、尿路结石、泌尿系结核及泌尿系良性或恶性肿瘤等。

【病机概要】　湿热聚于膀胱，热伤血络，血从下溢；或病延日久，肾阴不足，虚火灼络，络伤血溢。

【治法】　实证宜清热通淋，凉血止血；虚证宜滋阴清热，补虚止血。

【主方】　实证用小蓟饮子[31]合导赤散[120]；虚证用知柏地黄丸[160]以滋阴清热，并可加旱莲草、阿胶、小蓟等，以补虚止血。

【调护要点】　宜食甘凉清淡之品，忌食辛辣煎炸和肥甘厚味。

5. 膏淋

【症状】

实证　小便混浊如米泔水，置之沉淀如絮状，上有浮油如脂，或夹有凝块，或混有血液，尿道热涩疼痛。舌红，苔黄腻，脉濡数。

虚证　病久不已，反复发作，淋出如脂，涩痛反见减轻，形体消瘦，头昏无力，腰酸膝软。舌淡，苔腻，脉细弱无力。

【辨证要点】　实证小便混浊如米泔水，尿道涩痛；虚证久病反复，淋出如脂，尿道痛减。

本型常见于班氏丝虫病及结核感染、肿瘤引起的乳糜尿。

【病机概要】　湿热下注，气化不利，或肾虚下元不固，不能制约脂液，脂液下泄。

【治法】　实证宜清热利湿，分清泄浊；虚证宜补虚固涩。

【主方】　实证用程氏萆薢分清饮[272]加减；虚证用膏淋汤[281]。

若脾肾两虚，中气下陷，肾失固涩者，可用补中益气汤[140]合七味都气丸[8]，益气升陷，滋肾固涩。

【调护要点】　实证忌食辛辣肥甘；虚证宜食富含营养而易于消化的食物。

6. 劳淋

【症状】　小便不甚赤涩，但淋沥不已，时作时止，遇劳即发，腰酸膝软，神疲乏力。舌质淡，脉虚弱。

【辨证要点】　小便淋沥不已，遇劳即发。

本证可见于慢性肾盂肾炎、慢性前列腺炎等。

【病机概要】　劳伤过度，脾肾俱虚，湿浊留恋不去。

【治法】　健脾益肾。

【主方】　无比山药丸[34]加减。

如脾虚气陷，少腹坠胀，小便点滴而出，可配合补中益气汤[140]以益气升陷；如肾阴亏虚，面色潮红，五心烦热，可配合知柏地黄丸[160]以滋阴降火。

【调护要点】　宜食富含营养且不油腻、易消化的食品。慎房劳。

小结

淋证是指小便频数短涩，滴沥刺痛，欲出未尽，小腹拘急，或痛引腰腹的病证。

淋证分为热淋、石淋、血淋、气淋、膏淋、劳淋六种。在辨证时，除要辨明不同淋证的特征外，还要审察证候的虚实。各种淋证之间，彼此又有一定的关系，表现在转归上，一是虚实的相互转化，二是各种淋证之间的相互转化。认识并把握这种转化，对临床有实际指导意义。

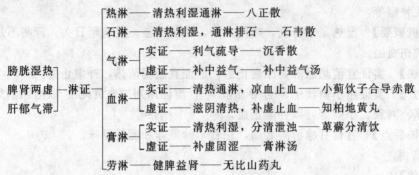

思考题

1. 如何区分血淋和尿血？
2. 如何辨别六种淋证？
3. 简述热淋、石淋的主证、治法和主方。

33 癃闭

概念

癃闭是指以小便量少,点滴而出,甚则小便闭塞不通为主症的一种疾病。其中又以小便不利,点滴而短少,病势较缓者称为"癃";以小便闭塞,点滴不通,病势较急者称为"闭"。

本病包括西医学中泌尿系梗阻之排尿困难和肾功能不全之少尿无尿等。

病因病机

癃闭的病位在膀胱,但与三焦、肺、脾、肾、肝均有着密切的关系,分述如下:

1. 湿热蕴积　膀胱湿热阻滞或肾热移于膀胱形成的湿热互结,均可以影响膀胱的气化,形成癃闭。

2. 肺热壅盛　肺为水之上源,热壅上焦,津液不布,致水道通调不利;又因热从上焦而下移于膀胱,则上、下焦均为热气所壅而成癃闭。

3. 脾气不升　脾主运化转输,若脾气亏虚,则升清降浊失常,而成癃闭。

4. 肝气郁滞　七情内伤,引起肝郁气滞,气机不调,致使水道的通调受阻,形成癃闭。

5. 尿道阻塞　瘀血凝聚,或尿路结石,停留不去阻塞于尿道膀胱之间,也可形成癃闭。

6. 肾气不充　肾阳不足,命门火衰,致膀胱气化不利,而成癃闭。

诊断与鉴别

癃闭与淋证的鉴别

病名 鉴别	癃　闭	淋　证
尿痛症状	无	滴沥刺痛
尿　量	少尿或无尿	小便频数短涩,但小便总量基本正常
排尿困难	有	有

辨证论治

癃闭的辨证,应先分清虚实。实证多病急,溲赤灼热,脉弦数;虚证多病缓,排溺无力,脉弱。

癃闭的治疗,应根据"腑以通为用"的原则,着眼于通。但是,引起癃闭的原因各有不同,临床必须审因论治,不可滥用通利小便之品。现分述如下:

1. 膀胱湿热

【症状】 小便不通或尿量极少、短赤灼热，小腹胀满，或大便不畅，口苦口粘。舌质红，苔黄腻，脉数。

【辨证要点】 尿闭或尿量极少、短赤灼热，舌红苔黄腻。

【病机概要】 素嗜醇酒或恣食肥甘，脾胃湿热蕴结，下注膀胱，气化不利。

【治法】 清利湿热，通利小便。

【主方】 八正散[12]加减。

热盛伤阴，口干舌红少津者，加生地、麦冬；心烦者加黄连、竹叶等。

【调护要点】 饮食宜清淡，忌食辛辣肥甘。

2. 肺热壅盛

【症状】 小便不通，或点滴不爽，咽干，烦渴欲饮，呼吸急促。舌苔薄黄，脉数。

【辨证要点】 小便不爽或闭而不通，气促烦渴，脉数。

【病机概要】 肺热气壅，失于肃降，不能通调水道，下输膀胱。

【治法】 清肺热，利水道。

【主方】 清肺饮[249]加减。

若热盛伤阴者，可酌加黄连、沙参、芦根等。

【调护要点】 忌食辛辣油腻，宜食清淡之品。

3. 肝郁气滞

【症状】 情志抑郁，多烦易怒，小便不通，或通而不爽，胁腹胀满。舌红，苔薄黄，脉弦。

【辨证要点】 小便不通或通而不爽，同时伴有情志抑郁，胸胁胀满。

【病机概要】 七情内伤，肝郁气滞，水液排泄受阻。

【治法】 疏肝理气，通利小便。

【主方】 沉香散[137]加减。

可酌加香附、郁金、青皮以增强理气作用；若气郁化火，加丹皮、山栀以清热解郁。

【调护要点】 忌忧思郁怒；忌辛辣助火食物。

4. 尿道阻塞

【症状】 小便点滴而下，或尿如细线，或阻塞不通，小腹胀满疼痛。舌色紫暗，或有瘀点，脉涩。

【辨证要点】 小便不通，或点滴而下，或尿如细线，小腹胀痛。

【病机概要】 瘀血败精或肿块结石，阻塞尿路，瘀阻气机。

【治法】 行瘀散结，通利水道。

【主方】 代抵当丸[87]加减。

5. 中气不足

【症状】 小腹坠胀，时欲小便而不得出，或量少而不畅，精神疲乏，纳差，气短。舌淡，苔薄，脉细弱。

【辨证要点】 时欲小便而不得出，小腹坠胀，纳差神疲。

【病机概要】 脾气虚弱，中气下陷，清气不升，浊阴不降。

【治法】 升清降浊，化气利水。

【主方】 补中益气汤[140]合春泽汤[171]。

【调护要点】 慎起居，戒劳作。调饮食，进补而不腻之品。

6. 肾阳衰惫

【症状】 小便不通或滴沥不畅，排出无力，面色㿠白，神气怯弱，畏寒，腰以下冷，膝软无力。舌质淡，苔白，脉沉细。

【辨证要点】 小便不通或排出无力，腰膝酸冷，脉沉细。

【病机概要】 肾阳不足，命门火衰，膀胱气化无力。

【治法】 温阳益气，补肾利尿。

【主方】 济生肾气丸[184]。

若阳虚甚者，酌加仙茅、淫羊藿等。

【调护要点】 应常食富于营养温补之品；节房事。

小结

癃闭的病位是在膀胱，但和三焦、肺、脾、肾、肝均有着密切的关系。引起癃闭的病因病机有湿热蕴结，肺热气壅，肝气郁滞，尿路阻塞，中气不足，肾元亏虚。癃闭的辨证首先应分清虚实，然后再权衡轻重缓急，进行辨证论治。

```
湿热蕴结 ┐                   ┌ 膀胱湿热—清利湿热，通利小便—八正散
肺热壅盛 │                   │ 肺热壅盛—清肺热，利水道—清肺饮
肝气郁滞 ├─膀胱气化不利—癃闭─┤ 肝郁气滞—疏肝理气，通利小便—沉香散
尿道阻塞 │                   │ 尿道阻塞—行瘀散结，通利水道—代抵当丸
脾气不升 │                   │ 中气不足—升清降浊，化气利水—补中益气汤合春泽汤
肾元亏虚 ┘                   └ 肾阳衰惫—温阳益气，补肾利尿—济生肾气丸
```

思考题

1. 如何区分癃闭与淋证？
2. 试述膀胱湿热、尿道阻塞、肾阳衰惫型癃闭的主证、治法及主方。

34 腰痛

概念

腰痛是指以腰部疼痛为主要症状的一类病证，可表现为腰部的一侧或两侧。因腰为肾之府，故腰痛与肾的关系最为密切。

西医学中的风湿病、强直性脊柱炎、腰肌劳损、急性腰部扭伤、腰椎间盘突出、腰椎骨质增生、腰椎结核和肿瘤、以及肾脏疾病、盆腔疾患等以腰痛为主症者，可参考本病辨证论治。

病因病机

1. 感受寒湿　坐卧湿地，或居处寒冷潮湿，或涉水冒雨，寒湿侵袭，以致经络阻滞，气血运行不畅，发为腰痛。

2. 湿热伤络　外感湿热，或湿热内蕴，或寒湿郁久化热，湿热蕴蒸，阻遏经脉，伤及腰府，发为腰痛。

3. 肾精亏损　平素过劳，或久病体弱，或年老精血亏虚，或房劳过度，以致肾精亏损，不能濡养经脉而发生腰痛；或肾气困惫，督脉不畅，也可引起腰痛。

4. 气滞血瘀　劳伤久病，或跌打外伤，气滞血凝，瘀血凝阻，脉络不和而发生腰痛。

诊断与鉴别

腰痛既是一种独立的疾病，又是多种疾病过程中的主要见症。因此，腰痛诊断易，而详细鉴别其病因病机、尤其是追究其原发疾病，则为不易。临证需谨守病机，治病求本。

辨证论治

腰痛辨证，首先要分辨标本缓急，虚实寒热。感受外邪所致者，其证多属表、属实，发病骤急，应根据寒湿、湿热的不同，祛邪通络，分别论治。由于肾精亏损所致者，其证多属里、属虚，常见慢性反复发作，治宜补肾益气。客邪久羁，损伤肾气，易成实中夹虚证；肾气久亏，卫阳不足，新感淫邪，则又常形成虚中夹实证，当细审邪正主次轻重，标本兼顾。气滞血瘀者，证多实中夹虚，治当活血行瘀，理气通络为主，善后还须调摄肾气，巩固疗效。

1. 寒湿腰痛

【症状】　腰部冷痛重着，转侧不利，逐渐加重，静卧痛不减，遇阴雨天加重。苔白腻，脉沉而迟缓。

【辨证要点】　腰部冷痛重着，阴雨天加重。

本证常见于风湿性腰痛、强直性脊柱炎、腰椎骨质增生等。

【病机概要】　寒湿之邪，侵袭腰部，痹阻经络。

【治法】　散寒利湿，温通经络。

【主方】 甘姜苓术汤[72]。

临证应用,可加桂枝、牛膝以温经通络,或加杜仲、寄生、续断以兼补肾壮腰;若腰痛左右不定,牵引两足,或连肩背,或关节游痛,是兼有风邪,宜独活寄生汤[195]加减,以祛风活络,补益肝肾。

【调护要点】 避风寒,宜热敷。

2. 湿热腰痛

【症状】 腰部胀痛,痛处有热感,热天或雨天加重,小便短赤。苔黄腻,脉濡数或弦数。

【辨证要点】 腰痛有热感,遇热加重,苔黄腻,脉数。

本型可见于肾盂肾炎、慢性盆腔炎等。

【病机概要】 湿热壅阻,经气不通。

【治法】 清热利湿,舒筋止痛。

【主方】 四妙丸[76]加减。

临证应用可酌加木瓜、络石藤,以加强舒筋通络止痛之功;若舌质红、口渴、小便短赤,脉弦数,则是热象偏重,可酌加栀子、泽泻、木通以助清利湿热。

【调护要点】 慎起居,避湿热,忌食辛辣肥甘等。

3. 瘀血腰痛

【症状】 腰痛如刺,痛有定处,痛处拒按,日轻夜重,轻者俯仰不便,重者不能转侧,常有外伤史。舌质紫暗或有瘀斑,脉涩。

【辨证要点】 腰痛如刺,痛处不移,舌质紫暗。

本证常见于腰椎肿瘤、急性腰扭挫伤、腰椎间盘突出症、腰肌劳损等。

【病机概要】 气滞血瘀,经脉阻塞。

【治法】 活血化瘀,理气止痛。

【主方】 身痛逐瘀汤[145]加减。

如外伤所致者,可加大黄,吞服三七粉;尿血者,加白茅根、丹皮、大小蓟。

【调护要点】 戒负重劳作。

4. 肾虚腰痛

【症状】 腰痛酸软,喜得揉按,腿膝无力,遇劳更甚,卧则减轻。偏阳虚者,则少腹拘急,面色㿠白,手足不温,舌淡,脉沉细;偏阴虚者,则心烦失眠,口燥咽干,面色潮红,手足心热,舌红少苔,脉细数。

【辨证要点】 腰酸膝软,遇劳更甚。偏阳虚兼有手足不温,脉沉细;偏阴虚兼有咽干失眠,舌红少苔。

本证常见于腰椎结核、肾脏疾病、慢性盆腔炎等。

【病机概要】 腰为肾府,肾气(精)亏虚,腰脊失养。

【治法】 偏肾阳虚者宜补肾助阳;偏肾阴虚者宜益肾滋阴。

【主方】 偏阳虚者以右归丸[68]为主;偏阴虚者以左归丸[65]为主。

如腰痛日久不愈,并无阳虚或阴虚症状者,可服用青娥丸[147]补肾以治腰痛。

【调护要点】 慎起居,节房事;宜食补而不腻之品。

小结

腰痛以肾虚为本，感受外邪、或跌打闪挫等为标。因此，临床上对寒湿、湿热及瘀血腰痛也常加用补肾强腰之品，以达到扶正祛邪的目的。

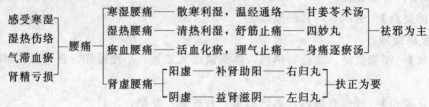

思考题

1. 临床上如何区分寒湿与湿热腰痛？
2. 肾虚腰痛的病因病机、辨证要点和治法、主方是什么？

35 消渴

概念

消渴是以多饮、多食、多尿、身体消瘦,或尿浊、尿有甜味为特征的病证。

西医学中的糖尿病、尿崩症、甲状腺功能亢进、精神性烦渴,可参考本病辨证论治。

病因病机

1. 饮食不节　长期过食肥甘、醇酒厚味,致脾胃运化失职,积热内蕴,化燥耗津,发为消渴。

2. 情志失调　长期精神刺激,导致气机郁结,进而化火,消烁肺胃阴津而发为消渴。

3. 劳欲过度　素体阴虚,房室不节,劳欲过度,损耗阴精,导致阴虚火旺,上蒸肺胃而发为消渴。

诊断与鉴别

本病以多饮、多食、多尿、形体消瘦为特征,需与某些疾病相鉴别:

1. 上消与温病伤津之烦渴多饮相鉴别:二者均有烦渴多饮症状,但后者有外感温热病史,并见卫气营血传变过程,而无上消常伴的多食多尿症状。

2. 中消与瘿病之善饥消瘦相鉴别:中消食量倍增,消谷善饥;瘿病饮量及饥饿情况不如中消严重。中消多伴上下消症状;瘿病常有颈前下部肿大,多伴指抖、多汗、目突等症状。

3. 下消与劳淋、尿浊相鉴别:下消为尿量多或兼浑;劳淋则尿频色清;尿浊为尿浑色白。劳淋与尿浊尿量均无明显增多,且其尿均无甜味。

辨证论治

本病虽有上、中、下三消之分,肺燥、胃热、肾虚之别,而临床上三多症状往往同时存在。治疗上,无论上、中、下三消均应立足于滋肾养阴,燥热较甚时可佐以清热,下消病久,阴损及阳者宜阴阳双补。

1. 上消　肺热津伤

【症状】　烦渴多饮,口干舌燥,尿频量多。舌边尖红,苔薄黄,脉洪数。

【辨证要点】　烦渴多饮,多尿。

本证常见于精神性烦渴、糖尿病、尿崩症等。

【病机概要】　肺热炽盛,肺阴耗伤,不能敷布。

【治法】　清热润肺,生津止渴。

【主方】　消渴方[216]加味。

如苔黄燥,烦渴引饮,脉洪大,为肺胃热炽,耗损气阴之候,可用白虎加人参汤[89]以清泄肺胃,生津止渴。

【调护要点】 忌辛辣烟酒动火之品，宜食清润生津、易于消化的食物。

2. 中消　胃热炽盛

【症状】 多食易饥，形体消瘦，大便干燥。苔黄，脉滑实有力。

【辨证要点】 多食善饥，形体消瘦，脉滑实。

本证常见于糖尿病、甲状腺功能亢进等。

【病机概要】 胃火炽盛，消谷烁津。

【治法】 清胃泻火，养阴增液。

【主方】 玉女煎[59]加黄连、栀子。

如大便秘结不行，可用增液承气汤[284]润燥通腑，待大便通后，再转用主方治疗。

【调护要点】 忌食肥甘醇酒厚味，节制谷麦食量；宜食苦瓜、冬瓜等蔬菜、豆类。

3. 下消

(1) 肾阴亏虚

【症状】 尿频量多，混浊如脂膏，或尿甜，口干唇燥，五心烦热。舌红苔少，脉沉细数。

【辨证要点】 尿频量多，混如脂膏，五心烦热，舌红苔少。

【病机概要】 肾阴亏耗，虚火内灼，肾失固摄，精微下注。

【治法】 滋阴固肾。

【主方】 六味地黄丸[46]。

若气阴两虚，伴见困倦、气短、舌淡红者，宜酌加党参、黄芪等益气之品。

【调护要点】 戒房劳。忌辛辣炙燥，宜食清淡滋阴，易消化之品。

(2) 阴阳两虚

【症状】 小便频数，混浊如膏，甚则饮一溲一，面色黧黑，耳轮焦干，腰膝酸软，形寒肢冷，阳痿不举。舌淡苔白，脉沉细无力。

【辨证要点】 小便频数，混浊如膏，腰酸形寒，脉沉细。

本证常见于尿崩症、糖尿病等。

【病机概要】 气阴被耗，下元虚惫，约束无权。

【治法】 温阳滋肾固摄。

【主方】 金匮肾气丸[163]。

如阴阳气血俱虚，可用鹿茸丸[239]。以上两方均可酌加覆盆子、桑螵蛸、金樱子等，以补肾固摄。

【调护要点】 节房事，慎起居。饮食宜补而不腻，忌食肥甘辛辣之品。猪胰、山药、茭白等对治疗有利，可常食。

小结

消渴是以多饮、多食、多尿，消瘦为特征的病症。饮食不节、情志失调、劳欲过度为其主要病因。其病机特点是阴虚为本，燥热为标；气阴两伤，阴阳俱虚；阴虚燥热，变证百出。此外，阴虚燥热，阴阳两虚等皆可致血行不畅，故消渴发病常与血瘀有关。因此，在治疗上，除滋阴治本，清热治标外，还应细察瘀血之征，酌加丹参、山楂、桃仁、红花等活血化瘀药，并在生活饮食上注意调理，以提高疗效。

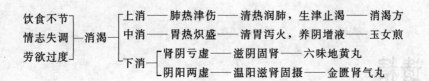

思考题

1. 消渴的病因病机特点是什么？
2. 消渴常分哪些证型辨证治疗？其辨证要点、病机概要和主方各是什么？
3. 消渴与瘀血在病因病机上有何关系？

36 遗精

概念

遗精是指不因性生活而精液遗泄的病证。若成年未婚男子，或婚后夫妻分居者，一个月遗精1~2次，则属于正常生理现象。

西医学中的神经官能症、慢性前列腺炎、精囊炎、后尿道炎、附睾炎以及某些慢性疾病出现的病理性遗精，可参考本病辨证论治。

病因病机

1. 心火亢盛，心肾不交　劳神太过或情志失调，则心阴暗耗，心阳独亢，心神不宁，淫梦泄精；心火偏亢，久伤肾水，水不济火，精室被扰，应梦而泄。

2. 湿热下注，热扰精室　由于醇酒厚味，损伤脾胃，湿浊内生，蕴而生热，湿热流注于下，扰动精室，使精液自遗。

3. 劳伤心脾，气不摄精　积劳损气，中气不足，心脾气虚者，每因劳伤太过或思虑太过，气虚更甚，清阳下陷，气不摄精而遗泄。

4. 肾虚精脱，精关不固　年少早婚，或恣情纵欲，或因手淫或因先天不足，秉赋素亏，肾虚精脱，精关不固。肾阴虚则阳亢，虚火扰动精室而梦遗；肾阳虚则精关不固而自遗。

病因病机概要：

```
劳神太过——心火亢盛，心肾不交——扰动精室 ┐
饮食不节——损伤脾胃，湿热内生——扰动精室 │
思虑劳倦——中气不足，心脾气虚——气不摄精 ├遗精
先天不足或房室不节——肾虚不藏——精关不固 ┘
```

诊断与鉴别

遗精常分梦遗、滑精二类。前者指夜有淫梦，精随梦泄；后者则不必有梦而遗精，其甚者精关不固，过力活动，或见闻感触，也会滑泄出精。此外，遗精还应与早泄相鉴别：早泄为性交时间过短，或一触即泄，或有性行为，未曾交合而精液排出，随之阴茎萎软，不能进行正常性交者。与不因性交而精液自动溢出的遗精、滑精不同。

辨证论治

遗精有梦遗、滑精之分。梦遗有虚有实，初起多因心火、肝郁、湿热、火热之邪，下扰精室，精气失位，应梦而泄，久遗则多致肾虚；滑精则多由梦遗发展而来，或秉赋素虚，或房劳、手淫而致，以虚证为多。

常见证型如下：

1. 君相火动，心肾不交。

【症状】 少寐多梦，梦中遗精，伴有心中烦热、心悸，头晕目眩，精神不振，体倦乏力，口干，小便短赤。舌红，脉细数。

【辨证要点】 少寐多梦，梦中遗精，心悸烦热，脉细数。

本型常见于神经官能症。

【病机概要】 心火内动，耗伤心血，火扰精室，精液走泄。

【治法】 清心安神，滋阴清热。

【主方】 黄连清心饮[232]。

若久遗伤肾、阴虚火旺者，可用知柏地黄丸[160]或大补阴丸[18]以滋阴泻火。

【调护要点】 调摄心神，排除杂念；适当运动；忌食辛辣醇酒。

2. 湿热下注，扰动精室。

【症状】 遗精频作，或尿时有少量精液外流，小便热赤浑浊或不爽，心烦，口苦，口舌生疮，大便溏臭、粘腻不爽，脘腹痞闷。苔黄腻，脉濡数。

【辨证要点】 遗精频作，小便热赤浑浊，大便溏臭不爽，苔黄腻。

本型常见于前列腺炎、精囊炎、后尿道炎等。

【病机概要】 湿浊流注于下，蕴而生热，扰动精室。

【治法】 清热利湿。

【主方】 程氏萆薢分清饮[272]或猪肚丸[256]。若脾湿下注，可用苍术二陈汤[126]加黄柏、柴胡、升麻。

【调护要点】 调情志；忌辛辣烟酒肥甘。

3. 劳伤心脾，气不摄精

【症状】 劳则遗精，心悸怔忡，失眠健忘，面色萎黄，肢体困倦，食少便溏。舌淡苔薄，脉弱。

【辨证要点】 劳则遗精，心悸怔忡，食少便溏，舌淡，脉弱。

本型常见于神经官能症。

【病机概要】 心脾气血不足，过劳更伤中气，气虚则神浮不摄而遗精。

【治法】 调补心脾，益气摄精。

【主方】 妙香散[132]或补中益气汤[140]。

若证属思虑伤脾致心脾两虚者，须重用补益心脾、益气升清药物，而不可清降收涩；若气虚阳浮导致心火不宁，需养气补血以宁潜心神，不可清心降火。临床可酌用归脾汤[95]、六味地黄丸[46]等，加减化裁。

【调护要点】 调摄心神，劳逸结合；宜食黄芪粥、莲子粥、扁豆粥等补而不腻之品；节房事。

4. 肾虚滑脱，精关不固。

【症状】 遗精频作，甚至滑精，腰膝酸软，眩晕耳鸣，咽干心烦，失眠健忘，低热颧红，形瘦，盗汗，发落齿摇。舌红少苔，脉细数。

若久病，可兼见形寒肢冷，阳痿早泄，尿少浮肿，溲色清白，或余沥不尽，面色㿠白。舌淡嫩有齿痕，脉沉细。

【辨证要点】 遗精频作、或滑精，腰膝酸软，神疲健忘。

本型常见于神经官能症，慢性前列腺炎及某些慢性疾病而出现遗精者。

【病机概要】 肾精失藏，阴损及阳，精关不固。

【治则】 补益肾精，固涩止遗。

【主方】 肾阴不足者用六味地黄丸[46]或左归丸[65]；阴损及阳者用右归丸[68]。

若肾失封藏，遗精严重者，需合用金锁固精丸[164]、水陆二仙丹[58]等；若心肾不交导致肾虚滑脱，还需酌加用桑螵蛸散[228]、斑龙丸[258]等交通心肾，宁神固精。

【调护要点】 饮食宜营养丰富，平素可食用核桃肉、五味子、鲜贝、甲鱼等滋阴壮阳之品。慎起居，调情志，节房事。

小结

遗精病多因情志失调、饮食不节、房劳过度等引起。其病与五脏均相关联，但其中与心肾关系最为密切。病始时心火亢盛、心肾不交，虚实夹杂者多见，治以清心安神、滋阴清热为先；久则肾精耗伤，转为虚证，病以肾虚不藏、精关不固者为多，治以补肾固精。若因湿热下注，影响疏泄，气虚下陷而致病者，多因脾胃功能失调，属虚实相兼，当立清热利湿、益气健脾之法。总的法则是：上则清心安神，中则调其脾胃、升举阳气，下则益肾固精。

```
君相火动，心肾不交 ┐       ┌ 心肾不交——治以清心安神，主方黄连清心饮
湿热下注，扰动精室 │       │ 湿热下注——治以清热利湿，主方萆薢分清饮
                    ├ 遗精 ┤
劳伤心脾，气不摄精 │       │ 劳伤心脾——治以调补心脾，主方妙香散或补中益气汤
肾虚滑脱，精关不固 ┘       └ 肾虚滑脱——治以补肾固精，主方六味地黄丸、左归丸、右归丸
```

思考题

1. 试述遗精的病因病机。
2. 何谓遗精、滑精、梦遗？
3. 遗精分几个证候类型？其辨证要点、治法、主方是什么？

37 痹证

概念

痹证是指风、寒、湿、热等外邪侵袭人体，闭阻经络，使气血运行不畅所导致的以肌肉、筋骨、关节发生酸痛、麻木、重着、屈伸不利、甚至关节肿大灼热等为主要临床表现的病证。

西医学中的风湿性关节炎、类风湿性关节炎、痛风、肩关节周围炎、骨性关节炎等，都可以参考本病辨证论治。

病因病机

1. 风寒湿邪，侵袭人体　　由于气候变化无常，冷热交错，或居处潮湿，涉水冒雨等原因，以致风寒湿邪侵袭人体，留着于经络、关节，使气血痹阻而为痹证。感邪偏盛不同，临床表现也就有所差别。

2. 感受热邪，或郁久化热　　感受风热之邪，与湿相并，致风湿热合邪为害。或素体阳盛或阴虚有热，感受外邪易从热化；或风寒湿痹，郁久化热，都可以形成风湿热痹。

病因病机要点：

```
内因——素体虚弱,正气不足,卫外不固 ┐
                                  ├ 肌肉、关节、经络痹阻 —— 痹证
外因——感受风、寒、湿、热之邪       ┘
```

诊断与鉴别

痹证是由于感受风、寒、湿、热等外邪所致，以肌肉、关节，筋骨等处的酸痛、麻木，甚或关节肿大灼热为主要特征。

本病与痿证的病变部位都在肢体、关节。应予鉴别：

鉴别\病名	痹　证	痿　证
临床特点	筋骨、肌肉、关节酸痛、重着、屈伸不利	肢体痿弱不用，肌肉瘦削
肢体关节疼痛	有	无

辨证论治

对于痹证的辨证，首先应辨清风寒湿痹与热痹的不同。热痹以关节红肿灼热疼痛为特点；风寒湿痹则虽有关节酸痛，但无局部红肿灼热。

```
        ┌ 关节红肿灼热疼痛 —— 热痹
        │ 关节酸痛游走不定 —— 行痹
痹证 ───┤
        │ 痛有定处，疼痛剧烈 —— 痛痹
        └ 肢体酸痛重着，肌肤不仁 —— 着痹
```

常见证型如下：

风寒湿痹

1. 行痹

【症状】 肢体关节酸痛，游走不定，关节屈伸不利，或见恶风发热。苔薄白，脉浮。

【辨证要点】 关节酸痛，游走不定。

本型常见于风湿性关节炎。

【病机概要】 风寒湿邪留滞经络，风邪偏盛，善行而数变，阻痹气血。

【治法】 祛风通络，散风除湿。

【主方】 防风汤[123]。

若酸痛以肩肘上肢关节为主者，加羌活、姜黄、白芷、川芎，以祛风通络止痛；若酸痛以膝踝等下肢关节为主者，加牛膝、防己、木瓜通经活络，祛湿止痛；若酸痛以腰膝为主者，加杜仲、桑寄生、续断、巴戟天、淫羊藿以温补肾气，强腰壮筋；若见关节肿大，苔薄黄，邪有化热之象者，宜寒热并施，用桂枝芍药知母汤[203]。

【调护要点】 避风寒，切勿汗出当风；饮食宜温热。

2. 痛痹

【症状】 肢体关节疼痛较剧，痛有定处，得热痛减，遇寒痛增，关节不可屈伸，痛处皮色不红，触之不热。苔薄白，脉弦紧。

【辨证要点】 关节疼痛较剧，痛有定处，遇寒痛增。

本型常见于类风湿性关节炎、肩关节周围炎初期。

【病机概要】 风寒湿邪内侵，寒邪偏盛，寒为阴邪，其性凝滞，闭阻经络。

【治法】 温经散寒，祛风除湿。

【主方】 乌头汤[53]。

痛剧者，酌加附子、干姜、桂枝、细辛等，散寒止痛；病久寒凝多兼血瘀，宜加制乳香、没药、蜈蚣、炒山甲、鸡血藤等，以活血通络止痛。

【调护要点】 注意防寒保暖；饮食宜温热。

3. 着痹

【症状】 肢体关节重着，酸痛，痛有定处，手足沉重，活动不便，或有肌肤麻木不仁，关节肿胀。苔白腻，脉濡缓。

【辨证要点】 肢体关节酸痛重着，肌肤不仁，苔白腻。

本型可见于类风湿性关节炎、肩关节周围炎、骨性关节炎等。

【病机概要】 风寒湿邪留滞经络、肌肉、关节，湿邪偏盛，湿性重浊粘滞，经络不畅。

【治法】 除湿通络，祛风散寒。

【主方】 薏苡仁汤[285]。

若肌肤不仁，症状较重，加海桐皮、豨莶草祛风通络；关节肿胀者，加草薢、木通、姜黄利水通络。

【调护要点】 避免居处湿冷；忌食生冷肥甘。

风湿热痹

【症状】 关节疼痛，局部灼热红肿，痛不可触，得热益甚，得冷稍舒，可病及一个或多个关节，多兼有发热恶风，汗出心烦，口渴思冷饮等症。舌苔黄燥，脉滑数。

【辨证要点】 关节红肿灼热疼痛，得热益甚，脉滑数。

本型常见于风湿性关节炎、痛风等。

【病机概要】 邪热壅郁经络、关节，气血郁滞不通。

【治法】 清热通络，祛风除湿。

【主方】 白虎加桂枝汤[90]。

可加银藤、连翘、黄柏、威灵仙、防己、桑枝清热祛风，活血通络。皮肤有红斑者，可加丹皮、生地、赤芍、忍冬藤等凉血散风；热痹化火伤津，症见关节红肿，痛如刀割，入夜尤甚，壮热烦渴，舌红少津，脉弦数者，治以清热解毒，凉血止痛，选用犀角散[274]，酌加生地、玄参、麦冬等养阴生津之品。

【调护要点】 居室要清爽通风，忌食辛辣、肥甘、醇酒等物。

各种痹证迁延不愈，正虚邪恋，瘀阻于络，津凝为痰，痰瘀痹阻，而出现疼痛时轻时重、关节肿大变形、屈伸不利、舌质暗紫，苔白腻，脉弦涩等症，治宜化痰祛痰，搜风通络，用桃红饮[204]加穿山甲、地龙、土鳖、全蝎等搜剔络道之品；亦可加白芥子、胆南星祛痰散结。

痹证日久，除有肢体、关节的症状外，还常出现气血不足及肝肾亏虚的症状。此时应祛邪扶正，攻补兼施，在祛风散寒除湿的同时，加以补益气血，滋养肝肾，选用独活寄生汤[195]加减。

在痹证的治疗中，风寒湿痹疼痛剧烈者，常用川乌、附子、细辛等祛风除湿、温经止痛的药物。应用这些药物时，剂量应由小量开始，再逐渐增加。久煎或与甘草同煎可以缓解其毒性。服药后若有舌唇发麻、手足麻木、恶心、心慌、脉迟等中毒症状时，应酌情减少剂量，或立即停药，并及时采取补救措施。

小结

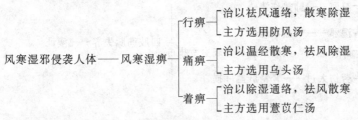

感受热邪或郁久化热——风湿热痹——治以清热通络，祛风除湿——主方选用白虎桂枝汤

思考题

1. 试述痹证发生与风湿寒三气的关系。
2. 痹证分为哪几个证候类型？其辨证要点、治法和主方是什么？

38 痿证

概念

痿证是指肢体筋脉弛缓、软弱无力,日久因不能随意运动而致肌肉萎缩的一种病证。

西医学中的多发性神经炎、急性脊髓炎、重症肌无力、肌营养不良症、周期性麻痹、进行性肌萎缩和表现为软瘫的中枢神经系统感染后遗症等,可参考本病辨证论治。

病因病机

1. 肺热伤津 感受温热邪毒,高热不退,或病后余热未尽,皆令肺受热灼,不能布送津液以润泽五脏,导致四肢筋脉失养,痿弱不用。

2. 湿热浸淫 久处湿地,冒雨涉水,湿淫经脉,郁久化热;或饮食不节,或过食肥甘、或嗜酒、或多食辛辣,损伤脾胃,内生湿热,以致湿热浸淫筋脉,影响气血运行,筋脉肌肉失于濡养而松弛不收,成为痿证。

3. 脾胃虚弱 脾为后天之本,平素脾胃虚弱,或久病中气受损,则受纳运化功能失常,津液气血生化之源不足,无以濡养五脏、运行气血,宗筋失养,关节不利,肌肉削瘦,成为痿证。如果原有痿证,经久不愈,导致脾胃虚弱,则痿证更加严重。

4. 肝肾亏虚 禀赋不足,或房室太过,精损难复,或因劳役太过,阴精亏损,均导致肾中水亏火旺,筋脉失养,成为痿证;若五志化火,肾水虚不能制火,以致火灼肺金,肺失治节,不能通调津液以溉五脏,脏气伤则肢体失养,亦可产生痿证。

此外,湿热下注,亦能损及肝肾,导致筋脉失养。

病因病机要点:

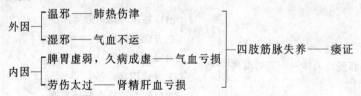

诊断与鉴别

痿证是以脏气内伤引起肢体失养,痿软不能随意任用的一种疾病。

本病应与痹证作鉴别。痹证亦有类似痿证之瘦削枯萎者,是由于痹证后期,肢体关节疼痛,不能运动,肢体长期废用所致。此外,痿证肢体关节一般不痛,痹证均有疼痛,其病因病机均有异,治法也各不相同,二者不能混淆。

辨证论治

本病以下肢痿躄最为多见,亦有手足均见痿弱者,严重者甚至足不能站立、手不能握物,久则肌肉痿削,甚至瘫痪。

痿证临床辨证应分为虚实两种。凡起病急,发展快,属于肺热伤津,或湿热浸淫者,多属实证；病史较久，起病与发展较慢，以脾胃及肝肾亏虚为多者，属于虚证。临床还须注意实中有虚，虚中有实之证。在临床治疗时，不论选方用药，针灸取穴，一般都重视调理脾胃这一治疗原则，但不能单以"独取阳明"的法则统疗各种类型的痿证，仍须辨证论治。

常见证型如下：

1. 肺热津伤，筋失濡润

【症状】 病起发热，或热退后突然出现肢体软弱无力，皮肤干燥，心烦口渴，咳呛痰少，小便黄少，大便燥结。舌质红，苔少，脉细数。

【辨证要点】 病起发热，或热后突然出现肢体软弱无力，咳呛咽干，舌红，苔少。

本型可见于急性脊髓炎、周期性麻痹、急性感染性多发性神经炎。

【病机概要】 温热犯肺，肺热伤津，津液不布，筋脉失养。

【治法】 清热润燥，养肺生津。

【主方】 清燥救肺汤[254]。

若热蒸气分，高热、口渴、有汗，可重用石膏，并加银花、知母，连翘清热祛邪；若咳呛少痰，酌加栝楼、桑白皮、枇杷叶等清润肃肺；若见身热虽退而食欲减退，口燥咽干较甚者，证属肺胃阴伤，宜用益胃汤[217]加苡仁、山药、谷芽之类益胃生津。

【调护要点】 居室宜清爽润湿；饮食忌辛辣、煎炸，宜清淡、甘润。

2. 湿热浸淫，气血不运

【症状】 四肢痿软，身体困重，或兼微肿、麻木，尤以下肢多见，或有发热，胸痞脘闷，小便短赤涩痛。苔黄腻，脉濡数。

【辨证要点】 四肢痿软，脘闷溲赤，苔黄腻。

本型常见于急性骨髓炎、急性感染性多发性神经炎、周期性麻痹。

【病机概要】 湿热浸淫四肢筋脉，气血运行受阻，筋脉肌肉失养。

【治法】 清热利湿，通利筋脉。

【主方】 加味二妙散[96]。

上方可加木通、薏仁、蚕砂、木瓜、牛膝等利湿通络之品。若湿偏盛，胸脘痞闷、肢重且肿者，可酌加厚朴、茯苓、泽泻理气化湿，夏秋季可加藿香、佩兰芳香化湿；如肢体麻木，关节运动不利，舌质紫暗，脉细涩，为夹瘀之证，酌加桃仁、红花、丹参、赤芍等，以活血通络；如形体瘦削，下肢有热感，心烦，舌红或中剥，脉细数，为热甚伤阴，上方去苍术，酌加生地、龟板、麦冬等，以养阴清热。

【调护要点】 居室应清爽通风干燥；饮食宜清淡，忌食辛辣酒类、肥甘等助湿生热之品。

3. 脾胃亏虚，精微不运

【症状】 肢体痿软无力，逐渐加重，食少腹胀，便溏，面浮而色不华，气短，神疲乏力。舌质淡，苔薄白，脉细。

【辨证要点】 肢体痿弱无力，逐渐加重，食少便溏，舌淡。

本型常见于重症肌无力、肌营养不良症、进行性肌萎缩和表现为软瘫的中枢神经系统感染后遗症。

【病机概要】 脾胃虚弱，气血化源不足，筋脉肌肉失养。

【治法】 补脾益气,健运升清。

【主方】 参苓白术散[169]。

若病久体弱,气血两虚者,宜重用党参、山药、白术,加黄芪、当归等,以补益气血;若体虚胖痰多者,可用六君子汤[45]补脾化痰。

【调护要点】 宜食益气健脾易于消化之品,如扁豆粥、山药粥、薏仁粥等。

4. 肝肾亏损,髓枯筋痿

【症状】 起病较缓,下肢痿软无力,腰脊酸软,不能久立,或伴目眩发落,咽干耳鸣,遗精或遗尿,或妇女月经不调,甚至步履全废,腿胫大肉渐脱。舌红少苔,脉细数。

【辨证要点】 起病较缓,下肢痿软,腰酸耳鸣,舌红少苔。

本型亦常见于重症肌无力、肌营养不良症、进行性肌萎缩和表现为软瘫的中枢神经系统感染后遗症。

【病机概要】 肝肾亏虚,精血不能濡养筋骨经脉。

【治法】 补益肝肾,滋阴清热。

【主方】 虎潜丸[151]。

本方治肝肾阴亏有热的痿证,为临床所常用。若热盛者,宜去锁阳、干姜;若兼见面色萎黄无华、心悸怔忡,舌淡红,脉细弱者,酌加黄芪、党参、当归、鸡血藤以补养气血;若久病阴损及阳,症见畏寒、阳痿,小便清长,舌淡,脉沉细无力者,则虎潜丸去黄柏、知母,酌加鹿角片、补骨脂、仙灵脾、巴戟天、肉桂、附子等补肾助阳之品。

此外,也可配用紫河车粉,或用猪、牛骨髓煮热,捣烂和入米粉、白糖调服。

【调护要点】 适当锻炼,戒房劳;宜食养阴补益之品,忌食辛辣。

痿证的治疗,除内服药物外,还可配用针灸、推拿或气功等综合疗法,并适当加强肢体的活动。这对痿证的恢复甚为重要,并有助于提高临床疗效。

痿证的预后,与病之虚实、病程之长短有关。实证多见于早期急性病例,病情较轻浅,疗效较好,功能较易恢复;虚证及慢性病例,病情缠绵,短期不易获效,功能恢复也较困难;年老体衰者,预后较差。

小结

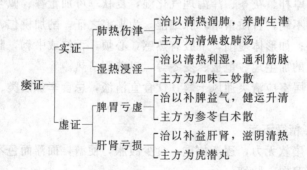

痿证
- 实证
  - 肺热伤津
    - 治以清热润肺,养肺生津
    - 主方为清燥救肺汤
  - 湿热浸淫
    - 治以清热利湿,通利筋脉
    - 主方为加味二妙散
- 虚证
  - 脾胃亏虚
    - 治以补脾益气,健运升清
    - 主方为参苓白术散
  - 肝肾亏损
    - 治以补益肝肾,滋阴清热
    - 主方为虎潜丸

思考题

1. 痿证的概念是什么?
2. 痿证分为哪几个证候类型?其辨证要点、治法和主方各是什么?
3. 痿证和痹证如何鉴别?

39 内伤发热

概念

内伤发热是指以内伤为病因，气血阴精亏虚、脏腑功能失调为基本病机所导致的发热病症。一般起病较缓，病程较长。临床上多表现为低热，仅少数可出现高热。此外，有些仅自觉发热或五心烦热，但测体温并不升高者，亦属于内伤发热的范畴。

西医学中的神经功能性低热、风湿热、结核病、甲状腺功能亢进、慢性感染性发热、恶性肿瘤之发热等，可参考本病辨证论治。

病因病机

1. 肝经郁热　情志抑郁，肝气不能疏达，气郁化火而致发热；或因恼怒过度，肝火内盛而致发热。这种发热和情志有密切关系，故又称"五志化火"。

2. 瘀血阻滞　由于气滞、劳倦、外伤、出血等原因导致瘀血产生，瘀血阻滞经络，气血运行不畅，郁遏不通，因而引起发热。

3. 阴精亏虚　素体阴虚，或热病日久，或因久泻伤阴，或误用、过用温燥药，导致阴精亏虚，水不制火，阳气相对偏盛而引起发热。

4. 血虚失养　久病心肝血虚、或脾虚不能生血，或因出血及产后、手术后失血过多，造成血虚失于濡养，不足以敛阴以致发热。

5. 中气不足　劳累过度，饮食失调，或久病失于调理，以致中焦脾胃气虚，中气不足，阴火自内而生并引起发热，称为"气虚发热"。

病因病机要点：

情志抑郁
瘀血阻滞
阴精亏虚 ——气血阴精亏虚，脏腑功能失调——内伤发热
血虚失养
中气不足

诊断与鉴别

内伤发热是以内伤为病因，导致气血阴精亏虚、脏腑功能失调所致的发热。

本病与外感发热都有发热症状，临床上应予鉴别：

病证\鉴别	内 伤 发 热	外 感 发 热
病　因	劳倦、饮食、情志等内伤而致	感受外邪
起病特点	起病缓慢，病程较长，或反复发作	起病较急，病程较短

(续表)

病证鉴别	内伤发热	外感发热
发热特点	以低热为主,发热而不恶寒,或虽感觉冷但得衣被则减。其热时作时止,或发无定时,或仅自觉发热,且多感觉手足心热	发热多表现为高热,发热初期常伴有恶寒,其寒虽得衣被而不减。外邪不除则发热不退
兼症	头晕神倦,自汗盗汗,脉弱无力等虚证	头身疼痛、鼻塞、咳嗽、脉浮等表证

辨证论治

对内伤发热的辨证,首先应辨明病因病机及证候虚实。气郁、血瘀属实;气虚、血虚、阴虚所致者属虚。应根据不同情况确立解郁、活血、益气、养血、滋阴的基本治法,切不可一见发热便用辛散或苦寒之剂。对内伤发热来说,发散易伤津耗气,苦寒易损伤脾阳或化燥伤阴,不但热不退,反而促使病情加重。

常见证型如下:

1. 肝郁发热

【症状】 时觉身热心烦,热势常随患者的情绪波动而起伏,精神抑郁或烦躁易怒,胸胁胀闷,善叹息,口苦而干,妇女常伴月经不调,经来腹痛或乳房发胀。舌苔黄,脉弦数。

【辨证要点】 身热心烦,热势随情志变化而起伏,胁胀口苦,脉弦数。

本型常见于甲状腺功能亢进、神经功能性低热。

【病机概要】 情志不畅,肝气郁结,气郁化火而致发热。

【治法】 疏肝解郁,清肝泻热。

【主方】 丹栀逍遥散[52]。

若热象较重,口干便秘者,可去白术、茯苓,加黄芩、龙胆草以清肝泻火;胁痛者加川楝子、郁金以理气止痛;若气郁日久,热邪伤阴,或素体阴虚而兼肝郁为患,用滋水清肝饮[271]以滋养肝肾,疏肝清热;气郁化火,热象较重,见面红耳赤,心烦易怒,溲赤便秘,舌质红绛,脉数,宜用龙胆泻肝汤[64]以清肝热泻肝火。

【调护要点】 调情志,忌郁怒;忌食辛辣之品。

2. 瘀血发热

【症状】 午后或夜晚发热,口干咽燥而不欲饮,躯干或四肢有固定痛处或肿块,甚者肌肤甲错,面色黯黑或萎黄。舌质紫暗或有瘀点瘀斑,脉涩。

【辨证要点】 午后或夜晚发热,身体有固定痛处或肿块,舌质暗紫。

本型常见于恶性肿瘤、风湿病发热。

【病机概要】 瘀血阻滞,气血运行不畅,壅遏不通而发热。

【治法】 活血化瘀。

【主方】 血府逐瘀汤[119]。

热甚者加丹皮、郁金、丹参、大黄以活血凉血;疼痛明显者,加延胡索、五灵脂活血止痛。

【调护要点】 调情志；宜食温热，忌食生冷；戒劳作。

3. 阴虚发热

【症状】 午后或夜间发热，或手足心发热，或骨蒸潮热，心烦盗汗，少寐多梦，口干咽燥，大便干结，尿少色黄。舌质红干或舌有裂纹，无苔或少苔，脉细数。

【辨证要点】 午后或夜间发热，手足心热，盗汗多梦，舌质红干，无苔或少苔。

本型常见于神经功能性发热、结核病及恶性肿瘤发热。

【病机概要】 阴虚则阳亢，水不制火，阴虚火旺而发热。

【治法】 滋阴清热。

【主方】 清骨散[251]。

若失眠者加酸枣仁、柏子仁、夜交藤以养心安神；盗汗较甚者，可加煅牡蛎、浮小麦、糯稻根以固表敛汗；阴虚较甚者，加生地、玄参、首乌以加强其滋阴作用；若兼有气短头晕、体倦乏力等气虚症状者，为气阴两虚，可加党参、北沙参、麦冬、五味子益气养阴。

【调护要点】 忌食辛辣煎炸、温燥动火之品；宜食甘润生津之品。节房事，调情志，戒劳作。

4. 血虚发热

【症状】 发热多为低热，头晕眼花，面色无华，心悸不宁，身倦乏力，唇甲色淡。舌淡，脉细弱。

【辨证要点】 低热，头晕眼花，面色无华，唇甲色淡。

本型常见于恶性肿瘤、风湿热、神经功能性发热等。

【病机概要】 阴血亏虚，不足敛阳而致发热。

【治法】 益气养血。

【主方】 归脾汤[95]或当归补血汤[115]。

【调护要点】 宜食补而不腻之品，忌食辛辣；戒过劳。

5. 气虚发热

【症状】 发热常在劳累后发作或加重，热势或高或低，神倦乏力，气短懒言，头晕自汗，易于感冒，食少便溏。舌质淡，苔薄白，脉细弱。

【辨证要点】 发热常在劳累后发作或加重，食少便溏，气短懒言。

本型常见于恶性肿瘤及结核病、慢性肾盂肾炎等慢性感染性发热。

【病机概要】 脾胃气虚，中气下陷，虚火内生。

【治法】 益气健脾，甘温除热。

【主方】 补中益气汤[140]。

若自汗多者，可加煅牡蛎、煅龙骨、浮小麦以固表敛汗；胸闷脘痞，舌苔白腻者，为挟有湿邪，可加茯苓、苍术、藿香、砂仁以健脾燥湿；若时冷时热，汗出恶风者，可加桂枝、芍药以调和营卫。

【调护要点】 避免过劳；忌食辛辣肥甘。可服黄芪粥、莲子粥、麦片粥等健脾和胃。此外，尚有阳虚发热之证，症见发热，形寒怯冷，四肢不温或下肢发冷，面色㿠白，头晕嗜卧，腰膝酸痛，舌质胖润或有齿痕，苔白润，脉沉细而弱，或浮大无力。治宜温补肾阳，用金匮肾气丸[163]加减。属于阳虚发热的，尚有阴盛格阳、真寒假热的特殊类型，症见身热、面赤、不恶寒，四肢厥逆，下利清谷，脉微欲绝。属阴寒至盛，格阳于外的危急重症，宜施附子、干姜、甘草、人参，以回阳救逆。

小结

内伤发热一证，由于病情复杂，病程往往较长，因此必须从病史、发热的特点、兼证等方面认真细微地观察辨证，以冀逐步取得疗效。

内伤发热多由情志、饮食、劳倦等病因所引起，气血阴精亏虚及脏腑功能失调是其共同的病机。本证应注意与外感发热相鉴别。治疗上应针对肝郁、血瘀、阴虚、血虚、气虚等不同证候而立法遣方。但不同原因引起的发热，常相互关联或相互转化，彼此兼夹。如肝郁发热可逐渐伤阴耗津，则转为气郁阴虚之发热；气虚和血虚可以互相影响，混合出现；气虚发热日久，病损及阳，阳气虚衰，则发展为阳虚发热。因此必须用发展和互相联系的观点去审因论治，才能取得治疗上的主动权。精神愉快，避免过劳，注意饮食调节，则有利于内伤发热的治疗和康复。

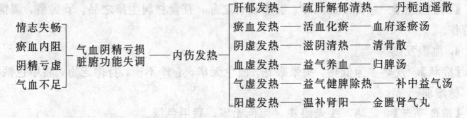

思考题

1. 内伤发热与外感发热如何鉴别？
2. 内伤发热常见哪几种证型？其辨证要点各是什么？

40 虚劳

概念

虚劳又称虚损，是由多种原因所致的，以脏腑亏损，气血阴阳不足为主要病机的多种慢性衰弱证候的总称。凡禀赋不足，后天失养，积劳内伤，久虚不复，而表现为各种亏损证候者，均属本证的范围。

西医学中的席汉综合征、阿狄森病、甲状腺功能减退症、再生障碍性贫血、慢性粒细胞性白血病等多种慢性或消耗性疾病，可参考本病辨证论治。

病因病机

1. 禀赋薄弱，体质虚羸　父母年老体弱，精血不旺；或妊娠期失于调摄，胎中失养；或出生后喂养不当，营养不良及遗传缺陷等因素，是造成禀赋薄弱，体质不强的主要原因。在体质不强的基础上，易于因劳致病，或因病致虚，久病难复而成为虚劳。

2. 烦劳过度，损及五脏　临床上以忧郁思虑，烦劳过度损及心脾或早婚多育、房劳伤肾最为多见。

3. 饮食不节，损伤脾胃　暴饮暴食，嗜欲偏食，营养不良，嗜酒过度等原因，都能损伤脾胃，影响其化生精微及生养气血的功能。若脾胃长期受损，必致气血来源不足，内不能和调于五脏六腑，外不能洒陈于营卫经脉，渐致虚劳。

4. 大病久病，失于调养　大病之后，因病邪过盛，脏气损伤；或热病日久，耗伤阴血；或寒邪久留，损阳伤正；或瘀血内结，新血不生；或病后失于调治，正气难复，都能损伤气血阴阳，逐渐发展，终成虚劳。

病因病机要点：

因虚致病，因病成劳　
因病致虚，久虚成劳　}—损及五脏——气、血、阴、阳亏损——虚劳

诊断与鉴别

虚劳是多种慢性衰弱性证候的总称。

本病与虚证及肺痨均表现有虚弱症状，应注意鉴别。

虚劳和内科其他病证中的虚证证型虽然在临床表现上、治疗方药方面有类似之处，但两者仍有区别。虚劳的各种证候，均以出现一系列精气不足的症状为特征，而其他病证的虚证，则各以其病证的主要症状为突出表现。例如眩晕一证的气血亏虚型及水肿一证的脾阳不振型，则分别以眩晕和水肿为最基本、最突出的表现。此外，虚劳一般都有较长的病程，病势缠绵，这也是有别于其它病虚证之处。

虚劳与肺痨的区别：肺痨为痨虫侵袭所致，病变部位主要在肺，具有传染性，以阴虚火旺为其病理特点，以咳嗽、咳血、潮热、盗汗、消瘦为主要的临床表现；而虚劳则由多种原因所致，其病损部位主要在五脏，一般不传染，以气、血、阴、阳亏耗为其病

机特点，分别出现五脏气、血、阴、阳亏虚的临床症状。

辨证论治

对虚劳的辨证，可归纳为气、血、阴、阳亏虚四大类

```
         ┌气虚——短气乏力，自汗，食少，便溏，舌淡，脉弱——益气
         │血虚——面色不华，唇舌色淡，脉细弱——养血
虚劳─────┤阴虚——五心烦热，颧红，口干咽燥，舌红少津，脉细数——滋阴
         └阳虚——倦怠嗜卧，形寒肢冷，肠鸣泄泻，舌质淡胖，脉虚弱或沉迟——温阳
```

在辨证过程中，应注意各种原因所致的虚损常相互影响，一脏有病，可以累及他脏；一虚而渐致多虚。如脾病可以及肺，肺病可以及肾，气虚不能生血，血虚无以生气，气虚者阳亦渐衰，血虚者阴亦不足，阴损及阳，阳损及阴等。故在临证时，要善于掌握病情的发展和归转，做到辨证明晰。

在虚劳的治疗方面，应以补益为基本原则。根据病理属性的不同，分别采取益气、养血、滋阴、温阳的治法并密切结合五脏病位的不同而选用方药，以增加治疗的针对性。由于人体的气血来源于先天，滋生给养于后天，故在虚劳的治疗中补益脾肾始终具有较重要的意义。

常见证型如下：

气虚

1. 肺气虚

【症状】 短气自汗，声音低怯，时寒时热，平素易于感冒，面色㿠白。舌质淡，脉弱。

【辨证要点】 短气自汗，易于感冒。

【病机概要】 肺气亏虚，卫表不固，营卫失和。

【治法】 补益肺气。

【主方】 补肺汤[143]。

若自汗较多者，合牡蛎散[144]益气固表以敛汗；若气阴两虚，兼见潮热盗汗者，加银柴胡、地骨皮、秦艽等养阴清热。

【调护要点】 避风寒，慎起居，忌食生冷。

2. 脾气虚

【症状】 饮食减少，食后胃脘不舒，倦怠乏力，大便溏薄，面色萎黄。舌淡苔薄，脉弱。

【辨证要点】 食少便溏，面色萎黄。

【病机概要】 脾不健运，胃肠传化失常，气血来源不足。

【治法】 健脾益气。

【主方】 加味四君子汤[97]。

若兼胃脘胀满，呕吐嗳气者，加半夏、陈皮以和胃降逆；兼食滞者，加莱菔子、神曲、麦芽、鸡内金、山楂消食健胃；若气虚及阳，脾阳渐虚，腹痛泄泻，手足欠温者，加肉桂、炮姜温中散寒；若脾气亏虚而主要表现为气虚下陷者，可用补中益气汤[140]以补益中气、升阳举陷。

【调护要点】 宜食补而不腻之品,忌生冷。

在气、血、阴、阳的亏虚中,气虚是临床上最常见的一类。尤以肺、脾气虚为多见,而心、肾气虚亦属不少,可参考心肾阳虚治法。

血虚

1. 心血虚

【症状】 心悸怔忡,健忘,失眠多梦,面色不华。舌质淡,脉细或结代。

【辨证要点】 心悸怔忡,面色不华,脉结代。

【病机概要】 心血亏虚,心失所养,血脉不充。

【治法】 养血安神。

【主方】 养心汤[185]。

若心动悸、脉结代者,可用炙甘草汤[165]以复脉定悸。

【调护要点】 宜食补益之品,勿暴食暴饮;慎起居,调情志,戒劳作。

2. 肝血虚

【症状】 头晕、目眩,胁痛,肢体麻木,筋脉拘急或惊惕肉瞤,妇女月经不调或闭经,面色不华。舌质淡,脉弦细或细涩。

【辨证要点】 头晕目眩,筋脉拘急。

【病机概要】 血不养肝,肝血亏虚,血脉不充,经脉失养。

【治法】 补血养肝。

【主方】 四物汤[79]。

可加制首乌、枸杞子、鸡血藤以增强补养肝血的作用。若眩晕耳鸣者,加女贞子、磁石、牡蛎等,以育阴潜阳;胁痛者,加柴胡、郁金、香附、川楝子理气通络。

【调护要点】 宜食补益之品,调情志,戒劳作。

血虚之中,以心、脾、肝的血虚较多见。气血同源,故血虚常伴有不同程度的气虚症状。因此,在补血的同时,应适当配伍益气药,以达到益气生血的目的。

阴虚

1. 肺阴虚

【症状】 干咳,咳血,咽燥,甚则失音,潮热盗汗,面色潮红。舌红少津,脉细数。

【辨证要点】 干咳、咽燥,潮热盗汗,舌红少津。

【病机概要】 肺阴亏损,肺失濡润,虚热内生,耗灼肺金。

【治法】 养阴润肺。

【主方】 沙参麦门冬汤[138]。

若咳嗽甚者,加百部、款冬花、紫菀以肃肺止咳;咳血者加白及、仙鹤草、鲜茅根凉血止血;潮热者加地骨皮、银柴胡、秦艽滋阴退热;盗汗者加牡蛎、浮小麦、麻黄根以固表敛汗。

【调护要点】 饮食忌辛辣、煎炸等助热伤阴之品;宜食果蔬、百合、鲜藕等甘凉滋润之品。

2. 心阴虚

【症状】 心悸、失眠、烦躁,潮热盗汗,面色潮红,口舌生疮。舌红少津,脉细数。

【辨证要点】 心悸、失眠、潮热盗汗，舌红少津。

【病机概要】 心阴亏虚，心失濡养，阴虚内热，津液不足。

【治法】 滋阴养心。

【主方】 天王补心丹[32]。

若见烦躁不安，口舌生疮者，可加黄连、木通、竹叶以清心泻火，导热下行。

【调护要点】 忌食辛辣、煎炸等助火伤阴之品；宜食滋阴养心之品，如五味子、麦门冬等水煎代茶饮。

3. 脾胃阴虚

【症状】 口舌干燥，不思饮食，大便秘结，甚至干呕，呃逆，面色潮红。舌干，苔少或无苔，脉细数。

【辨证要点】 不思饮食，口干唇燥，大便秘结，舌干苔少。

【病机概要】 脾胃阴虚，运化失常，阴虚内热，耗伤津液。

【治法】 养阴和胃。

【主方】 益胃汤[217]。

不思饮食者，加谷芽、麦芽、茯苓、山药益胃健脾；口干唇燥甚者加石斛、花粉以滋养胃阴；呃逆加刀豆、柿蒂、竹茹降逆止呃。

【调护要点】 调情志；忌辛辣煎炸之品，宜服用滋阴甘润之品，如玉竹、石斛等水煎代茶饮。

4. 肝阴虚

【症状】 头痛，眩晕，耳鸣，目干畏光，视物不清，急躁易怒，或肢体麻木，筋惕肉瞤，面色潮红。舌干红、少苔，脉弦细数。

【辨证要点】 目干畏光，筋惕肉瞤，舌干红少苔。

【病机概要】 肝阴不足，阴亏火旺，筋脉失养，虚风内动。

【治法】 滋养肝阴。

【主方】 补肝汤[142]。

若头痛、眩晕、耳鸣较重，或筋惕肉瞤者，加石决明、菊花、钩藤等平肝潜阳；目干涩、畏光、视物不清者，加女贞子、草决明、以养肝明目；若急躁易怒，尿赤便秘，舌红脉数者，加龙胆草、黄芩、栀子清肝泻火；胁痛者加川楝子、郁金以疏肝理气止痛。

【调护要点】 调情志，忌郁怒；忌辛辣、燥热之品。

5. 肾阴虚

【症状】 腰酸，遗精，两足痿弱，眩晕耳鸣，甚则耳聋，口干咽痛，潮热颧红。舌红少津，脉沉细。

【辨证要点】 腰酸遗精，潮热咽干，舌红少津。

【病机概要】 肾阴亏损，虚火内动，精关不固，髓海失充。

【治法】 滋补肾阴。

【主方】 左归丸[65]。

若腰酸遗精甚者,加煅牡蛎、金樱子、芡实、莲须,以固肾涩精。

【调护要点】 慎起居,节房事,戒劳作;忌食辛辣煎炸之品,宜进甘润补益之食。

阳虚

1. 心阳虚

【症状】 心悸,自汗,神倦嗜卧,心胸憋闷疼痛,形寒肢冷,面色苍白。舌淡或紫暗,脉细弱或沉迟。

【辨证要点】 心悸,自汗,形寒胸闷。

【病机概要】 心阳不足,阳虚气弱,鼓动无力,气机滞塞。

【治法】 益气温阳。

【主方】 拯阳理劳汤[180]。

若心胸憋闷疼痛者,加三七、红花、丹参、郁金活血化瘀,理气止痛。

【调护要点】 慎避风寒,忌食生冷,调理情志。

2. 脾阳虚

【症状】 面色萎黄,食少便溏,肠鸣腹痛,每因受寒或饮食不慎而加剧,形寒,神疲乏力,气少懒言。舌淡苔白,脉虚弱。

【辨证要点】 食少便溏,形寒乏力,舌淡脉虚。

【病机概要】 脾阳亏虚,运化失常,气虚中寒。

【治法】 温中健脾。

【主方】 附子理中丸[146]。

若腹中冷痛,便溏不止者,加良姜、吴茱萸、肉豆蔻、补骨脂以温中散寒,固肠止泻。

【调护要点】 宜食温热之品,忌食生冷油腻。

3. 肾阳虚

【症状】 腰背酸痛,遗精阳痿,多尿或尿失禁,面色苍白,恶寒肢冷,下利清谷或五更泄泻。舌淡胖有齿痕,苔白,脉沉迟。

【辨证要点】 腰酸肢冷,遗精阳痿,五更泄泻。

【病机概要】 肾阳虚衰,命门火衰,阴寒内盛。

【治法】 温补肾阳,兼养精血。

【主方】 右归丸[68]。

若遗精者,加金樱子、桑螵蛸、莲须或合金锁固精丸[164]以收涩固精;五更泄泻者,可合用四神丸[82]以温肾固肠止泻;若见喘促,短气,动则更甚,为肾不纳气,可加补骨脂、五味子、蛤蚧补肾纳气。

【调护要点】 适劳逸,节房事;调饮食,忌生冷;平素可选用核桃肉、紫河车等做成米粥、羹食用。

阳虚之证,大多由气虚逐渐发展而来。阳虚生寒,症状比气虚为重。由于肾阳为人身之元阳,故心、脾阳虚日久,常累及于肾,而出现心肾阳虚或脾肾阳虚病变,临证必须详察而兼治之。

小结

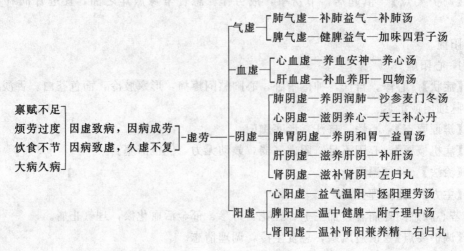

思考题

1. 肺劳与虚劳在病因、病位、临床表现方面有何不同？
2. 试述心血虚、肝血虚、肺气虚、脾阳虚、肾阴阳两虚的辨证要点、治法和主方。

附 录

1. 方剂索引

一 画

[1] 一贯煎（《柳州医话》）：沙参　麦冬　当归　生地黄　枸杞子　川楝子

二 画

[2] 二陈汤（《太平惠民和剂局方》）：半夏　陈皮　茯苓　炙甘草

[3] 二阴煎（《景岳全书》）：生地黄　麦冬　枣仁　生甘草　玄参　茯苓　黄连　木通　灯心　竹叶

[4] 二神散（《杂病源流犀烛》）：海金砂　滑石

[5] 十灰散（《十药神书》）：大蓟　小蓟　侧柏叶　荷叶　茜草根　山栀　茅根　大黄　丹皮　棕榈皮

[6] 十枣汤（《伤寒论》）：大戟　芫花　甘遂　大枣

[7] 丁香散（《古今医统》）：丁香　柿蒂　良姜　炙甘草

[8] 七味都气丸（《医宗己任篇》）：地黄　山茱萸　山药　茯苓　丹皮　泽泻　五味子

[9] 七厘散（《良方集腋》）：血竭　麝香　冰片　乳香　没药　红花　朱砂　儿茶

[10] 人参胡桃汤（《济生方》）：新罗人参　胡桃　生姜

[11] 人参养营汤（《太平惠民和剂局方》）：人参　甘草　当归　白芍　熟地黄　肉桂　大枣　黄芪　白术　茯苓　五味子　远志　橘皮　生姜

[12] 八正散（《太平惠民和剂局方》）：木通　车前子　扁蓄　瞿麦　滑石　甘草梢　大黄　山栀　灯心

[13] 八珍汤（《正体类要》）：人参　白术　茯苓　甘草　当归　白芍药　川芎　熟地黄　生姜　大枣

三 画

[14] 三子养亲汤（《韩氏医通》）：苏子　白芥子　莱菔子

[15] 三仁汤（《温病条辨》）：杏仁　白蔻仁　薏苡仁　厚朴　半夏　通草　滑石　竹叶

[16] 大七气汤（《医学入门》）：青皮　陈皮　桔梗　藿香　官桂　甘草　三棱　莪术　香附　益智仁　姜　枣

[17] 大补元煎（《景岳全书》）：人参　炒山药　熟地黄　杜仲　枸杞子　当归　山茱萸　炙甘草

[18] 大补阴丸（《丹溪心法》）：知母　黄柏　熟地黄　龟版　猪脊髓

[19] 大定风珠（《温病条辨》）：白芍药　阿胶　生龟板　生地黄　火麻仁　五味子　生

牡蛎 麦冬 炙甘草 鸡子黄 生鳖甲

[20] 大建中汤（《金匮要略》）：川椒 干姜 人参 饴糖

[21] 大承气汤（《伤寒论》）：大黄 厚朴 枳实 芒硝

[22] 大秦艽汤（《素问病机气宜保命集》）：秦艽 当归 甘草 羌活 防风 白芷 熟地黄 茯苓 石膏 川芎 白芍药 独活 黄芩 生地黄 白术 细辛

[23] 川芎茶调散（《太平惠民和剂局方》）：川芎 荆芥 薄荷 羌活 细辛（或香附） 白芷 甘草 防风

[24] 己椒苈黄丸（《金匮要略》）：防己 椒目 葶苈子 大黄

[25] 小半夏加茯苓汤（《金匮要略》）：半夏 生姜 茯苓

[26] 小半夏汤（《金匮要略》）：半夏 生姜

[27] 小青龙汤（《伤寒论》）：麻黄 桂枝 芍药 甘草 干姜 细辛 半夏 五味子

[28] 小建中汤（《伤寒论》）：桂枝 白芍 甘草 生姜 大枣 饴糖

[29] 小承气汤（《伤寒论》）：大黄 厚朴 枳实

[30] 小柴胡汤（《伤寒论》）：柴胡 黄芩 半夏 人参 甘草 生姜 大枣

[31] 小蓟饮子（《济生方》）：生地黄 小蓟 滑石 通草 炒蒲黄 淡竹叶 藕节 当归 山栀 甘草

四　画

[32] 天王补心丹（《摄生秘剂》）：人参 玄参 丹参 茯苓 五味子 远志 桔梗 当归身 天冬 麦冬 柏子仁 酸枣仁 生地黄 辰砂

[33] 天麻钩藤饮（《杂病诊治新义》）：天麻 钩藤 生石决明 川牛膝 桑寄生 杜仲 山栀 黄芩 益母草 朱茯神 夜交藤

[34] 无比山药丸（《太平惠民和剂局方》）：山药 肉苁蓉 熟地黄 山茱萸 茯神 菟丝子 五味子 赤石脂 巴戟天 泽泻 杜仲 牛膝

[35] 木防己汤（《金匮要略》）：木防己 石膏 桂枝 人参

[36] 木香顺气散（《沈氏尊生书》）：木香 青皮 橘皮 甘草 枳壳 川朴 乌药 香附 苍术 砂仁 桂心 川芎

[37] 止嗽散（《医学心悟》）：荆芥 桔梗 甘草 白前 陈皮 百部 紫菀

[38] 中满分消丸（《兰室秘藏》）：厚朴 枳实 黄连 黄芩 知母 半夏 陈皮 茯苓 猪苓 泽泻 砂仁 干姜 姜黄 人参 白术 炙甘草

[39] 五仁丸（《世医得效方》）：桃仁 杏仁 柏子仁 松子仁 郁李仁 橘皮

[40] 五皮散（《中藏经》）：桑白皮 橘皮 生姜皮 大腹皮 茯苓皮

[41] 五苓散（《伤寒论》）：桂枝 白术 茯苓 猪苓 泽泻

[42] 五积散（《太平惠民和剂局方》）：白芷 橘皮 厚朴 当归 川芎 白芍药 茯苓 桔梗 苍术 枳壳 半夏 麻黄 干姜 肉桂 甘草 姜

[43] 五磨饮子（《医方集解》）：乌药 沉香 槟榔 枳实 木香

[44] 六一散（《伤寒标本心法类萃》）：滑石 甘草

[45] 六君子汤（《医学正传》）：人参 炙甘草 茯苓 白术 陈皮 制半夏

[46] 六味地黄丸（《小儿药证直诀》）：熟地黄 山药 茯苓 丹皮 泽泻 山茱萸

[47] 六磨汤（《证治准绳》）：沉香　木香　槟榔　乌药　枳实　大黄
[48] 化虫丸（《医方集解》）：槟榔　鹤虱　苦楝根　枯矾　炒胡粉　使君子　芜荑
[49] 化肝煎（《景岳全书》）：青皮　陈皮　芍药　丹皮　栀子　泽泻　贝母
[50] 化积丸（《类证治裁》）：三棱　莪术　阿魏　海浮石　香附　雄黄　槟榔　苏木　瓦楞子　五灵脂
[51] 丹参饮（《医学金鉴》）：丹参　檀香　砂仁
[52] 丹栀逍遥散（《医统》）：当归　白芍药　白术　柴胡　茯苓　甘草　煨姜　薄荷　丹皮　山栀
[53] 乌头汤（《金匮要略》）：川乌　麻黄　芍药　黄芪　甘草
[54] 乌头赤石脂丸（《金匮要略》）：蜀椒　乌头　炮附子　干姜　赤石脂
[55] 乌头桂枝汤（《金匮要略》）：川乌　桂枝　生白芍　炙甘草　生姜　大枣　蜂蜜
[56] 乌梅丸（《伤寒论》）：乌梅　黄连　黄柏　人参　当归　附子　桂枝　蜀椒　干姜　细辛
[57] 少腹逐瘀汤（《医林改错》）：小茴香　干姜　延胡索　没药　当归　川芎　肉桂　赤芍药　蒲黄　五灵脂
[58] 水陆二仙丹（《证治准绳》）：金樱子　芡实

五　画

[59] 玉女煎（《景岳全书》）：石膏　熟地黄　麦冬　知母　牛膝
[60] 玉枢丹（《百一选方》）：山慈菇　续随子　大戟　麝香　腰黄　朱砂　五倍子
[61] 玉屏风散（《世医得效方》）：黄芪　白术　防风
[62] 正气天香散（《证治准绳》）：乌药　香附　干姜　紫苏　陈皮
[63] 石韦散（《证治汇补》）：石韦　冬葵子　瞿麦　滑石　车前子
[64] 龙胆泻肝汤（《兰室秘藏》）：龙胆草　泽泻　木通　车前子　当归　柴胡　生地黄（近代方有黄芩　栀子）
[65] 左归丸（《景岳全书》）：熟地黄　山药　山茱萸　菟丝子　枸杞子　川牛膝　鹿角胶　龟版胶
[66] 左归饮（《景岳全书》）：熟地　山萸肉　杞子　山药　茯苓　甘草
[67] 左金丸（《丹溪心法》）：黄连　吴茱萸
[68] 右归丸（《景岳全书》）：熟地黄　山药　山茱萸　枸杞子　杜仲　菟丝子　附子　肉桂　当归　鹿角胶
[69] 右归饮（《景岳全书》）：熟地　山萸肉　杞子　山药　杜仲　甘草　附子　肉桂
[70] 平胃散（《太平惠民和剂局方》）：苍术　厚朴　橘皮　甘草　生姜　大枣
[71] 甘麦大枣汤（《金匮要略》）：甘草　淮小麦　大枣
[72] 甘姜苓术汤（《金匮要略》）：甘草　干姜　茯苓　白术
[73] 甘遂半夏汤（《金匮要略》）：甘遂　半夏　芍药　甘草
[74] 甘露消毒丹（《温热经纬》）：滑石　茵陈　黄芩　石菖蒲　川贝母　木通　藿香　射干　连翘　薄荷　白蔻仁
[75] 四七汤（《太平惠民和剂局方》引《简易方》）：苏叶　制半夏　厚朴　茯苓　生姜

大枣

[76] 四妙丸（《成方便读》）：苍术　黄柏　牛膝　苡仁
[77] 四君子汤（《太平惠民和剂局方》）：党参　白术　茯苓　甘草
[78] 四味回阳饮（《景岳全书》）：人参　制附子　炮姜　炙甘草
[79] 四物汤（《太平惠民和剂局方》）：当归　白芍药　川芎　熟地黄
[80] 四逆汤（《伤寒论》）：附子　干姜　炙甘草
[81] 四逆散（《伤寒论》）：炙甘草　枳实　柴胡　芍药
[82] 四神丸（《证治准绳》）：补骨脂　肉豆蔻　吴茱萸　五味子　生姜　大枣
[83] 四海舒郁丸（《疡医大全》）：海蛤粉　海带　海藻　海螵蛸　昆布　陈皮　青木香
[84] 生脉散（《备急千金要方》）：人参　麦冬　五味子
[85] 生铁落饮（《医学心悟》）：天冬　麦冬　贝母　胆星　橘红　远志　石菖蒲　连翘　茯苓　茯神　玄参　钩藤　丹参　辰砂　生铁落
[86] 失笑散（《太平惠民和剂局方》）：五灵脂　蒲黄
[87] 代抵当丸（《证治准绳》）：大黄　当归尾　生地　穿山甲　芒硝　桃仁　肉桂
[88] 白头翁汤（《伤寒论》）：白头翁　秦皮　黄连　黄柏
[89] 白虎加人参汤（《伤寒论》）：知母　石膏　甘草　粳米　人参
[90] 白虎加桂枝汤（《金匮要略》）：知母　石膏　甘草　粳米　桂枝
[91] 白虎汤（《伤寒论》）：知母　石膏　甘草　粳米
[92] 半夏白术天麻汤（《医学心悟》）：半夏　白术　天麻　陈皮　茯苓　甘草　生姜　大枣
[93] 半夏厚朴汤（《金匮要略》）：半夏　厚朴　紫苏　茯苓　生姜
[94] 半硫丸（《太平惠民和剂局方》）：半夏　硫黄
[95] 归脾汤（《济生方》）：党参　黄芪　白术　茯神　酸枣仁　龙眼　木香　炙甘草　当归　远志　生姜　大枣
[96] 加味二妙散（《丹溪心法》）：黄柏　苍术　当归　牛膝　防己　萆薢　龟版
[97] 加味四君子汤（《三因方》）：人参　茯苓　白术　炙甘草　黄芪　白扁豆
[98] 加味四物汤（《金匮翼》）：白芍　当归　生地　川芎　蔓荆子　菊花　黄芩　甘草
[99] 加味清胃散（《张氏医通》）：生地　丹皮　当归　黄连　连翘　犀角　升麻　生甘草
[100] 加减承气汤（验方）：大黄　风化硝　枳实　礞石　皂角　猪胆汁　醋
[101] 加减复脉汤（《温病条辨》）：炙甘草　干地黄　生白芍　麦冬　阿胶　麻仁
[102] 加减葳蕤汤（《通俗伤寒论》）：玉竹　葱白　桔梗　白薇　豆豉　薄荷　炙甘草　大枣

六　画

[103] 百合固金丸（《医方集解》）：生地黄　熟地黄　麦冬　贝母　百合　当归　炒芍药　甘草　玄参　桔梗
[104] 地黄饮子（《宣明论》）：生地黄　巴戟天　山萸肉　石斛　肉苁蓉　五味子　肉桂　茯苓　麦冬　炮附子　石菖蒲　远志　生姜　大枣　薄荷

[105] 地榆散（验方）：地榆　茜草　黄芩　黄连　山栀　茯苓
[106] 芎芷石膏汤（《医宗金鉴》）：川芎　白芷　石膏　菊花　藁本　羌活
[107] 芍药汤（《素问病机气宜保命集》）：黄芩　芍药　炙甘草　黄连　大黄　槟榔　当归　木香　肉桂
[108] 芍药甘草汤（《伤寒论》）：白芍药　炙甘草
[109] 至宝丹（《太平惠民和剂局方》）：朱砂　麝香　安息香　金银箔　犀角　牛黄　琥珀　雄黄　玳瑁　龙脑
[110] 交泰丸（《韩氏医通》）：黄连　肉桂
[111] 安宫牛黄丸（《温病条辨》）：牛黄　郁金　犀角　黄连　朱砂　冰片　珍珠　山栀　雄黄　黄芩　麝香　金箔衣
[112] 安神定志丸（《医学心悟》）：茯苓　茯神　远志　人参　石菖蒲　龙齿
[113] 当归六黄汤（《兰室秘藏》）：当归　生地黄　熟地黄　黄连　黄芩　黄柏　黄芪
[114] 当归龙荟丸（《宣明论方》）：当归　龙胆草　栀子　黄连　黄芩　黄柏　大黄　青黛　芦荟　木香　麝香
[115] 当归补血汤（《内外伤辨惑论》）：黄芪　当归
[116] 竹叶石膏汤（《伤寒论》）：竹叶　石膏　麦冬　人参　半夏　粳米　炙甘草
[117] 竹沥达痰丸（《古今医鉴》）：青礞石　沉香　大黄　黄芩　竹沥　半夏　橘红　甘草　姜汁　茯苓　人参
[118] 竹茹汤（《本事方》）：竹茹　半夏　干姜　甘草　生姜　大枣
[119] 血府逐瘀汤（《医林改错》）：当归　生地黄　桃仁　红花　枳壳　赤芍药　柴胡　甘草　桔梗　川芎　牛膝
[120] 导赤散（《小儿药证直诀》）：生地黄　木通　竹叶　甘草
[121] 导痰汤（《济生方》）：半夏　陈皮　枳实　茯苓　甘草　制南星
[122] 防己黄芪汤（《金匮要略》）：防己　白术　黄芪　甘草　生姜　大枣
[123] 防风汤（《宣明论方》）：防风　当归　赤茯苓　杏仁　黄芩　秦艽　葛根　麻黄　肉桂　生姜　甘草　大枣

七　画

[124] 麦门冬汤（《金匮要略》）：麦冬　人参　半夏　甘草　粳米　大枣
[125] 麦味地黄丸（《医级》）：熟地黄　山萸肉　山药　丹皮　泽泻　茯苓　麦冬　五味子
[126] 苍术二陈汤（《杂病源流犀烛》）：苍术　白术　茯苓　陈皮　甘草　半夏
[127] 苏子降气汤（《太平惠民和剂局方》）：苏子　橘皮　半夏　当归　前胡　厚朴　肉桂　甘草　生姜
[128] 苏合香丸（《太平惠民和剂局方》）：白术　青木香　犀角　香附　朱砂　诃子　檀香　安息香　沉香　麝香　丁香　荜拨　苏合香油　熏陆香　冰片
[129] 杞菊地黄丸（《医级》）：枸杞子　菊花　熟地黄　山茱萸　山药　泽泻　丹皮　茯苓
[130] 杏苏散（《温病条辨》）：杏仁　紫苏叶　橘皮　半夏　生姜　枳壳　桔梗　前胡

茯苓　甘草　大枣
[131] 更衣丸（《先醒斋医学广笔记》）：芦荟　朱砂
[132] 妙香散（《沈氏尊生书》）：山药　茯苓　茯神　远志　黄芪　人参　桔梗　甘草　木香　辰砂　麝香
[133] 连朴饮（《霍乱论》）：制厚朴　黄连　石菖蒲　制半夏　香豉　焦山栀　芦根
[134] 连理汤（《张氏医通》）：人参　白术　干姜　炙甘草　黄连　茯苓
[135] 吴茱萸汤（《伤寒论》）：吴茱萸　人参　生姜　大枣
[136] 沉香降气散（《张氏医通》）：沉香　砂仁　甘草　香附　川楝子　延胡索
[137] 沉香散（《金匮翼》）：沉香　石韦　滑石　当归　橘皮　白芍　冬葵子　甘草　王不留行
[138] 沙参麦冬汤（《温病条辨》）：沙参　麦冬　玉竹　桑叶　甘草　天花粉　生扁豆
[139] 良附丸（《良方集腋》）：高良姜　香附
[140] 补中益气汤（《脾胃论》）：人参　黄芪　白术　甘草　当归　陈皮　升麻　柴胡
[141] 补阳还五汤（《医林改错》）：当归尾　川芎　黄芪　桃仁　地龙　赤芍　红花
[142] 补肝汤（《医宗金鉴》）：当归　白芍　川芎　熟地　酸枣仁　木瓜　炙甘草
[143] 补肺汤（《永类钤方》）：人参　黄芪　熟地　五味子　紫菀　桑白皮
[144] 牡蛎散（《太平惠民和剂局方》）：煅牡蛎　黄芪　麻黄根　浮小麦
[145] 身痛逐瘀汤（《医林改错》）：秦艽　川芎　桃仁　红花　甘草　羌活　没药　香附　五灵脂　牛膝　地龙　当归
[146] 附子理中丸（《太平惠民和剂局方》）：炮附子　人参　白术　炮姜　炙甘草

八　画

[147] 青娥丸（《太平惠民和剂局方》）：补骨脂　杜仲　胡桃肉　大蒜头
[148] 青麟丸（《邵氏经验良方》）：大黄20斤，用鲜侧柏叶　绿豆芽　黄豆芽　槐枝　桑叶　桃叶　柳叶　车前　鲜茴香　陈皮　荷叶　银花　苏叶　冬术　艾叶　半夏　厚朴　黄芩　香附　砂仁　甘草　泽泻　猪苓　煎汤蒸制，研末，牛乳　苏叶　梨汁　姜汁　童便　陈酒和丸
[149] 苓甘五味姜辛汤（《金匮要略》）：茯苓　甘草　五味子　干姜　细辛
[150] 苓桂术甘汤（《金匮要略》）：茯苓　桂枝　白术　甘草
[151] 虎潜丸（《丹溪心法》）：龟版　黄柏　知母　熟地黄　白芍药　锁阳　陈皮　虎骨　干姜
[152] 河车大造丸（《扶寿精方》）：紫河车　熟地黄　杜仲　天冬　麦冬　龟版　黄柏　牛膝
[153] 泻心汤（《金匮要略》）：大黄　黄芩　黄连
[154] 泻白散（《小儿药证直诀》）：桑白皮　地骨皮　生甘草　粳米
[155] 羌活胜湿汤（《内外伤辨惑论》）：羌活　独活　川芎　蔓荆子　甘草　防风　藁本
[156] 定志丸（《备急千金要方》）：党参　茯神　石菖蒲　远志　甘草汤泡，一方有茯苓　白术　麦冬
[157] 定痫丸（《医学心悟》）：天麻　川贝　胆南星　姜半夏

[158] 定喘汤（《摄生众妙方》）：白果　麻黄　桑白皮　款冬花　半夏　杏仁　苏子　黄芩　甘草

[159] 实脾饮（《济生方》）：附子　干姜　白术　甘草　厚朴　木香　草果　槟榔　木瓜　生姜　大枣　茯苓

[160] 知柏地黄丸（《医宗金鉴》）：知母　黄柏　熟地黄　山萸肉　山药　茯苓　丹皮　泽泻

[161] 金水六君煎（《景岳全书》）：当归　熟地黄　陈皮　半夏　茯苓　炙甘草　生姜

[162] 金铃子散（《素问病机气宜保命集》）：金铃子　延胡索

[163] 金匮肾气丸（《金匮要略》）：桂枝　附子　熟地黄　山萸肉　山药　茯苓　丹皮　泽泻

[164] 金锁固精丸（《医方集解》）：沙苑蒺藜　芡实　莲须　龙骨　牡蛎　莲肉

[165] 炙甘草汤（《伤寒论》）：炙甘草　人参　桂枝　生姜　阿胶　生地黄　麦冬　火麻仁　大枣

[166] 驻车丸（《备急千金要方》）：黄连　阿胶　当归　干姜

[167] 参附汤（《妇人良方》）：人参　熟附子　姜　枣

[168] 参苏饮（《太平惠民和剂局方》）：人参　苏叶　葛根　前胡　法半夏　茯苓　橘红　甘草　桔梗　枳壳　木通　陈皮　姜　枣

[169] 参苓白术散（《太平惠民和剂局方》）：人参　茯苓　白术　桔梗　山药　甘草　白扁豆　莲子肉　砂仁　薏苡仁

[170] 参蛤散（《济生方》）：人参　蛤蚧

九　画

[171] 春泽汤（《医方集解》）：白术　桂枝　猪苓　泽泻　茯苓　人参

[172] 枳实导滞丸（《内外伤辨惑论》）：大黄　枳实　黄芩　黄连　神曲　白术　茯苓　泽泻

[173] 荆防败毒散（《外科理例》）：荆芥　防风　羌活　独活　柴胡　前胡　川芎　枳壳　茯苓　桔梗　甘草

[174] 茯苓甘草汤（《伤寒论》）：茯苓　桂枝　炙甘草　生姜

[175] 茵陈五苓散（《金匮要略》）：茵陈蒿　桂枝　茯苓　白术　泽泻　猪苓

[176] 茵陈术附汤（《医学心悟》）：茵陈蒿　白术　附子　干姜　肉桂　炙甘草

[177] 茵陈蒿汤（《伤寒论》）：茵陈蒿　山栀　大黄

[178] 茜根散（《景岳全书》）：茜草根　黄芩　阿胶　侧柏叶　生地黄　甘草

[179] 指迷茯苓丸（《全生指迷方》）：茯苓　枳壳　半夏　风化硝　生姜

[180] 拯阳理劳汤（《医宗必读》）：人参　黄芪　肉桂　当归　白术　甘草　陈皮　五味子　生姜　大枣

[181] 牵正散（《杨氏家藏方》）：白附子　僵蚕　全蝎

[182] 胃苓汤（《丹溪心法》）：苍术　厚朴　陈皮　甘草　生姜　大枣　桂枝　白术　泽泻　茯苓　猪苓

[183] 济川煎（《景岳全书》）：当归　牛膝　肉苁蓉　泽泻　升麻　枳壳

[184] 济生肾气丸（《济生方》）：地黄　山药　山茱萸　丹皮　茯苓　泽泻　炮附子　桂枝　牛膝　车前子
[185] 养心汤（《证治准绳》）：黄芪　茯苓　茯神　当归　川芎　炙甘草　半夏曲　柏子仁　远志　五味子　人参　肉桂　酸枣仁
[186] 神术散（《医学心悟》）：苍术　陈皮　厚朴　甘草　藿香　砂仁
[187] 神犀丹（《温热经纬》）：犀角　石菖蒲　黄芩　生地黄　银花　金汁　连翘　板蓝根　豆豉　玄参　紫草　天花粉
[188] 香附旋覆花汤（《温病条辨》）：生香附　旋覆花　苡仁　半夏　橘皮　茯苓　苏子霜
[189] 香砂六君子汤（《时方歌括》）：木香　砂仁　陈皮　半夏　党参　白术　茯苓　甘草
[190] 复元活血汤（《医学发明》）：柴胡　栝楼根　当归　红花　甘草　穿山甲　大黄　桃仁
[191] 顺气导痰汤（验方）：半夏　陈皮　茯苓　甘草　生姜　胆星　枳实　木香　香附
[192] 保元汤（《情爱心鉴》）：人参　黄芪　肉桂　甘草　生姜
[193] 保和丸（《丹溪心法》）：神曲　山楂　茯苓　半夏　陈皮　连翘　莱菔子
[194] 独参汤（《景岳全书》）：人参
[195] 独活寄生汤（《备急千金要方》）：独活　桑寄生　秦艽　防风　细辛　当归　芍药　川芎　干地黄　杜仲　牛膝　人参　茯苓　甘草　桂心
[196] 追虫丸（《证治准绳》）：槟榔　雷丸　南木香　苦楝根　皂荚　黑丑　茵陈

十　画

[197] 秦艽鳖甲散（《卫生宝鉴》）：地骨皮　柴胡　秦艽　知母　当归　鳖甲　青蒿　乌梅
[198] 真人养脏汤（《证治准绳》）：诃子　罂粟壳　肉豆蔻　白术　人参　木香　官桂　炙甘草　生姜　大枣
[199] 真武汤（《伤寒论》）：炮附子　白术　茯苓　芍药　生姜
[200] 桂枝汤（《伤寒论》）：桂枝　芍药　生姜　炙甘草　大枣
[201] 桂枝甘草龙骨牡蛎汤（《伤寒论》）：桂枝　炙甘草　龙骨　牡蛎
[202] 桂枝加附子汤（《伤寒论》）：桂枝　芍药　炙甘草　生姜　大枣　附子
[203] 桂枝芍药知母汤（《金匮要略》）：桂枝　芍药　炙甘草　麻黄　白术　知母　防风　炮附子　生姜
[204] 桃红饮（《类证治裁》）：桃仁　红花　川芎　当归尾　威灵仙
[205] 桃花汤（《伤寒论》）：赤石脂　干姜　粳米
[206] 桃仁红花煎（《素庵医案》）：丹参　赤芍　桃仁　红花　制香附　延胡索　青皮　当归　川芎　生地
[207] 栝楼桂枝汤（《金匮要略》）：栝楼根　桂枝　芍药　甘草　生姜　大枣
[208] 栝楼薤白半夏汤（《金匮要略》）：栝楼　薤白　白酒　半夏

[209] 栝楼薤白白酒汤（《金匮要略》）：栝楼　薤白　白酒
[210] 栝楼薤白桂枝汤（《金匮要略》）：栝楼　薤白　桂枝　厚朴　枳实
[211] 柴胡疏肝散（《景岳全书》）：柴胡　枳壳　芍药　甘草　香附　川芎
[212] 柴枳半夏汤（《医学入门》）：柴胡　黄芩　半夏　枳壳　桔梗　杏仁　栝楼仁　青皮　甘草
[213] 凉膈散（《太平惠民和剂局方》）：川大黄　朴硝　甘草　山栀子仁　薄荷　黄芩　连翘
[214] 润肠丸（《沈氏尊生书》）：当归　生地　麻仁　桃仁　枳壳
[215] 涤痰汤（《济生方》）：制半夏　制南星　陈皮　枳实　茯苓　人参　石菖蒲　竹茹　甘草　生姜
[216] 消渴方（《丹溪心法》）：黄连末　天花粉末　生地汁　藕汁　人乳汁　姜汁　蜂蜜
[217] 益胃汤（《温病条辨》）：沙参　麦冬　生地黄　玉竹　冰糖
[218] 调胃承气汤（《伤寒论》）：大黄　芒硝　炙甘草
[219] 调营饮（《证治准绳》）：莪术　川芎　当归　延胡索　赤芍药　瞿麦　大黄　槟榔　陈皮　大腹皮　葶苈　赤茯苓　桑白皮　细辛　官桂　白芷　炙甘草　姜　枣
[220] 秘精丸（《济生方》）：菟丝子　家韭子　牡蛎　龙骨　桑螵蛸　茯苓　五味子　白石脂
[221] 射干麻黄汤（《金匮要略》）：射干　麻黄　细辛　紫菀　款冬花　半夏　五味子　生姜　大枣
[222] 逍遥散（《太平惠民和剂局方》）：柴胡　白术　白芍药　当归　茯苓　炙甘草　薄荷　煨姜
[223] 通窍活血汤（《医林改错》）：赤芍药　川芎　桃仁　红花　麝香　老葱　鲜姜　大枣　酒
[224] 通瘀煎（《景岳全书》）：当归尾　山楂　香附　红花　乌药　青皮　木香　泽泻
[225] 桑白皮汤（《景岳全书》）：桑白皮　半夏　苏子　杏仁　贝母　黄芩　黄连　栀子
[226] 桑杏汤（《温病条辨》）：桑叶　杏仁　沙参　浙贝母　豆豉　山栀　梨皮
[227] 桑菊饮（《温病条辨》）：桑叶　菊花　连翘　薄荷　桔梗　杏仁　芦根　甘草
[228] 桑螵蛸散（《本草衍义》）：桑螵蛸　远志　菖蒲　龙骨　人参　茯神　当归　龟版

十一　画

[229] 理中丸（《伤寒论》）：人参　白术　干姜　炙甘草
[230] 黄土汤（《金匮要略》）：灶心黄土　甘草　干地黄　白术　炮附子　阿胶　黄芩
[231] 黄连阿胶汤（《伤寒论》）：黄连　阿胶　黄芩　鸡子黄　芍药
[232] 黄连清心饮（《沈氏尊生书》）：黄连　生地黄　当归　甘草　酸枣仁　茯神　远志　人参　莲子肉
[233] 黄连温胆汤（《千金方》）：半夏　陈皮　茯苓　甘草　枳实　竹茹　黄连　大枣
[234] 黄芪汤（《金匮翼》）：黄芪　陈皮　火麻仁　白蜜
[235] 黄芪建中汤（《金匮要略》）：黄芪　白芍　桂枝　炙甘草　生姜　大枣　饴糖
[236] 黄病绛矾丸(验方)：厚朴　茅术　陈皮　甘草　绛矾　红枣

[237] 栀子豉汤（《伤寒论》）：栀子　豆豉

[238] 控涎丹（《三因极一病证方论》）：甘遂　大戟　白芥子

[239] 鹿茸丸（《沈氏尊生书》）：鹿茸　麦冬　熟地黄　黄芪　五味子　肉苁蓉　鸡内金　山萸肉　人参　牛膝　补骨脂　玄参　茯苓　地骨皮

[240] 麻子仁丸（《伤寒论》）：麻子仁　芍药　炙枳实　大黄　炙厚朴　杏仁

[241] 麻杏石甘汤（《伤寒论》）：麻黄　杏仁　石膏　炙甘草

[242] 麻黄汤（《伤寒论》）：麻黄　桂枝　杏仁　炙甘草

[243] 麻黄连翘赤小豆汤（《伤寒论》）：麻黄　杏仁　生梓白皮　连翘　赤小豆　甘草　生姜　大枣

[244] 旋覆代赭汤（《伤寒论》）：旋覆花　代赭石　人参　半夏　炙甘草　生姜　大枣

[245] 旋覆花汤（《金匮要略》）：旋覆花　新绛　葱

[246] 羚羊角汤（《医醇賸义》）：羚羊角　龟版　生地　丹皮　白芍　柴胡　薄荷　蝉衣　菊花　夏枯草　石决明

[247] 羚羊钩藤汤（《通俗伤寒论》）：羚羊角　桑叶　川贝　鲜生地　钩藤　菊花　白芍药　生甘草　鲜竹茹　茯神

[248] 清金化痰汤（《统旨方》）：黄芩　山栀　桔梗　麦冬　桑白皮　贝母　知母　栝楼仁　橘红　茯苓　甘草

[249] 清肺饮（《证治汇补》）：茯苓　黄芩　桑白皮　麦冬　车前子　山栀　木通

[250] 清胃散（《兰室秘藏》）：当归　生地黄　牡丹皮　升麻　黄连

[251] 清骨散（《证治准绳》）：银柴胡　胡黄连　秦艽　鳖甲　地骨皮　青蒿　知母　甘草

[252] 清营汤（《温病条辨》）：犀角　生地黄　元参　竹叶心　麦冬　丹参　黄连　银花　连翘

[253] 清瘟败毒饮（《疫疹一得》）：生石膏　小生地　乌犀角　真川连　栀子　桔梗　黄芩　知母　赤芍　玄参　连翘　甘草　丹皮　鲜竹叶

[254] 清燥救肺汤（《医门法律》）：桑叶　石膏　杏仁　甘草　麦冬　人参　阿胶　炒胡麻仁　炙枇杷叶

[255] 银翘散（《温病条辨》）：金银花　连翘　豆豉　牛蒡子　薄荷　桔梗　荆芥穗　甘草　竹叶　鲜芦根

[256] 猪肚丸（《金匮翼》）：白术　苦参　牡蛎　猪肚

[257] 猪苓汤（《伤寒论》）：猪苓　茯苓　泽泻　阿胶　滑石

十二画

[258] 斑龙丸（《景岳全书》）：熟地黄　菟丝子　补骨脂　柏子仁　茯苓　鹿角胶　鹿角霜

[259] 葛根汤（《伤寒论》）：葛根　麻黄　桂枝　生姜　甘草　芍药　大枣

[260] 葛根芩连汤（《伤寒论》）：葛根　黄芩　黄连　炙甘草

[261] 葶苈大枣泻肺汤（《金匮要略》）：葶苈子　大枣

[262] 越婢加术汤（《金匮要略》）：麻黄　石膏　甘草　大枣　白术　生姜

[263] 越婢加半夏汤（《金匮要略》）：麻黄　石膏　生姜　大枣　甘草　半夏
[264] 越鞠丸（《丹溪心法》）：川芎　苍术　香附　炒山栀　神曲
[265] 椒目栝楼汤（《医醇賸义》）：川椒目　栝楼仁　葶苈子　桑白皮　苏子　半夏　茯苓　橘红　蒺藜　生姜
[266] 硝石矾石散（《金匮要略》）：硝石　矾石
[267] 紫雪丹（《太平惠民和剂局方》）：滑石　石膏　寒水石　磁石　羚羊角　青木香　犀角　沉香　丁香　升麻　玄参　甘草　朴硝　朱砂　麝香　黄金　硝石
[268] 黑锡丹（《太平惠民和剂局方》）：黑锡　硫黄　川楝子　葫芦巴　木香　炮附子　肉豆蔻　阳起石　沉香　茴香　肉桂　补骨脂
[269] 痛泻要方（《景岳全书》引刘草窗方）：白术　白芍　防风　炒陈皮
[270] 温胆汤（《备急千金要方》）：半夏　橘皮　甘草　枳实　竹茹　生姜　茯苓
[271] 滋水清肝饮（《医宗已任篇》）：生地黄　山茱萸　茯苓　当归身　山药　丹皮　泽泻　白芍　柴胡　山栀　酸枣仁
[272] 程氏萆薢分清饮（《医学心悟》）：萆薢　车前子　茯苓　莲子心　菖蒲　黄柏　丹参　白术
[273] 犀角地黄汤（《备急千金要方》）：犀角　生地黄　丹皮　芍药
[274] 犀角散（《备急千金要方》）：犀角　黄连　升麻　山栀　茵陈
[275] 疏凿饮子（《世医得效方》）：商陆　泽泻　赤小豆　椒目　木通　茯苓皮　大腹皮　槟榔　生姜　羌活　秦艽

十三画

[276] 蒿芩清胆汤（《重订通俗伤寒论》）：青蒿　淡竹茹　仙半夏　赤茯苓　黄芩　生枳壳　陈广皮　碧玉散（滑石　甘草　青黛）
[277] 暖肝煎（《景岳全书》）：肉桂　小茴香　茯苓　乌药　枸杞子　当归　沉香　生姜
[278] 新加香薷饮（《温病条辨》）：香薷　鲜扁豆花　厚朴　金银花　连翘
[279] 解语丹（《医学心悟》）：白附子　石菖蒲　远志　天麻　全蝎　羌活　南星　木香　甘草

十四画

[280] 酸枣仁汤（《金匮要略》）：酸枣仁　知母　川芎　茯苓　甘草
[281] 膏淋汤（《医学衷中参西录》）：山药　芡实　龙骨　牡蛎　生地黄　党参　白芍
[282] 膈下逐瘀汤（《医林改错》）：五灵脂　当归　川芎　桃仁　丹皮　赤芍药　乌药　延胡索　甘草　香附　红花　枳壳

十五画以上

[283] 增液汤（《温病条辨》）：玄参　麦冬　生地
[284] 增液承气汤（《温病条辨》）：大黄　芒硝　玄参　麦冬　生地黄
[285] 薏苡仁汤（《类证治裁》）：薏苡仁　川芎　当归　麻黄　桂枝　羌活　独活　防风　川乌　苍术　甘草　生姜

[286] 橘皮竹茹汤（《金匮要略》）：人参　橘皮　竹茹　甘草　生姜　大枣

[287] 黛蛤散（验方）：青黛　海蛤壳

[288] 藿香正气散（《太平惠民和剂局方》）：藿香　紫苏　白芷　桔梗　白术　厚朴　半夏曲　大腹皮　茯苓　橘皮　甘草　大枣

[289] 礞石滚痰丸（《养生主论》）：青礞石　沉香　大黄　黄芩　朴硝

[290] 鳖甲煎丸（《金匮要略》）：鳖甲　乌扇　黄芩　柴胡　鼠妇　干姜　大黄　芍药　桂枝　葶苈子　石韦　厚朴　丹皮　瞿麦　紫葳　半夏　人参　䗪虫　阿胶　蜂房　赤硝　蜣螂　桃仁

[291] 镇肝熄风汤（《医学衷中参西录》）：怀牛膝　龙骨　生白芍　天冬　麦芽　代赭石　牡蛎　玄参　川楝子　茵陈蒿　甘草　龟版

2. 西医病名索引

一画

一过性脑缺血	(71)

三画

三叉神经痛	(78)
上呼吸道感染	(37)(38)
门脉性肝硬化	(137)
习惯性便秘	(115)

四画

支气管扩张	(37)(137)
支气管炎	(37)
支气管肺癌	(137)
支气管哮喘	(41)
不完全性幽门梗阻	(50)
中毒性痢疾	(112)
手足搐搦症	(75)
风湿性心脏病	(63)
风湿性关节炎	(165)
风湿热	(55)(171)
风湿病	(156)
心因性反应	(92)
心肌病	(63)
心肌梗死	(64)
心律失常	(59)
心绞痛	(64)
心脏神经官能症	(59)(63)
心源性水肿	(145)
心源性休克	(67)
心源性哮喘	(41)

五画

甲状腺功能亢进	(55)(59)(159)(171)
甲状腺功能减退	(175)
出血性休克	(67)

六画

老年性便秘	(115)
老年性眩晕	(82)
耳性眩晕	(102)
再生障碍性贫血	(137)(175)
肋间神经炎	(124)
休克	(55)
血小板减少性紫癜	(137)
血吸虫病	(111)
血管抑制性晕厥	(67)
血管性头痛	(78)
多发性神经炎	(168)
充血性心力衰竭	(50)(59)
肌营养不良症	(168)

七　画

更年期综合征	(55)(88)
更年期精神病	(92)
肝脓疡	(124)
肝寄生虫病	(124)
肝硬化	(124)(130)
肝硬化腹水	(133)
肝脾肿大	(130)
肝癌	(124)
肠扭转	(130)
肠梗阻	(130)
肠套叠	(130)
肠神经官能症	(104)
肠系膜及腹膜病	(121)
低血糖	(55)(59)
低血糖休克	(68)
低血压	(82)
饮食性便秘	(115)
进行性肌萎缩	(168)
尿毒症	(105)
尿崩症	(159)
阿米巴痢疾	(111)
阿狄森病	(175)

八　画

青光眼	(78)
枕神经痛	(78)
矽肺	(47)
直肠癌	(111)
肾小球肾炎	(137)
肾功能不全	(153)
肾肿瘤	(137)
肾结核	(137)
肾病综合征	(133)(145)
周围性面神经麻痹	(71)
周期性麻痹	(168)
食管炎	(105)
贫血	(59)(78)(82)(175)
贫血性失眠	(85)
乳糜尿	(149)
肩关节周围炎	(165)
泌尿系肿瘤	(149)
泌尿系结石	(149)
泌尿系结核	(149)
泌尿系梗阻	(153)
泌尿系感染	(149)
细菌性痢疾	(111)

九　画

胃下垂	(97)
胃及十二指肠溃疡	(97)
胃扩张	(105)
胃肠功能紊乱	(50)
胃肠型流行性感冒	(102)
胃肠神经官能症	(97)(104)(107)(121)(130)
胃肠痉挛	(121)
胃炎	(101)
胃粘膜脱垂症	(97)
胃癌	(97)(137)
肺不张	(45)
肺心病	(45)
肺气肿	(41)(45)
肺性脑病	(67)
肺炎	(37)(137)
肺结核	(37)(45)(137)
胆石症	(124)(127)
胆道蛔虫病	(124)
胆囊炎	(124)(127)
咽喉炎	(37)
姜片虫病	(118)
前列腺炎	(149)(162)
药物中毒性肝损伤	(127)
骨性关节炎	(165)
冠心病	(63)
幽门梗阻	(50)(130)
钩虫病	(118)

钩端螺旋体病	(127)	脑震荡后遗症	(78)
盆腔疾病	(156)	胰腺炎	(121)
重症肌无力	(168)	胸膜炎	(50)(63)
急性白血病	(137)	绦虫病	(118)
急性肝炎	(124)		
急性肾炎	(145)	十一 画	
急性胃炎	(97)(101)	梅尼埃病	(82)
急性胆囊炎	(124)	渗出性胸膜炎	(50)
急性腰部扭伤	(156)	黄疸型传染性单核细胞增多症	(127)
急性胰腺炎	(121)	黄疸型病毒性肝炎	(127)
急性肠炎	(107)	粘连性肠梗阻	(121)
急性脊髓炎	(168)	粘液性水肿	(145)
结肠过敏	(111)		
结肠炎	(121)	十二 画	
结肠癌	(111)	痛风	(165)
结核性脑膜炎	(75)	植物神经功能紊乱	(55)
结核性腹膜炎	(133)	喘息性支气管炎	(41)
结核病	(55)(171)	腔隙性脑梗塞	(71)
类风湿性关节炎	(165)	蛛网膜下隙出血	(71)
神经功能性低热	(171)	蛔虫病	(118)
神经官能症	(78)(82)(88)(92)(162)	蛲虫病	(118)
		强直性脊柱炎	(156)
十 画			
		十三 画	
高血压性失眠	(85)		
高血压性脑溢血	(71)	瘀胆型肝炎	(127)
高血压病	(78)(82)	腰肌劳损	(156)
高血压脑病	(67)	腰椎间盘突出	(156)
高热惊厥	(75)	腰椎肿瘤	(156)
席汉综合征	(175)	腰椎骨质增生	(156)
病毒性心肌炎	(59)(63)	腰椎结核	(156)
恶性肿瘤所致发热	(171)	腹腔肿瘤	(130)
流行性乙型脑炎	(75)		
流行性脑脊髓膜炎	(75)	十四 画	
流行性感冒	(33)(38)(78)	慢性支气管炎	(45)(50)
消化不良性失眠	(85)	慢性肝炎	(124)
脑血管痉挛	(67)	慢性肾炎	(145)
脑血栓形成	(71)	慢性肠炎	(107)
脑肿瘤	(75)(78)	慢性非特异性溃疡性结肠炎	(107)(111)
脑栓塞	(71)	慢性胆囊炎	(124)

慢性胃炎	(97)(101)	精神性烦渴	(159)
慢性萎缩性胃炎	(99)(103)	精神神经性便秘	(115)
慢性粒细胞性白血病	(175)		
慢性喘息性支气管炎	(41)	**十五画以上**	
慢性感染性发热	(171)	糖尿病	(159)
慢性缩窄性心包炎	(133)	癔病性昏厥	(67)
鼻窦炎	(78)	癔病性喘息	(45)
精神分裂症	(92)	躁狂抑郁症	(92)
精神性呕吐	(101)	癫痫	(95)

General Programme

1 Introduction

1.1 The Definition and Scope of TCM Internal Medicine

TCM internal medicine is a clinical branch which, in accordance with TCM theories, expounds internal diseases, their etiology and pathogenesis and the laws of diagnosis and treatment. It reflects distinctive theoretical feature of TCM and has clear superiority in clinical practice of TCM, thus occupying an important place in TCM.

TCM internal medicine covers a wide scope of treatment. In TCM theory, diseases are classified into two main groups: diseases due to exopathogens and diseases caused by internal injury. The former mainly refers to such febrile diseases as typhoid, wind-warm syndrome, summer fever, damp-warm syndrome which were discussed in *Shang Han Lun* (Treatise on Febrile Diseases) and *Wen Bing Xue* (Doctrine of Epidemic Febrile Diseases). These diseases are syndromically classified in terms of the pathological changes of the six meridians, *wei*, *qi*, *ying* and *xue*, and *san-jiao*. The latter includes those of the *zang-fu* organs as well as the meridians and callaterals discussed in *Jin Gui Yao Lue* (Synopsis of Prescriptions of the Golden Chamber). The differentiation of the syndromes and the selection of the treatment of these diseases are made in light of the etiological theory about and the pathological changes of the *zang* and *fu*, *qi*, blood and body fluid, and the meridians and collaterals. Diseases due to exopathy and diseases caused by internal injury are different, but are related to each other at the same time. It is in this wide field and with the aid of TCM theory that TCM internal medicine deals with the causes, the mechanism, the diagnostic and therapeutic principles and methods of these diseases. In this book, a discussion is made mainly about the diseases caused by internal injury.

1.2 The Characteristics of TCM Internal Medicine

TCM internal medicine concentratively and prominently embodies the characteristics of the theoretical and practical systems of TCM. As a medical branch studying life phenomena, revealing the course of illness, exploring the therapeutic mechanism and trying to find the way to keep in good health and prevent disease, TCM has shown its peculiarity compared with the traditional medicine of some other regions and nationalities, and the modern Western Medicine as well.

TCM regards the human body as an organic whole, in which *zang-fu* and the body surface are coorperative, mental activities and the human body's physiology and pathology have effect on one another. Meanwhile, it also stresses that life activity is closely related to the natural and social environments and it looks upon life process and the course of illness as synthetical, macroscopical and dynamical. This is one of TCM's main characteristics known as the holistic concept. Such a holistic medical model is as scientifically advanced as biological – psychological – sociological model of modern Western Medicine, but the former came into being more than 2000 years earlier. TCM takes the essence of ancient Chinese philosophy —— the *yin – yang* theory, the five – element theory and the theory of correspondence between man and universe —— as its basic guiding ideology, with the theoretical system of selecting treatment by differentiating syndromes (STDS) embodying the gist of dialectic materialism. TCM internal medicine carries out such theoretical system and guiding ideology in clinical practice, thus reflecting the characteristics of TCM and its superiority.

1.2.1 Adhering to Pathogenesis and Searching for the Primary Causes of Disease in Treatment

Pathogenesis means the mechanism and regularity of the occurrence, the development and the changes of a disease. TCM theory holds that the development of pathogenesis reflects the nature of a disease and the state of human constitution as being excess or deficiency of *yin* or *yang*. Therefore, TCM attaches great importance to the strict adherence of pathogenesis in STDS.

There are various diseases which are of various clinical symptoms and, besides, the individual differences are notable. So diseases manifest themselves quite differently under pathological conditions. The symptoms are dispersive and local on most occasions and at a certain stage of illness some false appearance is likely to occur. That is why TCM objects to "treating the head when the head aches, treating the foot when the foot aches", but advocates grasping the syndrome, making a comprehensive analysis of the pathogenesis and tracing to its source, i. e., searching for the primary causes of a disease in treatment.

Every disease has different types of syndrome, and every syndrome is of its own pathogenesis. But, from the point of view of TCM theory, they can be summarized as three patterns. They are the excess or deficiency of the vital *qi* and the pathogenic factor, the imbalance of *yin* and *yang*, and the abnormality of *qi* and blood. In clinical practice, however intricately and unusually the patient's illness manifests itself, the goal of searching for the primary cause of the disease in treatment can certainly be attained as long as the doctor makes a clear distinction of the syndrome and strictly adheres to the pathogenesis.

The Excess or Deficiency of Vital – *qi* and the Pathogenic Factor

TCM pathogenic theory holds that, the pathogenic factor can not invade in when the vital *qi* is sufficient inside the body and that intrusion of the pathogenic factor certainly results from insufficiency of vital *qi*. The contrast of the forces and the struggle between the vital *qi* and the pathogenic factor are the basic causes of the development and conversion of illness. Hyperactivity of the pathogenic factor is certain to damage the vital *qi* and, therefore, the illness gets worse; wheras the illness will abate if the vital *qi* is strong enough to drive the pathogenic factor out of the body. So in differentiating syndrome and selecting treatment, it is the first priority to make a contrast between the vital *qi* and the pathogenic factor at a definite stage of an illness so as to decide whether the therapy of eliminating the pathogenic factor or strengthening the vital *qi* or the combination of both should be carried out.

The excess or deficiency of vital *qi* and pathogenic factor leads directly to the change of the nature of a disease. Hyperactivity of the pathogen will cause excess syndrome, i. e. hyperactivity of the pathogenic factor is the principal aspect of the pathological process. Exhaustion of essence *qi* brings about deficiency syndrome, which means that the overconsumption of the vital *qi* (*yin* and *yang*, *qi*, blood and body fluid) is the principal aspect during the process of disease. Excess – syndrome, deficiency – syndrome and excess in combination with deficiency syndrome are often found in TCM internal medicine. Syndromes mainly caused by overactivity of pathogenic factors are stagnation of phlegm, retention of indigested food, retention of water within the body, accumulation of blood stasis, overactivity of pathogenic heat, and obstruction of *fu* – *qi*, etc.. On the contrary, such syndromes as insufficient formation of *qi* and blood or their overconsumption, dysfunctions of the *zang* – *fu* organs, insufficient production of body fluid, hypoactivities of the channels and collaterals, etc. are all caused by the deficiency of vital *qi*. It is also worth noticing that the contrast of forces between vital *qi* and pathogenic factor runs through the whole process of illness, but manifests itself in different ways at various stages. Besides, illness itself results from the struggle between the vital *qi* and the pathogenic factor. Therefore in clinical practice, there is no pure deficiency – syndrome or excess – syndrome. Both of them are merely relative, not absolute. What must be emphasized is the principal aspect of the contradiction.

The excess or deficiency of vital *qi* and pathogenic factor during the illness is likely to cause false appearance, i.e., the symptoms are different from the nature of the disease. Cases in point are "appearance of deficiency in extreme excess" and "symptoms of excess in extreme deficiency". Deficiency in reality with pseudo – excess symptoms and excess in reality with pseudo – deficiency symptoms often occur at the critical stage of an illness. So the doctor must be expert at analysing the pathogenesis, mastering the nature, clarifying the false appearances and searching for the primary cause of the disease in treatment.

Imbalance between *yin* and *yang*

It is believed with TCM that *yin* and *yang* in equilibrium is the summary of a healthy mechanism. However, various pathogenic factors can cause *yin* and *yang* in the body to wane or wax so that the relative dynamic balance between *yin* and *yang* is destroyed, thus leading to the relative excessiveness or deficiency of *yin* or *yang*, or separation of *yin* and *yang* and further bringing about illness, or even deterioration of illness. So *yin* and *yang* are the internal cause of the occurrence and development of a disease and the imbalance between *yin* and *yang* is an important part of the pathogenesis theory of TCM. Life is dependent upon the body which can never for a moment separate from *yin - yang*. *Yin - yang* imbalance is a summary of the pathological relationships of the imbalances between *zang -* and *fu -* organs, channels and collaterals, *qi* and blood, and *ying* and *wei*, etc., and it shows the nature of the functional and organic pathological changes that take place in the course of life.

Yin - yang imbalance involves all the pathological changes in the body and, therefore, manifests itself in complicated ways, which, in general, can be summed up as follows.

① Relative execess of *yin* and *yang*.

Hyperactivity and overabundance of heat are known as excess of *yang*, which can lead to heat syndromes of excess type caused by the five emotions, the six pathogenic factors (i.e. wind, cold, summer - heat, dampness, dryness and fire), stagnancy of *qi* and blood stasis or dyspepsia. While the excess of *yin* means the relative excessiveness of *yin* pathogen shown in the pathological changes of the body manifested as functional disorders and overabundance of cold. The excess of *yin* is often found in such cold syndromes of excess type caused by the direct attack of pathogenic cold and its accumulation in the spleen and stomach or due to too much intake of cold or raw food, etc..

As *yin* and *yang* are interdependent, an excess of *yin* is certain to lead to deficiency of *yang*, and deficiency of *yang - qi* in different degrees is often found in cold syndromes of excess type. Similarly, an excess of *yang* will lead to deficiency of *yin*, and the body fluid is consumed by heat syndromes of excess type. However, the excess of *yin* or *yang* is the principal aspect of the pathogenesis.

② Relative deficiency of *yin* and *yang*

This includes the deficiency of *yin* and that of *yang*. *Yang* deficiency refers to such pathological changes as the abatement of the organic functions of the body and the consumption of *yang - qi*, which, in most cases, is caused by congenital defect, lack of proper nourishment after birth, internal injury due to over - exertion, and exhaustion due to prolonged illness. *Yang* deficiency causes relative *yin -* excess, so *yang* insufficiency will result in endogenous cold - syndrome, manifesting itself in deficiency - cold syndromes like intolerance of cold with cold extermities, and mental fatigue. *Yin* deficiency means the loss of *yin -* blood, body fluid and essence within the body, and the consequent abatement of the moistening and nourishing functions. In the case of *yin* deficiency, *yang - qi* is out of control and becomes relatively excessive. So deficiency of *yin* brings about interior heat - syndrome, manifesting itself in such deficient heat - syndromes as dysphoria with feverish sensation in the chest, palms and soles, steaming sensation in the bone with hectic fever, night sweat and dry throat.

The theory of *yin - yang* interdependence also suggests that the deficiency of *yin* affects *yang* and vice versa, and, therefore, a pathological state of the deficiency of both *yin* and *yang* is likely to be caused. In this case, the doctor must master the nature of the illness and select treatment in accordance with the cause. In addition, the *yin - yang* imbalance involves another special type of pathogenesis, namely, the inter - repellency between *yin* and *yang*, including two aspects: (1) *yang* being kept externally by *yin* - excess in the interior, and (2) *yin* being kept externally by *yang* - excess in the interior. The former clinically takes the form of cold syndrome with pseudo - heat symptoms, and the latter heat syndrome with pseudo - cold symptoms. *Yin - yang* inter - repellency originates from the hyperactivity of *yin* (or *yang*) which exists inside the body and, in time, drives *yang* (or *yin*) out.

While the pathogenesis changes, the *yin - yang* imbalance reaches its critical stage -the exhaustion of both *yin* and *yang* which is caused by *yin* or *yang* depletion. *Yin* depletion results from the excessive consumption of *yin* - blood and body fluid, and *yang* depletion from the exhaustion of the body's *yang - qi* or its prostration, which consequently causes the seriously declined functions of the whole mechanism. In this case, any failure of prompt and proper treatment will cause the patient to end in " the dissociation of *yin* and *yang* leading to exhaustion of the essence *qi*".

Abnormality of *Qi* and Blood

The relationship between *qi* and blood of the human body is the same as that between *yin* and *yang*. *Qi* is a part of *yang* and plays the role of warming, representing the functions of *zang - fu* organs and the vital *qi* of the body. Blood is a part of *yin* and takes charge of moistening and nourishing, being the material nutrition for life activity. *Qi* and blood physiologically promote and transform each other. So the pathogenesis change of the abnormality of *qi* and blood involves not only *qi* deficiency, exhaustion of *qi* brought about by insufficient production or excessive consumption of *qi*, but also such *qi* disorders as stagnation, reversed flow, retention of *qi* caused by the abnormal movement of *qi*; not only blood - deficiency caused by insufficient production or excessive consumption of blood, but also blood stasis, hemorrhage due to blood - heat, etc. that are caused by the obstructed circulation of blood. Besides, as *qi* and blood are interrelated, the changes of pathogenesis often seen in clinical practice are blood stasis due to *qi* stagnation, blood stasis due to *qi* deficiency, failure in retaining blood due to *qi* deficiency, exhaustion of *qi* resulting from hemorrhage, deficiency of both *qi* and blood, and so on.

The abnormality of *qi* and blood is closely and directly connected with the functions of *zang - fu* organs. This is because the lung dominates *qi*; the heart is in charge of blood; the spleen is the source of *qi* and blood and controls the flow of blood; the liver stores blood and takes charge of the dispersing function; the kidney governs the reception of air and stores essence which shares a common source with blood. So the abnormality of *qi* and blood is certain to have something to do with the debility or disorder of the function of a certain *zang* or *fu* - organ. As for the pathogenesis of *qi* and blood or *zang - fu* organs, please refer to 2.3 and 2.4.

In brief, various clinical manifestations reflect multiple pathogenesis changes; still, it is quite possible for the doctor to get hold of the crux and find out the primary cause of disease in treatment so long as he/she has a sound understanding and mastery of such essential principles of pathogenesis as the excess or deficiency of vital *qi* and the pathogenic factor, the imbalance between *yin* and *yang*, and the abnormality of *qi* and blood.

1.2.2 Differentiation of Both Disease and Syndromes

The basic principle in understanding and treating disease is selecting treatment by differentiating syndromes (*Bianzheng Lunzhi*), which is also one of the notable characteristics of TCM internal medicine.

TCM internal medicine covers a wide scope. Differentiating syndromes (*Bianzheng*) means analysing and synthesizing the symptoms and signs and relative information collected by the four diagnostic methods, identifying the cause, the nature, the location and the degree of seriousness of the illness so that a conclusion about the syndrome is drawn. Selecting treatment (*Lunzhi*) means, on the basis of the differentiation of the syndrome and in accordance with the pathogenesis, determining therapeutic principle and method. Differentiating syndrome is the basis, the premise of selecting treatment, while treatment is, of course, the means of curing the patient of his/her illness. The process of selecing treatment by differentiating syndromes is the process of understanding and dealing with the illness. The two are interrelated and inseparable from each other, which incarnate the combination of theory with practice.

TCM differentiates not only diseases (*Bing*) but also syndromes (*Zheng*), *Bian Bing* and *Bian Zheng* in Chinese. Syndrome (*Zheng*) is a summary of the pathological changes at a definite stage of a certain disease. It involves the location, nature and cause of a disease, the relationship between vital *qi* and the pathogenic factor, and the changes of the excess or deficiency of *qi*, blood, *yin* and *yang*, and comprehensively, profoundly and accurately reveals the nature of the pathological changes at a definate stage of the development of the illness. Disease (*Bing*) is the name of illness, such as dysentery, asthma and dyspnea, apoplexy and *Xiao Ke*. By differentiating disease is meant discriminating one disease from another, while differentiating syndromes means distinguishing different types of syndromes of the same disease so that the treatment selected is all the more objective. Cold, for example, is a kind of disease, but it involves different types of syndromes: wind-cold or wind-heat exterior syndrome, both of which are a summary of some concrete pathological changes in the disease, that is, its location is in the exterior and its cause pertains to either wind-cold or wind-heat, and, therefore, it must be treated by relieving the exterior syndrome with drugs pungent in flavor and warm in property or with drugs pungent in flavor but cool in property. So it can be seen that selecting treatment by differentiating syndrome is, on the one hand, different from the method of treating the head when the head aches and treating the foot when the foot aches and, and on the other, different from the method of suiting one prescription to one disease without making a distinction between the primary and the secondary or the different stages of the illness.

To sum up, one of the characteristics of TCM internal medicine is the combination of differentiating disease with differentiating syndromes. TCM has adopted this principle ever since *Han* and *Tang* Dynasties on the basis of differentiating disease. To study TCM internal medicine well, it is essential to make a thorough study of the relationship between disease and syndrome. In TCM internal medicine, it is often the case that the diseases are named after the most important and notable symptoms, some of which can indicate the principal contradictions of the diseases, but others are too macroscopic or general. It is syndrome that provides a concrete and exact summarization of the pathological mechanism at a definite stage of the development of a disease, which is of great and practical significance to the diagnosis and treatment of the disease. That is why TCM pays special attention to the differentiation of the syndromes.

1.2.3 Treating the Same Disease with Different Methods, and Treating Different Diseases with the Same Method

Another characteristic of TCM internal medicine, which is based on the selecting treatment by differentiating syndrome and stresses the combination of differentiatig both disease and syndrome, is to treat the same disease with different methods and to treat different diseases with the same method.

The same disease refers to such a disease which, though suffered by different patients, takes similar main symptoms as its basic pathologic change. But the syndrome of the disease is certain to vary on account of the differences of the patients' constitutions, different degrees of the excess or deficienty of *yin* and *yang*, different times, seasons and places of occurrence and different stages of the pathological change during the illness. And this diversity of syndrome becomes the premise of treating the same disease with different methods because the characteristic and superiority of the selecting treatment by differentiating syndrome are chiefly embodied by "syndrome". While diagnosing and treating disease, TCM internal medicine focuses on the difference of the pathogenesis, i. e. the syndrome, rather than the disease itself. As TCM sees it, syndrome reflects the concrete pathogenic change and coincides with the pathogenic change, too.

Those who suffer from the same disease may possibly bear very different syndromes, and to cope with these different syndromes, methods different in both therapeutic principle and technique must be adopted. Take the cold for example. As its occurrence is different in season, cause, pathogenesis, vital-qi of the human body, it can be classified into wind-cold syndrome, wind-heat syndrome, summer-heat and dampness syndrome, qi-deficiecy syndrome and yin-deficiency syndrome as well. To counter these different types of syndrome, a choice of therapeutic methods should be made: relieving the exterior syndrome with drugs pungent in flavor and warm in property, relieving the exterior syndrome with drugs pungent in flavor and cool in property, eliminating summer-heat and dampness from the superficies of the body by diaphoresis, supplementing qi and expelling the pathogenic factor from the body surface as well as nourishing yin and relieving the exterior syndrome. We call such a treatment as treating the same disease with different methods.

Reversely, different diseases, at a certain stage of the development or in a certain period of the pathological change of different patients, may manifest themselves in a similar syndromes. Pathological changes basically similar usually share something in common, and this is the premise of treating different diseases with the same method. Treating different diseases with the same method implies that the same principle and method may be applied for different diseases on condition that they share some pathological syndromes in common. For example, diarrhea, prolapse of rectum, hysteroptosis and gastroptosis are completely different diseases, but they are of the same pathological mechanism that the spleen-qi is too deficient to send up nutrients and to govern the blood flow, so they bear the similar syndrome and can be treated with a similar method of invigorating the spleen to replenish qi or elevating the spleen $yang$ to control the blood flow. We call such a treatment treating different diseases with the same method.

To take the selecting treatment by differentiating syndromes as the basic principle of diagnosis and treatment, it is important to have a sound understanding of the relationship between disease and syndrome, being aware of not only the fact that a disease may manifest itself in different syndromes but also the fact that different diseases may manifest themselves in the same syndrome in the course of their development. So it is evident that TCM puts great emphasis on the concept of syndrome because syndrome involves substantial pathological content and, therefore, is the core of the unique system of selecting treatment by differentiating syndrome. The premise, the basis of treating the same disease with different methods and treating different diseases with the same method, lies in the similarity or difference of the syndromes. The same treatment is performed if the syndromes are of the same type; different treatments are adopted in case the syndromes are different. Clearly enough, treating the same disease with different methods and treating different diseases with the same therapeutic principle give expression to the essence and advantage of the selecting treatment by differentiating syndrome which is a theoretical system of TCM internal medicine, and of the whole TCM as well.

1.3 Requirements and Methods in Studying TCM Internal Medicine

TCM internal medicine is an extremely important clinical branch of TCM, which, by making use of the basical TCM theories, expounds the causes and pathogeneses of various diseases as well as the laws of selecting treatment in the field of internal medicine, and explores concrete therapeutic methods and the curative effects.

The requirements of studying TCM internal medicine are to grasp the basic theories, the elementary knowledge and the basic skills, to understand and have a mastery of the characteristics of TCM internal medicine and the treatment of commonly encountered diseases and to improve the capability of doing clinical and scientific research.

The methods to study TCM internal medicine involves three stages: systematic theoretical studies (class education), on probation and clinical practice before graduation, with particular emphasis laid on each stage. At the first stage, the students are required to have a profound understanding of TCM theories and the essentials, master firmly the characteristics of TCM internal medicine and the system of selecting treatment by differentiating syndrome. At the second stage, the students are placed on probation, i.e., under the guidance of the teachers, they do practice in diagnosing, differentiating syndromes, prescribing on probation so as to get a deeper understanding of the theory they have studied in class, come into contact with clinical work, integrate theory with practice and improve their perceptual knowledge. And at the third stage, the students are to be instructed by senior doctors in clinical practice of internal medicine, serving the patients directly, making an overall application of the theories to clinical work, improving their basic skills and raising their comprehensive capacity of analysing and treating illness, i.e., improving their mastery and practical application of the selecting treatment by differentiating syndrome.

To study TCM internal medicine well, it is important for the students to review regularly the fundamental subjects that they have already studied so as to lay a solid foundation for the study of internal medicine. The students are expected to associate what they are studying with what they have studied, for some diseases discussed in interenal medicine are not only different but also related.

To study TCM internal medicine well, it is essential to integrate theory with practice, to be expert at synthesizing, analysing, making judgments and grasping the nature of disease, and to master excellent therapeutic skills. Only by collecting clinical data accurately through the four diagnostic methods, can it be possible to differentiate the syndrome correctly and treat the disease effectively.

To study TCM internal medicine well, it is equally important to have a grasp of the approaches most in use in selecting treatment by differentiating syndrome as well as the theories on pathogenesis and syndromes. After a process of repeated intensification of knowledge — practice — knowledge enriched — practice improved, the goal of improving the techniques of treatment will be attained.

To study TCM internal medicine well, it is necessary to always keep in mind the characteristics and advantages of TCM internal medicine: adhering to the etiology and searching for the primary cause of disease in treatment, combining the differentiation of disease with the differentiation of syndrome but pay special attention to the latter, treating the same disease with different methods and treating different diseases with the same therapeutic principle. Bring the unique superiority of TCM into full play, and we will make great contributions to the health of the whole mankind.

Discussions

1. Why is it a characteristic of TCM internal medicine to strictly adhere to the etiology and to search for the primary cause of disease in treatment?

2. How do you understand the combination of differentiating disease and differentiating syndrome? Which of the two aspects is emphasized by TCM internal medicine?

3. What is the theoretical core of treating the same disease with different methods and treating different diseases with the same method?

2 Therapeutic Principles and Methods of TCM Internal Medicine

The characteristics and superiority of the system of selecting treatment by differentiating syndrome are clearly seen in the therapeutic principles and methods of TCM internal medicine. The therapeutic principles consist of two main aspects: syndrome differentiation and principles of treatment. And the therapeutic methods can be grouped under twelve heads: diaphoresis, heat-clearing, purgation, mediation, warming, tonification, resolving, astringing, regulating the flow of *qi*, treating blood disorders, inducing resuscitation and spasmolysis.

The methods commonly used in syndrome differentiation in TCM internal medicine are involved in the chapter of "Syndrome Differentiation" in TCM Diagnostics. But when used in internal treatment, these methods have their own specific characteristics. In consideration of the connection between the elementary courses and clinical application, we are going to, in light of the basic concept and classification of pathogeneses and syndromes used in selecting treatment by differentiating syndrome about miscellaneous diseases, and in the hope that the students can gain new insights through restudying the old material and make constant progress in selecting treatment by differentiating syndrome, mainly discuss the basic concept of the pathogenesis and syndromes of the five pathogenic factors, of the six channels and the four systems (*wei*, *qi*, *ying*, and blood), of *qi* and blood, and that of the *zang-fu* organs.

2.1 Basic Concept of the Pathogenesis and Syndromes Caused by the Five Pathogenic Factors

The five pathogenic factors refer to the five pathological changes which are caused by the functional disorders of *zang-fu* organs and are similar to wind, cold, dampness, dryness and fire.

The wind, cold, dampness, dryness and fire syndromes may be caused by any of the six external etiological factors (wind, cold, summer-heat, dampness, dryness and fire) invading the body, or internally produced by the pathological changes of *zang* and *fu* organs. Syndromes that are due to the five internal pathogenic factors are called endogenous wind, endogenous cold, endogenous dampness, endogenous dryness and endogenous fire, so as to distinguish them from those caused by the six external etiological factors.

It must be pointed out that the pathogenesis by the five pathogenical factors is not only the product of the pathological changes of *zang* and *fu*-organs, but also the secondary cause that affects the functional activities of *zang-fu* organs. So it is necessary to find out its relationship with the functional activities of *zang* - *fu* organs so as to adhere to the pathogenesis and search for the primary cause of disease in treatment.

According to TCM theory, there are some specific relationships between the five *zang* - organs and the five pathogenic factors in terms of the five elements theory, which play an important guiding role in the whole process of selecting treatment by differentiating syndromes according to the pathological changes of *zang* and *fu*. The specific relationships suggest: Wind and the liver belong to wood, and wind is active, so endogenous wind is due to the disorder of the liver's function; cold and the kidney pertain to water, and water has a cold and stagnant nature, that's why endogenous cold are often caused by the deficiency of kidney - *yang*; dampness and the spleen belong to earth, and earth promotes growth, produces myriads of things and takes an aversion to stagnancy, therefore, endogenous dampness is closely related to the weakness of the spleen's *yang* - *qi*; dryness and the lung pertain to metal, endogenous dryness has something to do with the disorder of the lung's functions of dispersing, descending and distributing body fluids; fire - heat and the heart belong to fire, so hyperactivity of pathogenic fire and hyperactivity of fire due to *yin* deficiency are usually associated with the functional disorder of the heart.

Meanwhile, as the human body is a complex but systematic organic unity that takes the functional activities of the five *zang* - organs as its centre in its dynamic balance, the five *zang* organs, on account of the close relations and coordinations among *zang*, *fu*, *qi* and blood, are physiologically bound up with one another and pathologically affect and turn into each other. The pathogenic changes and syndromes caused by any of the endogenous wind, endogonous cold, endogenous dampness, endogenous dryness and endogenous fire tend to manifest themselves mainly in a certain *zang* - organ, then involve other relative *zang* - *fu* organs, leading to the disorders of the functions of two or more *zang* - organs. Therefore, to explore the pathogenesis and the syndromes caused by the five pathogenic factors, it is essential to strictly adhere to the pathogenesis, search for the primary cause of the disease, make a clear distinction between deficiency and excess, and the primary and secondary, identify the diseased part, and distinguish excess from deficiency of *yin*, *yang*, *qi* and blood.

2.1.1 Wind

Endogenous wind and pathogenic wind have similar properties: floating, changable, active and likely to occur in any season of the year. The saying "Wind is the chief of all diseases" sums up the multiplicity of wind syndromes.

Such clinical syndromes as dizziness, tremor, clonic convulsion, infantile convulsion, stiff - neck, tic of limbs, deviation of the eyes and mouth, opisthotonos, etc. are all wind syndromes.

Wind syndromes consist of two types: exopathic type and endogenous type. The former includes syndrome due to the invasion of wind, and is divided into wind-cold syndrome, wind-heat syndrome, wind-dampness syndrome, and wind edema; and the latter wind-syndrome caused by hyperactivity of the liver-*yang*, occurrence of wind syndrome in case of extreme heat, and endopathic wind due to blood deficiency.

This section is to mainly deal with the pathogenesis and syndromes of endopathic wind.

TCM theory holds that such syndromes as dizziness, blurred vision, tic of limbs, numbness of the body, tremor, rigidity, or even coma, unconsciousness, deviation of the eyes and mouth, hemiplegia or general limitedness of movement are mostly related to the liver and wind. This is because the liver has its opening in the eyes, controls the activity of the tendon, stores blood, bears the dispersive function and is responsible for anger. So endopathic wind syndromes from dysfunctions of *zang-fu* organs are likely to be related to the abnormality of the liver's function.

The characteristics of pathogenesis of endopathic wind syndromes are:

①Being apt to chiefly attack the head and cause pathological change;

②Being apt to be accompanied by the pathogen of phlegm;

③Being apt to cause "fire and wind to stir up each other", when combined with endopathic fire syndromes.

The causes for endogenous wind syndromes are as follows:

(1) Wind-syndrome caused by hyperactivity of the liver-*yang*.

[Pathogenesis] Consumption of liver-*yin* and kidney-*yin* causes water to fail in nourishing wood and *yin* unable to suppress the *yang* leading to the hyperactivity of liver-*yang* and wind stirring accompanied with phlegm. Therefore, the mentality is confused.

[Syndromes] Dizziness, tendency to fall, severe headache, numbness and tremor of the limbs, difficulty of speech, involuntary movement of the limbs, walking haltingly, red tongue, wiry, thready and rapid pulse or wiry and tense pulse; and in case of serious illness: sudden faint, stiff tongue and inability to speak, facial hemiparalysis, hemiplegia (apoplexy).

[Treatment] Nourishing *yin* and suppressing hyperactive *yang*, and calming the liver to stop the wind.

[Recipe] *Da Ding Feng Zhu*[19], *Zhen Gan Xi Feng Tong*[291], etc.

(2) Wind-syndrome caused by extreme heat

[Pathogenesis] Hyperactivity of pathogenic heat that injures *ying* and blood, burns the liver channel and attacks the heart, and the excessive heat stirs up the wind in the liver.

[Syndromes] Pyrexia with polydipsia, clonic convulsion with stiff neck, superduction of the eyes, apisthotonos, unconsciousness, crimson tongue, yellowish fur, wiry and rapid pulse.

[Treatment] Clearing away pathogenic heat from the liver, and calming the endopathic wind and restoring consciousness.

[Recipe] *Ling Yang Gou Teng Tang*[247], *An Gong Niu Huang Wan*[111], *Zi Xue Dan*[267].

(3) Wind stirring due to *yin* (blood) - deficiency

[Pathogenesis] The deficiency of *yin* - fluid and blood makes them unable to moisten and nourish the muscles, leading to the stirring - up of endopathic wind of deficiency type.

[Syndromes] Numbness of the limbs, muscular contracture, twitching and cramp, reddish tongue, or red tongue with insufficient fluid, thready pulse.

[Treatment] Nourishing *yin* and enriching blood, relieving wind and calming the liver.

[Recipe] *Jia Jian Fu Mai Tang*[101], *Bu Gan Tang*[142], *Di Huang Yin Zi*[104].

2.1.2 Cold

Endogenous cold and pathogenic cold have much in common in causing diseases: both of them are *yin* pathogens, impairing *yang - qi* and tending to bring about such painful syndromes as stagnation of *qi* and blood and obstruction of the functional activities of *qi*. Exopathic cold attacks the body mainly in winter, while endopathic cold syndromes from the hypofunction of the *zang - fu* organs, which are also known as *yang* deficiency or cold of insufficiency type, are likely to occur in any of the four seasons, though mainly in winter.

Clinical syndromes such as muscular twitching and cramp, warmlessness of the limbs, stagnation of *qi* and blood, pain and inability of the *zang - fu* functions, as well as deficiency of *yang - qi* all belong to cold syndromes.

Cold syndromes involve endopathic and exopathic cold syndromes: Exopathic syndroms generate from pathogenic cold attacking the superficial part of the body and pathogenic cold attacking *zang* and *fu*. Endopathic cold is chiefly due to the insufficiency of *yang - qi* inside the body and thereupon occurs internally the pathogenic *yin* cold. This is primarily attributable to the hypofunction of the kidney, the spleen or the heart.

TCM theory holds that endogenous cold from *yang* insufficiency is responsible for intolerance of cold and coldness of the limbs, pale complexion, vomiting and slobbering, diarrhea with undigested food in the stool, muscular twitching and cramp, local cold - pain, mental weariness and fatigue, and tendency for lying and warmth. This is because the kidney - *yang* is the root of the *yang - qi* of the whole body, the spleen - *yang* is the origin of the middle - *jiao yang*, and the heart - *yang* promotes blood flowing in the vessels. Meanwhile, the heart - *yang* and the spleen - *yang* are entirely dependent upon the kidney - *yang* for warmth and support. So the deficiency of the kidney - *yang* is the most important factor leading to the pathogenesis of cold of deficiency and many pathological changes such as edema due to *yang* insufficiency and *yang* short of warmth should be differentiated and treated according to the state of the kidney.

The pathogenetic characteristics of endogenous cold syndromes are:

① Doing damage to *yang-qi* of the body;

② Leading to the hypofunction or disorder of *zang* and *fu*;

③ Being likely to cause pain, fluid-retention and phlegm-retention.

Endogenous cold is often seen in the following syndromes:

(1) Excess of *yin*-cold

[Pathogenesis] *Yang-qi* being asthenic and short of warmth; *yang* asthenia leading to *yin* sthenia, and the excess of *yin* bringing about cold syndrome; *yang* being too weak to activate *qi* to promote diuresis, and the accumulated cold water in time becomes retention or edema.

[Syndromes] Coldness of the body and limbs; in case of severe illness: reversed coldness of the limbs, vomiting and slobbering, diarrhea with undigested food in the stool, edema of the face and limbs; whitish, moist and glossy fur, deep and wiry pulse or deep, thready and weak pulse.

[Treatment] Warming *yang* to dispel cold.

[Recipe] *Si Ni Tang*[80], *Ji Sheng Shen Qi Wan*[184], *Zhen Wu Tang*[199].

(2) Deficiency of *yang* of the spleen and kidney

[Pathogenesis] Middle-*jiao yang* being exhausted on various accounts, involving the kidney-*yang*, or the kidney-*yang* being too deficient to warm and nourish the spleen-*yang*, as a result, leading to the deficiency of both the kidney-*yang* and the spleen-*yang*.

[Syndromes] Pale complexion, cold-pain in the loins and knees or lower abdomen, intolerance of cold and tendency for warmth, diarrhea before dawn, long but thin micturition; pale and enlarged tongue, deep and weak pulse.

[Treatment] Warming and tonifying the spleen and kidney.

[Recipe] *Liang Fu Wan*[139], *Fu Zi Li Zhong Wan*[146].

(3) Deficiency of the heart-*yang*

[Pathogenesis] The heart-*yang* being damaged on account of prolonged illness or fulminant disease, *yang* being too weak to perform its warming function, leading to excess of *yin* cold and obstructing *yang* in the chest.

[Syndromes] Palpitation and oppressed feeling in the chest, dyspnea and chest pain, and the pain getting worse in case of being hit by cold, bluish lips and coldness of the limbs, pale complexion, spontaneous perspiration with a sensation of the body being cold, intermittent and uneven pulse.

[Treatment] Warming *yang* and supplementing *qi*, dispersing cold to remove obstruction in the collaterals.

[Recipe] *Gui Zhi Jia Fu Zi Tang*[202], *Gua Lou Xie Bai Gui Zhi Tang*[210], *Wu Tou*

Gui Zhi Tang[55].

2.1.3 **Dampness** (phlegm, fluid-retention)

Dampness, a kind of *yin* pathogen which tends to damage *yang-qi*, first attacks the lower part of the body in most cases. The disease caused by damp pathogen has prolonged course and is difficult to cure. Pathogenic dampness can be divided into endogenous dampness and exopathic dampness. Exopathic dampness invades the body on account of long residence in damp places or exposure to water, rain or damp weather. Endopathic dampness is caused by the deficiency of the spleen-*yang*, so that the spleen fails to perform its function of transport, distribution and discharge of body fluids, and in consequence, water metabolism in the body is out of order. It is worthy of notice that the exopathic dampness is very likely to cause the spleen-*yang* to be obstructed and lead to endogenous dampness. And the insufficiency of the spleen-*yang* to generate damp pathogen in the body, tends to incur in invasion of exopathic dampness. So, different as they are, endogenous dampness and exopathic dampness are closely related to each other in etiology. This is what is usually said.

Damp syndrome often clinically seen are aching, heaviness and swelling pain of the body, restriction of the movements of the joints, poor appetite, fullness of the stomach and diarrhea, heaviness and pain of the head and body, whitish fur and soft-floating pulse.

Exopathic dampness includes cold-dampness, wind-dampness, summer-heat dampness, and damp-heat, which invade the body mainly through the muscular striae on the surface, or enter the joints, or damage the spleen and stomach. In most cases, pathogenic dampness attacks the body together with other pathogenic factors. Besides, the invasion of pathogenic dampness may cause the pathological changes of either cold transformation or heat transformation because of the functional differences of *zang* and *fu* organs, the divergences of the constitutions as well as inadequate remedies.

Endogenous dampness is a pathological product, and it is a pathogenic factor, too. Endogenous dampness is mostly produced by improper diet —— excessive intake of cold and uncooked food, alcohol, fat and sweets, or irregular meals. Whatever the cause, it is certain to damage the functions of the spleen and the kidney, leading to the deficiency of *yang-qi*. The dysfunction of the spleen in transport and retention of water within the body will consequently accumulate and become retention of body fluid or phlegm.

This section mainly deals with endogen…. dampness.

Endog   us dampness primarily takes the following forms: poor appetite, fullness of the stomach and anorexia, loose stool and diarrhea, heaviness and edema of the limbs. As endogenous dampness and phlegm-retention, though different, are of the same origin, endogenous dampness is usually accompanied by phlegm-retention, stopping or accumulating in the chest or abdomen, spreading in the muscular striae, condensing into phlegm pathogen penetrating everywhere. In the meantime, endogenous dampness is brought about by the deficiency of the spleen-*yang*, i.e., deficiency in origin, but damp pathogens internally accumulated often manifest as excess in superficiality. So damp pathogens attack the body from both within and without, and the disease is lingering and hard to cure. When deficiency and excess occur simultaneously, attention must be paid to both the reinforcement and elimination, and it is especially important to differentiate what is primary from what is secondary in the differentiation of syndromes and selection of treatment so as to tonify the spleen and warm the kidney and to dispel dampness and remove the fluid retention.

The pathogenetic characteristics of endogenous dampness are:

①Being of causality with the deficiency of the spleen-*yang*, and causing lingering diseases;

②Being a pathological product, and a pathogenic factor, too;

③Being likely to damage *yang-qi*, obstruct *qi* and stop fluid, and produce phlegm from fluid retention; deficiency in the interior but excess in the exterior.

Endogenous dampness is mainly shown in the following syndrome types:

(1) Disturbance of the spleen due to cold-dampness

[Pathogenesis] Excessive cold food or irregular daily life resulting in the invasion of exopathic dampness accompanied by cold pathogen ; or usual excess of endogenous dampness causing the body to be hit by pathogenic cold dampness, thus afflicting middle-*jiao yang* and giving rise to cold-dampness inside the body.

[Syndromes] Abdominal and epigastric distention, poor appetite, nausea, abdominal pain and loose stool, tastelessness and thirstlessness, heaviness in the head as if it were bound, coldness of the limbs, or even heaviness sensation in the body or general edema; whitish, moist and glossy or greasy fur, soft and floating, moderate pulse.

[Treatment] Warming the middle-*jiao* to resolve dampness.

[Recipe] *Shi Pi Yin*[159], *Wei Ling Tang*[182].

(2) Retention of damp-heat in the middle-*jiao*

[Pathogenesis] Attack of the body by damp-heat or excessive intake of fat and sweets leading to damp-heat which accumulates in the spleen and stomach.

[Syndromes] Fullness in the stomach, nausea, anorexia and bitter taste, stickiness in the mouth, no desire for drink in case of thirst, scanty dark urine, or fever going up and down, fever being not relieved after sweating, or yellowish complexion and the skin, tickle on the skin, yellowish and greasy fur, soft and floating, rapid pulse.

[Treatment] Clearing away heat and eliminating dampness.

[Recipe] *Lian Pu Yin*[133], *Gan Lu Xiao Du Dan*[74].

(3) Retention of dampness due to the deficiency of the spleen

[Pathogenesis] Improper diet doing damage to the spleen and stomach, leading to the failure of their functions of transporting, descending and ascending, and, in consequence, the retention of water within the body.

[Syndromes] Sallow complexion, mental fatigue, tiredness and heaviness in the limbs, upset in the stomach and abdomen, aversion to greasy food, loss of appetite, loose stool and diarrhea; pale and enlarged tongue, thin but moist or greasy fur, soft and floating, thready pulse.

[Treatment] Invigorating the spleen for eliminating dampness.

[Recipe] *Xiang Sha Liu Jun Zi Tang*[189], *Shi Pi Yin*[159], etc.

Appendix 1: Phlegm

Many diseases are caused by phlegm pathogen. That is why people usually say: "The evil influence of phlegm may cause various diseases." By phlegm it is meant, on the one hand, the material sputum excreted, and on the other, the syndromes and symptoms in the form of phlegm, such as choking sensation in the chest and fullness in the stomach, nausea and diarrhea, dizziness and palpitation, numbness of the skin, swelling of the joints, subcutaneous mass, as well as manic-depressive psychosis. Owing to different contributing factors, there are cold, heat, dryness, dampness and wind types of phlegm; and in each type there are sub-types of excess and deficiency, occurring in different *zang-fu* organs.

Phlegm pathogen may cause various syndromes. But the pathogenesis, in general, lies in the dysfunctions of the lung, the spleen and the kidney. The spleen is the source of phlegm because it is in charge of transporting and transforming water. The lung is the organ that stores phlegm and the upper source of water, so in case the lung fails to perform its dispersing and descending functions, the body fluid is likely to accumulate and become phlegm. The kidney-*yang* is the motivation of the spleen-*yang* and the lung-*qi* and the root of vital-*qi* of the whole body, therefore the deficiency of the kidney-*yang* and kidney-*qi* may cause body fluid to accumulate inside the body and the obstruction of flow of *qi* and generation of phlegm. In addition, the insufficiency of *yin*-blood of *zang* and *fu* organs can also cause the flaring-up of fire of deficiency type and formation of phlegm from body fluids. Once phlegm is formed, it is brought up and down by *qi*, spreading everywhere inside the body —— filling the seven orifices on the face, or being detained in the channels and collaterals, thus leading to various disorders.

Classifications of Diagnosis and Treatment

(1) Phlegm stagnation in the lung

[Pathogenesis] The attatck by exopathogen or prolonged cough making the lung fail to spread body fluids which, consequently, accumulate into phlegm.

[Syndromes] Cough and dyspnea, rale, whitish abundant expectoration which is easily coughed up, or other cold and heat exterior syndromes seen at the same time, thin, whitish and greasy fur, floating or slippery pulse.

[Treatment] Ventilating the lung and resolving phlegm.

[Recipe] *Zhi Sou San*[37], *Xing Su San*[130].

(2) Mental confusion due to phlegm

[Pathogenesis] Injury due to seven emotions or the attack by damp and turbid pathogenic factors, which obstruct the functional activities of *qi*, leading to stagnation of *qi* and accumulation of phlegm, and the functional disorder of the heart.

[Syndromes] Coma and depressive psychosis, choking sensation in the chest and precordial pain, fainting and unconsciousness; whitish and greasy fur, slippery pulse.

[Treatment] Eliminating phlegm for resuscitation.

[Recipe] *Dao Tan Tang*[121], *Su He Xiang Wan*[128].

(3) Retention of phlegm in the spleen and stomach

[Pathogenesis] Improper diet or tiredness and anxiety doing damage to the spleen and stomach so that the spleen fails in performing its transporting and transforming function, thus causing dampness to become phlegm.

[Syndromes] Fullness in the stomach and poor appetite, nausea and vomiting, tiredness and weakness, heaviness in the body and drowsiness; whitish and greasy fur, enlarged tongue, soft and floating, moderate pulse.

[Treatment] Strengthening the spleen and reducing phlegm.

[Recipe] *Ping Wei San*[70], *Liu Jun Zi Tang*[45].

(4) Stagnancy of phlegm in the liver

[Pathogenesis] Stagnation of the liver-*qi* bringing about retention of *qi* and collection of phlegm, so that *qi* and phlegm hinder each other.

[Syndromes] Sensation of something stucking in the throat when swallowing, dull pain in the chest and hypochondrium, eructation, susceptibility to anger and depression; thin, whitish and greasy fur, wiry and slippery pulse.

[Treatment] Reducing phlegm by alleviation of mental depression.

[Recipe] *Si Qi Tang*[75].

(5) Stirring of phlegm in the kidney

[Pathogenesis] Protracted illness damaging the kidney, resulting in deficiency of the kidney-*yang*, the kidney failing to perform its steaming and ascending function, causing the retention of water within the body, which goes upward and becomes phlegm; or exhaustion of the kidney-*yin* leading to hyperactivity of fire, and fire of deficiency type scorching body fluids and turning them into phlegm.

[Syndromes] Dyspnea and shortness of breath, pale tongue, deep and thready pulse; or dizziness and tinnitus, lassitude in the loins and knees, red tongue with little fur, thready and rapid pulse.

[Treatment] Reducing phlegm by warming or nourishing the kidney.

[Recipe] *Ji Sheng Shen Qi Wan*[184], or *Jin Shui Liu Jun Jian*[161].

(6) Phlegm staying in the joints, meridians and collaterals.

[Pathogenesis] Phlegm stagnating in the joints, meridians and collaterals, resulting in stagnation of qi and blood, and obstruction of the collaterals.

[Syndromes] Pain and edema in the joints, numbness in the limbs, or hemiplegia, facial hemiparalysis, or scrofula, goiter, node and lump; whitish and greasy fur, wiry and slippery pulse.

[Treatment] Resolving the hard lumps; removing obstruction in the collaterals and reducing phlegm.

[Recipe] *Si Hai Shu Yu Wan*[83], *Zhi Mi Fu Ling Wan*[179].

In brief, both phlegm and dampness are due to the hypofunction of the spleen, the lung and the kidney, with weakened vital -qi as the origin. Phlegm retained in the body often leads to excess syndrome, typical of, clinically, excess in the secondary and deficiency in the primary. So it is essential to stick to the principle of relieving the secondary in an acute case, relieving the primary symptoms in a chronic case and relieving the primary and the secondary aspects at the same time. In acute cases, treatment must be first given to the retained phlegm, and in chronic cases, the functions of the spleen, the lung and the kidney must be recuperated. Meanwhile, it is necessary to take counter measures in accordance with the property of the pathogens which appear simultaneously with the phlegm pathogen. For example, dryness - phlegm syndrome should be removed by moisturizing, wetness - phlegm syndrome be eliminated by drying, and persistent phlegm be got rid of by softening.

Appendix 2: Fluid - Retention

The cause of fluid -retention is much of the same as dampness and phlegm, originating from the abnormal functions of the spleen, lung and kidney, the obstructed activity of qi as well as the abnormality of water metabolism. Fluid - retention can be divided into four kinds in accordance with the part where it is retained: fluid -retention in the stomach and intestines is called *Tan Yin* (retention of phlegm and fluid), fluid -retention under the hypochondrium is known as *Xuan Yin* (pleural effusion); generalized accumulation of fluid is called *Yi Yin* (anasarca); and excessive fluid in the lung and chest is known as *Zhi Yin*. Wherever it is retained, fluid -retention syndrome is always found to be deficient in origin and excessive in superficiality.

Fluid - retention may be brought about by various causes, but the general pathogenesis is always due to the fact that the spleen - *yang* is too insufficient to transport and transform nutrients, so that body fluid is retained and, then, accumulated into fluid -retention. As kidney - *yang* is insufficient, the functional activity of qi is in disorder and unable to warm the spleen - *yang* and, in consequence, fluid is accumulated inside and, then, flows to every part of the body. The lung is the upper source of water, in case the lung fails to disperse and distribute body fluid, it will be accumulated into fluid -retention. Therefore, the pathogenesis is alway found to be excess of *yin* due to *yang* insufficiency, abnormality of water metabolism, and the retention of body fluid.

Classifications of Diangnosis and Treatment

(1) *Tan Yin* (Phlegm retention)

[Pathogenesis] Failure of middle – *jiao yang* resulting in the retention of fluid in the stomach and intestines.

[Syndroms] Hardness, fullness and ache in the gastral cavity, sound of vibrated water in the stomach, vomit of the mixture of phlegm and saliva, loss of desire for water, dizziness, or sound of flowing water in the intestines; whitish and glossy fur; slippery pulse.

[Treatment] Warming *yang* to dispel retention of phlegm, or expelling accumulated water by purgation.

[Recipe] *Ling Gui Zhu Gan Tang*,[150] *Ji Jiao Li Huang Wan*,[24] etc.

(2) *Xuan Yin* (Pleural effusion)

[Pathogenesis] Body fluid flowing in hypochondrium causes the collaterals to be blocked, and failure of *qi* in ascending and descending.

[Syndroms] Distention and pain in the chest and hypochondrium, which get worse when coughing with spittle, turning the body and breathing, shortness of breath; whitish fur; wiry and deep pulse.

[Treatment] Expelling body fluid retention with potent purgatives.

[Recipe] *Shi Zao Tang*,[6] *Ting Li Da Zao Xie Fei Tang*,[261] etc.

(3) *Yi Yin* (Anasarca)

[Pathogenesis] The failure of the lung – *qi* and spleen – *qi* in distributing body fluid, leading to its spreading unchecked.

[Syndroms] Ache, heaviness or even edema in the limbs, difficulty in urination, fever with chills, anhidrosis and cough with dyspnea, phlegm with a lot of foams; whitish fur; wiry and tense pulse.

[Treatment] Warming and resolving phlegm and fluid retention.

[Recipe] *Xiao Qing Long Tang*[27].

(4) *Zhi Yin* (Excessive fluid in the hypochondrium and epigastrium)

[Pathogenesis] Fluid retained in the lung and chest resulting in the abnormal rising of the lung – *qi*.

[Syndroms] Cough with dyspnea, fullness sensation in the chest, difficulty in lying supine in severe cases, much phlegm in the form of white foams, edema on the face after prolonged cough; greasy and whitish fur; wiry and tense pulse.

[Treatment] Warming the lung and resolving fluid – retention in case cold fluid – retention is in the lungs; and warming and invigorating the spleen and kidney in case of the deficiency of the spleen – *yang* and kidney – *yang*.

[Recipe] To warm the lung and resolve fluid retention: *Xiao Qing Long Tang*[27]. To warm and invigorate the spleen and kidney: *Jin Gui Shen Qi Wan*[163], *Ling Gui Zhu*

Gan Tang[150].

2.1.4 Dryness

Pathogenic dryness is apt to harm the body fluid as well as the lung, resulting in such "dry symptoms" as dry mouth and nose, dryness of throat and thirst, dry cough with little phlegm or phlegm with blood, dryness and rhagades in the skin, wizened hair, rough and emaciated muscles and constipation. Dryness pathogen can be divided into two types: exopathic dryness and endogenous dryness. The former leads to disease on account of the attack of the dryness pathogen outside of the body. The exopathic dryness invades the body from the mouth and nose, and illness starts from the lung and *weifen*. As the body may be attacked either by the remaining *qi* of summer fire or by the cold *qi* of early winter, there are warm-dryness syndrome and cold-dryness syndrome in exopathic dryness. Endogenous dryness usually takes place after high fever, vomiting, diarrhea or too much of perspiration or hemorrhage. Exopathic dryness often occurs in autumn, while endogenous dryness in any season of the year. The latter is going to be detailed here.

The pathogenesis of endogenous dryness can be summed up as follows: the exhaustion of body fluid, the comsumption of *yin*-blood, and the pathologic change mainly involving the lung, stomach, kidney and liver.

The pathogenic features of endogenous dryness are:

① It is apt to cause the body fluid to be exhausted and *yin*-blood to be damaged;

② It is likely to stir up endogenous wind and endogenous fire (heat).

Endogenous dryness often manifests itself as the following types:

(1) Exhaustion of fluid in the lung and stomach

[Pathogenesis] Consumption of body fluid due to excessive heat, or caused by undue diaphoresis, emetic therapy or purgation.

[Syndroms] Dry nose, throat and mouth, thirst, dry cough without phlegm, constipation, brief discharge of little urine, dry and lustreless skin, and dry tongue with little fluid.

[Treatment] Promoting the production of body fluid to moisten dryness.

[Recipe] *Sha Shen Mai Dong Tang*[138], *Zeng Ye Tang*[283], etc.

(2) Deficiency of the liver-*yin* and kidney-*yin*

[Pathogenesis] Consumption of essense and blood after prolonged illness or massive hemorrhage.

[Syndroms] Dry mouth and throat, lassitude and soreness in the loins and knees, dysphoria with feverish sensation in the chest, palms and soles, dry and withered hair, emaciated muscles, emission and night sweat, and amenorrhea in females, reddened tongue with little fur; thready and rapid pulse.

[Treatment] Nourishing *yin* and blood.

[Recipe] *Mai Wei Di Huang Wan*[125], *Qi Ju Di Huang Wan*[129]

2.1.5 Fire

TCM theory holds that heat is a little amount of fire, and fire a large quantity of heat. That is why fire and heat are often clinically mentioned in the same breath. Any of the six exopathic factors (wind, cold, summer-heat, dampness, dryness and fire) may possibly turn into fire or heat when it enters the body. And any of the seven emotions (joy, anger, melancholy, anxiety, grief, fear and terror) may also be transmitted into heat or fire when it stagnates inside the body to cause disorder of *qi*. TCM theory always summarizes the extensiveness of pathogenic fire by "the excessive remainder of *qi* means fire".

Fire, a kind of *yang* pathogens, is apt to damage *yin*-fluid, disturb the seven orifices, stir blood and consume it, give rise to endogenous wind, and carry with it phlegm and turbid pathogen.

Pathogenic fire is devided into exopathic fire and endogenous fire when causing disease. Exopathic fire is mostly caused by affection of warm pathogen or heat pathogen, while endogenous fire originates from the imbalance of *yin* and *yang* of the *zang-fu* organs. In such an imbalance, an excess of *yang* leads to fire of excess type, and the pathological changes involve the lung and stomach, and, in particular, the heart and liver, with such symptoms as aphthous stomatitis, red eyes and bitter taste, dryness and pain in the throat, gingivitis, vexation and restlessness; deficiency of *yin* brings about fire of deficiency type, and affects the heart and liver and especially the lung and kidney, with such symptoms as dysphoria with feverish sensation in the chest, palms and soles, low fever and night sweat, flushing of the zygomatic region, xenophthalmia and dry throat, dizziness and tinnitus, and the like. So it can be seen that the disease caused by endogenous fire consists of excess type as well as deficiency type, which occur in different parts of the body, and are of different pathogenesis, and, therefore, must be treated in different ways.

This section mainly deals with endogenous fire.

The characteristics of pathogenic fire are as follows:

①The patient's condition changes rapidly, with blood consumed, wind stirred up and phlegm produced.

②Pathogenic fire tends to go upward so as to invade the seven orifices and disturb mentality.

③Pathogenic fire consumes *yin*-fluid, with noticeable heat symptoms.

④Pathogenic fire is often closely related to emotions, over-exertion and undue sexual desire.

Endogenous fire consists of the following types:

Fire of Excess Type

(1) Flaming of the heart-fire

[Pathogenesis] Irregular emotions is pent up and turned into pathogenic fire.

[Syndrome] Vexation and flushed face, thirst with desire for drink, aphtha and tongue sore, insomnia and restlessness; reddened tongue; rapid pulse.

[Treatment] Clearing away the heart-fire.

[Recipe] *Xie Xin Tang*[153], etc.

(2) Excess of the liver-fire

[Pathogenesis] Emotions are out of control; the liver fails to perform its dispersive function so that the liver-*qi* is stagnated and turned into pathogenic fire which makes upward invasion.

[Syndrome] Headache and dizziness, tide-like tinnitus, dysphoria and irritability, flushed face and conjunctival congestion, bitter taste and dry throat, burning pain in the chest and hypochondrium; reddened tongue with yellowish fur; wiry and rapid pulse.

[Treatment] Purging the live of pathogenic fire.

[Recipe] *Long Dan Xie Gan Tang*[64], etc.

Fire of Deficiency Type

(1) Deficiency of the kidney and the stir of fire

[Pathogenesis] Prolonged illness causes the impairment of *yin*, hemorrhage or loss of essence so that the consumption of the kidney-*yin* is brought about and pathogenic fire of deficiency type comes into being inside the body.

[Syndrome] Dizziness and tinnitus, lassitude in the loins and knees, dry mouth and throat, amnesia and diffcult sleep, dysphoria with feverish sensation in the chest, palms and soles, hectic fever and night sweat, physique emaciation, emission and premature ejaculation; red and dry tongue; thready and rapid pulse.

[Treatment] Nourishing the kidney and removing the fire.

[Recipe] *Zhi Bai Di Huang Wan*[160], etc.

(2) Lung-asthenia and fire-obstruction

[Pathogenesis] Exhaustion of the lung-*qi* due to over-exertion or consumption of *yin* caused by prolonged cough and, in consequence, deficiency of *yin* leading to hyperactivity of fire.

[Syndrome] Shortness of breath and dry cough, little but thick sputum or with blood streaks, dry mouth and throat, flushing of the zygomatic region and hoarseness, bone-heat and hectic fever, dysphoria with feverish sensation in the chest, palms and soles; red tongue with little saliva; thready and rapid pulse.

[Treatment] Nourishing *yin*, moistening the lung and clearing away the fire.

[Recipe] *Bai He Gu Jin Tang*[103], *Qin Jiu Bie Jia San*[197], etc.

Summary

The pathogenesis of the five pathogenic factors is directly associated with the *zang* and *fu* organs, *yin* and *yang*, and *qi* and blood. Of the internal diseases, those caused by the five pathogenic factors are the most commonly seen pathological changes. The five endogenous pathogenic factors, on the one hand, are caused by the pathological changes of the functions of the *zang - fu* organs, and, on the other, are the direct factors leading to new pathological changes, bringing about further disturbance to the dynamic equilibrium of *yin* and *yang* of *zang - fu'*s *qi* and blood, and causing the diseases even more complicated. So, in the realm of TCM internal medicine, it's impossible to direct correctly the selection of treatment by differentiating syndromes without a fundamental and accurate mastery of the pathagenesis and syndromes caused by the five pathogenic factors.

Discussions

1. What are the differences between the concept of the five pathogenic factors and that of the five endogenous pathogenic factors?

2. What are the pathological characteristics of each of the five endogenous pathogenic factors?

3. What syndrome types does each of the five endogenous pathogenic factors consist of? And what are the syndromes and treatments?

2. 2 Basic Concept of the Pathogenesis and Syndromes of the Six Meridians and *Wei*, *Qi*, *Ying* and *Xue*

The pathogenesis and the syndromes of the six meridians and those of *wei*, *qi*, *ying* and *xue* are two main categories, according to which the syndromes of epidemic febrile diseases caused by exopathogens are classified and dealt with, and, therefore, play a guiding role in clinical treatment in internal medicine and are of specific importance and value. But the analysing and differentiating of febrile disases in accordance with the theory of the six meridians and *wei*, *qi*, *ying* and *xue* must be applied to clinical practice in connection with the theory of analysing and differentiating pathological conditions in light of the eight principal syndromes as well as the differentiation of diseases according to the pathological changes of the *zang - fu* organs.

2. 2. 1 Introduction to the Pathogenesis and Syndromes of the Six Meridians

[Concept] The theory of the pathogenesis, syndromes and selection of treatment on the basis of the differentiation of syndromes in accordance with the theory of the six meridians originates from the theoretical system, established in the book Treatise on

Febrile Diseases, of analysing and differentiating epidemic febrile diseases caused by exopathogens. The pathogenesis, the syndromes and the treatment are respectively discussed as follows.

(1) *Taiyang* disease

[Pathogenesis] *Taiyang* dominates the superficiality of the six meridians, and, in case the superficiality is invaded by wind-cold pathogen, channel *qi* fails to flow smoothly.

[Syndrome] Aversion to wind and cold, headache, hidrosis or anhidrosis, arthralgia, neck rigidity, floating pulse.

[Treatment] For cases with exterior syndrome of excess and anhidrosis, relieving the exterior syndrome with drugs pungent in flavor and warm in property; for cases with exterior syndrome of deficiency and hidrosis, regulating *ying* and *wei*.

[Recipe] *Ma Huang Tang*[242] used to relieve the exterior syndrom; *Gui Zhi Tang*[200] used to regulate *ying* and *wei*.

(2) *Yangming* disease

[Pathogenesis] Pathogenic factor enters *Yangming qi* system, and excessive heat consumes the fluid in the stomach by burning it. Pathogenic factor enters *Yangming fu*-organ, and dyspepsia is caused and dryness-heat accumulated inside.

[Syndrome] *Yangming* meridian disease: sthenic fever, aversion to heat, profuse perspiration, extreme thirstiness, and full and large pulse. *Yangming fu*-organ disease: hectic fever and hidrosis, hardness and fullness and tenderness of the abdomen, constipation, delirium in severe cases, and dry fur.

[Treatment] Clearing away the heat and purging the fire for cases with *Yangming* meridian disease; dispelling the heat of excess type for cases with *Yangming fu*-organ disease.

[Recipe] *Bai Hu Tang*[91] to clear away the heat and purge the fire; *Da Cheng Qi Tang*[21], *Xiao Cheng Qi Tang*[29], or *Tiao Wei Cheng Qi Tang*[218] to dispel the excess-type heat.

(3) *Shaoyang* disease

[Pathogenesis] *Shaoyang*, the pivot of the six meridians, dominates the part between the interior and the exterior. The pathogenic factor that invades the body attacks the vital-*qi* between the interior and the exterior so that *qi* fails to ascend and descend and spread smoothly.

[Syndrome] Alternate spells of fever and chill, feeling of fullness and discomfort in the chest and hypochondrium, bitter taste and dry throat, taciturnity and loss of appetite, and wiry pulse.

[Treatment] Eliminating the pathogenic factor from *Shaoyang*.

[Recipe] *Xiao Chai Hu Tang*[30].

(4) *Taiyin* disease

[Pathogenesis] *Taiyin* is the chief of the three *yin* channels. Invasion of *Taiyin* by pathogenic factors causes the insufficiency of the spleen – *yang*, the stagnation of cold – dampness in the middle – *jiao* and direct attack of pathogenic cold on the *yin* channels, and, as a result, the failure of ascending and descending.

[Syndrome] Fullness of the abdomen with occasional pain, poor appetite, vomiting and diarrhea, tastelessness and thirstlessness, pale tongue and whitish fur, and slow or moderate pulse.

[Treatment] Warming the middle – *jiao* to dispel cold.

[Recipe] *Li Zhong Tang*[229], etc.

(5) *Shaoyin* disease

[Pathogenesis] The pathogenic factor entering *Shaoyin* does damage to the heart and the kidney. According to the excess or deficiency of *yin* and *yang* of the human body, *Shaoyin* diseases can be divided into two types: in case of *yin* – deficiency, heat – transmisson from *yang*, and, in case of *yang* – deficiency, cold – transmisson from *yin*.

[Syndrome] In case of cold of insufficiency type of *Shaoyin*: aversion to cold and coldness in the limbs, somnolence and mental fatigue, watery diarrhea with indigested food in the stool, and indistinct and thready pulse; in case of fever of deficiency type of *Shaoyin*: insomnia due to vexation, dry mouth and throat, and thready and rapid pulse.

[Treatment] In case of cold – transmission: recuperating the depleted *yang* and rescuing the patient from collapse; and in case of heat – transmission: nourishing *yin* and clearing away the heat.

[Recipe] *Si Ni Tang*[80] for cold – transmission, *Huang Lian E Jiao Tang*[231] for heat – transmission.

(6) *Jueyin* disease

[Pathogenesis] When *Jueyin* is diseased, excessive *Jue* – heat is brought about, *qi* is out of order and cold and heat syndromes occur simultaneously.

[Syndrome] Constant thirst, reflux of *qi* to the heart, pain and hotness sensation in the heart, anorexia, cold limbs and diarrhea, vomiting or vomiting of ascarides.

[Treatment] Combined therapy of warming with heat – clearing

[Recipe] *Wu Mei Wan*[56].

2.2.2 Introduction to the Pathogenesis and Syndromes of *Wei*, *Qi*, *Ying* and *Xue*

Theory of *wei*, *qi*, *ying* and *xue* is a TCM theoretical system of febrile diseases, which expounds the ways of syndrome differetiation and treatment of febrile diseases at different depths and stages, and, therefore, is mainly applied to the treatment of exopathic and infectious febrile diseases. Here is just a brief discussion of it.

(1) *Weifen* Syndrome

[Pathogenesis] Pathogenic warmth that invades the body from the exterior attacks the lung and is stagnated in *wei*, so that disorder of *qi* is caused, with the pathogen and the vital-*qi* struggling at *weifen*.

[Syndroms] Fever and dry mouth, slight aversion to wind and cold, occasional headache and pain in the throat, cough, red margin and tip of the tongue, and floating and rapid pulse.

[Treatment] Relieving the exterior syndrome with drugs pungent in flavour and cold in property.

[Recipe] *Yin Qiao San*[255], *Sang Ju Yin*[227], etc.

(2) *Qifen* syndrome

[Pathogenesis] Wind-warm pathogen invades the lung and stomach, or damp-heat lingers in *san-jiao*, thus leading to the struggle between the vital-*qi* and the pathogenic factor at *qifen*.

[Syndrome] High fever and aversion to heat, thirst with a bitter taste, vexation, cough, fever unrelieved with sweating, dark urine, full and large pulse or deep and replete pulse.

[Treatment] Clearing away the heat, expelling the pathogenic factor from the exterior and promoting the dispersing function of the lung.

[Recipe] *Zhi Zi Chi Tang*[237], *Ma Xing Shi Gan Tang*[241], *Bai Hu Tang*[91], and for damp-heat lingering in *san-jiao*, *Hao Qin Qing Dan Tang*[276], *Gan Lu Xiao Du Dan*[74], etc.

(3) *Yingfen* syndrome

[Pathogenesis] Constant invasion of pathogenic warmth consumes *ying-yin* and heat sinks into the pericardium and mentality is disturbed.

[Syndrome] Fever and vexation, dry mouth and sleeplessness, reddened or crimson tongue, and rapid pulse; or indistinct skin eruptions, or coma and delirium, rapid pulse.

[Treatment] Expelling heat from *yinfen* or removing the heat from the heart to restore consciousness.

[Recipe] *Qing Ying Tang*[252] or *An Gong Niu Huang Wan*[111], *Zi Xue Dan*[267].

(4) *Xuefen* syndrome

[Pathogenesis] Pathogenic warmth entering *xuefen* does damage to the heart and liver, causing consumption of genuine-*yin*, affecting the kidney, stirring up and consuming blood, and impairing *yin* and giving rise to wind.

[Syndrome] High fever, coma or mania, distinct skin eruptions, hematemesis, nose-bleeding, hemafecia, hematuria, tic or spasm of the limbs, crimson or red and bright mirror-like tongue, feeble and rapid or running pulse.

[Treatment] Removing heat from the blood and dissipating blood stasis, or removing heat from the liver and calming the endopathic wind, or nourishing *yin* and tranquilizing the endogenous wind.

[Recipe] *Xi Jiao Di Huang Tang*[273], *Ling Yang Gou Teng Tang*[247] for removing heat from the liver and calming the endopathic wind, *Da Ding Feng Zhu*[19] for nourishing *yin* and tranquilizing the endogenous wind.

Summary

The differentiation of syndromes of the six meridians are named after the channels, which is of profound implication, for channels, on the one hand are subordinate to *zang-fu* organs and, on the other, they are closely connected with the six kinds of natural factors and the eight principal syndromes serving as guidelines in diagnosis. By analyzing and differentiating of febrile diseases in accordance with the theory of the six meridians, it is meant that the occurrence and development of epidemic febrile diseases caused by exopathogens are classified into six main syndrome tpes so as to direct clinical practice, while analyzing and differentiating the development of epidemic febrile disease by studying the condition of the four systems (*wei*, *qi*, *ying* and *xue*) means that the whole process of the occurrence and development of a febrile disease is divided into four stages, or the four syndrome types defined in accordance with the severeness of a febrile disease and the depth of the part where it is.

Syndrome differentiation in light of the six-meridian theory and that in accordance with the condition of *wei*, *qi*, *ying* and *xue* have much in common. For example, they both take as their main task the differentiation and treatment of epidemic febrile diseases caused by exopathogens, they analyze and differentiate febrile diseases according to the rule of the development from the exterior to the interior and from the shallow to the deep. The "*weifen* syndrome" and "*qifen* syndrome" in the doctrine of epidemic febrile disease are quite similar to what are called "*taiyang* disease" and "*yangming* disease" in *Shang Han Lun*(Treatise on Febrile Diseases). These diseases, in most cases, are exterior syndromes at initial stage, interior and excess syndrome at excessive-heat stage, and deficiency syndromes at later stage. But syndrome differentiation in light of the six-meridian theory and that in accordance with the condition of *wei*, *qi*, *ying* and *xue* possess respective characteristics. For instance, the theory of exogenous febrile disease tends to treat coma and delirium with purgative therapy, while the doctrine of epidemic febrile disease adds to it the therapy of removing heat from the heart to resuscitate mentality, the former lays particular stress on recuperating depleted *yang*, with attention paid to *yang-qi*, while the latter attacks great importance to the recuperation of depleted *yin*, always taking care to preserve *yin*-fluid. Generally speaking, however, both of them take the eight principal syndromes as their general principles and *zang-fu* and channels and collaterals as their bases. It's important to have a comprehensive knowledge of their similarities and differences, and, from the point of view of holistic concept, combine them together and make flexible use of them so as to differentiate syndromes and select treatment correctly.

Discussions

1. What's the concept of syndrome differentiation according to the six-meridian theory? To what field is it applicable?

2. What is the concept of syndrome differentiation in accordunce with the condition of *wei*, *qi*, *ying* and *xue*? And the syndrome types?

3. What's the relationship between syndrome differentiation according to the six-meridian theory and that in accordance with the condition of *wei*, *qi*, *ying* and *xue*? And what's the relationship between the two and syndrome differentiation in accordance with the eight principal syndromes as well as the *zang-fu* theory?

2.3 Basic Concept of the Pathogenesis and Syndromes of *Qi* and Blood

In TCM theory, *qi* and blood are regarded as the source and motive force of life activity. *Qi* belongs to *yang*, and blood to *yin*. So they always accompany, generate, promote and depend upon each other. *Qi* plays the role of warming, transmitting, promoting and controlling blood, while blood takes it as its task to nourish and carry *qi*. Thus it can be seen that the two are closely related to each other.

Qi and blood, on the one hand, are the substances produced when *zang-fu* organs are performing their functions, and, on the other, being the material base indispensable to *zang-fu* functions, are constantly consumed by life activities. It is this dynamic equilibrium of mutual transformation and wane and wax of *qi* and blood that keeps the body healthy. Should the relations, between *qi* and blood or their dynamic equilibrium, be broken up, their pathological changes would be brought about, such as deficiency of *qi* and blood, *qi*'s failure in controlling blood, exhaustion of *qi* resulting from hemorrhea, and stagnancy of *qi* and blood stasis.

The pathological changes of *qi* and blood not only affect *qi* and blood themselves but also affect the functional activities of the *zang-fu* organs. So, to discuss the pathogenesis and syndromes of *qi* and blood, it's necessary to take *zang-fu* into account, and to deal with the differentiation of syndromes according to the pathological changes of the *zang-fu* organs, it's essential to have a good mastery of the pathogenesis of *qi* and blood. Only in this way, can it be possible to get a correct command of the dialectical ideology of TCM internal medicine.

2.3.1 *Qi* Disease

In TCM theoretical system, *qi* implies, first, the refined substances that form and keep alive life activity, such as *ying-qi* and *zong-qi*, and, second, the activities and manifestations of the various functions of the body, such as *zang-qi* and *jing-qi*. The two implications mentioned above are different, but each of them may sometimes contain the other. This is one of the main characteristics of TCM theory.

To sum up, *qi* is responsible for warming, promoting, defending, astringing and transforming. *Qi* belongs to *yang*. That's why deficiency of *qi* is mostly manifested as various symptoms of consumptiveness and cold of deficiency type. And hyperfunction of *qi* may lead to fire-syndrome. Any disorder of the movement of *qi* may cause it to accumulate and become fire so that heat comes into being inside.

The movement of *qi* is known as *qi ji* (functional activities of *qi*), generally referring to the functional manifestions of the tissues and organs (*zang-fu* organs, channels and collaterals, etc.) of the body in the whole process of life. The basic forms of the movement of *qi* are ascending, descending, in-going and out-going, which depend directly on and reflect the functional activities of the *zang-fu* organs.

The pathological changes of *qi* can be grouped under two heads: insufficiency of formation and abnormality of movement. Types commonly seen are discussed below.

Deficiency syndromes

(1) Deficiency of *qi*

[Pathogenesis] Weakness after prolonged illness, improper diet and many other causes leading to the insufficient formation of *yuan qi* (primordial *qi*) or its excessive consumption, and, in consequence, the decline of the functions of *zang-fu* organs.

[Syndromes] Dizziness, fatigue, listlessness and wordlessness, spontaneous perspiration, pale tongue and feeble pulse.

[Treatment] Invigorating *qi*.

[Recipe] *Si Jun Zi Tang*[77].

(2) *Qi* collapse

[Pathogenesis] Deficiency of *qi* leading to the abnormality of *qi*'s ascent and descent, *qi* being too weak to go up.

[Syndromes] Dizziness, fatigue and listlessness, sensation of fullness and straining in the abdomen, proctoptosis, pale tongue and white fur, and weak pulse.

[Treatment] Invigorating *qi* and lifting it.

[Recipe] *Bu Zhong Yi Qi Tang*[140].

Excess syndromes

(3) Stagnation of *qi*

[Pathogenesis] Tense emotions, improper diet, invassion by exopathic factors, etc. making *qi* unable to move smoothly and leading to *qi* stagnation.

[Syndroms] Distending pain in the hypochondrium and abdomen, shifting pain varying in severeness, thin fur and taut pulse.

[Treatment] Promoting the flow of *qi* and dredging the stagnation.

[Recipe] *Jin Ling Zi San*[162], *Wu Mo Yin Zi*[43], etc.

(4) Reversed flow of *qi*

[Pathogenesis] Abnormal ascent and descent of *qi*, which often refers to the reversed upward flow of *qi* and fire caused by the adverse rising of the lung-*qi* and the stomach - *qi* or by the undue ascent of the liver - *qi*.

[Syndromes] The stomach: hiccup, eructation, vomiting; the liver: headache, dizziness and syncope, hematemesis; the lung: cough and dyspnea.

[Treatment] Lowering the adverse flow of *qi* and relieving asthma.

[Recipe] *Su Zi Jiang Qi Tang*[127], *Xuan Fu Dai Zhe Tang*[244], etc.

2.3.2 Blood Disease

Blood, the most essential nutrient of life activity, pertains to *yin* and plays the role of nourishing. The spleen produces blood and keeps it flowing; the liver stores blood; the heart controls the circulation of blood and the heart - *yang* serves as the dynamic force keeping blood running in the vessels so that nutritious substances are distributed to every part of the body.

Blood diseases are usually marked by deficiency of blood, blood stasis as well as hemorrhage, which are different and related to one another at the same time. Blood deficiency may lead to hemorrhage and hemorrhage may be the pathogenesis of blood stasis. Blood stasis is likely to result in continual bleeding, and before the removal of blood stasis, new blood can't be possibly produced, thus leading to blood deficiency.

The main types of blood disease are:

(1) Deficiency of blood

[Pathogenesis] Various causes that bring about insufficient formation and consumption of blood may lead to deficiency of blood.

[Syndromes] Pale complexion, pale lips and nails, dizziness, palpitation and insomnia, numbness of the hands and feet, pale tongue, and weak and thready pulse.

[Treatment] Enriching the blood.

[Recipe] *Si Wu Tang*[79].

(2) Blood stasis

[Pathogenesis] Deficiency of *qi*, *qi* stasis, accumulation of cold, or accumulation of heat preventing blood from flowing smoothly and leading to blood stasis.

[Syndromes] Stabbing pain which is localized, tenderness, local purpura, tumour, purplish and dim lips and nails, squamous and dry skin, blood stasis that occurs in a definite *zang* or *fu* organ is likely to affect its functions, thus causing such corresponding symptoms as chest pain, hemoptysis, hematemesis and hemafecia.

[Treatment] Promoting blood circulation to remove blood stasis.

[Recipe] *Xue Fu Zhu Yu Tang*[119].

(3) Hemorrhage

[Pathogenesis] Hemorrhage is often caused by pathogenic fire that makes blood flow preposterously, or by failure of controlling blood as a result of deficiency of *qi*, or by deficiency of kidney -*yin* because *yin* deficiency leads to hyperactivity of fire and fire of deficiency type does damage to the collaterals.

[Syndromes] Hemoptysis, hematemesis, hemafecia, hematuria, and epistaxis.

[Treatment] For those with preposterous blood flow: purging away the heat and arresting bleeding; for those with failure of controlling blood due to *qi* deficiency: invigorating *qi* to control blood ; and for those with hyperactivity of fire and *yin* deficiency: nourishing *yin* to reduce pathogenic fire.

[Recipe] *Xi Jiao Di Huang Tang*[273] for purging away the heat and arresting bleeding, *Gui Pi Tang*[95] for invigorating *qi* to control blood , and *Qian Gen San*[178] for nourishing *yin* to reduce pathogenic fire.

Summary

The main points of the treatment of the diseases of *qi* and blood are summed up below.

1. Illness of deficiency type should be treated by tonifying method. Illness of *qi* deficiency should be treated by invigorating *qi*, mainly, the *qi* of the lung, spleen and kidney. Illness of blood deficiency be treated by enriching blood; as *qi* and blood transform each other, enriching blood and invigorating *qi* should be performed simultaneously so as to attain the goal of supplementing *qi* and promoting the production of blood.

2. Stasis syndrome should be treated with dissipating method, and stagnancy syndrome by promoting the circulation of *qi* or blood. Excess syndromes of *qi* and blood should be treated by regulating the flow of *qi* , sending down the abnormally ascending *qi*, promoting the flow of *qi*, activating blood flow and removing blood stasis.

3. Hemorrhage must be arrested as soon as possible, treatment must be adopted in accordance with the cause, such as removing heat from the blood to stop bleeding, and nourishing *yin* and reducing pathogenic fire to stop bleeding. In treating those with failure of controlling blood due to deficiency of *qi*, it is especially important to keep in mind the principle of treating acute and severe hemorrhage: blood, which is visible, can't be possibly produced soon, and *qi*, which is invisible, must be reinforced at any time.

Simultaneous diseases of *qi* and blood are grouped under the following heads:

1. *Qi* stagnancy and blood stasis, *qi* stagnancy preventing blood from flowing freely, treated by promoting the circulation of *qi* to remove blood stasis.

2. *Qi* deficiency and blood stasis, *qi* being too weak to promote blood flow, treated by invigorating *qi* and promoting the circulation of blood.

3. Deficiency of both *qi* and blood, caused by insufficient formation or excessive consumption of *qi* and blood, treated by invigorating *qi* and enriching blood.

4. *Qi* deficiency and hemorrhage, *qi* being too weak to control blood and thus leading to hemorrhage, treated by invigorating *qi* to control blood.

5. Exhaustion of *qi* resulting from hemorrhea, hemorrhage leading to exhaustion of *qi* on account of *qi* losing its prop, treated by arresting bleeding and reinforcing *qi*.

Discussions

1. The physiological relationship between *qi* and blood and their pathological interaction.
2. What are the main types of the pathogenesis and syndromes of blood disease?

2.4 Basic Concept of the Pathogenesis and Syndromes of *Zang* – *Fu* Organs

Zang – *fu* diseases are the pathological changes of the functions of the *zang* – *fu* organs that manifest themselves in various clinical syndromes. And the abnormal functions of the *zang* – *fu* organs and the consequent pathological changes are known as *zang* – *fu* pathogenesis.

Differentiating syndromes according to the theory of *zang* – *fu*, the core of selecting of treatment by differentiating syndromes in TCM internal medicine, is based on the mastery of *zang* – *fu* diseases and the understanding of *zang* – *fu* pathogonesis, and, therefore, a dialectical method to make clear the location and nature of the pathological changes. The pathogenesis and syndromes of the five pathogenic factors, the six channels, *wei*, *qi*, *ying* and *xue* as well as *qi* and blood must be centered on *zang* and *fu*, for one of the important guiding principles of diagnosing in light of TCM theory is the holistic concept that takes the five *zang* – organs as its center.

Zang –*fu* organs are closely related to each other, and a unity of the whole body. The five *zang* – organs generate, restrict, encroach and counter – restrict one another, *zang* and *fu* are exterior –interiorly related, and meridians and collaterals integrate the body into a whole by connecting closely together the five *zang* – organs and six *fu* – organs, the limbs and bones, the five sense organs and nine orifices, and the skin and muscles and tendons. *Qi*, blood and body fluid are produced and distributed by *zang* and *fu*, which, in turn, depend on *qi*, blood and body fluid for performing their physiological activities. That's why *zang* – *fu* pathogenesis and syndromes are certain to involve *qi*, blood and fluid as well as meridians and collaterals. Complicated as the relations are, they can still be summed up by the eight principal syndromes serving as guidelines in diagnosis, namely, *yin* and *yang*, exterior and interior, cold and heat, and deficiency and excess syndromes. So differentiating syndromes by the theory of the eight principal syndromes must be taken as the basis of syndrome differentiation according to the theory of *zang* and *fu* organs. These two ways of differentiating syndromes are the basis, and the core of selecting treatment by differentiating syndromes in TCM internal medicine.

2.4.1 Introduction to the Pathogenesis and Syndromes of the Pulmonary (Large Intestine) System

Characteristics of Pathogenesis:

(1) The lung controls *qi* and is responsible for respiration. So the pathological

changes of the lung are mainly manifested in the abnormal in-going, out-going, ascending and descending of qi.

(2) The lung, a tender organ, has its orifice in the nose and is exteriorly related to the skin and hair. So the lung is the first to be affected once the body is invaded by exopathic factors.

(3) The lung-qi must be kept flowing freely. Any obstruction of the lung-qi will lead to cough with dyspnea.

(4) The blood vessels converge in the lung, and the lung is responsible for the coordination of functional activities. So abnormal flow of the lung-qi will cause abnormal flow of the heart-blood.

(5) The lung regulates water metabolism and transports water into the bladder. So once the lung-qi fails to descend, stagnancy of body fluid will be brought about.

(6) The lung and the large intestine are interior-exteriorly related. The purifying and descending function of the lung and the transporting function of the large intestine have effect on each other.

The diseases commonly seen in clinical practice are common cold, cough, asthma with wheezing, syndrome characterized by dyspnea, pulmonary abscess, tuberculosis hemoptysis, epistaxis, and so on.

Classifications of Diagnosis and Treatment

Excess syndromes

(1) Invasion of the pathogenic cold to the lung

[Pathogenesis] Affection by pathogenic cold leading to obstruction of the lung qi and cold fluid-retention inside the body causing impairment of the purifying and descending function of the lung.

[Syndrome] In cases with tachypnea due to attack of pathogenic wind-cold: aversion to cold and fever, anhidrosis, headache and body discomfort, stuffy nose and watery nasal discharge, cough with thin sputum, thin and white fur, and floating and tense pulse; in cases with cold fluid-retention: severe cough, shortness of breath and heaviness sensation in the body, whitish and frothy sputum and large quantity of sputum, whitish and moist and glossy fur, floating or slippery pulse.

[Treatment] Ventilating the lung and dispelling the cold, or warming and resolving phlegm-retention.

[Recipe] *Ma Huang Tang*[242], *Xiao Qing Long Tang*[27].

(2) The encroachment of the lung by pathogenic heat

[Pathogenesis] Wind-heat affecting the upper-*jiao* or stagnated cold turning into heat, so that phlegm and heat are accumulated and the lung fails to perform its purifying and descending function.

[Syndromes] In cases with invasion of the lung by wind-heat: cough with yellowish sputum, or thick nasal discharge or aversion to wind and fever, sore-throat, thin and yellowish fur, and floating and rapid pulse; in cases with accumulation of phlegm and heat in the lung: cough with large quantity of thick and yellowish sputum, or with stench or pus and blood, dyspnea with bronchial wheezing, cough with pain in the chest, extreme thirst and desire for drinking, dark urine and constipation, red tongue and dry and yellowish fur, slippery and rapid pulse.

[Treatment] Dispelling wind and removing heat, or removing heat from the lung and dissolving phlegm.

[Recipe] *Sang Ju Yin*[227], *Yin Qiao San*[255], or *Qing Jin Hua Tan Tang*[248], etc.

(3) Stagnation of phlegm in the lung

[Pathogenesis] Invasion by exopathic factors or prolonged dyspnea causing the lung to be unable to distribute body fluid, leading to accumulation of phlegm-dampness in the lung; or the spleen being too weak to perform its transporting function, and accumulated dampness turning into phlegm which goes upward and soils the lung.

[Syndromes] In cases with stagnation of phlegm-dampness in the lung: cough with much thick and sticky, whitish or grey sputum, shortness of breath, thick and whitish and greasy fur, and soft-floating and slippery pulse; in cases with stagnation of excessive fluid in the lung: dyspnea with bronchial wheezing, pain and fullness sensation in the chest and hypochondrium, sleeplessness due to the dyspnea, greasy and yellowish fur, and taut and slippery or rapid pulse.

[Treatment] Removing dampness from the lung to reduce phlegm, or removing heat from the lung to clear away phlegm stagnation.

[Recipe] *Er Chen Tang*[2], *Ping Wei San*[70] or *Ting Li Da Zao Xie Fei Tang*[261], *Kong Xian Dan*[238], etc.

Deficiency syndromes

(1) Lung-dryness due to *yin*-deficiency

[Pathogenesis] Invasion by exopathic dryness leading to consumption of the lung-fluid, or pathogenic wind, pathogenic warm, etc., causing impairment of body fluid and dryness-transformation; or attack on the lung by other pathogenic factors, impairment of the lung caused by prolonged cough and the consumption of both *qi* and blood resulting in the deficiency of the lung-*yin* and fever of deficiency type that bums and consumes the lung-*yin*.

[Syndromes] In cases with invasion of the lung by pathogenic dryness: cough with dyspnea, little but sticky phlegm sometimes with blood streak, dry mouth and sore throat, or sensation of slight cold and fever, thin and dry fur, red tip and margin of the tongue, and thready and rapid pulse; in cases with fever of deficiency type: dry cough with little phlegm or phlegm with blood, hoarseness and red throat, hectic fever and night sweat, emaciation, red tongue and thin fur, and thready and rapid pulse.

[Treatment] Clearing away the lung-heat and moisturizing dryness, or nourishing *yin* and moisturizing the lung.

[Recipe] *Sang Xing Tang*[226], *Qing Zao Jiu Fei Tang*[254], or *Bai He Gu Jin Tang*[103], *Sha Shen Mai Dong Tang*[138], etc.

(2) Deficiency of the lung – *qi*

[Pathogenesis] Overstrain, impairment of the lung due to prolonged cough, or insufficient transformation of *qi*.

[Syndromes] Cough with shortness of breath, fatigue and dislike of speech, weak and low voice, intolerance of wind and spontaneous perspiration, pale tongue and thin and whitish fur, weak and feeble pulse.

[Treatment] Replenishing and restoring the lung – *qi*.

[Recipe] *Bu Fei Tang*[143], etc.

Accompanying syndromes

(1) Insufficiency of the spleen involving the lung: insufficiency of the spleen – *qi* accompanied by insufficiency of the lung – *qi*, treated by strengthening the lung by way of reinforcing the spleen, or invigorating the spleen to benefit the lung, with *Liu Jun Zi Tang*[45], etc.

(2) Deficiency of *Yin* of both the lung and the kidney: deficiency of the lung – *yin* accompanied by deficiency of the kidney – *yin*, treated by nourishing the kidney and the lung, with *Liu Wei Di Huang Wan*[46], *Sheng Mai San*[84], etc.

(3) The liver – fire affecting the lung: stagnation of the liver – *qi* accompanied by retention of pathogenic heat in the lung, treated by removing heat from the liver and purging the lung of pathogenic fire, with *Dai Ge San*[287], and *Xie Bai San*[154], and so on.

Main Points of Diagnosis and Treatment

① The lung is a tender organ with little tolerance to cold and heat. So, in treatment, drugs used should be of mild action, acrid and sweet in taste and have calming and moistening effect, and heavy drugs that are hot in nature and have drying effect must be avoided.

② There are two different methods to treat pulmonary diseases: direct treatment and indirect treatment. The former means that, in light of the cause and pathogenesis, such methods are adopted as promoting the dispersing function of the lung, removing heat from the lung, warming the lung, moistening the lung, tonifying the lung, astringing the lung, etc. The latter means that, in accordance with the inter – restriction and inter – generation of the five *zang* – organs, such methods are used as strengthening the lung (i.e. metal) by way of reinforcing the spleen (earth) so as to regulate the relations between the lung and other *zang* – organs.

③ Diseases of the pulmonary system are divided into two categories: those caused by exopathogen and those caused by internal injury. In most cases, the former are excess syndromes, and the latter are deficiency in primary but excess in the secondary; and the former occur at the lung and *wei*, and the latter mainly inside the lung, being related to the heart, liver, spleen and kidney, which should be given an overall consideration in clinical practice.

Appendix: Introduction to the Pathogenesis and Syndromes of the Large Intestine

Characteristics of Pathogenesis

The lung and the large intestine are exterior - interiorly related and correspond to each other. Any obstruction of the lung -*qi* will lead to the stagnation of the large intestine -*qi*. The large intestine is in charge of transporting waste matter and is dominated by the spleen, so the insufficiency of the spleen -*yang* is likely to cause disorder of the large intestine's transporting function. As the large intestine is also responsible for the further absorption of body fluid, the insufficiency of the spleen -*yin* will bring about the insufficiency of fluid in the large intestine, thus leading to difficulty in defecation.

Diseases of the large intestine commonly found are constipation, diarrhea, dysentery, abdominal pain, and what not.

Classification of Diagnosis and Treatment

(1) Excess heat of the large intestine

[Pathogenesis] Pathogenic heat of excess type accumulating in the *yangming fu* - organ leading to obstruction.

[Syndromes] Constipation, abdominal pain and tenderness, or fever and vomiting, or loose stool, or fecal impaction due to heat with watery discharge, or dysphoria and delirium, dry and yellowish or sallow and prickled fur, deep and forceful pulse.

[Treatment] Clearing away heat and resolving stagnation.

[Recipe] *Da Cheng Qi Tang*[21], etc.

(2) Damp -heat of the large intestine

[Pathogenesis] Invasion of summer - heat and dampness and improper or dirty diet leading to the accumulation of damp - heat in the large intestine.

[Syndromes] Diarrhea, or dysentery with bloody stool or with mucus or purulent discharge, tenesmus, burning sensation in the anus, abdominal pain, fever and heaviness sensation in the body, greasy and yellowish fur, and slippery and rapid pulse.

[Treatment] Clearing away heat and eliminating dampness.

[Recipe] *Ge Gen Qin Lian Tang*[260] or *Bai Tou Weng Tang*[88], etc.

(3) Deficiency cold of the large intestine

[Pathogenesis] Insufficiency of both the spleen and the kidney, or impairment of *yang* caused by extreme cold, or pathogenic cold entering the intestines directly.

[Syndromes] Loose stool or constant diarrhea, fullness in the abdomen and occasional pain relieved by warming and pressing, or proctoptosis, coldness in the limbs, pale tongue, thin and whitish fur, and thready and weak pulse.

[Treatment] Warming *yang* and dispelling cold.

[Recipe] *Fu Zi Li Zhong Tang*[146], etc.

(4) Insufficiency of body fluid in the large intestine

[Pathogenesis] Impairment of the large intestines fluid caused by dryness-heat, or the spleen-yin being too deficient to go down into the large intestine, thus leading to the insufficiency of fluid.

[Syndromes] Dry and hard stool at a few days' interval, foul breath and dry throat, or dizziness and abdominal distention, reddened tongue with little saliva, dry and yellowish fur, and thready pulse.

[Treatment] Loosening the bowel to relieve constipation.

[Recipe] *Ma Zi Ren Wan*[240], *Zeng Ye Cheng Qi Tang* [284].

2.4.2 Introduction to the Pathogenesis and Syndromes of the Heart (Small Intestine) System

Characteristics of Pathogenesis

(1) The heart controls blood circulation as well as mental and emtional activities. So the pathological changes of the heart are mainly seen in the disorder of blood flow and the abnormality of mental and emotional activities.

(2) The pericardium is the periphery of the heart, and so it is the first to be attacked in case of the reverse transmission of pathogenic warmth.

(3) The diseases of the heart are mainly caused by internal injury. The deficiency of the heart-yin is mostly caused by the insufficiency of heart blood, and the deficiency of the heart-yang by the insufficiency of the heart-qi.

(4) Excess syndrome and heat syndrome of the heart are mostly caused by emotional depression, fire-transmission and phlegm-production, phlegm-fire disturbing the heart, or stagnancy of qi and blood stasis, blockage of the meridians, or fluid retention blocking the heart-yang.

Classification of Diagnosis and Treatment

Deficiency Syndromes

(1) Insufficiency of the heart-yang (-qi)

[Pathogenesis] Delicate constitution, weakness due to prolonged illness, impairment of yang caused by sudden attack of a serious illness.

[Syndromes] Palpitation, shortness of breath, oppressed feeling in the chest, precordial pain, or pale complexion, chillness in the body and spontaneous perspiration, feeble or knotted and intermitted pulse.

[Treatment] Warming the heart-yang, supplementing the heart-qi.

[Recipe] *Gui Zhi Jia Fu Zi Tang*[202], *Yang Xin Tang*[185].

(2) Insufficiency of the heart-yin (-blood)

[Pathogenesis] Impairment of yin after hemorrhage or due to febrile disease, or excessive anxiety leading to the consumption of yin-blood; or insufficient transformation of blood.

[Syndromes] Palpitation, vexation, fear and restlessness, dreamy sleep, reddened tongue and little fur, and thready and rapid pulse.

[Treatment] Nourishing *yin*, nourishing the heart and tranquilizing the mind.

[Recipe] *Tian Wang Bu Xin Dan* [32], *Si Wu Tang* [79], etc.

Excess Syndromes

(1) Internal disturbance by phlegm-fire

[Pathogenesis] Emotional depression leading to stagnation of *qi* and fire-transmission that boils fluid and turns it into phlegm and phlegm-fire disturbs the heart and impairs the pericardium.

[Syndromes] Palpitation, maniac-depressive psychosis, insomnia due to dysphoria, reddened or chapped tongue, little fur, and slippery and rapid pulse.

[Treatment] Clearing away the heart-fire, dissolving phlegm and purging intense heat.

[Recipe] *Meng Shi Gun Tan Wan* [289].

(2) Blockage of the heart-yang by fluid-retention

[Pathogenesis] The stagnation of phlegm and fluid retention blocking the heart-*yang*, thus leading to the disorder of *qi*.

[Syndromes] Palpitation, oppressed feeling in the chest, paroxysmal dizziness, vomiting with phlegm and saliva, greasy and whitish fur, taut and slippery or deep and tense pulse.

[Treatment] Removing fluid retention and eliminating phlegm.

[Recipe] *Fu Ling Gan Cao Tang* [174], *Dao Tan Tang* [121].

(3) Stagnation of the heart blood

[Pathogenesis] The heart-*qi* or the heart-*yang* being too insufficient to promote blood flow vigorously, thus leading to *qi* stagnation and blood stasis as well as collaterals blockage.

[Syndromes] Severe palpitation, oppressed feeling in the chest with stabbing pain, sharp pain in the chest in severe cases, bluish purple lips, coma and coldness of limbs, dark tongue or with ecchymosis, thready and uneven or knotted and intermitted pulse.

[Treatment] Promoting blood circulation to remove obstruction in the collaterals and blood stasis.

[Recipe] *Xue Fu Zhu Yu Tang* [119], etc.

Accompanying syndromes

(1) Deficiency of both the heart and the spleen: accompanied by the deficiency of the heart-*qi* and the deficiency of the spleen-*qi*. Treatment: tonifying the heart and the spleen with *Gui Pi Tang* [95].

(2) Breakdown of the normal physiological coordination between the heart and the kidney: the deficiency of the heart-*yin* leading to the stir of fire of deficiency type in the kidney, accompanied by the deficiency of both the heart-*yin* and the kidney-*yin* and

hyperactivity of fire due to *yin* deficiency, treated by restoring the normal coordination between the heart and the kidney with *Huang Lian E Jiao Tang* [231], *Jiao Tai Wan* [110], etc.

(3) Insufficiency of both the heart-*qi* and the lung-*qi*: accompanied by the insufficiency of the heart-*yang* and lung-*yang*, treated by tonifying the heart and the lung with *Bao Yuan Tang* [192].

Main Points of Diagnosis and Treatment

①*Qi* belongs to *yang*, and blood to *yin*. They depend on each other. So the deficiency of the heart-*yang* is certain to be accompanied by the deficiency of the heart-*qi*, and the deficiency of the heart-*yin* by the deficiency of the heart-blood. In clinical practice, attention must be paid to this kind of relationship to find the *yang* aspect of *yin* and the *yin* aspect of *yang* and to give consideration to both of them.

② In treating diseases of the heart system, consideration must be given to the relations between the heart and the spleen, the lung, the liver and the kidney. For example, the deficiency of the heart-*yang* and the blockage of the heart-*yang* by fluid retention are related to the dysfunction of the spleen-*yang* in transport; and the deficiency of the heart-*yin* and the disturbance of the heart by phlegm-fire are connected with the deficiency of both the liver-*yin* and the kidney-*yin* and the hyperactivity of fire. All these must be coped with in an integrative way.

③ Diseases of the heart system are divided into deficiency and excess syndromes, but one of them is often found in the other. For example, any obstruction by blood stasis is usually excess syndrome caused by deficiency, manifested as deficiency in origin and excess in superficiality. So it is important to distinguish between superficiality and origin, and deal with them in order of urgency.

④ The heart controls mental activities. Any imbalance between *qi* and blood or between *yin* and *yang* of the heart will cause disturbance of mental and emotional activities. In treatment, drugs that are effective in relieving mental stress or tranquilizing the mentality should be made use of.

Appendix: Introduction to the Pathogenesis and Syndromes of the Small Intestine

Characteristics of Pathogenesis

The heart and the small intestine are connected exterior-interiorly. The small intestine is responsible for receiving the food stuff from the stomach and separating the useful substances from the waste ones. Diseases of the small intestine are mostly caused by improper diet thus leading to the impairment of the spleen and stomach, which affects the small intestine downward. The pathogenesis lies in the small intestine's failure in separating the useful from the waste and transporting them. Deficiency and cold syndromes of the small intestine are often related to the impairment of the spleen and stomach, and the excess and heat syndromes are usually brought about by the heart-fire that comes down to the small intestine.

The diseases of the small intestine commonly found in clinical practice are diarrhea, abdominal pain, hematuria and so on.

Classification of Diagnosis and Treatment

(1) Cold of deficiency of the small intestine

[Pathogenesis] Improper diet leading to the impairment of the spleen and stomach and, then, the dysfunction of the small intestine in separating the useful substances from the waste ones.

[Syndromes] Diarrhea with bowel sound, vague abdominal pain relieved by pressing, pale tongue, thin and whitish fur, and thready and moderate pulse.

[Treatment] Warming and promoting the small intestine.

[Recipe] *Wu Zhu Yu Tang*[135].

(2) Heat of excess of the small intestine

[Pathogenesis] The heart-fire descending to the small intestine.

[Syndromes] Vexation and insomnia, aphtha and tongue sore, dark urine with pain or even hematuria, reddened tongue and yellowish fur, and slippery and rapid pulse.

[Treatment] Clearing away the heart-fire and promoting the heat to descend.

[Recipe] *Dao Chi San*[120], *Liang Ge San*[213].

2.4.3 Introduction to the Pathogenesis and Syndromes of the Spleen (Stomach) System

Characteristics of Pathogenesis

(1) The spleen and stomach are related exterior-interiorly, with the spleen in charge of sending up essential substances and the stomach in charge of sending digested food downward and, thus, dryness and dampness supplemented each ofter. Any disturbance in ascending and descending of the spleen and stomach will lead to the dysfunction in receiving and transforming food into chyme and transporting it, so that vomiting, diarrhea, etc, are caused.

(2) As the spleen has the function of transporting and transforming nutrients and the stomach has the function to receive food and transform it into chyme, they are the source of the growth and development of *qi* and blood. Should the functions of the spleen and stomach be out of order, the source would be weakened and the body would be short of nutrients.

(3) The spleen controls blood flow. In case of deficiency of the spleen-*qi*, *qi* fails to keep blood flowing within the vessels so as to prevent its extravasation, so that blood troubles are caused.

(4) The spleen is in charge of transportation and transformation. Dysfunction of the spleen in transport will lead to abnormal distribution of body fluid and the stagnancy and accumulation of fluid will result in fluid retention and swelling. So the diseases of

the spleen often have to do with dampness, characterized by being deficiency in origin but excess in superficiality.

Diseases of the spleen (stomach) system often clinically found are: diarrhea, stomachache, hiccup, vomiting, phlegm stagnation, spitting blood, hemafecia, etc.

Classifications of Diagnosis and Treatment

Deficiency syndromes

(1) Insufficiency of the spleen – *yang*

[Pathogenesis] Excessive cold and uncooked food, weaknesss due to prolonged illness as well as excessive medicine of cool property leading to impairment of the spleen – *yang* and the dysfunction of the spleen in transportation and transformation.

[Syndromes] Sallow complexion and coldness in the gastric cavity, vomiting with watery fluid, anorexia and loose stool, or coldness of the limbs, pale tongue, whitish fur, and soft – floating and weak pulse.

[Treatment] Warming the middle – *jiao yang*.

[Recipe] *Li Zhong Wan*[229].

(2) Deficiency of *qi* in middle – *jiao*

[Pathogenesis] Delicate constitution, overstrain, impairment due to prolonged illness; dysfunction in transportation and transformation due to the deficiency of the spleen, as well as the spleen's incompetence in sending up essential substances.

[Syndromes] Anorexia and abdominal distention, fatigue and dislike of speech, loose stool with bowel sound, tenesmus or even proctoptosis in severe cases, pale tongue, thin and whitish fur, and weak and moderate pulse.

[Treatment] Invigorating the spleen and replenishing *qi*.

[Recipe] *Bu Zhong Yi Qi Tang*[140].

Excess syndromes

(1) Cold – dampness retention in the spleen

[Pathogenesis] Affection by exopathic cold – dampness or excessive endogenous pathogenic dampness causing the middle – *jiao yang* to be blocked and the spleen to fail in transporting and transforming essential substances.

[Syndromes] Fullness in the gastric cavity and anorexia, fatigue and heaviness sensation of the head and body, stickiness of the mouth and thirstlessness, loose stool or diarrhea, greasy and whitish fur, and soft – floating pulse.

[Treatment] Activating the spleen and resolving dampness.

[Recipe] *Wei Ling Tang*[182].

(2) Retention of damp – heat in the interior

[Pathogenesis] Affection of seasonal pathogens or excessive alcohol and sweets leading to the impairment of both the spleen and stomach and the dysfunction in transportation and transformation, so that dampness and heat are both stagnated or even steam the liver and gallbladder.

[Syndromes] Distention of the hypochondrium and gastic cavity, anorexia and bitter taste, fever and heaviness sensation in the body, dark urine and loose stool, and sallow complexion and itch of the skin if serious, greasy and yellowish fur, and soft-floating and rapid pulse.

[Treatment] Clearing away heat and promoting diuresis.

[Recipe] *Yin Chen Hao Tang*[177], *Wu Ling San*[41].

Accompanying syndromes

(1) Incoordination between the spleen and the stomach: insufficiency of the spleen and hypofunction of the stomach accompanied by disturbance in ascending and descending, treated by replenishing *qi* and activating the middle - *jiao*, or regulating the function of the spleen and the stomach, with *Xiang Sha Liu Jun Zi Tang*[189], etc.

(2) Deficiency of both the spleen - *yang* and the kidney - *yang*: the insufficiency of the *yang - qi* of the spleen accompanied by that of the kidney, treated by strengthening the spleen and warming the kidney, with *Fu Zi Li Zhong Tang*[146], *Si Shen Wan*[82], etc.

(3) Affection of the lung by dampness in the spleen: hypofunction of transportation due to the insufficiency of the spleen accompanied by the affection of the lung by phlegm -dampness, treated by eliminating dampness and removing phlegm, with *Er Chen Tang*[2], etc.

(4) Insufficiency of both the heart and the spleen: see the accompanying syndromes of the heart system.

Main Points of Diagnosis and Treatment

①The pathogenesis and syndromes of the spleen system are mostly deficiency in origin and excess in superficiality, a distinction between the origin and superficiality should be made so as to carry out treatment in order of urgency.

②The spleen tends to be benefited by dryness and damaged by dampness, therefore, exopathic dampness is likely to be trapped in the spleen, thus leading to endo - genous dampness because of the spleen's being deficiency. So the spleen diseases are closely related to pathogenic dampness, and damp syndrome is always found in the diseases caused by cold, heat, deficiency or excess. And in treatment, drugs effective in eliminating, drying dampness and promoting diuresis should be used.

③The diseases of the spleen are mostly caused by deficiency and cold, while those of the stomach by excess and heat, as the old saying goes, *yangming* disease occurring in strong persons while *taiyin* disease in weak persons. So the spleen can be strengthened and reinforced by ascending and the stomach can be regulated and put right by descending.

④The spleen and stomach lie in the middle - *jiao*, and are the pivot of the ascending and descending *qi* within the whole body. So they interact on other *zang* and *fu* organs, and are especially related to the liver and the kidney. Treatment, therefore, must be carried out from the point of view of holistic concept and with all of them taken into account.

Appendix: Introduction to the Pathogenesis and Syndromes of the Stomach

Characteristics of Pathogenesis

The stomach receives food and transforms it into chyme. Any improper or unclean diet will affect the stomach, which tends to be benefited by moisture, impaired by dryness and regulated by descending. The diseases of the stomach include dryness syndrome caused by heat accumulation from indigested food and that manifested as the stomach's failure in descending, such as hiccup and vomiting.

The diseases of the stomach commonly met with in clinical practice are stomachache, gastric discomfort, vomiting, hiccup, constipation, and so on.

Classifications of Diagnosis and Theatment

(1) Cold syndromes of the stomach

[Pathogenesis] Constant insufficiency of the stomach - *yang* or excessive cold and uncooked food leading to the invasion of pathogenic cold and its accumulation in the stomach.

[Syndromes] Pain and coldness in the gastric cavity, which, in slight cases, lingers, and, in severe cases, causes a subjective sensation of contraction, and gets more serious in cold and relieved in warmth, vomiting of watery fluid, pale tongue, whitish and glossy fur, and slow pulse.

[Treatment] Warming the stomach and dispelling cold.

[Recipe] *Liang Fu Wan*[139], etc.

(2) Heat syndrome of the stomach

[Pathogenesis] Affection of the stomach by pathogenic heat, excessive pungent food, or constant excessive stomach - heat combined with stagnation of fire due to uncontrolled emotions.

[Syndromes] Burning pain in the gastric cavity, gastric discomfort with regurgitation of saliva, polyorexia, desire for cold drinks or foul breath, girgival swelling pain and bleeding, reddened tongue with little saliva, yellowish fur, and slippery and rapid pulse.

[Treatment] Clearing away the stomach - heat.

[Recipe] *Qing Wei San*[250].

(3) Deficiency syndrome of the stomach

[Pathogenesis] Exhaustion of the stomach - *yin* caused by pathogenic fire.

[Syndromes] Dry mouth and lips, anorexia, retching and hiccup, dry stool, reddened tongue with little fur or glossy and reddish tongue, and thready and rapid pulse.

[Treatment] Nourishing the stomach to promote the production of body fluid.

[Recipe] *Yi Wei Tang*[217], etc.

(4) Excess syndrome of the stomach

[Pathogenesis] Improper diet leading to food stagnation.

[Syndromes] Distending pain in the gastric cavity, anorexia, eructation, vomiting of sour and foul indigested food, dyschesia, greasy fur, and slippery pulse.

[Treatment] Promoting digestion and eliminating indigested food.

[Recipe] *Bao He Wan*[193], etc.

2.4.4 Introduction to the Pathogenesis and Syndromes of the Liver (Gallbladder) System

Characteristics of Pathogenesis

(1) The liver governs normal flow of *qi*, like to spread out freely and is averse to depression. It adjusts emotional activities, which are closely related to the liver. Depression of the liver - *qi* will lead to obstruction of the hepatic vessels and collaterals. Repeated or persistent emotional abnormality may cause the abdominal mass. Blood stasis and retention of water may bring about the tympanites. The jaundice is caused by stagnation of dampness and heat in the liver and the gallbladder as well as bile to overflow to muscle and skin. The hernia is produced by the retention of cold and the stagnation of *qi*.

(2) The liver has the function of storing blood and regulating its amount. If the liver fails to function properly in storing blood, various bleeding syndromes will ensue. If the liver - blood fails to nourish the tendons due to deficiency, numbness of limbs and flaccidity syndrome will appear.

(3) The liver corresponds to wood in the five elements and is characterized by ascending - spreading movement. Liver -*yin* deficiency and liver -*yang* excess will result in headache and dizziness. Deficiency of the liver -*yin* and kidney - *yin* due to the exuberant *yang* of the liver will bring about apoplectic stroke.

Liver diseases common in clinic: apoplectic stroke, vertigo, headache, convulsive diseases, mania -depressive syndrome, *jue* - syndrome, abdominal mass, tympanites, hematemesis, bleeding, tinnitus, etc.

Classifications of Diagnosis and Treatment

Excess -syndrome

(1) Liver - *qi* stagnation

[Pathogenesis] Depression and anger impair the liver and cause its abnormal dispersing function further leading to obstructed flow of *qi* and block blood circulation.

[Syndromes] Fullness and distending pain in the hypochondriac regions, nausea, regurgitation, abdominal pain, diarrhea, which come on or get aggravated with emotional disorders; or abdominal mass, menstrual irregularity; thin fur and wiry pulse.

[Treatment] Removing stagnation of liver - *qi* and eliminating abdominal mass.

[Recipe] *Chai Hu Shu Gan San*[211], *Shi Xiao San*[86].

(2) Flaming - up of liver - fire

[Pathogenesis] The failure of the liver and gallbladder in dispersion, leading to fire transmission from *qi* stagnation, which goes upward and disturb the head.

[Syndromes] Burning pain in the hypochondrium, vomiting of bitter saliva, distending pain in the head, dizziness, tinnitus, congested eyes, irritability, hematemesis, dark urine, constipation, reddened tongue with yellowish fur and taut, rapid pulse.

[Treatment] Clearing away fire in the liver and gallbladder.

[Recipe] *Long Dan Xie Gan Tang*[64].

(3) Liver-wind stirring internally

[Pathogenesis] Liver-*qi* producing fire, excessive *yang* leading to fire rising upward to disturb the head.

[Syndromes] Coma, convulsions, vertigo, numbness, headache, sometimes with deviated mouth and eyes, tongue rigidity, and hemiplegia.

[Treatment] Calming the liver to stop the wind and restraining the *yang*.

[Recipe] *Tian Ma Gou Teng Yin*[33], etc.

(4) Accumulation of cold in the liver meridian

[Pathogenesis] The liver meridian affected by *yin*-cold causing disturbance of the liver-*qi*, and obstruction of the collaterals.

[Syndromes] Lower abdominal distention, dragging sensation and pain in testes, contracture of the scrota, emaciation, aggravated by cold and alleviated by warmth, moist tongue with whitish fur, deep, wiry pulse.

[Treatment] Warming the meridian and the liver.

[Recipe] *Nuan Gan Jian*[277], etc.

Deficiency-Syndrome

Deficiency of the liver-*yin*

[Pathogenesis] Deficiency of kidney-*yin* will make water fail to nourish wood. When stagnated liver-*qi* turns into fire, the excessive fire will impair *yin* and make it fail to arrest *yang*, leading to deficiency-wind stirring inside the body.

[Syndromes] Dizziness, headache, tinnitus, deafness, numbness of the limbs, mild trembling of the muscles, dryness and uneasy feeling of the eyes, less sleep, dry throat, reddened tongue with scanty saliva, little fur, and thready rapid pulse.

[Treatment] Nourishing kidney-*yin* and liver-*yin* to suppress the *yang*.

[Recipe] *Yi Guan Jian*[1], *Qi Ju Di Huang Wan*[129].

Acompanying symptoms

Liver-*qi* attacking the stomach: Accompanied with stagnation of liver-*qi* and disorder of stomach-*qi*, treated by purging liver-fire and regulating the stomach; recipe: *Si Ni San*[81] and *Zuo Jin Wan*[67].

Disharmony between the liver and spleen: Accompanied with liver-*qi* stagnation and spleen-deficiency, treated by regulating the liver and spleen; recipe: *Xiao Yao San*[222].

Disharmony of the liver and gallbladder: Accompanied with deficiency of liver-blood, flaming up of the deficient – *yang*, the failure of blood to nourish the heart, treated by nourishing the liver, removing fire from the gallbladder and easing the mind; recipe: *Suan Zao Ren Tang*[280].

Yin – deficiency of the liver and kidney: Accompanied with deficiency of the liver and kidney *yin* – essence and deficiency – fire attacking internally, treated by nourishing *yin* and sending down fire; recipe: *Da Bu Yin Wan*[18].

Main Points of Diagnosis and Treatment

①The liver syndrome is divided into deficiency and excess types. The liver is a solid visceral organ responsible for ascending – spreading movements and often seen in excess –syndromes with *yang* – excess. Lingering excess – syndrome is apt to consume and impair the liver – *yin*, resulting in the syndrome of the interior – deficiency and the exterior – excess, to which special attention must be paid.

②In excess – syndromes, liver – *qi* stagnation, liver – fire flaring up and up – stirring of liver – wind have the same cause. They appear at the different stages of the same course of pathology and can not be completely separated. The doctor must be able to recognize the cause at the sight of the syndromes and select treatment by differentiating syndromes.

③In deficiency – syndromes, deficiency of liver – *yin* and upward disturbance by hyperactive *yang* result from deficiency of kidney – *yin* and essence failing to produce blood. That is why the liver and kidney must be treated at the same time for the syndromes of hyperactivities of dificiency – *yang* and liver – wind stirring internally.

Appendix: Pathogenesis and Syndromes of the Gallbladder

Characteristics of Pathogenesis

(1) The gallbladder is attached to the liver and is exterior – interiorly related to the liver. So liver – *qi* stagnation usually affects the excretion of the bile, manifested as the occurrence of the liver disease and that of the gallbladder simultaneously.

(2) The gallbladder is of the fortitudinous nature, therefore, pathologically it is liable to excess of fire.

(3) Fire and heat may produce phlegm from body fluid, so the syndrome of the gallbladder is usually accompanied with phlegm. As phlegm – fire often attacks the heart, the doctor should give attention not only to purging away heat in the gallbladder to resolve phlegm but to clearing away heart – fire and tranquilizing the mind.

Gallbladder diseases common in clinic are frighting, insomnia, tinitus, dizziness.

Classification of Diagnosis and Treatment

(1) Deficiency syndrome of the gallbladder (see Disharmony of the Liver and Gallbladder)

(2) Excess – syndrome of the gallbladder

[Pathogenesis] Emotional upsets causes functional disorder of *qi* and generation of phlegm. Inner accumulation of phlegm-heat will lead to dysfunction of the gallbladder and the stomach.

[Syndromes] Blurred vision, deafness, fullness in the chest and hypochondriac pain, irritability, insomnia, vomiting of bitter saliva, palpitation, and restleness; yellowish and greasy fur, wiry and slippery pulse.

[Treatment] Clearing away phlegm-heat and regulating the stomach to descend the adverse *qi*.

[Recipe] *Huang Lian Wen Dan Tang*[233].

2.4.5 Introduction to Syndrome and Pathogenesis of the Renal (Bladder) System

Characteristics of Pathogenesis

(1) The kidney is called "the origin of congenital constitution", and stores genuine *yin* and primordial *yang*, so vital essence stored by the kidney is preserved without being unnecessarily eliminated. All syndromes of the kidney are asthenic ones due to the impaired essence-*qi* resulting from congenital weakness, overwork and prolonged illness. TCM believes "When diseases of all the other *zang* organs are too severe, they are certain to involve the kidney".

(2) Essence stored by the kidney is the major material foundation for the growth, development and reproduction of the human being. Insufficiency of the kidney or deficiency of vital portal -fire may lead to impotence and morning diarrhea; deficiency of the kidney-*qi* and its failure in astringing function may lead to noctural emission, premature ejaculation.

(3) The kidney is in charge of the body fluid and maintains its normal metabolism. In case of deficient kidney-*yang*, the kidney will fail to send downward the body fluid, causing accumulation of water-dampness in the body or spreading over the superficies, thus, fluid retention or edema follows.

Such symptoms of the kidney are often seen in clinic as *Xiao Ke* (*XiaXiao*), edema, uroschesis, spermatorrhea, impotence, lumbage, vertigo, tinnitus and diarrhea.

Classifications of Diagnosis and Treatment

(1) Unconsolidation of the kidney-*qi*

[Pathogenesis] Insufficiency of the kidney-*qi* with decline of its reserving function due to overstrain or protracted illness.

[Syndromes] Weakness and soreness of the loins and back, nocturnal emission, premature ejaculation, nocturia, frequent clear and dribbling urination, even incontinence of urine, pale tongue with thin whitish fur, weak pulse.

[Treatment] Consolidating and regulating kidney-*qi*

[Recipe] *Da Bu Yuan Jian*[17], *Mi Jing Wan*[220].

(2) Failure of the kidney to receive inspiration

[Pathogenesis] Impairment of the kidney – *qi* due to overwork or *qi* – deficiency after protracted illness and failure of the kidney in receiving.

[Syndromes] Shortness of breath, and severe panting aggravated on slight exertion, cough with sweating, even incontinence of urine due to severe cough, pale complexion, pale tongue with thin fur, weak pulse.

[Treatment] Promoting inspiration and reinforcing the kidney.

[Recipe] *Ren Shen Hu Tao Tang*[10], *Shen Jie San*[170].

(3) Deficiency of the kidney – *yang*

[Pathogenesis] Insufficiency of the kidney and the vital portal – fire resulting from intemperance in sexual life or protracted illness.

[Syndromes] Soreness and weakness of the loins and knees, aversion to cold, nocturia, impotence, dizziness, tinnitus, pale tongue, deep and weak pulse.

[Treatment] Warming and reinforcing kidney – *yang*.

[Recipe] *You Gui Wan*[68], *Jin Gui Sheng Qi Wan*[163].

(4) Edema due to the kidney – insufficiency

[Pathogenesis] Deficiency of kidney – *yang* can not warm and transform fluid, causing overflow of pathogenic fluid.

[Syndromes] Generalized pitting edema due to overflow of fluid in the skin, specially over the lower limbs, scanty urination; in case of phlegm converted from the fluid: cough with much sputum, and dyspnea on moving, pale tongue with whitish fur, deep and slippery pulse.

[Treatment] Warming *yang* to promote diuresis.

[Recipe] *Zhen Wu Tang*[199], *Ji Sheng Shen Qi Wan*[184].

(5) Deficiency of the kidney – *yin*

[Pathogenesis] Impairment of the kidney – *yin* due to overstrain from sexual intercourse or prolonged illness.

[Syndromes] Lassitude in the loins and knees, dizziness, tinnitus, insomnia, amnsia, seminal emission, premature ejaculation, and emaciation, reddened tongue with little fur and thready pulse.

[Treatment] Nourishing the kidney – *yin*.

[Recipe] *Liu Wei Di Huang Wan*[46]

(6) Hyperactivity of fire due to *yin* – deficiency

[Pathogenesis] Internal heat – syndrome caused by deficiency of the kidney – *yin*.

[Syndromes] Hectic fever, night sweat, dry mouth, sore throat, nocturnal emission, flushed zygomatic region, congested lips, red tongue with little fur, thready and rapid pulse.

[Treatment] Nourishing *yin* and expelling fire.

[Recipe] *Zhi Bai Di Huang Wan*[160].

Accompanying syndromes

(1) Deficiency of the kidney and the spleen: Accompanied with kidney – *yang* deficiency, spleen – *qi* deficiency. It can be treated by invigorating the heart to benifit the spleen with *Fu Zi Li Zhong Tang*[146], *Si Shen Wan*[82].

(2) Kidney fluid attacking the heart: Accompanied with *yang* – deficiency of the kidney and heart, and blockage of the heart – *yang*. It can be treated by warming *yang* to promote urination with *Zhen Wu Tang*[199].

Main Points of Diagnosis and Treatment

①There is no exterior or excess syndrome for the kidney. Heat syndrome of the kidney is caused by *yin* – deficiency and cold syndrome caused by *yang* – deficiency.

②The kidney – deficiency syndrome is divided into *yin* – deficiency and *yang* – deficiency. It can be treated by reinforcement, not purgation.

③The kidney is closely related to other *zang* – *fu* organs. For example, failure of water to nourish wood may causes hyperactivity of the liver – *yang*; child – organs affecting mother – ogans may impair the lung – *yin*; failure of water to flow upward may lead to disharmony between the heart and kidney; failure of fire to generate earth may lead to insufficiency of the spleen – *yang*. Therefore, the physician must pay attention to the syndromes of the kidney system in clinical practice, especially, the mutual influence among *zang* – *fu* organs.

Appendix: Pathogenesis and Syndrome of the Urinary Bladder

Characteristics of Pathogenesis

The urinary bladder communicates directly with the kidney to which it is exterior – interiorly related. The kidney regulates water metabolism and the urinary bladder stores and excretes urine. Therefore, they have a close relationship. The pathologic change of the kidney may involve the bladder directly, manifested as dysfunction of *qi* activity.

Bladder diseases common in clinic: dysuria, enuresis, incontinent urine.

Classifications of Diagnosis and Treatment

(1) Deficiency – cold syndrome

[Pathogenesis] Deficiency of the kidney – *qi*, dysfunction of consolidating of the bladder.

[Syndrome] Frequent micturition, polyuria or aconuresis, sleek and smooth tongue with whitish fur, deep and thready pulse.

[Treatment] Consolidating and governing the kidney – *qi*.

[Recipe] *Sang Piao Xiao San*[228].

(2) Excess (Dampness) – heat syndrome

[Pathogenesis] Dampness–heat attacking the bladder.

[Syndrome] Frequent micturition, urgency of micturition, uridynia and pain, yellowish and turbid urine, hematuria or uronary calculus, accompanied with fever and lumbago, red tongue with yellowish greasy fur, rapid pulse.

[Treatment] Clearing away dampness and heat.
[Recipe] *Ba Zheng San*[12].

Summary

The pathogenesis and syndromes of *zang - fu* organs occupy the most important place in the therapeutic principles and differentiating methods in TCM internal medicine, and are the kernel of selecting treatment by differentiating syndromes. Differentiating syndromes and pathogenesis of the *zang - fu* organs may directly influence and dominate the changes of deficiency, excess, *qi*, blood, *yin* and *yang* in the body, and help the physicians to understand the location and nature of a disease and to understand how the *zang - fu* organs interact in the pathological process. Complicated and changeable as the pathogenesis and syndromes of *zang - fu* diseases are, they can never be separated from the *yin - yang* and five - element theories, and display definitely the eight principal syndromes as *yin* and *yang*, the exterior and the interior, cold and heat, deficiency and excess, which should be emphasized always in studying TCM internal medicine.

Discussions

1. What is the concept of the pathogenesis and syndromes of the *zang - fu* organs? What functions have they in the internal medicine of TCM?

2. Which types and therapeutic principles have the pathogenesis and syndrome of the five *zang* organs?

3. What are the characteristics of the pathogenesis of the five *zang* organs?

2.5 Medical Treatment

2.5.1 Therapeutic Principles

Therapeutic principles, or the principles of treatment, are an important component of TCM clinical theories. They are the guide to TCM clinical treatment, the basis of therapeutic methods and prescriptions as well as the rules of selecting treatment on the basis of a thorough analysis of the pathogenesis and syndromes of the disease. Therapeutic principles are different from therapeutic methods: the former being the macroscopic, holistic and strategic mastery and guide, and the latter the microscopic, concrete and tactical means or measures. Therefore, therapeutic principles form a link between the preceding and the following in the system of selecting treatment by differentiating the syndromes in TCM.

The five main therapeutic principles of TCM are discussed below.

1. Routine Treatment and Treatment Contrary to the Routine

Routine treatment is one that is most commonly used in clinical practice, such as the treatment of cold - syndrome with drugs of warm nature, treatment of heat - syndrome with drugs of cold nature, treatment of deficiency - syndrome by reinforcement and that of excess - syndrome by purgation. It is fit for these cases in which the pathogenesis and the symptoms are in coordination and the condition of illness is simple. The nature of the drugs to be used must be just opposite to that of the syndrome. For example, syndromes caused by wind - cold pathogen are treated by relieving the exterior syndrome with drugs pungent in flavour and warm in property, and syndromes due to the invasion of the lung by warm and heat pathogen treated by relieving fever with drugs of pungent flavor and cool nature.

Treatment contrary to the routine is a kind of treatment that is applied on the basis of the nature of the pathogenesis to special cases in which false appearances of cold, heat, deficiency or excess syndromes are found. Examples of these treatments are treatment of pseudo - cold syndrome with drugs of cold nature, treatment of pseudo - heat syndrome with drugs of hot nature, treatment of obstructive diseases with tonic drugs, treatment of purgation diseases with purgatives, etc.. The treatment contrary to the routine is characterized by using such drugs, the nature of which is in coordination with the nature of the symptoms. For example, coldness of the extremities varying with the virulence of the pathogenic heat is treated with *Bai Hu Tang*, and diarrhea and delirium are treated with *Cheng Qi Tang*, etc.

2. The Primary (*Ben*) and the Secondary (*Biao*) in a Chronic or Acute Case

The secondary means the main clinical symptoms of a disease; the primary refers to its cause and pathogenesis. In the process of the changes of a disease, the therapeutic principle is to relieve the secondary in an acute case, to remove the primary in a chronic case, to treat both the primary and secondary symptoms at the same time if they are in combination and to treat one of them if it dominates the rest.

Relieving the secondary in an acute case means that the secondary symptom that occurs abruptly with a rapid progress and is harmful to the patient must be first got rid of. By removing the primary (the root) in an insidious case is meant that in these cases in which the condition of illness develops slowly the treatment must proceed from the nature of the disease. Dealing with a mild case with the treatment of aiming at both the primary and the secondary symptoms means relieving the primary and secondary symptoms at the same time when both of them are getting serious. And by treating a severe case with potent drugs of specific action is meant that the secondary symptoms or the primary symptoms are first aimed at according to their severity.

3. Supporting Vital - *Qi* and Eliminating Pathogens

As TCM theory sees it, when vital - *qi* is full inside the body, pathogens can not invade in; and whenever the body is exposed to pathogens, it must be the result of deficiency of *qi*. The process of illness, in a sense, is the process of the fighting between the vital - *qi* of the body and the pathogenic factors. When the former gets the upper hand of the latter, disease will be wiped out, but in case the latter defeats the former, disease will occur or deteriorate. Supporting the vital – *qi* means invigorating, which is applied to the treatment of deficiency of the vital – *qi*; and eliminating pathogenic factors means purgation and is applied for the excess of pathogens. Therefore, supporting the vital – *qi* and eliminating pathogens actually is to change the relative strength of the vital –*qi* and pathogenic factors so as to cure a disease.

Most frequently adopted in practice are the combination of the above two methods, for they are supplementary to each other and have their own particular emphasis as well. Generally a physician should follow the principle of strengthening the vital – *qi* with pathogenic factors repelled out and eliminating the pathogenic factors without hurting the vital – *qi*.

4. Invigoration and Purgation of *Zang* and *Fu* Organs

The human body is an organic whole, and the *zang* and *fu* organs are physiologically related to and pathologically affect one another. Therefore, the interrestricting, inter – generating and exterior – interior relations of the *zang* – *fu* organs are taken as the therapeutic principle of invigoration and purgation in clinical practice, which is summarized as follows:

(1) Reinforcing the mother – organ in case of deficiency – syndrome, and in case of excess – syndrome, reducing the child – organ.

This is a therapautic principle clinically in accordance with the interrestricting and intergenerating relations of the *zang* – *fu* organs. The so – called mother – and son – organs are named in the order of the intergenerating relations of the five elements. For example, there's a mother – and – son relationship between the kidney and the liver. In treating the deficiency of the liver – blood, the kidney – essence is indirectly invigorated while the liver – blood is reinforced, so that essence and blood transform into each other and the goal of nourishing the liver – blood is attained. This is what is called reinforcing the mother in treating cases of deficiency. Similarly, the excess of the liver – fire, which affects the storing function of the kidney and thus leads to emission or nocturnal emission, can be treated by removing heat from the liver so that the pathogenic factor of excess type is dispelled and the disease of the kidney is cured. This is what is called treating excess syndrome by reducing the child – organ.

(2) Strengthening water to restrict *yang* and benefiting fire to weaken *yin*.

This is a treatment of interior syndrome that takes the pathogenesis of the *zang* – *fu* organs as the point of departure. By strengthening water to restrict *yang* is meant that syndromes due to deficiency of the kidney – *yin* or upward floating of *yang* in deficiency condition must be treated with recipes that are effective in nourishing the kidney – *yin*, i. e. strengthening water. And benefiting fire to weaken *yin* means that syndromes caused by deficiency of the kidney – *yang* or excess of *yin* – cold in the interior must be treated by warming the kidney – *yang*, or benefiting fire.

(3) Purging the exterior and calming the interior, opening the interior and activat-

ing the exterior, and clearing the interior and moistening the exterior.

These therapeutic methods are based on the exterior - interior relations of the *zang -fu* organs, and applicable to these cases in which both a *zang* - organ and a *fu* - organ that are exterior - interiorly related to each other get diseased. For instance, the lung and the large intestine are exterior - interiorly related, when the heat of excess type of *Yangming* or constipation leads to the stagnation of the lung - *qi*, good result will be obtained by using *Liang Ge San* to purge the exterior (the large intestine) and calm the interior (the lung) rather than the treatment of the lung itself.

5. Treatment in Accordance with Three Conditions

The three conditions refer to the seasonal conditions, local conditions and the constitution of the patient. The treatment herein means that proper treatment must be carried out in accordance with the seasonal and local conditions, and the physique, sex and age of an individual as well. This therapeutic principle clearly reflects the holistic concept of TCM as well as the characteristics and the superiority of selecting treatment by syndrome differentiation, therefore, is the important guarantee of the improvement of curative effect.

2.5.2 Therapeutic Methods

The therapeutic methods commonly used under the guidance of the therapeutic principles are as follows.

Relieving Exterior Syndrome Method

This therapy is used to induce sweat and dispel exopathogens, also known as diaphoretic therapy, which includes relieving the exterior syndrome with drugs pungent in flavor and cool in property, relieving the exterior syndrome with drugs pungent in flavor and warm in property, supplementing *qi* and expelling the pathogenic factors from the body surface, letting eruptions with drugs of acid flavor and cool nature, dispelling dampness with drugs of pungent flavor, as well as ventilating the lung and inducing diuresis, etc. In clinical practice, it is worthy of notice that this therapy must be avoided in cases with exhaustion of blood and essence due to vomiting or diarrhea, or with open sores, or with dribbing urination or difficulty in urination. To prevent *yin* from impairment and *yang* from over - consumption, excessive diaphoresis should be avoided. Attention must also be paid to the local conditions and the physical differences of the patients. And in case accompanying syndromes are found, this therapy should be used in combination with other therapeutic methods.

Heat - Clearing Method

This method is used to treat heat syndromes, known as clearing away heat or purging fire or removing pathogenic heat from the blood and toxic substances from the *zang -fu* organs, including clearing away heat from *qifen* and clearing away heat from *yingfen*. But a distinction must be made between the appearance and nature as well as the deficiency and excess of cold and heat before it is put to use. Cases with interior heat due to deficiency of *yin* must be treated by nourishing *yin* so as to clear away heat instead of a direct treatment with drugs of bitter taste and cold nature. This method must not be applied to those cases in which the invassion of pathogenic factors still remains. But heat syndrome with pseudo-cold symptoms can be treated with treatment contrary to the rout-ine.

Purgative Method

This therapy is used in removing material pathogens of excess type, relaxing the bowels and purging the turbid, dispelling the retained water and clearing phlegm, including purgation with drugs of cold nature, purgation with drugs of warm nature, laxation with drugs of loosening nature and excreting accumulated water with hydrogogue. If pathogens is still in the exterior or between the exterior and the interior, purgation cannot be used so as to avoid the invasion of exopathogen. And as for those who are old and weak, or pregnant, or have suffered from prolonged illness, purgation must be used with great caution or avoided. Purgative method mustn't be overused lest the impairment of the vital-*qi* should be caused.

Regulating Method

This method is used to mediate symptoms in the *Shaoyang* meridian. It is mostly used to treat half-exterior and half-interior syndrome, and to regulate the functional activities of the *zang - fu* organs to drive the pathogens out, including relieving *Shaoyang* disease by mediation, regulating the functional activities of the liver and spleen, as well as regulating the functional activities of the stomach and intestines. The therapy is mainly used when *Shaoyang* gets diseased. A distinction between the exterior and the interior of *Shaoyang* and between the excess of cold and that of heat is essential so as to make appropriate adaptations in applying it.

Interior-Warming Method

This method is used to treat interior cold syndromes, it is effective in replenishing and restoring *yang-qi* and dispelling pathogenic cold, also called warming method, including warming the middle-*jiao* to dispel cold, expelling pathogenic cold from meridians, as well as helping recover *yang* and rescuing the patient from collapse, etc. In clinical practice, a distinction between the appearance and the nature of cold and heat must be made so as not to be misled by a pseudo-cold syndrome in which the coldness of the extremities varies with the virulence of pathogenic heat. Besides, in recuperating depleted *yang* to rescue the patient from collapse, excessive warmth and dryness must be avoided lest blood consumption and impairment of fluid and *qi* should be brought about. And cases with cold of deficiency type should be treated by restoring *qi* with drugs of sweet taste and warm nature.

Tonification

This method is applied to deficiency syndromes, effective in treating deficiency syndromes of *qi* and blood, *yin* and *yang*, and *zang* and *fu*, including invigorating *qi*, enriching blood, and invigorating *yin* and *yang*. In clinical practice, it's important to be on guard against such false appearances as "symptoms of excess in extreme deficiency" and "appearance of deficiency in extreme excess". In addition, attention must be paid to such relations as *qi* and blood being of the same origin, and interdependence between *yin* and *yang*, tonifying *yang* by nourishing *yin* and nourishing *yin* by tonifying *yang*, supplementing *qi* and promoting the production of blood. This therapy must never be applied to excess syndromes.

Elimination (Dispelling Therapy)

The method is used to resolve accumulation or stagnation of pathogenic factors of excess type, such as removing food retention and promoting digestion, resolving goister and scrofula, eliminating swelling, inducing decomposition of calculi, etc. This method, also a method of eliminating pathogenic factors, must never be misused in treating deficiency syndromes, and, on the other hand, should be used in combination with therapy for invigoration: eliminating undigested food or swelling must be carried out at the same time of reinforcing the spleen, inducing decomposition of calculi or resolving goister and scrofula must be performed in combination with soothing the liver or normalizing the function of the gallbladder, etc.

Regulating *Qi*

This method is used to treat disorders of *qi*, including promoting the circulation of *qi*, sending down abnormally ascending *qi*, etc., mainly used in dealing with reversed flow of *qi* and *qi* stagnation caused by stagnation of the liver – *qi*, obstruction of the lung –*qi* and failure of descending of the stomach – *qi*. Cases that belong to excess syndrome can all be treated with this method but the excess or deficiency of *qi* must first be made clear. As the drugs used in regulating the flow of *qi* are of pungent or bitter taste and dry or warm nature, undue use of the method should be prevented so as not to impair *yin* and consume the fluid.

Regulating Blood

This method is used to treat blood stasis, accumulation of blood stasis and bleeding, including promoting blood circulation to remove blood stasis, arresting bleeding, etc., applied to such blood disorders as irregular flow of blood, obstruction of blood stasis, hemoptysis, hematemesis, nose – bleeding, hemafecia, hematuria, etc. Attention must be paid to the relations between *qi* and blood in applying this method, for both *qi* stagnation and deficiency of *qi* are all likely to lead to blood stasis. The therapy may be used in combination with warming *yang* to dispel cold, removing pathogenic heat from blood, supplementing *qi* and activating blood circulation, and so on, but must be applied with caution to pregnant women. It's also worthy of notice that proper drugs that are effective in removing blood stasis and activating blood circulation should also be used so as to arrest bleeding without any blood stasis left.

Astringency

This therapy, being effective in consolidating the superficial resistance to stop perspiration, astringing the intestines to relieve diarrhea and arresting seminal emission, is applied to prostraction syndromes such as unconsolidation of the lung – qi, spontaneous perspiration, unconsolidation of the kidney – qi, seminal emission and spermatorrhea and enuresis, unconsolidation of the spleen – qi, diarrhea, proctoptosis, etc. Therapy for inducing astringency, which is part of the therapy for invigoration, should not be used to treat heat syndromes, excess syndromes or hyperactivity of fire due to *yin* deficiency. Besides, this is not a method aiming at the primary cause of a disease, therefore, it's important to find out and take into consideration the actual cause and make use of it in combination with invigorating qi, warming *yang*, etc.

Resuscitation

This therapy is used to resuscitate consciousness, including waking up the patient from unconsciousness by clearing away heat and eliminating cold – phlegm for resuscitation. The former is applied to heat – blockage syndromes due to the invassion of the pericardium by pathogenic heat, and the latter to wind – stroke syndrome (of *Taiyang*), excessive – syndrome of coma accompanied with cold manifestations, phlegm syncope, syncope resulting from disorder of qi, etc. This therapy, intended merely to cause resuscitation, should be, according to the pathogenesis and symptoms, accompanied with such methods as clearing away heat, relaxing the bowels, tranquilizing the endogenous wind, or resolving phlegm. Drugs effective in causing resuscitation shouldn't be decocted too much as they are aromatic and volatile.

Spasmolysis

This therapy is applied to the treatment of clonic convulsion, infantile convulsion, coma and so on caused by various factors, including clearing away heat to tranquilize the endogenous wind, calming the liver and the endogenous wind, nourishing the blood to stop wind, expelling endogenous wind to relieve convulsion, etc. But in actual application of this method, endogenous wind must be differentiated from exopathic wind, with the former treated in combination with nourishing *yin* to soften the liver, checking exuburant *yang* to clear heat. etc. , and the latter treated by means of expelling. Drugs to remove mind are usually of a pungent flavor and dry nature, so they should be used with care lest *yin* should be impaired.

Summary

In TCM internal treatment, under the guidance of the therapeutic principles, the twelve therapeutic methods discussed above may be put to use either individually or in a combined way, depending on the different stages of the development of the disease. Only in this way, can it be possible to make good use of the characteristics and the superiority of the theory of selecting treatment on the basis of syndrome differentiation.

Discussions

1. What are the five main therapeutic principles of TCM internal medicine?
2. What are the therapeutic methods commonly used in internal medicine?

Each Exposition

1 Cold

General

Cold is an exogenous ailment caused by wind or seasonal pathogenes. It occurs in any season, esp. in spring and winter, manifested by nasal obstruction, rhinorrhea, cough, sneezing, aversion to wind and cold, fever and general pain or malaise, and is classified into mild, severe, cold and heat syndromes.

Treatment of common cold and flu in Western Medicine may be conducted with reference herein.

Etiology and Pathogenesis

1. Attack by exogenous wind   Pathogenic wind, the most common factor for diseases, often attacks the human body and causes disorder of the lung - *qi*, *wei - qi* and *ying - qi* in combination with cold, heat, and dampness pathogens.

2. Unconsolidated *wei - yang*   It is due to constant climatic variations and irregular temperature in winter and spring, *wei - qi* (defensive *qi*) fails to keep the skin warm and nourished to control sweat, to regulate the body temperature, leading to the invasion of exopathic factors.

3. Usual weak constitution   Patients with deficient vital - *qi*, or weakness due to chronic illness, or imbalanced *yin* and *yang* are susceptible to wind pathogen and bear uniqueness in the course of disease.

4. Disease due to seasonal pathogen   Cold due to seasonal pathogens bears infectiousness of various degrees and results in prevalence of pestilence and diseases of other kinds if serious.

The pathogen first attacks the upper - *jiao*, esp. such pulmonary parts as the mouth, nose, skin and hair marked by nasal obstruction, cough, general pain, aversion to wind and cold, and fever.

Key Points:

Exopathic cause	Exteriorly attacked by wind - cold, wind - heat and seasonal pathogens	Stagnated exopathogen on the body surface resulting in disorder of lung - *qi* and *wei - qi* (classified into cold, heat, deficiency and excess forms) → cold
Endopathic cause	Weakened lung - *qi* and *wei - qi* and insufficiency of vital - *qi*	

Diagnosis and Discrimination

Cold is seen in fever and aversion to wind (cold) simultaneously, and is manifested by pulmonary symptoms and general malaise. When discriminated from other interior syndromes it features fulminant occurrence, short course, and mild symptom. It should specially be distinguished from pestilence at early stage, generally the former involving slight or no fever but the latter inevitably high fever. Besides cold has a short course and is of mild symptom which will be relieved by the application of diaphoretics manifested by calm pulse and normal body temperature. Whereas the pestilence symptoms get aggravated progressively manifested by sweating and rapid pulse, and as long as the heat remains not expelled, epidemic factors will go inward with complex progress. Close observation and careful discrimination of the patients are necessary particularly in winter and spring.

Selecting Treatment by Differentiating Syndromes (STDS)

Confirmed diagnosis shall be followed immediately by differentiating syndromes to favor treatment. Here are the main points:

Cold:
- Wind–cold: Attack by wind–cold pathogen manifested by badly aversion to wind and cold, slight fever, anhidrosis, general pain, floating and tense pulse
- Wind–heat: Attack by wind–heat pathogen manifested by aversion to wind, perspiration with fever, slight thirstiness, red margin and tip of tongue, itching throat, floating and rapid pulse
- Summer–heat and dampness: Seasonal occurrence manifested by fever, less sweat, sluggishness and distending pain in the head and body, thin yellowish greasy fur, soft and floating pulse or soft-floating and rapid pulse
- General deficiency with exopathic factor: Usual deficiency of yin–yang and qi–blood concomitant with different symptoms and signs when attacked by exopathic factors and manifested by feeble pulse
- Seasonal cold: Fulminant occurrence manifested by aversion to cold with high fever, thirstiness, rapid and strong pulse, marked general symptom with quick progress of disease

Common syndromes:

1. Cold due to wind–cold

[Symptoms] Badly aversion to cold, mild fever, anhidrosis, headache, bodily pain or malaise, nasal obstruction, coarse voice, cough, sneezing, watery nasal discharge, itching throat, thin whitish sputum, non–thirstiness or preference for hot drinks, normal tongue with thin whitish fur, floating and tense pulse.

[Main Points of Differentiation] Badly aversion to cold, mild fever, anhidrosis, clear nasal discharge, and bodily pain.

It is often seen in common cold.

[Pathogenesis] Exopathic factors retain in the lung and *weifen* and cause the failure of the lung to release lung-*qi* and keep it descendant resulting in counteraction between vital-*qi* and pathogen in the striae.

[Treatment] Dispel the pathogen from the superficies and release stagnated lung-*qi* with drugs of acrid taste and warm nature.

[Recipe] *Jing Fang Bai Du San*[173].

In case of severe cold in the superficies and bodily pain and headache, add *Herba Ephedrae* and *Ramulus Cinnamomi* to facilitate the flow of lung-*qi* and dispel cold as well as to warm and activate superficies-*yang*.

[Nursing Points] Take proper rest, avoid cold and uncooked food, and avoid wind-cold.

2. Cold due to wind-heat

[Symptoms] Marked fever, slight aversion to wind-cold, sweating, distending pain in the head, cough with little thick yellowish sputum, dry or reddened or painful throat, nasal obstruction with thick yellowish discharge, thirstiness with preference for drinks; normal tongue or reddish tip of tongue with dry thin yellowish fur, floating and rapid pulse.

[Main Points of Differentiation] Marked fever, slight aversion to wind-cold, sweating, thick nasal discharge, sore throat.

[Pathogenesis] Exopathic wind-heat invades the lung and impairs the body fluid, resulting in heat stagnation in the striae and pulmonary system and disorder of dispersing function of defensive *qi* of lung.

[Treatment] Dispel the pathogen in the superficies and clear away heat from the lung with drugs of acrid taste and cool nature.

[Recipe] *Yin Qiao San*[255].

In case of severe headache, add *Folium Mori* and *Flos Chrysanthem Xi Indici* to clear away heat pathogen and activate the mind; of sore throat, add *Rhizoma Belamcandae*, *Radix Scrophulariae* and crude *Radix Glycyrrhizae*; of thick yellowish sputum, add *Radix Scutellariae*, *Fructus Trichosanthis* and *Rhizoma Anemarrhenae* to release lung-heat, eliminate phlegm and stop coughing.

[Nursing Points] Take proper rest, drink much water, and avoid pungent and fried food.

3. Cold due to summer-heat and dampness

[Symptoms] Fever, slight aversion to wind, little sweat, lassitude or pain of the body, dizziness and distending pain of the head, thick nasal discharge, cough with thick sputum, mouthful greasiness, thirstiness without preference for drinks, vexation, chest fullness and nausea, scanty dark urine; thin yellowish and greasy fur, soft-floating and rapid pulse.

[Main Points of Differentiation] It occurs in summer manifested as fever and lassitude, dizziness and distention of the head, vexation and nausea.

[Pathogenesis] Summer-heat pathogen in combination with dampness pathogen is likely to violate the superficies - *yang* and obstruct the seven orifices, impair the lung - *qi* and inhibit the flow of *yang - qi* in the middle - *jiao* as well.

[Treatment] Relieve exterior syndrome by clearing away summer - heat and dampness.

[Recipe] *Xin Jia Xiang Ru Yin*[278].

In case summer - heat overpowers dampness with marked heat syndrome, add *Rhizoma Coptidis*, *Herba Artemisiae*, *Folium Nelumbinis* and *Rhizoma Phragmitis* to eliminate summer - heat; in case summer - heat is overpowered by dampness sticking around the superficies, add *Herba Agastachis* and *Herba Eupatorii* to eliminate dampness and dispel exterior syndrome; in case of severe internal dampness, add *Rhizoma Atractylodis*, *Rhizoma Pinelliae* and *Pericarpium Citri Reticulatae* to regulate the middle - *jiao* and eliminate dampness; in case of scanty dark urine or difficulty in urination, add *Liu Yi San*[44], *Cortex Phellodendri* and *Poria Rubra* to clear away heat and promote diuresis.

[Nursing Points] Take light meal, avoid fruit and cold uncooked food as well as greasy food.

4. Cold due to deficiency of *qi*

[Symptoms] Marked aversion to cold, mild fever, anhidrosis or continuously spontaneous perspiration, lassitude and soreness of the body, weak cough with low voice and slight dyspnea which are to be aggravated on slight exertion; pale and large tongue with thin whitish fur, weak pulse.

[Main Points of Differentiation] General deficiency constitution, marked aversion to cold, mild fever, weak cough, lassitude, feeble pulse.

[Pathogenesis] Deficient *yang* leads to lowered superficial resistance and prevailing pathogenic factors, which is recurrent and difficult to recover.

[Treatment] Strengthen the body resistance to eliminate pathogenic factors.

[Recipe] *Shen Su Yin*[168] or *Yu Ping Feng San*[61].

[Nursing Points] Lead a regular life; avoid wind - cold; refrain from cold and uncooked food, take nutrious and easily - digested food.

5. Cold due to deficient *yin*

[Symptoms] Fever, slight aversion to wind - cold, less sweat, dizziness, dry mouth and dysphoria, dry cough with little sputum, reddened tongue with little fur, thready and rapid pulse.

[Main Points of Differentiation] Fever with little sweat, dysphoria and dry cough, reddened tongue with little fur.

[Pathogenesis] Failure of the body fluid to sweat and eliminate pathogen while in general deficiency of *yin* and body fluid and attacked by exopathic factors.

[Treatment] Nourish *yin* to relieve exterior syndromes.

[Recipe] *Jia Jian Wei Rui Tang*[102].

In case of severe thirstiness and dry throat, add *Radix Adenophorae Strictae* and *Radix Ophiopogonis* to mourish *yin* and promote the production of body fluid.

[Nursing Points] Take light and digestible food instead of pungent, fried or greasy food.

6. Epidemic cold

[Symptoms] Abrupt aversion to cold with trembling and high fever if serious, general aching pain, acute headache, flushed cheeks, red eyes, lassitude and lack of strength, congestion of throat or sometimes with anorexia, nausea, constipation, no cough or slight cough with rare nasal obstruction or discharge; rapid pulse.

[Main Points of Differentiation] Epidemic and abrupt occurrence manifested as aversion to cold and high fever, acute headache and bodily pain, lack of strength, mild respiratory symptoms but severe constitutional ones.

It may be seen in influenza.

[Pathogenesis] Seasonal pathogen invades the *wei* and retains in the lung with quick progress, resulting in the impairment of body fluid and *yang* respectively by heat pathogen and seasonal one.

[Treatment] Clear away heat and toxic material.

[Recipe] *Qing Wen Bai Du Yin*[253].

In case of marked symptoms due to epidemic heat, add *Folium Isatidis*, *Radix Isatidis*, *Rhizoma Polygoni Cuspidati*, and *Herba Taraxaci*; of cough with dyspnea due to heat retention in the lung, add *Gypsum Fibrosum* and *Radix Scutellariae* to clear away heat in the lung; if the symptoms herein are accompanied with deficiency or impairment of vital - *qi*, add discretionarily drugs for supplementing *qi* and arresting prostration, promoting the production of body fluid and nourishing *yin*. Changeable as this syndrome is, close and careful observation is necessary to prevent pathogens and toxic material from penetrating inward.

[Nursing Points] Prevention is the first priority; reduce social activities during the epidemic season; take orally the *Radix Isatidis* granule preparation after its being infused in boiling water; and fumigation with vinegar may be applied indoors for detoxification. The patient needs to take proper rest and reduce activities, to take medicines as required and coordinate with doctors and nurses promptly for observation and prevention of disease progress.

Summary

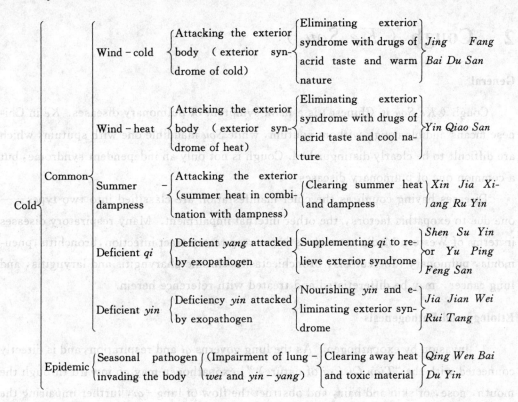

Discussions

1. Tell the difference between common cold and epidemic cold.
2. How many types is cold classified into? What are the differentiation main points, therapeutic methods and recipes of each?

2 Cough (*Ke Sou*)

General

Cough (*Ke Sou* in Chinese) is a main symptom of pulmonary diseases. *Ke* in Chinese means audible cough without sputum, while *Sou* inaudible one with sputum, which are difficult to be clearly distinguished. Cough is not only an independent syndrome, but a common one of pulmonary diseases.

Diseases having cough as the chief manifestation are classified into two types——one due to exopathic factors, the other internal impairment. Many respiratory diseases in terms of Western Medicine, such as upper respiratory tract infection, bronchitis, pneumonia, pulmonary tuberculosis, bronchiectasis, chronic pharyngitis and laryngitis, and lung cancer, may be differetiated and treated with reference herein.

Etiology and Pathogenesis

1. Invasion by exopathogen   As the lung governs *qi* and respiration, and is directly connected with the *"Tian Qi* (*qi* of nature)", exopathogen may go inward through the mouth, nose, or skin and hair, and obstruct the flow of lung -*qi*, further impairing the lung - *yin* and bringing about cough. Of all the exopathic factors, wind, cold, dryness and heat (fire) are most likely to generate cough.

2. Disorder of the *zang - fu* function   The functional disorder of the five *zang* and six *fu* organs may all hold up the ascent and descent of vital -*qi*, and further affect the function of the lung to control *qi*, resulting in cough, which is clinically known as "endopathogens impairing the lung". Commonly seen in practice is cough due to impairment of the lung, respectively inclusive of phlegm transformed from spleen -dampness, transformed fire from stagnated liver - *qi*, and failure of the kidney in reception of air.

3. Spontaneous pulmonary disease   Protracted course of pulmonary disease may impair the lung -*qi* and further cause the disorder of the lung's function to govern *qi* and its dispersing, purifying and descending function resulting in cough. It is the same case with chronic consumption of lung - *yin* and its failure in purifying and moistening function.

All in all, the attack by exopathogen or disorder of the *zang - fu* organs will not generate cough unless the lung is impaired. Hence, the etiology and pathogenesis of cough are not confined to the lung, nor is it dispensable from the lung.

Key Points:

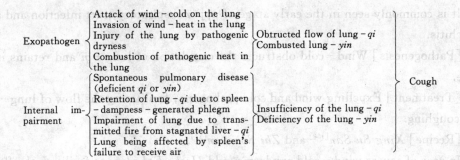

Diagnosis and Discrimination

Disease with cough as the chief manifestation may be diagnosed as such in practice. The traditional definition of *Ke* and *Sou*, little as its practical significance is, may be neglected for it is difficult to separate them. Cough is a relatively independent syndrome as well as one of several pulmonary diseases. Therefore, inspection of symptoms and causes and selection of treatment for different types are required clinically on the basis of definite diagnosis.

Selecting Treatment by Differentiating Syndromes

The clear diagnosis of cough is comparatively easy, but the accurate treatment in accordance with classification is critical for exopathogen, internal impairment, and the diseased *zang - fu* organs may all lead to cough, showing various causes and complex pathogeneses. Whether it is due to the attack by exopathogen or due to internal impairment depends on the duration, rhythm, property, predisposing cause and concomitant signs of cough, which should be followed by differentiation and inspection of causes to distinguish between cold, heat, sthenia or asthenia syndromes and guide their treatments.

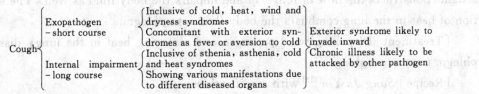

Common Syndromes:

1. Cough due to attack by exopathogen

(1) Obstructed lung - *qi* due to wind - cold

[Symptoms] Cough with coarse voice and thin whitish sputum, shortness of breath, and itching throat concomitant with headache, nasal obstruction and clear discharge, bodily soreness, aversion to cold, fever, and anhidrosis; pale tongue with thin whitish fur, floating pulse or floating tense pulse.

[Main Points of Differentiation] Cough with thin whitish sputum concomitant with exterior syndrome of wind - cold.

It is commonly seen in the early stage of upper respiratory tract infection and acute bronchitis.

[Pathogenesis] Wind – cold obstructs the circulation of lung – qi and retains in the striae.

[Treatment] Expelling wind and cold pathogens; facilitating the flow of lung – qi to stop coughing.

[Recipe] *Xing Su San*[130] and *Zhi Sou San*[37].

In case of severe wind – cold syndrome, add *Herba Ephedrae* to facilitate the flow of the lung – qi and expel cold pathogen; of severe phlegm – dampness syndrome, add *Rhizoma Pinelliae*, *Cortex Magnoliae Officinalis* and *Poria* to dissolve phlegm and dry dampness; of exterior cold and interior heat syndrome with shortness of breath and fever, add *Gypsum Fibrosum*, *Radix Scutellariae* and *Cortex Mori Radicis* to remove exterior syndrome and heat pathogen.

[Nursing Points] Avoid wind and cold pathogen; restrain from irritative food as cold, uncooked or acrid in nature.

(2) Invasion of wind – heat pathogen in the lung

[Symptoms] Frequent cough with rude respiration and coarse voice; sore throat, thick yellowish sputum with difficulty in expectoration, and slight thirstiness concomitant with headache, fever, aversion to wind, sweating, bodily soreness, and yellowish nasal discharge; thin yellowish fur, floating rapid pulse.

[Main Points of Differentiation] Cough with rude respiration, yellowish sputum, sorethroat, fever, sweating, and floating rapid pulse.

It is commonly seen in upper respiratory tract infection, acute bronchitis, the early stage of pneumonia, influenza, and concurrent infection of chronic bronchitis.

[Pathogenesis] The wind – heat pathogen invades the lung and affects the body resistance, obstructs the flow of lung – qi and impairs the body fluid as well. The stagnation of heat in the lung combusts the body fluid into phlegm.

[Treatment] Dispelling wind pathogen and removing heat in the lung; dissolving phlegm to stop coughing.

[Recipe] *Sang Ju Yin*[227] with modification.

In case of stagnation of heat pathogen in the lung, add *Rhizoma Anemarrhenae* and *Radix Scutellariae* to clear away heat in the lung; of sharp sore throat, add Rhizoma Belamcandae and *Radix Sophorae ubprostratae* to clear away heat and relieve the sore throat; of short breath similiar to dyspnea, add *Radix Peucedani* and *Rructus Arctii* to facilitate the flow of lung – qi; of severe *yin* impairment, add *Radix Adenophorae Strictae* and *Radix Trichosanthis* to promote the production of body fluid and dispel heat pathogen.

[Nursing Points] Refrain from fried, pungent, or greasy food; take regular meals; and quit drinking and smoking.

(3) Impairment of the lung by wind and dryness pathogens

[Symptoms] Dry cough or irritated cough, itching and dry throat, and little thick sputum with spitting difficulty or blood streaks concomitant with dry nose and lips, and even chest pain after coughing, nasal obstruction, and headache with mild fever and chills; reddened tip of tongue with dry thin yellowish fur; thready and somewhat rapid pulse.

[Main Points of Differentiation] Dry cough, itching throat, little thick sputum with spitting difficulty or blood streaks.

It may be seen in pulmonary tuberculosis, chronic bronchitis, chronic pharyngitis and lung cancer.

[Pathogenesis] The dryness pathogen combusts the lung and impairs the body fluid, leading to disorder of qi and disharmony of superficial wei - qi.

[Treatment] Dispelling wind and lung - heat; moistening dryness to stop coughing.

[Recipe] *Sang Xing Tang*[226].

In case of great loss of the body fluid, add *Rhizoma Polygonati Odoratic* and *Radix Ophiopogonis* to nourish lung - yin; of severe heat syndrome, add *Gypsum Fibrosum* and *Rhizoma Anemarrhenae* to remove heat from the lung; of dryness pathogen with cold nature, apply drugs of warming and moistening nature, e. g. *Xing Su San*[130] plus *Flos Farfarae*, *Radix Stemonae* and *Radix Asteris*, to stop coughing.

[Nursing Points] Refrain from pungent and fried food; quit drinking and smoking.

2. Cough due to internal impairment

(1) Stagnation of phlegm - dampness in the lung

[Symptoms] Repeated cough with coarse voice and thick whitish sputum or sputum stasis; fullness in the stomach, poor appetite, weariness and lack of strength, vomitting, nausea and loose stool; greasy whitish fur, soft and floating, slippery pulse.

[Main Points of Differentiation] Coarse cough with much sputum; fullness in the stomach, nausea, vomitting and anorexia; greasy whitish fur.

It is seen in chronic bronchitis and pulmonary emphysema.

[Pathogenesis] The phlegm generated from spleen - dampness invades upward and obstructs the flow of lung - qi, affecting the dispersing, purifying and descending function of the lung.

[Treatment] Invigorating the spleen and eliminating dampness; resolving phlegm to stop coughing.

[Recipe] *Er Chen Tang*[2] or *San Zi Yang Qin Tang*[14] with modification

In case of extreme deficiency of middle - jiao yang and stagnation of cold phlegm in the lung, add *Herba Asari* and *Rhizoma Zingiberis* to warm the lung and reduce phlegm; of excessive facial weariness due to deficient spleen, add *Radix Codonopsis Pilosulae*, *Rhizoma Atractylodis Maerocephalae* and prepared *Radix Glycyrrhizae* to warm the middle - jiao yang and invigorate the spleen. Take *Liu Jun Zi Tang*[45] at the remission stage.

[Nursing Points] Take light diet of warm nature; avoid internal injury due to overstrain or sexual intemperance; refrain from cold, uncooked or greasy food; quit smoking and drinking.

(2) Accumulation of phlegm and heat in the lung

[Symptoms] Cough with dyspnea and rude respiration or rale in the throat; much thick yellowish sputum with difficulty in expectoration, fish-stench smell or even blood stain; fullness in the chest and hypochondrium which is aggravated while coughing; flushed cheeks and fever with thirstiness and preference for drinks; reddened tongue with greasy yellowish fur, slippery and rapid pulse.

[Main Points of Differentiation] Cough with dyspnea and rude respiration, chest fullness, yellowish sputum, flushed cheeks, fever, reddened tongue with yellowish fur, slippery and rapid pulse.

It is seen in pulmonary abscess, concurrent infection of bronchiectasis, lobar pneumonia, and lung cancer.

[Pathogenesis] Heat pathogen obstructs the flow of lung-qi and converts the body fluid into phlegm, leading to impairment of the vessels and collaterals and disorder of qi's functional activities.

[Treatment] Removing heat pathogen to resolve phlegm; purifying the lung-qi to stop coughing.

[Recipe] *Qing Jin Hua Tan Tang*[248] with modification.

In case of pus-like fish-stench sputum, add *Herba Honttuyniae*, *Semen Coicis* and *Semen Benincasaeq*; of chest fullness with dyspnea, add *Semen Lepidii seu Descuruiniae*; in case of impairment of body fluid due to phlegm-fire, add *Radix Asparagi*, *Radix Ophiopogonis*, *Radix Trichosanthis*, and *Radix Adenophorae Strictae* to nourish *yin* and generate body fluid.

[Nursing Points] Quit smoking and drinking; refrain from pungent, greasy food and food likely to generate heat and phlegm pathogen.

(3) Invasion of the lung by liver-fire

[Symptoms] Paroxysmal cough, flushed cheeks and dry throat while coughing with a feeling of difficulty in expectoration, little thick sputum; pain in the chest and hypochondrium induced from coughing, bitter taste, varied symptoms and signs due to emotional changes; thin yellowish fur with little saliva; wiry and rapid pulse.

[Main Points of Differentiation] Varied cough or upward flow of qi due to emotional changes; pain in the chest and hypochondrium induced from coughing; wiry and rapid pulse.

It is seen in tuberculous pleurisy, chronic laryngopharyngitis and trachitis.

[Pathogenesis] The liver-qi gets stagnated and converts into fire pathogen which goes upward and affects the purifying and descending function of the lung. It is also known as "the wood-fire impairing metal", and converting body fluid into phlegm.

[Treatment] Removing liver-fire and clearing away lung-heat to stop coughing.

[Recipe] *Dai Ge San*[287] plus *Xie Bai San*[154].

In case of excessive liver-fire, add *Cortex Moutan Radicis* and *Fructus Gardeniae*; of frequent spitting due to adverse flow of *qi*, add *Fructus Perillae*, *Caulis Bambusae in Taeniam*, *Folium Eriobotryae*, *Fructus Aurantii* and *Flos Inulae*; of thick sputum and dry throat, add *Flos Fritillariae Thunbergii*, *Os Costaziae*, *Radix Trichosanthis* and *Radix Ophiopogonis* to resolve phlegm and promote the production of body fluid, and astringe the lung to stop coughing.

[Nursing Points] Adjust feelings and emotions; quit smoking and drinking; refrain from pungent food and food likely to generate fire pathogen and to consume *qi*.

(4) Deficiency of lung-*qi*

[Symptoms] Weak cough with dyspnea to be aggravated on slight exertion; little thin sputum, weariness, aversion to wind-cold, cold limbs, spontaneous perspiration, dim complexion; pale fur, thready deep week pulse.

[Main points of Differentiation] Cough with short breath to be aggravated on slight exertion; cold limbs, spontaneous perspiration, thready deep weak pulse.

It is seen in pulmonary emphysema, cor pulmonale, chronic bronchitis and lung cancer.

[Pathogenesis] Deficient lung-*qi* causes disorder of reception of air, *qi*'s failure in descending and ascending function, resulting in frequent coughing.

[Treatment] Tonifying the lung and *qi* to relieve cough and dyspnea.

[Recipe] *Bu Fei Tang*[143] with modification.

In case of excessive cold-phlegm, add *Fructus Perillae*, *Herba Asari* and *Ramulus Cinnamomi*; in case of dyspnea due to kidney deficiency, add *Gecko*, *Magnetitum*, and *Lignum Aquilariae Resinatum*. Cough due to deficient lung-*qi* is often accompanied by dyspnea, the treatment of which should base on careful differentiation and center on regulating *yin* and *yang* of the lung and kidney.

[Nursing Points] Lead a regular life; avoid cold-wind; quit smoking and drinking; refrain from irritative, cold and uncooked food and food likely to impair *yang*, and take nutritious but ungreasy food.

(5) Deficiency of lung-*yin*

[Symptoms] Dry cough with shortness of breath, little sputum or blood-stained sputum or even hemoptysis, dry mouth and throat with hoarse voice, afternoon fever, dysphoria, flushed face, night sweat, insomnia, slimness and loss of vitality; reddened tongue with little fur, thready rapid pulse.

[Main Points of Differentiation] Dry cough and dry throat, hemoptysis or blood-stained sputum, hectic fever, night sweat, reddened tongue with little fur.

It is commonly seen in pulmonary tuberculosis, chronic bronchitis, tuberculous pleurisy and lung cancer.

[Pathogenesis] Deficient lung-*yin* causes the internal accumulation of heat of deficiency type, and the failure of lung's purifying and moistening function, which further lead to consumption of the body fluid and injured collaterals respectively resulting in cough and hemoptysis.

[Treatment] Nourishing *yin* and moistening the lung to relieve cough and resolve phlegm.

[Recipe] *Sha Shen Mai Dong Tang*[138] with modification.

In case of cough with dyspnea, add *Fructus Schisandrae*, and *Fructus Chebulae* to astringe the lung - *qi*; of marked hectic fever and deficient *yin*, add *Herba Artemisiae Chinghao*, *Carapax Trionycis*, *Cortex Lycii Radicis*, *Radix Stellariae* and *Rhizoma Picrorhizae* to remove heat of deficiency type; of sputum with hemoptysis, add *Nodus Nelumbinis Rhizomatis*, *Cortex Moutan Radicis* and *Fructus Gardeniae* to clear away heat and stop bleeding; of slow recovery, add *Radix Rehmanniae Praeparata*, *Fructus Schisandrae* and *Fructus Corni* to nourish *yin* and invigorate kidney.

[Nursing Points] Quit smoking and drinking; refrain from pungent food and food likely to generate fire pathogen and injure *yin*.

Summary

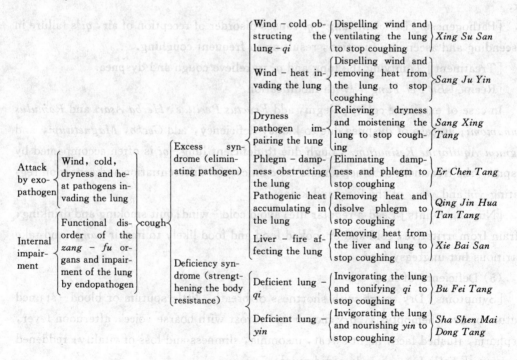

Discussions

1. How is cough classified? How is cough due to attack by exopathic factors distinguished from that due to internal impairment?

2. List the symptoms and signs, main points for diagnosis, therapeutic methods and recipes for each syndrome of cough due to attack by exopathic factors.

3. What are the *zang - fu* organs related to cough? And what is the pathogenesis?

3 Asthma with Wheezing

General

Asthma with wheezing is a morbid condition marked by paroxysmal rale and shortness of breath, featuring shortness and difficulty in breathing, wheezing, and even inability to keep horizontal position.

Since bronchial wheezing is always accompanied by dyspnea, it is also known as asthma, specially referring to paroxysmal dyspnea and rale in the throat. Although such is excluded in this chapter as pulmonary diseases and other syndromes characterized by dyspnea, the differentiation and treatment of which may be conducted on this basis.

This may also serve as a reference in treating bronchial asthma (endogenous, exogenous and mixed types), chronic asthmatic bronchitis, and pulmonary emphysema.

Etiology and Pathogenesis

Asthma with wheezing belongs to paroxysmal diseases, the causes of which comprise endopathic and exopathic ones.

1. The endopathic cause is also known as "root", which is usually the result of retention of phlegm in the lung. Phlegm retention is roughly divided into syndrome of cold type and that of heat type.

(1) Cold - phlegm: It is the result of frequent and repeated attack by wind - cold pathogen, which fails to evade and retains in the lung. It may also result from long - term intake of cold or uncooked food, which impairs the lung - qi, and prevents it from circulating body fluid. Besides the deficient *yang* due to chronic illness, aversion to cold and cold limbs may likewise impair the lung - qi, hence generating cold - phlegm internally.

(2) Heat - phlegm: Excessive intake of pungent or greasy food will produce phlegm and heat, which go upward and invade the lung. The accumulation of heat - phlegm may also be the result of chronic retention of cold - phlegm converting into heat syndrome, or the result of impaired *yin* due to chronic illness or usual excess of *yang*.

2. The exopathic cause is also called predisposing cause, the direct factor for the attack of asthma with wheezing. It generally includes the invasion by exopathogen, improper diet, emotional variation, and overstrain.

Invasion by exopathogen: When the organism fails to adapt to sudden climatic changes, wind, cold, summer - heat and dampness may all induce asthma with wheezing. So may the inhalation of pollen, smoke and dust, and irritative smells.

Improper diet: Partiality for a particular kind of food, or excessive intake of greasy and sweet or fish - stench or mutton food may all induce asthma with wheezing.

Emotional variation: The drastic variation of the seven emotions may obstruct the ascending and descending function of qi, and the stagnated lung-qi will further enliven the endopathic cause, thus asthma is induced.

Overstrain: Overstrain may consume and injure the qi of the spleen, kidney and lung, which enlivens the internally latent pathogen, thus leading to asthma with wheezing.

Key Points:

Endopathic cause: Usual retention of cold or heat-phlegm in the lung, or general deficiency of qi due to chronic illness or deficient lung-qi
Exopathic cause: Invasion by exopathogen, improper diet, emotional variation, or overstrain inducing the endopathogen
} Inducing latent phlegm to uprise with qi { Domination of pathogen and deficiency of vital-qi } Asthma with wheezing

Diagnosis and Discrimination

At the stage of attack, it's easily discriminated from other diseases for its obvious symptoms and signs manifested as paroxysmal shortness of breath and wheezing. The enquiry of medical history will reveal evident predisposing cause and history of attack. It usually has premonitory, e.g. itching throat, rhinocnesmus, choking sensation in the chest, etc.

Differences between asthma and dyspnea may center on the medical history and symptoms: the latter referring to breathing difficulty as short or faint breathing without repeated attack and wheezing, while the former necessarily involving dyspnea.

Differences between asthma and cough may also resort to the medical history: asthma reveals abrupt attack and rapid remission, and the patient looks normal during the intermission; while cough may sometimes involve rale and shortness of breath, which is easily distinguished from paroxysmal asthma with wheezing.

Asthma with wheezing, from the view-point of Western Medicine, is the hypersensitivity of organism (the lung) to certain sensitinogen, and hence shows paroxysmal quality. But in terms of TCM, it belongs to syndrome of dominating pathogen and deficient vital-qi, demonstrating the former character at the stage of attack and the latter during intermission.

Discrimination between Asthma, Dyspnea and Cough

Discrimination \ Disease	Asthma	Dyspnea	Cough
Illness history	Repeated inter-mittent attack	Progressive aggravation & continuity	Progressive aggravation & continuity
Symptom & sign	Wheezing short breath	Difficult breathing, short breath, dyspnea	Cough accompanied sometimes by dyspnea, asthma
Predisposing cause	Evident	Unclear	Unclear

Selecting Treatment by Differentiating Syndromes

Clear diagnosis should be followed by differentiation and treatment in accordance with the different conditions at the stage of attack and intermission, and a clear distinction between cold, heat, deficiency and excess syndromes as well.

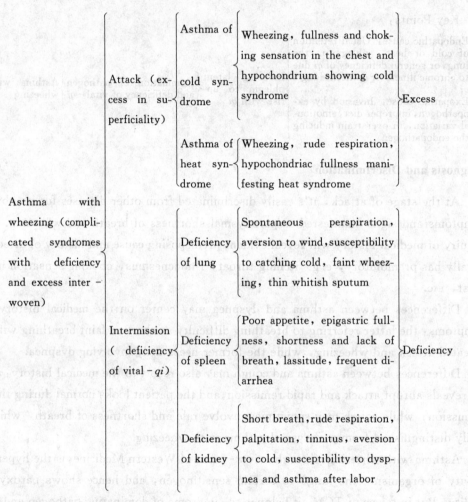

Common Syndromes:

1. At the stage of attack

(1) Asthma of cold syndrome

[Symptoms] Short breath with wheezing, white sputum, choking sensation in the chest and hypochondrium, slight cough, dark blue complexion, non-thirstiness or preference for hot drinks which are to be induced by cold pathogen and manifested as aversion to cold and cold limbs or headache and fever; whitish moist and glossy fur, wiry tense pulse or floating tense pulse.

[Main Points of Differentiation] Wheezing and dyspnea to be induced at the attack of cold, and bearing premonitory as itching nose and throat; whitish moist and glossy fur.

[Pathogenesis] The accumulation of cold - phlegm in the lung is induced by pathogen and causes obstructed circulation of *qi*. The counteraction between phlegm and *qi* further leads to stagnated upper - *jiao yang*.

[Treatment] Warm the lung to dispel cold pathogen; relieve phlegm to stop asthma with wheezing.

[Recipe] *She Gan Ma Huang Tang*[221] and *Xiao Qing Long Tang*[27].

Both decoctions are applicable to this syndrome. In case of much sputum and unsmooth throat, use, in the first place, the former decoction; in case of excessive cold pathogen, apply the latter decoction to dispel both external and internal cold by warming therapy. If the syndrome is gradually relieved post treatment, therapies of restoring *qi* and strengthening the body resistance should be adopted to solidify the effect. If the syndrome remains not remitted and instead, is accompanied by weariness, sweating, difficulty in breathing which impairs the heart - *yang* and is likely to develop into prostration syndrome, rescue work must be conducted with combined Western and Chinese therapy. And drugs to tonify the kidney, improve inspiration and arrest prostration must be added.

[Nursing Points] Lead a regular life; avoid wind - cold; refrain from overstrain, uncooked and cold food.

(2) Asthma of heat syndrome

[Symptoms] Short breath and rude respiration, roaring rale, frequent cough, fullness in the chest and hypochondrium, dysphoria and restlessness, yellowish or white thick sputum with difficult spitting; persperation, thirstiness and preference for cold drinks, flushed face and bitter taste, nonaversion to cold, or fever and headache sometimes; reddened tongue with yellowish greasy fur; slippery and rapid pulse or taut and slippery pulse.

[Main Points of Differentiation] Short breath and rude respiration, roaring rale, thick sputum, dysphoria, reddened tongue with yellowish greasy fur.

[Pathogenesis] The accumulation of phlegm - heat is induced by the exopathogen, causing the counteraction between phlegm and heat, obstruction of the air passage, and excessive accumulation of heat.

[Treatment] Facilitating the flow of lung - *qi* to clear away heat; removing phlegm to stop asthma.

[Recipe] *Ding Chuan Tang*[158], *Yue Bi Jia Ban Xia Tang*[263].

Both include the colding and warming therapy. As asthma of heat syndrome mostly results from fire pathogen which is transformed from the accumulation of cold, it is not advisable to apply cold therapy only. In case of exterior cold and interior heat, add *Gypsum Fibrosum*, *Ramulus Cinnamomi* and *Rhizoma Anemarrhenae*; in case of slimness and dry throat due to the impaired *yin* by heat pathogen, of night sweat and fidget due to deficiency, add discretionally *Radix Ophiopogonis*, *Radix Adenophorae Strictae*, and *Cordyceps* to clear away heat and nourish *yin*, to resolve phlegm and relieve asthma. If the syndromes get aggravated and tend to generate prostration syndrome, rescue work must be conducted with combined Western and Chinese medicine.

[Nursing Points] Refrain from pungent and greasy food; lead a regular life.

2. At the stage of intermission

(1) Deficiency of the lung

[Symptoms] The patient is aversive to wind with spontaneous perspiration, and susceptible to catching cold. Usually asthma is induced by climatic changes and manifested as stuffy nose with clear discharge, short breath and low voice, faint wheezing and clear whitish sputum, pale complexion and pale tongue with thin whitish fur, thready weak pulse or feeble large pulse.

[Main Points of Differentiation] Spontaneous perspiration, aversion to wind, susceptibility to catching cold, faint wheezing, and repeated attack due to climatic changes.

[Pathogenesis] Deficient lung-*qi* and lowered resistance lead to failure of the dispersing function of the superficies and accumulation of phlegm in the lung.

[Treatment] Tonifying the lung-*qi* and strengthening the body resistence.

[Recipe] *Yu Ping Feng San*[61].

In case of marked exterior deficiency and aversion to cold and wind, add *Ramulus Cinnamomi*, *Radix Paeoniae Alba*, *Rhizoma Zingiberis Recens*, and *Fructus Ziziphi Jujubae* to regulate *ying-qi* and *wei-qi* and strengthen the body resistance; in case of deficiency of both *qi* and *yin* marked by dry mouth, reddened throat and little sputum, apply *Sheng Mai San*[84] in combination to supplement *qi* and nourish *yin*.

[Nursing Points] Avoid irritation by sensitinogen; refrain from cold and uncooked food; lead a regular life.

(2) Deficiency of the spleen

[Symptoms] Poor appetite, epigastric fullness, loose stool, diarrhea after intake of greasy food, asthma frequently induced by improper diet and manifested as much sputum, short breath and lassitude; pale tongue with whitish moist and glossy fur or greasy fur; thready weak pulse.

[Main Points of Differentiation] Poor appetite, epigastric fullness, loose stool, lassitude, asthma frequently induced by improper diet.

[Pathogenesis] Deficient spleen-*qi* results in the spleen's failure in transport, deficiency of the middle-*jiao qi*, as well as the accumulation of phlegm-dampness in the body.

[Treatment] Strengthening the spleen to reduce phlegm.

[Recipe] *Liu Jun Zi Tang*[45] with modification.

In case of insufficiency of the spleen - *yang* and marked cold syndrome, add *Rhizoma Zingiberis* and *Semen Myristicae* to warm and invigorate the spleen - *yang*.

[Nursing Points] Lead a regular life; avoid cold pathogen; refrain from greasy or cold or uncooked food; and avoid eating and drinking too much at one meal.

(3) Deficiency of the kidney

[Symptoms] The usual short breath and rude respiration is likely to aggravate on slight exertion manifested as unsmooth inhalation, palpitation, dizziness, tinnitus, weakness and soreness of the loins and knees, weariness and lassitude, and asthma due to overstrain as well as aversion to cold and cold limbs, spontaneous perspiration, pale complexion, large pale tongue, deep thready pulse; while the deficiency of kidney - *yin* reveals a state of vexation, flushed cheeks, greasy sweating, reddened tongue with little fluid, thready and rapid pulse.

[Main Points of Differentiation] Short breath and rude respiration likely to aggravate on slight exertion; waist soreness and weariness; or vexation and flushed cheeks ready to induce asthma due to overstrain.

[Pathogenesis] Deficiency of both kidney *yin* and *yang* leads to failure of respiration, *qi*'s loss of its governor.

[Treatment] Tonifying the kidney to promote respiration.

[Recipe] *Jin Gui Shen Qi Wan*[163] or *Qi Wei Du Qi Wan*[8].

The former is applicable to patients of deficient kidney - *qi* and *yang*, the latter is to tonify the kidney and promote respiration. For patients of marked deficiency of *yin*, subtract drugs of warming nature and add *Radix Ophiopogonis*, *Radix Angelicae Sinensis*, and *Colla Plastri Testudinis*.

[Nursing Points] Avoid overstrain or sexual intemperance; take nutritious and easily - digested food.

Summary

A paroxysmal pulmonary disease as asthma with wheezing is, the predisposing cause matters much in the course of attack, of which the prevention, reduction or extinction must be given priority to. During the intermission it is necessary to strengthen the lung, spleen, and kidney *qi*. As the endopathic cause, pathogenic accumulation due to weakened body resistance is the main one for this syndrome, the principle of "interior syndrome coming after the exterior one" should be observed in treatment.

Being obstinate and of repeated attack and protracted course, spontaneous remission may be seen in some teengae patients after they acquire sufficient kidney - *qi* as adults. In case of drastic attack and dangerous condition with an indication of prostration syndrome, rescue work must be conducted immediately with combined Western and Chinese Medicine.

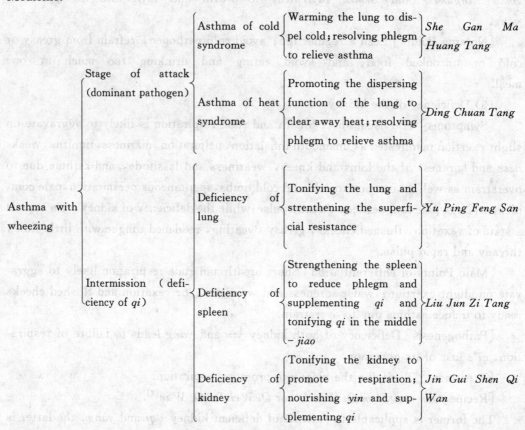

Discussions

1. How is asthma of cold syndrome distinguished from that of heat syndrome?

2. What are the different types of asthma to be differentiated during intermission?

3. How many types are included of asthma at the satge of attack? And what are the differentiation main points, therapeutic methods and recipes for each?

4 Dyspnea

General

It is a pulmonary disease featuring dyspneic respiration. The patient demonstrates a morbid condition manifested as open mouth, lifted shoulders, nares flaring and failure in staying horizontally due to breathing difficulty, which leads to prostration syndrome if serious.

It relates to many acute or chronic diseases and is the chief manifestation of pulmonary diseases. But it may also result from pathologic changes of other organs which affect the lung. Hence treatment should base on the differentiation of both diseases and symptoms and signs.

Differentiation and treatment herein are referential to such diseases in Western Medicine as chronic asthmatic bronchitis, acute bronchitis, pulmonary emphysema, cor pulmonale, pulmonary tuberculosis, atelectasis, hysterical gasp, lung cancer, and mediastinal tumor which all have dyspnea as the chief manifestation.

Etiology and Pathogenesis

Its causes are inclusive of attack by exopathic factors and internal impairment. No matter which organ is involved first, dyspnea will not be generated until it affects the lung's function to govern *qi* and respiration.

1. Attack by exopathic factors   Severe wind - cold or wind - heat pathogen will obstruct the flow of lung - *qi* and retain in the skin, hair or striae. The accumulated pathogen may impair the lung or convert the body fluid into phlegm, which all lead to failure of the lung in its purigying and descending function and adverse flow of *qi*. Thus dyspnea occurs.

2. Improper diet   Indulgence in greasy or cold or uncooked or pungent food, or excessive alcohol will result in dysfunction of the spleen in transportation and transformation and occurrence of thick phlegm which invade upward, obstruct the flow of lung - *qi*, and cause *qi*'s failure in its ascending and descending function. Thus dyspnea occurs. Likewise, the combined phlegm and fire derived from chronic accumulation of phlegm - dampness may cause the upward invasion of lung - *qi*, generating dyspnea.

3. Emotional abnormality   Emotional depression and anxiety will cause stagnation of *qi*, the upward flow of liver - *qi*, and failure of the lung in its purifying and descending function, further resulting in dyspnea syndrome.

4. Overstrain, sexual intemperance or chronic illness   Chronic illness in combination with overstrain will consume and damage the lung - *qi* and lung - *yin*, leading to

dyspnea due to *qi* 's loss of its governor. Chronic illness will damage the spleen and sexual intemperance will impair the kidney. As the spleen is the source of phlegm and the kidney the organ to receive air, impairment of both will inevitably affect the lung, bringing about dyspnea.

The occurrence of dyspnea chiefly lies in the lung and kidney, the former being the governor of *qi*, the latter the root. Dyspnea is classified into deficiency and excess types, the former originating from the kidney and the latter the lung. In general, dyspnea derives from *qi* 's disorder in ascending, descending, ingoing and outgoing.

Key Points:

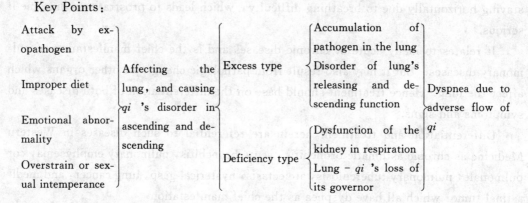

Diagnosis and Discrimination

Dyspnea is a pulmonary disease featuring dyspneic respiration, open mouth, lifted shoulders and nares flaring, which should be distinguished clinically from cough, asthma and shortness of breath. See the table in Chapter 3 for discrimination from asthma with wheezing and cough.

Discrimination between Dyspnea & Short Breath

Discrimination \ Disease	Dyspnea	Short breath
Symptoms & signs	Dyspneic respiration, open mouth, lifted shoulders, nares flaring	Deficiency *qi*, feeble and short breath similar to dyspnea but without voice
Posture	Inability to keep horizontal position	Lying in bed, and ability to keep horizontal position
Quality	Classified into deficiency and excess types	Deficiency syndrome on the whole

Selecting Treatment by Differentiating Syndromes

Confirmed diagnosis should be followed by differentiation between deficiency or excess types.

Symptoms	Syndrome	Type
Dyspnea and cough with short breath, chest fullness and tense pulse, headache and anhidrosis	Attack of wind-cold in the lung	Excess type (inclusive of combination of excess and deficiency)
Dyspnea and uprising of *qi*, chest fullness and pain, rude respiration, slippery and rapid pulse	Exterior cold and interior heat	
Dyspnea and cough with upwelling of *qi*, chest pain, yellowish sputum with blood streaks, fever and thirstiness, rapid pulse	Stagnation of phlegm-heat in the lung	
Dyspnea and chest fullness, much thick sputum, vomiting and nausea, anorexia, slippery pulse	Obstructed lung-*qi* by phlegm	
Dyspnea due to emotional variations, suffocated feeling, fullness and pain in the chest and hypochondrium, taut pulse	Obstructed lung-*qi*	Syndrome characterized by dyspnea
Low dyspnea with faint breath, feeble cough, spontaneous perspiration, aversion to wind, or hectic fever and reddened throat	Deficiency of the lung	
Chronic dyspnea to be aggravated on slight exertion, exhalation over-powering inhalation, weariness, cold limbs or dysphoria with feverish sensation in chest, palms and soles	Deficiency of the kidney	Deficiency type
Drastic dyspnea with open mouth and lifted shoulders, upright posture, rale, palpitation, sweating, and rootless pulse	Prostration syndrome	

Common Syndromes:

1. Dyspnea of excess type

(1) Attack of wind-cold in the lung

[Symptoms] Dyspnea with short breath, chest fullness and cough, much thin sputum concomitant with aversion to cold, headache, anhidrosis, non-thirstiness and fever sometimes; thin whitish fur; floating and tense pulse.

[Main Points of Differentiation] Dyspnea and short breath, much thin sputum concomitant with exterior syndrome of wind-cold of excess type.

It is commonly seen in asthmatic bronchitis, dyspnea due to acute bronchitis, and pulmonary emphysema.

[Pathogenesis] Accumulation of wind-cold in the superficies will invade the lung, causing lung's failure in dispersing function. The cold pathogen will convert the body fluid into phlegm, leading to dyspnea.

[Treatment] Promoting the dispersing function of the lung and dispelling cold to relieve dyspnea.

[Recipe] *Ma Huang Tang*[242] with modification.

In case of sweating but unrelieved dyspnea, add *Radix Paeoniae Alba*, *Cortex Mag-*

noliae Officinali* and *Prepared Licorice*; of severe attack by cold pathogen and much thin frothy sputum, apply *Xiao Qing Long Tang*[27] to disperse exopathogens from superficies and warm the interior.

[Nursing Points] Avoid wind and cold pathogen; refrain from cold or uncooked or greasy food.

(2) Exterior cold and interior heat

[Symptoms] Dyspnea, short breath and rude respiration, distending pain of the chest, nares flaring, thick sputum with difficulty in spitting concomitant with aversion to cold, fever, dysphoria, bodily pain, or sweating or anhidrosis with thirstiness, reddened tongue with thin whitish or yellowish fur, floating rapid pulse or slippery rapid pulse.

[Main Points of Differentiation] Dyspnea and rude respiration with loud voice, aversion to cold, fever, floating rapid pulse or slippery rapid pulse.

It is commonly seen in pneumonia, concurrent infection of bronchiectasis, pulmonary emphysena, and concurrent infection of cor pulmonale.

[Pathogenesis] The unrelieved cold pathogen in the superficies goes inward and turns into heat, which obstructs the flow of lung-qi and causes adverse flow of qi. Thus dyspnea occurs.

[Treatment] Promoting the dispersing function of the lung and purging away heat to relieve dyspnea.

[Recipe] *Ma Xing Shi Gan Tang*[241].

In case of severe heat syndrome, add *Radix Scutellariae*, *Cortex Mori Radicis* and *Fructus Trichosanthis*; of excessive sputum, add *Semen Lepidiiseu Descurainiae* and *Rhizoma Belamcandae*.

[Nursing Points] Refrain from pungent, sweet and greasy food; quit smoking and drinking; take in light meal.

(3) Accumulation of phlegm-heat in the lung

[Symptoms] Dyspnea, cough and upwelling of qi, distending pain of the chest, much yellowish thick sputum or blood-stained sputum concomitant with dysphoria, fever, sweating, thirstiness and preference for cold drinks, dry throat, flushed face, dark urine, or constipation; yellowish greasy fur, slippery rapid pulse.

[Main Points of Differentiation] Dyspnea, cough and upwelling of qi, dysphoria, distending pain in the chest, yellowish sputum with yellowish greasy fur.

It is commonly seen in pneumonia, concurrent infection of bronchiectasis, pulmonary emphysema, and concurrent infection of cor pulmonale, lung cancer, and mediastinal tumor.

[Pathogenesis] The accumulation of pathogenic heat in the lung converts the body fluid into phlegm, and obstructs the functional activity of qi, hence generates the disorder of the lung in its purifying and descending function.

[Treatment] Clearing away heat and phlegm to relieve dyspnea.

[Recipe] *Sang Bai Pi Tang*[225].

In case of severe heat syndrome and fever, add *Gupsum Fibrosum* and *Rhizoma Anemarrhenae* to clear *qi* and purge away heat; of dry throat with thirstiness, add *Radix Trichosanthis* to promote the production of body fluid and clear away heat; of dyspnea and upwelling of *qi* as well as inability to keep horizontal posture, add *Semen Lepidii seu Descurainiae*, *Radix et Rhizoma Rhei* and *Natrii Sulfas* to relax the bowels, purge wastes and send down abnormally ascending *qi*; of smelly sputum, add *Herba Houttuyniae* and *Semen Coicis*.

[Nursing Points] Refrain from pungent and greasy food; quit smoking and drinking.

(4) Stagnation of phlegm in the lung

[Symptoms] Dyspnea, cough, fullness and choking sensation in the chest and respiration with uprising head on aggravation, much white thick sputum with difficulty in spitting, sticky mouth and tastelessness, anorexia and nausea; thick whitish greasy fur, slippery pulse.

[Main Points of Differentiation] Dyspnea, cough, chocking sensation in the chest, respiration with uprising head, much white thick sputum, anorexia and nausea, thick whitish greasy fur.

It is commonly seen in atelectasis, pulmonary emphysema, cor pulmonale, chronic asthmatic bronchitis and silicosis.

[Pathogenesis] Dysfunction of the middle – *jiao yang* produces phlegm and causes it to retain in the lung. This further result in lung's failure in descending function, thus dyspnea arises.

[Treatment] Resolving phlegm to relieve asthma.

[Recipe] *Er Chen Tang*[2] plus *San Zi Yang Qin Tang*[14].

In case of severe dysfunction of the spleen, add *Rhizoma Atractylodis* and *Cortex Magnoliae Officinalis* to dry dampness and regulate the spleen's function; of adverse flow of *qi* and fierce dyspnea and cough, add *Flos Fritillariae Thunbergii* and *Herba Ephedrae* to disperse the lung – *qi* and relieve dyspnea.

[Nursing Points] Take in light and easily – digested food; refrain from greasy, sweet or fried food.

(5) Retention of lung – *qi*

[Symptoms] Dyspnea on emotional irritation or abnormality manifested as sudden shortness of breath, faint rale, suffocated feeling and pain in the chest, choking feeling in the throat, or insomnia, hypochondriac pain, and palpitation; wiry pulse.

[Main Pints of Differentiation] The attack of dyspnea is in close connection with emotional variations, specially depression and anger, and manifested as suffocated and oppressed feeling in the chest, strong choking sensation in the throat, and wiry pulse.

It can be seen in hysterical dyspnea.

[Pathogenesis] The stagnation and adverse flow of liver -qi affect the lung and further cause dyspnea.

[Treatment] Relieving stagnated liver -qi and sending dowm abnormally ascending qi to stop dyspnea.

[Recipe] *Wu Mo Yin Zi*[43] with modification.

In case of marked palpitation and insomnia, add *Semen Ziziphi Spinosae* and *Radix Polygalae*.

[Nursing Points] Regulate emotions and avoid depression and anger; refrain from pungent or greasy food.

2. Dyspnea of deficiency type

(1) Deficiency of the lung

[Symptoms] Dyspnea with fright due to deficient *qi*, snore, feeble cough, faint voice, thin sputum, spontaneous perspiration, aversion to wind; or dry cough, unsmooth throat, dysphoria with smothery sensation, flushed face; reddish tongue or reddened tongue with peeling fur; soft weak pulse or thready rapid pulse.

[Main Points of Differentiation] Dyspnea, shortness of breath, fright due to deficient *qi*, faint voice; weak pulse.

It is commonly seen in chronic asthmatic bronchitis, atelectasis, pulmonary enphysema, and cor pulmonale.

[Pthogenesis] Deficiency of the lung is inclusive of deficiecy of lung -qi and that of lung - yin. Deficiency of the lung -qi causes weakened body resistance, and the deficiency of lung - yin will lead to upward flaming of fire of deficiency type.

[Treatment] Invigorating the lung -qi and nourishing yin to relieve dyspnea.

[Recipe] *Sheng Mai San*[84] plus *Bu Fei Tang*[143].

In case of accumulation of cold -phlegm due to deficient *qi* and *yang*, add *Rhizoma Zingiberis*, *Radix Glycyrrhizae* and *Stalactium* to warm the lung and resolve phlegm so to relieve dyspnea; in case of the excessive deficiency of *yin*, add *Rhizoma Polygonati Odorati*, *Radix Adenophorae Strictae* and *Bulbus Lili* to mourish *yin* and relieve dyspnea; in case of inappetence, loose stool, or bearingdown feeling in the abdomen, which is thought to be the result of deficiency of both lung and spleen, add discretionally such drugs as *Bu Zhong Yi Qi Tang*[140] to invigorate *qi* and relieve dyspnea.

[Nursing Points] Avoid wind and cold; refrain from overstrain and pungent food.

(2) Deficiency of the kidney

[Symptoms] Chronic dyspnea and exhalation overpowering inhalation likely to aggravate on slight exertion, incontinence of breath, weariness, cold limbs and instep swelling, sweating, dark blue complexion with purple or pale lips, pale tongue with white fur or black but moist fur, indistinct and thready pulse or deep weak one; or dyspnea and cough, dry throat, flushed face, dysphoria, cold feet, greasy sweating, dry reddened tongue, thready rapid pulse.

[Main Points of Differentiation] Chronic dyspnea, exhalation overpowering inhalation, cold limbs and instep swelling, indistinct thready pulse or deep weak one; or dyspnea, cough, dry throat, flushed face, cold feet, dry reddened tongue.

It can be seen in cor pulmonale, pulmonary emphysema, atelectasis and pulmonary tuberculosis.

[Pathogenesis] Deficiency of the kidney is also inclusive of deficiency of kidney – qi and that of kidney – yin. The former will cause the kidney's failure in respiration, and qi's loss of its governor; the latter will lead to the uprising of single – $yang$ and qi's failure in respiration as well. Both will involve dyspnea.

[Treatment] Tonifying the kidney and improving its respiration; nourishing yin to relieve dyspnea.

[Recipe] *Jin Gui Shen Qi Wan*[163], *Shen Jie San*[170] or *Qi Wei Du Qi Wan*[8].

In case of deficiency of kidney – qi, apply *Jin Gui Shen Qi Wan* to warm the kidney – $yang$; in case of dyspnea with upwelling of qi, and mobile sensation under the navel, apply *Shen Jie San* to improve respiration; in case of dyspnea due to deficient kidney – yin, apply *Qi Wei Du Qi Wan* with modification to nourish yin; in case of flushed cheeks and sweating over forehead known as floating $yang$, add *Os Draconis*, *Concha Ostreae* to suppress $yang$ for relieving dyspnea.

Dyspnea due to kidney deficiency usually has a long course of illness which is commonly manifested as $yang$ impairment affecting yin. Hence during the recuperation *Placenta Hominis* powder and *Semen Juglandis* should be taken regularly to strengthen the body resistance for consolidating the constitution.

[Nursing Points] Avoid cold and wind; refrain from overstrain or sexual intemperance.

(3) Prostration syndrome

[Symptoms] Violent dyspnea, open mouth, lifted shoulders, fanning of the nostrils, upright posture and inability to keep horizontal posture, or rale, dysphoria, palpitation, dark blue face with purple lips, beady sweating, cold limbs, weariness, floating large pulse or intermittent pause of pulse, or vague pulse; or dysphoria and interior heat, dry throat and flushed cheeks, sticky sweating, thready, rapid and rootless pulse.

[Main Points of Differentiation] Violent dyspnea, inability to keep horizontal posture, sweating, cold limbs, scattered pulse; or dysphoria and flushed cheeks, sticky sweating, thready rapid and rootless pulse.

It is seen in cor pulmonale, heart failure, lung cancer, mediastinal tumor.

[Pathogenesis] Exhausting lung – qi and the decline of heart – $yang$ and kidney – $yang$ lead to the exhaustion of yin and $yang$ and vital – qi; genuine – yin causes the single – $yang$ uncontrolled and qi to rise upward.

[Treatmen] Strengthening $yang$ and tonifying yin; suppressing the prostration syndrome and relieving dyspnea.

[Recipe] *Shen Fu Tang*[167] to be used for oral administration of *Hei Xi Dan*[268].

Or apply *Du Shen Tang*[194] with *Os Draconis*, *Concha Ostreae*, *Radix Panacis Quinquefolii* and *Fructus Schisandrae* added to it.

[Nursing Points] Prostration syndrome, the most dangerous stage of dyspnea, needs emergency treatment by combined Chinese and Western therapy apart from strengthening the body resistance with Chinese drugs to prevent delayed chance of treatment. Besides it needs careful attendence and close observation.

Summary

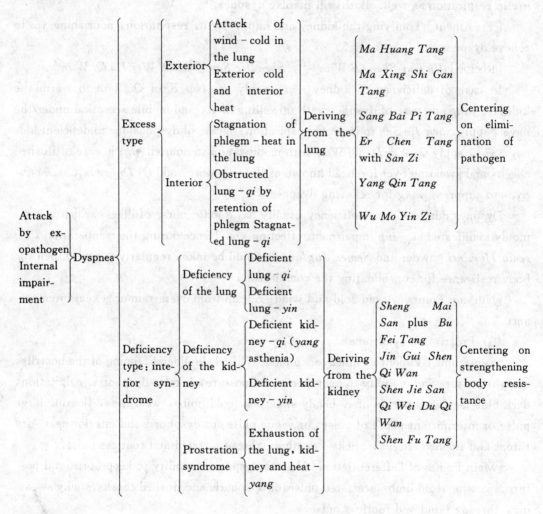

Discussions

1. How is asthma with wheezing related to and distinguished from dyspnea?

2. How is dyspnea of excess type discriminated from that of deficiency type? And how many types are they respectively classified?

3. List the differentiation main points, therapeutic methods, and recipes for different syndromes of dyspnea.

5 Fluid Retention

General

Fluid retention is a morbid condition marked by retention of body fluid in some regions of the human body due to abnormal fluid circulation and transportation.

Fluid retention bears a concept in broad sense and one in narrow sense. The former is as mentioned above, being the generalization of different fluid retention syndromes; while the latter refers only to one of them, specially the morbid condition due to retention of body fluid in the spleen, stomach and intestines.

Differentiation and treatment herein are applicable to certain stage of such diseases as chronic bronchitis, bronchial asthma, exudative pleurisy, tuberculous pleurisy, gastrointestinal functional disturbance, incomplete pylorochesis, congestive heart-failure and acute glomerulonephritis in Western Medicine.

Etiology and Pathogenesis

1. Attack by cold-dampness Wading, walking in the rain, lying on wet land, sharp cold climate may all affect the defensive energy of the body, and further cause obstruction of the lung-*qi*, invasion of pathogenic cold-dampness from the exterior to the interior, and disturbance of the spleen and stomach. Consequently the exopathic dampness induces the endopathic dampness, resulting in water retention within the body.

2. Improper diet Intake in large quantity of cold water, tea, and uncooked food leads to counteraction between cold and heat, weakened function of middle-*jiao yang*, and dysfunction of the spleen in transport and transformation. Hence pathogenic water arises internally and retention syndrome occurs due to abnormal metabolism of the body fluid.

3. Internal injury by overstrain or sexual intemprance Internal retention of the body fluid may be the result of injury of the spleen and kidney respectively due to overstrain and sexual intemprance, leading to *yang* deficiency or disturbed transport and transformation.

TCM holds that *san-jiao* is the site of *qi* activity, of which the upper-*jiao* (the lung) has the function to disperse body fluid and keep water pure and descendant; the middle-*jiao* (the spleen) bears the function to transport and transform food stuff and fluid; the lower-*jiao* (the kidney) the function to evaporate and transform water and separate the clear from the turbid. Therefore dysfunction of any one of the three and obstruction of *qi* activity will necessarily affect the normal process of fluid absorption, transport and discharge, and retention of pathogenic water at any part of the body is called fluid retention syndrome.

Key Points:

Attack by exogenous cold -dampness—Impairing defensive energy and damaging the lung - *qi*

Improper diet—Impairing the spleen - *yang*

Overstrain or sexual intemperance—Impairing the kidney - *yang* and spleen- *yang*

⎫ Deficient *yang* and excessive *yin* leading to disturbance of *san - jiao* in *qi* transformation ⎬ Fluid retention

Diagnosis and Discrimination

Discrimination between Phlegm, Fluid Retention, Water & Dampness

Disease	Pathogenesis	Characteristics
Phlegm	Retention of the body fluid due to metabolism disorder	Thick, located everywhere, changeable, usu. the result of heat evaporation, belonging to pathogenic *yang*
Fluid retention		Thin, usu. retaining locally within the body, the result of cold accumulation, belonging to pathogenic *yin*
Water		Clear secretion, often suffusing the surface of the body and the whole body, belonging to pathogenic *yin* and further classified into *yin* and *yang* type
Dampness		Thick and greasy, chronic occurrence of disease, difficult to die out, belonging to pathogenic *yin*, often accompanied by other pathogen

Besides fluid retention needs to be distinguished from other syndromes as asthma with wheezing, syndrome characterized by dyspnea, and edema. The various types of fluid retention (phlegm retention, pleural effusion, anasarca, and excessive fluid in the hypochondrium and epigastrium) are named pathologically in accordance with the location of pathogenic water; while asthma with wheezing, syndrome characterized by dyspnea and edema are named in accordance with the characteristics of signs of disease. Fluid retention and edema both are the result of diseased body fluid, but the former only sees fluid in some part of the body while the latter all over the body. Hence, they have differences and some internal relations as well.

Selecting Treatment by Differentiating Syndromes

The differentiation of fluid retention should follow a classification of it in accordance with the different locations into phlegm retention, pleural effusion, anasarca, and excessive fluid in the hypochondrium and epigastrium. See the following table for discrimination.

Discrimination / Disease	Location	Pathogenesis	Chief signs
Phlegm retention	Stomach & intestines	Deficiency of the spleen - *yang*	Epigastric fullness, viberating sound of water in the stomach and intestines; vomiting of sputum foams
Pleural effusion	Hypochondrium	Dysfunction of the lung	Twinge in the chest and hypochondrium, epigastric fullness and rigidity, retching
Anasarca	Overall body	Dysfunction of the lung and spleen	Edema and pain over the body, anhidrosis, dyspnea and cough
Excessive fluid in the hypochondrium and epigastrium	Chest lung	Deficiency of the lung - *qi*	Cough and dyspnea, inability to keep horizontal posture, white sputum in large amount

The treatment of fluid retention should follow the principle of relieving symptoms by warming therapy. It chiefly manifests a state of *yang* deficiency and *yin* excess as well as exterior syndrome of excess type and interior syndrome of deficiency type. Therefore, the treatment should center on tonifying the spleen and warming the kidney, and sometimes the therapies as inducing sweating, promoting diuresis and purgation may be applied for the treatment of the symptoms.

1. Phlegm retention

(1) Deficiency of spleen - *yang*

[Symptoms] Fullness in the chest and hypochondrium, epigastric fullness, viberating sound of water in the stomach, gastrointestinal preference for warmth and aversion to cold, slight dorsal aversion to cold, vomit of clear water or sputum, thirstiness without preference for drinks, often vomit after drinking water; palpitation, shortness of breath, poor appetite, loose stool, gradual slimness of the body; white slippery fur, wiry thready and slippery pulse.

[Main Points of Differentiation] Eeigastric fullness, viberating sound of water in the stomach, aversion to cold with preference for warmth, poor appetite, and loose stool.

It is commonly seen in gastrointestinal dysfunction, incomplete pylorochesis, and congestive heart - failure.

[Pathogenesis] Phlegm retention in the middle - *jiao* will cause deficient spleen - *yang* and further bring about internal accumulation of cold - dampness and failure of lucid *yang* to rise.

[Treatment] Warming and invigorating the spleen - *yang*; removing retention and making the adverse flow of *qi* normal.

[Recipe] *Ling Gui Zhu Gan Tang*[150] or *Xiao Ban Xia Jia Fu Ling Tang*[26].

In case of severe fluid-retention syndrome due to deficient spleen-*yang*, apply the first decoction; in case of retention in epigastrium and failure of descending of the stomach-*qi*, apply the other decoction; in case of difficulty in urination, palpitation and dizziness, add *Rhizoma Alismatis* and *Polyporus Umbellatus*; in case of cold-pain in the gastric cavity, and frequent spitting of saliva, add *Cortex Cinnamimi*, *Rhizoma Zingiberis* and *Fructus Euodiae* to warm the middle-*jiao* and making the adverse flow of *qi* normal; in case of severe epigastric fullness, add *Fructus Aurantii Inmaturus* to promote the circulation of *qi* and relieve fullness.

[Nursing Points] Avoid wind and cold; refrain from cold or uncooked or greasy food.

(2) Retention of fluid in the stomach and intestines

[Symptoms] Fullness or pain in the stomach and abdomen, diarrhea, relieved symptoms after diarrhea but followed by aggravation; viberating sound of water through the intestines, or constipation, abdominal fullness, dry mouth without preference for water; yellowish or thick whitish fur; deep and wiry pulse or deep-sited pulse which is unavailable until repeated effort.

[Main Points of Differentiation] Abdominal fullness, diarrhea or constipation, dry mouth without preference for water, viberating sound of water through the intestines, deep wiry pulse.

It is commonly seen in gastrointestinal neurosis.

[Pathogenesis] Fluid-retention in the stomach and intestines causes the obstruction of *yang* when newly accumulated retention adds to the unrelieved original one.

[Treatment] Eliminating retention by means of purgation.

[Recipe] *Ji Jiao Li Huang Wan*[24] or *Gan Sui Ban Xia Tang*[73].

In case of heat pathogen derived from retention of fluid in the intestines, apply the former recipe to eliminate it; in case of retention of fluid in the stomach and intestines, apply the latter for the purpose of reinforcement and elimination in combination; in case of upward invasion of fluid and severe chest fullness, add *Fructus Aurantii Immaturus* and *Cortex Magnoliae Officinalis* to promote the circulation of *qi* and fluid. But the elimination of fluid must be conducted in combination with reinforcement of vital energy lest excessive purgation would impair the middle-*jiao yang* even more seriously.

[Nursing Points] Refrain from cold, uncooked, greasy or sweet food.

2. Pleural effusion

(1) Pathogens invading the chest and lung

[Symptoms] Twinge in the chest and hypochondrium likely to aggravate on breathing or movement, epigastric fullness and rigidity, alternate spells of fever and chill or fever without aversion to cold, lack of sweat or sweating without relief of fever, cough, retching, shortness of breath, bitter taste and dry throat; whitish or yellowish thin fur;

wiry and rapid pulse.

[Main Points of Differentiation] Twinge in the chest and hypochondrium likely to aggravate due to breathing or movement, epigastric fullness and rigidity, retching and bitter taste; wiry and rapid pulse.

It is commonly seen in pleurisy, pneumonia, bronchitis, and bronchial asthma.

[Pathogenesis] When attacked by seasonal pathogen, heat will get accumulated in the chest and lung, resulting in the dispersing failure of lung - qi and retainment of pathogenic factors in *Shaoyang* .

[Treatment] Dispersing the lung - qi by mediation method.

[Recipe] *Chai Zhi Ban Xia Tang*[212].

In case of cough with rude respiration and sharp hypochondriac pain, add *Cortex Mori Radicis* and *Semen Sinapis Albae* to this recipe; in case of marked epigastric fullness and rigidity, bitter taste and retching, add *Rhizoma Pinelliae* and *Fructus Trichosanthis*; in case of marked heat syndrome and excessive perspiration, apply this recipe plus *Ma Xing Shi Gan Tang*[241].

[Nursing Points] Refrain from greasy or pungent food; lead a regular daily life; avoid exopathogens.

(2) Fluid in the chest and hypochondrium

[Symptoms] Cough and spitting will induce pain, difficulty in breathing, cough, dyspnea, and inability to keep horizontal posture or ability to keep lateral position on the side of retention, where is seen hypochondriac fullness or even bulge of the chest. Also manifested are thin whitish greasy fur, deep and wiry pulse or wiry and slippery pulse.

[Main Points of Differentiation] Cough and dyspnea, adverse flow of qi, inability to keep horizontal posture, pain in the chest and hypochondrium, wiry and slippery pulse.

It is commonly seen in exudative pleurisy, pneumonia and bronchial asthma.

[Pathogenesis] Fluid retention and obstructed qi will lead to obstructed channels and collaterals as well as the lung - qi, resulting in uprising of fluid retention.

[Treatment] Eliminating retained fluid.

[Recipe] *Shi Zao Tang*[6].

This recipe is mainly applicable to fluid retention in the chest, domination of pathogen without general deficiency of qi, and excessive accumulation of water pathogen. In case of pathogenic factor of excess type and general deficiency of qi, apply *Kong Xian Dan*[238] to promote the dispersing function of the lung and regulate the circulation of qi for eliminating fluid in slow action. If drastic vomiting and diarrhea occur after the administration of *Shi Zao Tang* and *Kong Xian Dan*, stop for two or three days and apply *Jiao Mu Gua Lou Tang*[265] instead to purge away fluid retention. In case of excessive sputum and saliva, add *Bulbus Allii Macrostemi* and *Semen Armeniacae Amarum*; in case of general deficiency of qi and poor appetite, as well as chronic fluid retention, add *Ramulus Cinnamomi*, *Rhizoma Atractylodis Macrocephalae*, and *Radix Glycyrrhizae* to activate *yang* and relieve fluid. For patients of chronic illness or general weakness, drastic purgation is not advisable.

[Nursing Points] Refrain from cold or uncooked or greasy food. Be well attended and keep away from exopathogen.

(3) Disharmony of collateral-*qi*

[Symptoms] Fullness, pain or malaise in the chest and hypochondrium with twinge or burning sensation, unsmooth breathing or oppressed cough; protracted course if serious and aggravation on wet weather; dark tongue with thin fur, wiry pulse.

[Main Points of Differentiation] Pain in the chest and hypochondrium with twinge or burning sensation, oppressed cough, fullness of the chest, dark tongue and wiry pulse.

It is commonly seen in old pleurisy.

[Pathogenesis] Chronic retention of fluid causes obstructed flow of *qi* and obstruction of collaterals.

[Treatment] Regulating the flow of *qi* to regulate the function of collaterals.

[Recipe] *Xiang Fu Xuan Fu Hua Tang*[188] with modification

In case of chest fullness, greasy fur due to excessive accumulation of phlegm, add *Fructus Trichosanthis* and *Fructus Aurantii*; if chronic illness gets into the collaterals with marked pain, add *Radix Angelicae Einensis*, *Semen Persicae*, *Flos Carthami*, and *Resina Commiphorae Myrrhae*; in case of productive cough with thin sputum known as the result of unrelieved fluid retention, add *Exocarpium Benincasae*, *Cortex Mori Radicis* and *Medulla Tetrapanacis*.

[Nursing Points] Refrain from pungent or fried or greasy food. Regulate emotions.

(4) Interior heat due to deficient *yin*

[Symptoms] Paroxysmal cough, dry mouth and throat, non-productive cough with little thick sputum, or afternoon fever, flushed cheeks, night sweat, dysphoria, insomnia, fullness and pain in the chest and hypochondrium, long course of disease, slim figure; reddened tongue with little fur, thready rapid pulse.

[Main Points of Differentiation] Cough, dry throat, little thick sputum, flushed cheeks, night sweat, reddened tongue with little fur.

It is commonly seen in tuberculous pleurisy.

[Pathogenesis] Fluid retention and *qi* obstruction turn into heat pathogen and impair *yin*, causing deficient *yin* and dryness of the lung, as well as disharmony of the collaterals.

[Treatment] Nourishing *yin* to remove heat; clearing collaterals to dispel fluid retention.

[Recipe] *Sha Shen Mai Dong Tang*[138] plus *Xie Bai San*[154].

In case of dry cough with little sputum and dry throat with chest pain and reddened tongue, apply the former decoction; in case of cough due to adverse flow of *qi* and burning heat over the skin, apply the latter; in case of severe hectic fever suggesting seriously injured *yin*, add *Carapax Trionycis*, *Radix Cynanchi Atrati*, and *Radix Scrophulariae*; in case of drastic cough, add *Bulbus Fritillariae Cirrhosae* and *Radix Stemonae*; in case of sharp pain and fullness in the chest and hypochondrium, add *Retinervus Luffae Fructus*, *Pericartium Trichosanthis*, *Radix Curcumae*, and *Fructus Aurantii*; in case of deficient vital -*qi*, weariness and shortness of breath due to chronic illness, add discretionally *Radix Astragali seu Hedysari*, *Rhizoma Atractylodis Macrocephalae*, *Fructus Schisandrae* and *Radix Pseudostellariae*.

[Nursing Points] Refrain from pungent food and alcohol; avoid sexual activity.

3. Anasarca

[Symptoms] Bodily pain and heaviness, puffy limbs, aversion to cold, anhidrosis; or cough and dyspnea, much frothy white sputum, chest fullness, retching without preference for drinks, whitish fur, wiry and tense pulse.

[Main Points of Differentiation] Heaviness and pain, puffy limbs, aversion to cold, anhidrosis, cough and dyspnea, much frothy white sputum.

It is commonly seen in bronchitis.

[Pathogenesis] Attack by exopathic wind-cold and stagnated function of the superficies will cause dysfunction of the lung and spleen, resulting in suffusion of water over the limbs and body surface.

[Treatment] Relieving superficial syndromes to remove fluid.

[Recipe] *Xiao Qing Long Tang*[27].

In case of oliguria and severe limb edema, add *Poria*, *Polyporus Umbellatus* and *Rhizoma Alismatis*; of heat and upset due to retention, and whitish and yellowish fur in combination, add *Gypsum Fibrosum*; in case of indistinct cold syndrome, subtract *Rhizoma Zingiberis*, and *Herba Asari*.

[Nursing Points] Avoid wind and cold; refrain from cold, uncooked and greasy food.

4. Excessive fluid in the hypochondrium and epigastrium

(1) Location of cold-fluid in the lung

[Symptoms] The patient shows cough, dyspnea, adverse flow of *qi*, and inability to keep horizontal posture with much frothy sputum and of protracted course, which are likely to aggravate in cold weather or when attacked by cold. Worse still are facial edema and instep swelling. Or the symptoms are invisible on usual occasions but break out when attacked by cold manifested as pain in the waist and back, trembling with fever and chills and accompanied by whitish slippery or greasy fur, wiry and tense pulse.

[Main Points of Differentiation] Cough, dyspnea, and adverse flow of *qi*, and inability to keep horizontal posture, much white sputum, immediate outbreak when attacked by cold.

It is commonly seen in chronic bronchitis, pulmonary emphysema, cor pulmonale, congestive heart – failure and renal failure.

[Pathogenesis] Fluid retention will attack the lung, resulting in excessive cold – fluid and the stagnation of phlegm and *qi*, and overflow of fluid.

[Treatment] Warming the lung to relieve fluid retention.

[Recipe] *Xiao Qing Long Tang*[27].

In case of excessive fluid retention and indistinct cold and exterior syndrome, apply *Ting Li Da Zao Xie Fei Tang*[261]; in case of general deficiency of *qi* without marked exterior syndrome, apply *Ling Gan Wu Wei Jiang Xin Tang*[149]; in case of chest fullness and adverse flow of *qi* with turbid fur, apply the above recipe plus *Semen Sinapis Albae* and *Semen Raphani*; in case of excessive fluid retention manifested as chest pain and dysphoria, apply the above recipe in combination with *Radix Euphorbiae Kansui* and *Radix Knoxiae*; in case of domination of pathogen and deficiency in lower – *jiao* and conversion of stagnated fluid retention into heat manifested as epigastric fullness and rigidity, dark complexion, polydipsia, cough and dyspnea, apply *Mu Fang Ji Tang*[35] to promote the circulatoin of fluid and dissolve stangation, as well as to restore *qi* and remove heat; if long standing accumulation of cold fluid retention converts into heat manifested as thick sputum and dry throat, reddened tongue and lack of saliva, apply *Mai Men Dong Tang*[124] plus *Fructus Trichosanthis*, *Radix Stephaniae Tetrandrae* and *Bulbus Fritillariae Cirrhosae* to promote the production of body fluid, remove retention and clear away heat.

[Nursing Points] Avoid wind and cold; regulate diet, and refrain from cold or uncooked or greasy food.

(2) Deficient *yang* of the spleen and kidney

[Symptoms] Dyspnea and shortness of breath likely to aggravate on slight exertion; or cough with fright due to deficient *qi*, much sputum, poor appetite, chest fullness and weariness, aversion to cold and cold limbs, abdominal contracture or subjunctive sensation of contraction, sub – umbilical convulsion, instep swelling, difficult urination, or frothy saliva and dizziness, blurred vision; enlarged tongue with whitish moist fur or grayish greasy fur, deep and thready pulse.

[Main Points of Differentiation] Dyspnea and shortness of breath, aversion to cold and cold limbs, instep swelling, poor appetite, much sputum, dizziness, blurred vision; enlarged tongue, deep and thready pulse.

It is commonly seen in pulmonary emphysema, bronchial asthma, and congestive heart – failure.

[Pathogenesis] Chronic fluid retention will invade the spleen and kidney, and make them fail in warming and transforming function, resulting in suffusion of water.

[Treatment] Warming and invigorating the spleen and kidney to remove fluid retention.

[Recipe] *Jin Gui Shen Qi Wan*[163], *Ling Gui Zhu Gan Tang*[150].

In case of excessive deficiency of spleen, apply first of all the latter decoction to strengthen the spleen and eliminate fluid retention; in case of excessive deficiency of kidney, apply the former to warm the kidney for elimination of fluid retention; in case of poor appetite and much sputum, add *Rhizoma Pinelliae* and *Pericarpium Citri Reticulatae*, *Fructus Amomi*, *Semen Amomi Cardamomi*; in case of sub-umbilical convulsion, dizziness and blurred vision, apply *Wu Ling San*[41] or *Zhen Wu Tang*[199] to check the adverse flow of *qi* for relieving fluid retention.

[Nursing Points] Avoid wind and cold; refrain from cold or uncooked food; and refrain from overstrain and excessive sexual activity.

Summary

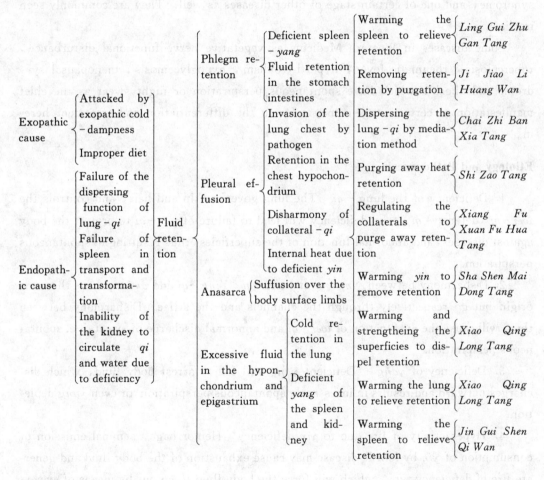

Cause	Mechanism		Type	Subtype	Treatment	Formula
Exopathic cause	Attacked by exopathic cold-dampness; Improper diet	Fluid retention	Phlegm retention	Deficient spleen-*yang*	Warming the spleen to relieve retention	*Ling Gui Zhu Gan Tang*
				Fluid retention in the stomach intestines	Removing retention by purgation	*Ji Jiao Li Huang Wan*
Endopathic cause	Failure of the dispersing function of lung-*qi*; Failure of spleen in transport and transformation; Inability of the kidney to circulate *qi* and water due to deficiency		Pleural effusion	Invasion of the lung chest by pathogen	Dispersing the lung-*qi* by mediation method	*Chai Zhi Ban Xia Tang*
				Retention in the chest hypochondrium	Purging away heat retention	*Shi Zao Tang*
				Disharmony of collateral-*qi*	Regulating the collaterals to purge away retention	*Xiang Fu Xuan Fu Hua Tang*
				Internal heat due to deficient *yin*	Warming *yin* to remove retention	*Sha Shen Mai Dong Tang*
			Anasarca	Suffusion over the body surface limbs	Warming and strengtheing the superficies to dispel retention	*Xiao Qing Long Tang*
			Excessive fluid in the hypon-chondrium and epigastrium	Cold retention in the lung	Warming the lung to relieve retention	*Xiao Qing Long Tang*
				Deficient *yang* of the spleen and kidney	Warming the spleen to relieve retention	*Jin Gui Shen Qi Wan*

Discussions

1. How is fluid retention classified in a broad sense? And how are they discriminated?
2. What are the similarities and differences of phlegm, fluid, water and dampness?
3. How is excessive fluid in the hypochondrium and epigastrium differentiated and treated clinically?

6 Spontaneous Perspiration & Night Sweat

General

Spontaneous perspiration and night sweat belong to abnormal discharge of sweat due to imbalance of *yin* and *yang* or lowered superficial resistance. The former refers to perspiration while awake and aggravation on slight exertion; whereas the latter denotes sweating while asleep and spontaneous stop post sleep. Either is a relatively independent syndrome, and one of certain stage of other diseases as well. They are commonly seen in clinic.

Some diseases in Western Medicine as vegetative nerve functional disturbance, tuberculosis, rheumatic fever, hyperthyroidism, hypoglycemosis, menopausal syndrome and shock, which have spontaneous perspiration or night sweat as the chief manifestation at certain stage, may refer to the differentiation and treatment herein.

Etiology and Pathogenesis

1. Deficiency of the lung - *qi* The lung governs skin and hair, and controls the *wei - qi* (defensive *qi*). Its deficiency will lead to failure of *wei - qi* to protect the body against diseases, and abnormal function of the superficies, thus resulting in spontaneous perspiration.

2. Disharmony between *ying - qi* and *wei - qi* *Ying - qi* and *wei - qi* have the same origin but go respectively through the channels and the striae. Disharmony between them will cause the dysfunction of *wei - qi* and abnormal discharge of sweat, i.e. spontaneous perspiration.

3. Deficiency of *yang* Deficient *yang* will fail to arrest body fluid, which discharges outward and results in incessantly spontaneous perspiration, or even *yang* depletion.

4. Hyperactivity of fire due to *yin* deficiency Hemorrhage, seminal emission or consumption of *yin* by febrile disease may cause exhaustion of the body fluid and generate fire of deficiency type, which will force the body fluid to go out by means of sweat, resulting in night sweat.

5. Stagnation of pathogenic heat When liver - fire and damp - heat retain interiorly, they will force the body fluid to discharge and thus lead to spontaneous perspiration.

Key Points:

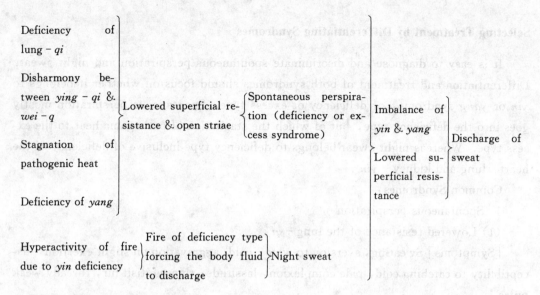

Diagnosis and Discrimination

Spontaneous perspiration features sweating while awake, but night sweat is characterized by sweating while asleep and spontaneous stop post sleep. Hence it is easy to diagnose and discriminate them.

Spontaneous perspiration and night sweat should be distinguished from prostration syndrome and perspiration after shivering.

The discrimination is listed in the following diagram:

Discrimination \ Name	Spontaneous perspiration	Prostration syndrome	Perspiration after shivering	Night sweat
Etiology pathogenesis	Deficient lung-*qi* Disharmony between *ying-qi* & *wei-qi* Deficient *yang* Stagnation of pathogenic heat	Prostrate vital-*qi* and *yang* depletion often seen in emergency cases	Febrile disease due to exogenous attack Counteraction between vital-*qi* & pathogenic factors, often seen in acute febrile diseases	Excessive consumption of premordial essence Internal accumulation of fire of deficiency type Injured body fluid and its inability to stay inside
Symptoms	Sweating while awake, usually accompanied by exterior syndrome, bearing slight, constitutional symptoms	Sweating while awake or fast asleep, profuse sweating, cold limbs, critical condition	Fever, listlessness, thirstiness, sudden aversion to cold and shivering followed by sweating	Sweating while asleep, and spontaneous stop post sleep

Selecting Treatment by Differentiating Syndromes

It is easy to diagnose and discriminate spontaneous perspiration and night sweat. Differentiation and treatment of both syndromes should focus on whether it belongs to *yin* or *yang* syndrome, or deficiency or excess type. Spontaneous perspiration mostly goes into the deficiency type, but of which the stagnation of pathogenic heat to the excess type. Whereas night sweat belongs to deficiency type inclusive of deficiency of the heart, lung and kidney - *yin*.

Common Syndromes:

1. Spontaneous perspiration

(1) Lowered resistance of the lung - *qi*

[Symptoms] Sweating, aversion to wind - cold, aggravation on slight exertion, susceptibility to catching cold, pale complexion, lassitude; thin whitish fur, thready weak pulse.

[Main Points of Differentiation] Sweating, aversion to wind - cold, susceptibility to catching cold.

It is commonly seen in vegetative nerve functional disturbance and hypoglycemosis.

[Pathogenesis] Deficiency of lung - *qi* due to general deficiency of *qi* resulting in lowered superficial resistance.

[Treatment] Invigorating *qi* and strengthening the superficial resistance to stop sweating.

[Recipe] *Yu Ping Feng San* [61].

In case of profuse sweating, add *Radix Ephedrae*, *Fructus Tritici Levis* and calcined *Concha Ostreae* to arrest *yin* and sweat.

[Nursing Points] Avoid wind and cold, esp. while sweating.

(2) Disharmony between *ying - qi* and *wei - qi*

[Symptoms] Sweating, aversion to wind, general malaise, occasional fever and chills, or sweating over half - length or certain parts of the body, thin whitish fur, moderate pulse.

[Main Points of Differentiation] Spontaneous perspiration, aversion to wind, abrupt fever and chills, sweating over certain parts of the body.

It may be seen in certain stage of vegetative nerve functional disturbance, hyperthyroidism and rheumatic fever.

[Pathogenesis] General deficiency of vital - *qi* causes imbalance of *yin* and *yang*, disharmony between *ying - qi* and *wei - qi*, lowered superficial resistance.

[Treatment] Regulating *ying - qi* and *wei - qi*.

[Recipe] *Gui Zhi Tang* [200] with modification.

In case of excessive sweating, add calcined *Os Draconis* and calcined *Concha Ostreae* to arrest sweat by consolidating and governing action; of deficient *qi*, add *Radix Scutel-*

lariae to invigorate *qi* and strengthen the superficial resistance; of aversion to cold due to deficient *yang*, add *Radix Aconiti Praeparata* to warm *yang*; in case of insomnia or sweating over half-length, apply *Gan Mai Da Zao Tang* [71].

[Nursing Points] Avoid wind and cold; refrain from greasy and sweet food.

(3) Deficiency of *yang*

[Symptoms] Patients of deficient *yang* due to chronic illness or patients with serious disease will show abruptly incessant perspiration, faint voice, weariness and lassitude, short breath, cool limbs, and weak pulse.

[Main Points of Differentiation] Abruptly incessant perspiration following chronic or serious illness.

It is commonly seen in hypoglycemosis and shock.

[Pathogenesis] Deficient *yang* due to chronic or serious illness causes *yang*'s failure to arrest *yin*.

[Treatment] Invigorating *qi* and warming *yang* to arrest sweating.

[Recipe] *Sheng Mai San*[84] with modification.

This syndrome needs immediate treatment to stop sweating and relieve the constitutional deficiency lest it should aggravate and turn into prostration syndrome due to *yang* or *yin* depletion.

In case of incessant sweating and distinct cool limbs, add *Radix Scutellariae* and *Radix Ginseng* to invigorate *qi* and strengthen *yang*; or add calcined *Os Draconis* and *Concha Ostreae* to arrest sweat and consolidate the body resistance; in case of aggravated condition, apply *Shen Fu Tang*[167] to recuperate depleted *yang* and rescue the patient from collapse, to arrest sweat and relieve prostration syndrome.

[Nursing Points] Take rest for close observation of the condition; replenish body fluid and avoid uncooked or cold food; keep away from wind and cold pathogen; take comprehensive measures if necessary.

(4) Stagnation of pathogenic heat

[Symptoms] Incessant perspiration, flushed face as if baked, restlessness, limb pain, no fever subsidance post sweating, bitter taste, yellowish urine and dry stool; reddened tongue with yellowish fur; rapid and strong pulse.

[Main Points of Differentiation] Incessant perspiration, no fever subsidance, bitter taste, yellowish urine, reddened tongue with yellowish fur, rapid pulse.

It can be seen in rheumatic fever, menopausal syndrome, and hyperthyroidism.

[Pathogenesis] Excessive accumulation of liver-fire or damp-heat inside combusts the body fluid and causes it to discharge.

[Treatment] Removing heat from the liver, and removing dampness to restore *ying-qi*.

[Recipe] *Long Dan Xie Gan Tang* [64].

In case of impaired body fluid due to excessive sweating, thirstiness and preference for drinks, add *Radix Trichosanthis*, fresh *Rhizoma Phragmitis* and *Herba Dendrobii*; in case of constipation due to pathogenic heat, add *Radix et Rhizoma Rhei Recens* and *Natrii Sulfas* to relax the bowels and purge wastes; in case of indistinct heat but distinct damp-heat, apply *Si Miao Wan*[76] and *Folium Bambusae*, *Fructus Gardeniae* and *Rhizoma Coptidis* at discretion to eliminate heart-fire and relieve anxiety.

[Nursing Points] Drink appropriate amount of water to replenish body fluid; refrain from pungent or greasy food; keep emotional balance and avoid depression and anger.

2. Night sweat

(1) Deficiency of the heart blood

[Symptoms] Sweating while asleep and immediate stop of sweating after waking up; palpitation, less sleep and dreaminess, malaise, shortness of breath, lack of strength, pale complexion; pale tongue with thin fur; feeble pulse.

[Main Points of Differentiation] Night sweat, palpitation, dreaminess, pale tongue.

It may be seen in tuberculosis, vegetative functional disturbance and menopausal syndrome.

[Pathogenesis] The deficiency and consumption of heart blood causes the body fluid to overflow and discharge as sweat due to interior disturbance by fire of deficiency type.

[Treatment] Enriching the blood and nourishing the heart to arrest sweat.

[Recipe] *Gui Pi Tang* [95].

In case of excessive sweat, add calcined *Os Draconis*, calcined *Concha Ostreae*, *Fructus Schisandrae* and *Fructus Tritici Levis*; in case of *yin* impairment in combination with heat syndrome, add *Herba Artemisiae*, *Rhizoma Anemarrhenae*, and *Cortex Lycii Radici*.

[Nursing Points] Refrain from pungent food and food likely to consume *qi* and impair *yin*; lead a regular life; avoid wind and cold; regulate emotions.

(2) Deficiency of lung-*yin* and kidney-*yin*

[Symptoms] Night sweat, hectic fever, dysphoria and sleeplessness, chronic dry cough, lassitude in loins and knees, dysphoria with feverish sensation in chest, palms and soles, slim figure; of females, menstruation of small amount and bright red colour, irregular menstruation, and somnial coitus; of males, nocturnal emission; reddened tongue with little fur; thready rapid pulse.

[Main Points of Differentiation] Night sweat, hectic fever, dry cough, slim figure, lassitude in loins, nocturnal emission; reddened tongue with little fur.

It may be seen in certain stage of tuberculosis, hyperthyroidism and menopausal syndrome.

[Pathogenesis] Hemorrhage or nocturnal emission will lead to *yin* deficiency of the lung and kidney and combustion of fire of deficiency type, forcing sweat to discharge.

[Treatment] Nourishing *yin* and removing heat to arrest sweat.

[Recipe] *Dang Gui Liu Huang Tang* [113].

In case of severe hectic fever, add *Radix Anemarrhenae*, *Cortex Lycii Radici* and

Plastrum Testudinis; of severe night sweat, add calcined *Os Draconis*, calcined *Concha Ostreae* and *Radix Ephedrae*; in case of severe heat syndrome of deficiency type, add *Herba Artemisiae*, *Carapax Trionycis* and *Radix Stellariae* apart from application of *Cortex Phellodendri* with large amount.

[Nursing Points] Lead a regular life and avoid sexual intemperance; refrain from pungent food and take light meal to nourish *yin* instead.

Summary

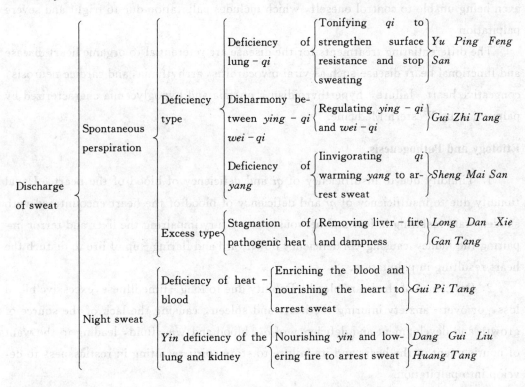

Discussions

1. How is spontaneous perspiration distinguished from night sweat, sweating from exhaustion and sweating with rigor?

2. How many syndromes is spontaneous perspiration classified into? Why do the deficiency dyndrome and excess syndrom both result in spontaneous sweating?

3. List the differentiation main points, pathogenesis outline, therapeutic methods and recipes for each type of night sweat.

7 Palpitation

General

Palpitation is a morbid condition marked by self-feeling palpitation and anxiety, even being unable to control oneself, which includes palpitation due to fright and severe palpitation.

The differentiating treatments for the disease are referential to organic heart disease and functional heart disease such as viral myocarditis, arrhythmia, and cardiac neurosis, congestive heart-failure, hyperthyroidism, anemia and hypoglycemia characterized by palpitation by Western Medicine.

Etiology and Pathogenesis

1. Timidity due to insufficiency of *qi* and deficiency of blood of the heart   Usual timidity due to insufficiency of *qi* and deficiency of blood of the heart encountered with sudden start resulting in fear and nervousness; or fury impairing the liver and terror impairing the kidney, causing *yin* deficiency downward and flaring-up of fire to disturb the heart resulting in palpitation.

2. Deficiency of the heart blood   Debility due to long-time illness, excessive blood loss, or over-anxiety injuring the heart and spleen, causing the lack of the source of growth and development and deficiency of *qi*, blood and *yin*-fluid, leading to the want of nourishment of the heart and its failure to store spirit resulting in restlessness to develop into palpitation.

3. Hyperactivity of fire due to *yin* deficiency   Debility due to long illness impairing the kidney-*yin*; or usual deficiency of the kidney-*yin* causing flaring-up of fire of deficiency type to disturb the heart resulting in palpitation.

4. Advanced hypofunction of the heart   Severe and long illness making insufficiency of *yang* unable to warm and nourish the heart vessels resulting in palpitation.

5. Excessive fluid invading the heart   Insufficiency of both the spleen and the kidney-*yang* failing in transforming and excreting fluid so that fluid accumulates in the body and inhibits the heart-*yang* resulting in palpitation.

6. Blood stasis obstructing collaterals   Advanced hypofunction of the heart and impeded circulation of blood; or wind-cold-dampness fighting against blood vessels to invade the heart causing the obstruction in heart channels and impeded circulation of *ying* blood resulting in palpitation.

Key Points:

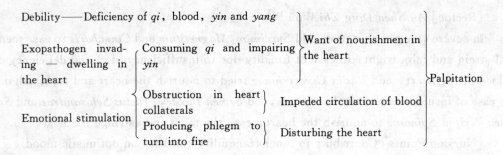

Diagnosis and Discrimination

Palpitation is manifested as self-feeling palpitation and anxiety. Both palpitation due to fright and severe palpitation will display the same symptoms of nervousness and palpitation, but there are some differences in their etiologies and states of illness.

Discrimination \ Disease	Palpitation due to fright	Severe palpitation
Etiologies	Caused by external factors: either by fright, or by fury	Caused by internal factors, or by deficiency of yin and blood, or due to insufficiency of the heart-yang
States of illness	Sudden and rapid onset of palpitation by fits and starts, but with light degree of seriousness and short period	Slow onset with slight tiredness, but with heavy degree of seriousness

Selecting Treatment by Differentiating Syndromes

In differentiating syndromes of palpitation, firstly, one should make sure whether the patient feels involuntary palpitation and nervousness; secondly, it is necessary to distinguish excess syndrome from deficiency syndrome, and deficient heart-yang from deficient heart-yin and to make certain whether it is complicated with phlegm or stasis; and thirdly, severe palpitation should be distincted from palpitation due to fright in their etiologies and states of illness.

Common Syndromes:

1. Timidity due to insufficiency of qi and deficiency of blood of the heart

[Symptoms] Palpitation, susceptible to fright, fidgeting, insomnia and dreamful sleep, whitish and thin fur or ordinary fur, tremulous and rapid pulse or feeble and wiry pulse.

[Main Points of Differentiation] Palpitation and susceptible to fright.

This type is common in cardiac neurosis.

[Pathogenesis] Fright causing disorder of qi making the heart fail to store spirit, resulting in adverse flow of qi and blood.

[Treatment] Tranquilizing the mind and calming the fright by nourishing the heart.

— 301 —

[Recipe] *An Shen Ding Zhi Wan*[112].

In severe case of palpitation, add *Succinum*, *Magnetitum* and *Cinnabaris* to ease mental strain and calm fright; in case of timidity due to insufficiency of *qi* and deficiency of blood of the heart, add *Radix Glycyrrhizae* fried to nourish the heart and replenish *qi*; in case of insufficiency of the heart-*yin*, add *Semen Biotae*, *Fructus Schisandrae* and *Semen Ziziphi Spinosae* to nourish the heart, ease the mind and astringe the heart-*qi*.

[Nursing Points] Contribute to inner tranquility and keep an optimistic mood.

2. Insufficiency of blood of the heart

[Symptoms] Palpitation, dizziness, pale complexion, tiredness, pink tongue, thready and weak pulse.

[Main Points of Differentiation] Palpitation accompanied with dizziness, dim complexion and thready pulse.

This type is seen in anemia, hypoglycemosis, viral myocarditis and arrhythmia.

[Pathogenesis] Deficiency of blood of the heart making a pale complexion, a malnourished heart and brain, and unfilled vessels.

[Treatment] Enriching the blood to nourish the heart and supplementing *qi* to ease the mind.

[Recipe] *Gui Pi Tang*[95].

In case of severe palpitation with intermittent pulse, use *Zhi Gan Cao Tang*[165] to replenish *qi* and blood, nourish *yin* and restore pulse; At the late stage of febrile disease which has impaired the heart-*yin* resulting in palpitation, adopt *Sheng Mai San*[84] to supplement *qi* and *yin*.

[Nursing Points] Eat more nourishing food; Avoid over-working.

3. Hyperactivity of fire due to *yin* deficiency

[Symptoms] Palpitation, restlessness, vexation, insomnia, dizziness, blurred vision, feverish sensation in the palms and soles, tinnitus, soreness of the loins, red tongue with little fur or without fur, thready and rapid pulse.

[Main Points of Differentiation] Palpitation, vexation, insomnia, feverish sensation in the palms and soles, red tongue with little fur.

This type can be observed in cardiac neurosis, arrhythmia and hyperthyroidism.

[Pathogenesis] Insufficiency of the kidney-*yin* and discordance between water and fire causing flaming of the heart-fire to disturb the heart.

[Treatment] Nourishing *yin* to remove pathogenic fire and nourishing the heart to calm the mind.

[Recipe] *Tian Wang Bu Xin Dan*[32].

If complicated with soreness of the waist and nocturnal emission, use *Zhi Bai Di Huang Wan*[160].

[Nursing Points] Do not have pungent food; Avoid smoking and drinking, and sexual intemperance as well.

4. Insufficiency of the heart – *yang*

[Symptoms] Palpitation, restlessness, oppressed feeling in chest, short breath, pale complexion, chilliness and cold limbs, pale tongue, feeble pulse or deep and thready pulse.

[Main Points of Differentiation] Palpitation accompanied with short breath, chilliness and cold limbs, pale tongue, and deep and feeble pulse.

This type is observable in viral myocarditis, congestive heart – failure, arrhythmia, cardiac neurosis, anemia and hypoglycemosis.

[Pathogenesis] Insufficiency of the heart – *yang* due to lasting illness or poor health weakening the function of the heart as the dynamic force of blood circulation.

[Treatment] Warming and recuperating the heart – *yang*, and tranquilizing the mind and arresting palpitation.

[Recipe] *Gui Zhi Gan Cao Long Gu Mu Li Tang*[201].

If the case is in serious state with symptoms of sweating and cold limbs, add *Radix Ginseng* and *Radix Aconiti praeparata* to recuperate depleted *yang* and rescue the patient from collapse.

[Nursing Points] Avoid over – working; refrain from uncooked or cold food; keep away from wind and cold.

5. Excessive fluid invading the heart

[Symptoms] Palpitation, dizziness, feeling of stuffiness in chest and epigastrium, chills and cold limbs, oliguria, or edema of lower extremity, thirst but no desire for drinking, nausea, salivating, whitish and slippery fur, and wiry and slippery pulse.

[Main Points of Differentiation] Palpitation with feeling of stuffiness in epigastrium, cold limbs, nausea, salivating, whitish and slippery fur.

This type is common in congestive heart – failure, viral myocarditis and anemia.

[Pathogenesis] Insufficiency of *yang* unable to transform the fluid, causing water – retention in the body to invade the heart; stagnation of excessive fluid obstructing the middle – *jiao* making lucid *yang* fail to distribute.

[Treatment] Inspiring the heart – *yang* and promoting the circulation of *qi* to induce diuresis.

[Recipe] *Ling Gui Zhu Gan Tang*[150].

In case of upward adverse flow of excessive fluid with symptoms of nausea and vomiting, add *Rhizoma Pinelliae*, *Pericarpium Citri Reticulatae* and *Rhizoma Zingiberis Recens* to regulate the stomach and lower the adverse flow of *qi*; In case of insufficiency of the kidney – *yang* making the kidney fail to regulate water metabolism leading to excessive fluid invading the heart, adopt *Zhen Wu Tang*[199].

[Nursing Points] Do not eat uncooked, cold, fat or sweet food. In severe case of edema, have low salt diet.

6. Stagnation of the heart blood

[Symptoms] Palpitation, restlessness, chest tightness, intermittent heartache, or bluish purple lips, dark purple tongue or with ecchymoses, uneven pulse or intermittent pulse.

[Main Points of Differentiation] Palpitation with chest tightness and heartache, dark purple tongue or with ecchymoses.

This type is seen in coronary heart disease and cardiac neurosis.

[Pathogenesis] Stagnated heart vessels making a malnourished heart and causing stagnated heart-yang and the obstructed collaterals and vessels.

[Treatment] Promoting blood circulation to remove blood stasis and regulating the flow of qi to clear away the obstruction from the vessels.

[Recipe] *Tao Ren Hong Hua Jian*[206].

In serious case of palpitation, add *Os Draconis* and *Concha Ostreae* at discretion to relieve palpitation and tranquilize the mind.

[Nursing Points] Do not take part in strenuous exercise. Avoid anxiety and fury.

Summary

Cause	Category	Type	Treatment
Exopathogen invading (stagnating the heart vessels); Emotional stimulation (turning into fire to attack the heart); Usual debility (making a malnourished heart) → Palpitation	Deficiency complicated with excess (reinforcement and elimination in combination)	Excessive fluid invading the heart	Treated by inspiring the heart-yang and promoting the circulation of qi to induce diuresis; recipe: *Ling Gui Zhu Gan Tang*
		Stagnation of the heart blood	Treated by promoting blood circulation to remove blood stasis and regulating the flow of qi to clear away the obstruction from the collaterals; recipe: *Tao Ren Hong Hua Jian*
	Deficiency syndrome (mainly reinforcement)	Insufficiency of the heart blood	Treated by enriching the blood to nourish the heart and supplementing qi to ease the mind; recipe: *Gui Pi Tang*
		Insufficiency of the heart-yang	Treated by warming and recuperating the heart-yang, and tranquilizing the mind and arresting palpitation; recipe: *Gui Gan Long Mu Tang*
		Timidity due to insufficiency of qi and deficiency of blood of the heart	Treated by tranquilizing the mind and calming the fright by nourishing the heart; recipe: *An Shen Ding Zhi Wan*
		Hyperactivity of fire due to yin deficiency	Treated by nourishing yin to remove pathogenic fire and nourishing the heart to calm the mind; recipe: *Tian Wang Bu Xin Dan*

Discussions

    1. Retell the pathogenesis of palpitation.

    2. What are the types of palpitation of deficiency type? What are their respective points of differentiation, treatments and recipes?

    3. How do you distinguish palpitation from severe palpitation?

8 Pectoral Pain with Stuffiness

General

Pectoral pain with stuffiness is a morbid condition marked by chest pain and stuffiness, sometimes the pain spreading to the whole back, short breath and dyspnea causing difficulty in lying.

The differentiating treatments for the disease are referential to coronary atherosclerotic cardiopathy, viral myocarditis and cardiomyopathy as well as cardiac neurosis and pleurisy showing the symptoms of obstruction of *qi* in the chest by Western Medicine.

Etiology and Pathogenesis

1. Cold invading the body   Usual insufficiency of *yang* in the chest causes pathogenic cold to invade the body and stagnation of *qi* and accumulation of cold to obstruct the chest - *yang* resulting in obstruction of *qi* in the chest.

2. Improper diet   Improper diet such as over-eating of fat, sweet or cold, uncooked food, or having an addiction for drinking that makes the impairment of the spleen and stomach causing their dysfunction in transport and the accumulation of dampness to turn into phlegm; phlegm obstructing channels and collaterals will lead to stagnation of *qi* and stasis of blood to obstruct the chest - *yang* resulting in pectoral pain with stuffiness.

3. Emotional irregulation   Axiety will injure the spleen causing stagnation of *qi* due to hypofunction of the spleen and further bringing on failure of the spleen to transport the body fluid which will accumulate to turn into phlegm; depression and fury will impair the liver causing its failure in governing normal flow of *qi* and stagnation of the liver - *qi* which sometimes will turn into fire and convert the body fluid into phlegm; stagnancy of *qi* and phlegm will lead to smoothless flow of blood, obstruction of vessels and collaterals and dysfunction of the chest - *yang* and stagnated heart - vessels resulting in obstruction of *qi* in the chest.

4. Senile decay   In the senile, gradual decay of the kidney - *qi* will appear, insufficiency of the kidney - *yang* will make the kidney fail to inspire the *yang* of five *zang* - organs causing insufficiency of the heart - *qi* and hypofunction of the heart-*yang*; deficiency of the kidney - *yin* will make the kidney fail to nourish the *yin* of five *zang* - organs bringing about the consumption of the heart - *yin*; interior deficiency and exterior excess lead to stagnancy of *qi* and blood stasis to check the moving of the chest - *yang* causing obstruction of the heart vessels and thus resulting in obstruction of *qi* in the chest.

The above etiologies and pathogeneses will sometimes take on by twos, or by threes, or crossingly. Generally, they all belong to interior deficiency and exterior excess.

Key Points:

Cold invading the body
Improper diet
Emotional irregulation
Senile decay
} Deficiency of the chest-*yang* and stagnancy of *qi* and blood stasis } Obstruction of *qi* in the chest

Diagnosis and Discrimination

Pectoral pain with stuffiness is characterized by chest pain and stuffiness, sometimes the pain may spread to the back. Angina pectoris is the dangerous stage of pectoral pain with stuffiness, while epigastralgia and pleural effusion will also display the symptom of chest pain, therefore, discrimination between the four should be made.

Discrimination \ Disease	Pectoral pain with stuffiness	Pleural effusion	Angina pectoris	Epigastralgia
Aching point	In the chest	In the sternocostal part	In the chest (occasionally on the stomach or the back and shoulders)	In the stomach
Aching features	Choking pain with short period relieved by rest or drugs	Continuous distent pain aggravated with respiration	Continuous severe pain not to be relieved	Distent and vague pain
Accompanied symptoms	The pain spreading to the left shoulder and back, sudden onset after excitement or over-working	Cough, spitting phlegm, fullness in ribs	Sweating, cold limbs, purplish lips, bluish color extending from nails to the joints, intermittent pulse	Eructation, nausea, acid regurgitation

Selecting Treatment by Differentiating Syndromes

In differentiating syndromes of pectoral pain with stuffiness, one should distinguish deficiency syndrome from excess syndrome and exterior syndrome from the interior one.

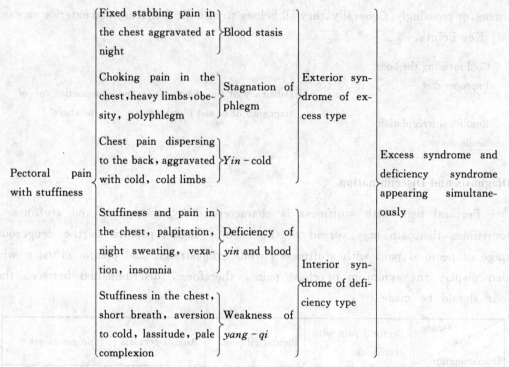

Common Syndromes:

1. Stagnation of the heart blood

[Symptoms] Fixed stabbing pain in the chest aggravated at night, intermittent palpitation and restlessness, dark - purple tongue, deep and uneven pulse.

[Main Points of Differentiation] Stabbing pain in the chest aggravated at night, dark - purple tongue.

This type is seen in acute myocardial infarction and angina pectoris.

[Pathogenesis] Long stagnation of qi causes blood stasis to obstruct collaterals.

[Treatment] Removing blood stasis by promoting blood circulation and removing obstruction in the collaterals to relieve pain.

[Recipe] *Xue Fu Zhu Yu Tang*[119].

In case of severe pectoal pain with stuffiness, add *Lignum Dalbergiae Odoriferae*, *Radix Curcumae* and *Rhizoma Corydalis*; In case of mild blood stasis, *Dan Shen Yin*[51] may be adopted.

[Nursing Points] Avoid mental stimulation, depression and anger; lead a regular daily life and guard against wind and cold; refrain from uncooked, cold, greasy and sweet food; do not smoke or drink.

2. Stagnation of phlegm

[Symptoms] Choking pain in the chest spreading to the shoulder and back, short breath, heavy limbs, obesity, polyphlegm, greasy fur and slippery pulse.

[Main Points of Differentiation] Choking pain in the chest, polyphlegm, greasy fur and slippery pulse.

This type is commonly seen in angina pectoris due to coronary heart disease and myocardiac infarction.

[Pathogenesis] Stagnation of phlegm obstructing the chest - *yang*, and channels and collaterals.

[Treatment] Activating *yang* to remove obstruction and eliminating phlegm.

[Recipe] *Gua Lou Xie Bai Ban Xia Tang*[208].

In case of serious stagnation of phlegm, add *Rhizoma Zingiberis*, *Pericarpium Citri Reticulatae* and *Semen Amomi Cardamomi* to activate *yang* for eliminating phlegm and warm the middle - *jiao* for promoting the flow of *qi*.

[Nursing Points] Avoid smoking, drinking, and fat, sweet and greasy food.

3. Stagnation of *yin* - cold

[Symptoms] Chest pain dispersing to the back aggravated with cold, stuffiness of chest, short breath, palpitation, inability to lie evenly due to dyspnea if serious, pale complexion, cold limbs, whitish fur, and deep and thready pulse.

[Main Points of Differentiation] Chest pain dispersing to the back aggravated with cold, pale complexion, cold limbs, whitish fur, deep and thready pulse.

This type is observable in angina pectoris due to coronary heart disease, pleurisy, and cardiomyopathy.

[Pathogenesis] Cold invading the body leads to deficiency of *yang* - *qi* and obstructed functional activities of *qi*.

[Treatment] Activating *yang* with drugs pungent in flavor and warm in property and expelling cold by removing obstruction.

[Recipe] *Gua Lou Xie Bai Bai Jiu Tang*[209].

Fructus Aurantii Immaturus, *Ramulus Cinnamomi*, *Radix Aconiti praeparata*, *Radix Salviae Miltiorrhizae* and *Lignum Santali* may be added to strengthen the effect of activating *yang* and removing obsruction, dispelling cold to smooth the collaterals. In case of excessive phlegm - dampness, chest pain with coughing of saliva, add *Rhizoma Zingiberis Recens*, *Pericarpium Citri Reticulatae*, *Poria* and *Semen Armeniacae Amarum* to promote circulation of *qi* and eliminate phlegm; in case of dominant *yin* - cold and serious state of illness manifested as continuous heartache spreading to the back and vice versa, chilliness, cold limbs, inability to lie because of dyspnea, deep and tense pulse, use *Wu Tou Chi Shi Zhi Wan*[54] and *Su He Xiang Wan*[128] to relieve pain.

[Nursing Points] Keep warm; take proper rest; avoid uncooked and cold food.

4. Deficiency of the heart - *yin* and the kidney - *yin*

[Symptoms] Stuffiness and pain in the chest, palpitation, night sweating, vexation, insomnia, soreness of loins and knees, tinnitus, dizziness, red tongue or tongue with ecchymosis, little fur, thready and rapid pulse or thready and uneven pulse.

[Main Points of Differentiation] Stuffiness and pain in the chest, palpitation, night sweating, soreness of loins, tinnitus, red tongue with little fur.

This type can be observed in coronary heart disease and cardiac neurosis.

[Pathogenesis] Debility due to lasting illness will impair the heart – *yin* and kidney – *yin*, which further causes inadequate supply of nutrients for the vessels and stagnation of *qi* and blood.

[Treatment] Nourishing *yin* to strengthen the kidney and nourishing the heart to ease the mind.

[Recipe] *Zuo Gui Yin*[66]

In severe case of deficiency of the heart – *yin* with vexation and insomnia, add *Radix Ophiopogonis*, *Fructus Schisandrae*, *Semen Biotae* and *Semen Zizyphi Spinosae* to nourish the heart for easing the mind; in serious case of stuffiness and pain in the chest, add *Radix Angelicae Sinensis*, *Radix Salviae Miltiorrhizae*, *Rhizoma Ligustici Chuanxiong* and *Radix Curcumae* to nourish the blood and remove obstruction in the collaterals; in case of hyperactivity of *yang* due to *yin* deficiency with dizziness, blurred vision, and numb tongue, add *Radix Polygoni Multiflori praeparata*, *Fructus Ligustri Lucidi*, *Ramulus Uncariae cum Uncis*, *Concha Haliotidis Recens*, *Concha Ostreae Recens* and *Carapax Trionycis* to nourish *yin* and subdue over – abundant *yang*.

[Nursing Points] Refrain from sexual intemperance; avoid over – working; keep emotional balance; do not eat pungent food.

5. Deficiency of *qi* and *yin*

[Symptoms] Stuffiness and dull pain in the chest by fits and starts, palpitation, short breath, lassitude, no desire to talk, dim complexion, dizziness and blurred vision aggravated with over – working, red tongue or teeth – printed tongue, thready and weak pulse or intermittent pulse.

[Main Points of Differentiation] Stuffiness and dull pain in the chest, palpitation, short breath aggravated with over – working, thready and weak pulse.

This type is seen in cardiomyopathy, cardiac neurosis, latent coronary heart disease and remote myocardial infarction.

[Pathogenesis] Long period of obstruction of *qi* in the chest leads to deficiency of *qi* and *yin*, which further causes *qi*'s failure in promoting the flow of blood, and obstruction of channels and collaterals.

[Treatment] Supplementing *qi* and nourishing *yin*, and promoting blood circulation to remove obstruction in the collaterals.

[Recipe] *Sheng Mai San*[84] with *Ren Shen Yang Ying Tang*[11]

In serious case of chest pain, add *Radix Salviae Miltiorrhizae*, *Radix Notoginseng*,

Herba Leonuri, *Radix Curcumae* and *Faeces Trogopterorum* to remove obstruction in the collaterals by promoting blood circulation; in case of intermittent pulse caused by deficiency of *qi* and blood unable to nourish the heart, adopt *Zhi Gan Cao Tang*[165] as a synergist to nourish *qi* and blood, replenish *yin* and get the pulse back to normal.

[Nursing Points] Avoid over-working; do not eat pungent food.

6. Deficiency of *yang-qi*

[Symptoms] Stuffiness in the chest, short breath, the chest pain radiating to the back if serious, palpitation, sweating, aversion to cold, cold limbs, soreness of the loins, lassitude, pale complexion, pale or blue purple lips and nails, pale tongue or dark purple tongue, deep and thready pulse or thready and feeble pulse almost unable to feel.

[Main Points of Differentiation] Stuffiness in the chest, short breath, aversion to cold, cold limbs, sweating, lassitude, deep, thready pulse.

This type is common in angina pectoris due to coronary heart disease, cardiomyopathy and viral myocarditis.

[Pathogenesis] Deficiency of *yang-qi* stagnating the chest-*yang* and obstructing functional activities of *qi* and blood circulation.

[Treatment] Supplementing *qi* and warming *yang*, and promoting blood circulation to remove obstruction in the collaterals.

[Recipe] *Shen Fu Tang*[167] with *You Gui Yin*[69]

In case of prostration of the heart-*yang* manifested as blue purple complexion, lips and nails, profuse sweating, cold limbs, and feeble pulse almost unable to feel, use larger amount of *Radix Ginseng Rubra* and *Radix Aconiti praeparata*, and add calcined *Os Draconis* and *Concha Ostreae* to recuperate depleted *yang* and rescue the patient from collapse; in case of deficiency of *yang* affecting *yin* and deficiency of both *yang* and *yin*, add *Radix Ophiopogonis* and *Fructus Schisandrae* to warm *yang* and nourish *yin*.

[Nursing Points] Keep warm; do not overwork; avoid cold and uncooked food.

Summary

Causes	Pathogenesis		Syndrome	Treatment	Principle
Cold invading the body; Improper diet; Emotional irregulation; Senile decay	Deficiency of the chest-yang; Stagnation of phlegm; Stagnancy of qi and blood stasis	Obstruction of qi in the chest	Exterior syndrome of excess type — Stagnation of the heart blood	Treated by promoting blood circulation to remove blood stasis and removing obstruction in the collaterals to relieve pain; recipe: *Xue Fu Zhu Yu Tang*	Treating exterior syndrome first
			Stagnation of phlegm	Treated by activating *yang* to remove obstruction and eliminating phlegm; recipe: *Gua Lou Xie Bai Ban Xia Tang*	
			Stagnation of *yin*-cold	Terated by activating *yang* with drugs pungent in flavor and warm in property and expelling cold to treat stagnation syndrome of *qi* and blood; recipe: *Gua Lou Xie Bai Bai Jiu Tang*	
			Interior syndrome of deficiency type — Deficiency of the heart-*yin* and the kidney-*yin*	Treated by replenishing *yin* to strengthen the kidney and nourishing the heart to calm the mind; recipe: *Zuo Gui Yin*	Mainly strengthening the body resistance
			Deficiency of *qi* and *yin*	Treated by supplementing *qi* and nourishing *yin*, and promoting blood circulation to remove obstruction in the collaterals; recipe: *Sheng Mai San* plus *Ren Shen Yang Ying Tang*	
			Deficiency of *yang-qi*	Treated by supplementing *qi* and activating *yang*, and promoting blood circulation to remove obstruction in the collaterals; recipe: *Shen Fu Tang* with *You Gui Yin*	

It is as important to deal with the deficiency type as the excess type for cases manifesting interior syndrome of deficiency type, exterior syndrome of excess type, and syndrome of deficiency and excess in combination.

Discussions

1. How many clinical types are there in pectoral pain with stuffiness?
2. Retell the respective main points of differentiation and treatments of stagnation of *yin* - cold, stagnation of phlegm and stagnancy of the heart blood.

9 Syncope (*Jue* Syndrome)

General

Syncope is a disease marked by sudden fainting, loss of consciousness and cold limbs.

The differentiating treatments for the disease are referential to the faintings by hysteria, vasodepress, hypertensive cerebral diseases, cerebro-vascular spasm, hypoglycemosis, hemorrhagic shock, cardiogenic shock and pulmonary encephalopathy by Western Medicine.

Etiology and Pathogenesis

1. Syncope from disorder of *qi*   This is one type of syncopes caused by anger, panic and excessive passion, which will result in the disorder of *qi* leading to the stuffiness in the chest and the blocking of the routes between apertures. Or it can be brought about by the deficiency of primordial *qi* accompanied with fright, or by excessive fatigue resulting in the want of *yang - qi*, the deficiency and descent of *qi* and lucid *yang* failing to rise.

2. Syncope due to excessive bleeding   The long-lasting hyperactivity of the liver -*yang* in combination with fury will bring about the upward movement of blood due to adverse flow of *qi*, whose accumulation will block the seven orifices resulting in syncope. And there is another possibility for this type of syncopes, that is massive bleeding as the result of persistent illness resulting in the deficiency of blood, or excessive postpartum hemorrhage or some other diseases.

3. Syncope due to phlegm stagnation   This takes place on those persons who are in the state of deficiency of *qi* due to obesity on condition that they have spirit, butter or fat and sweet food, which will be harmful to their spleens and stomachs resulting in the dysfunction of those organs and causing the retention of dampness to produce sputum which will stagnate within the body and bring about the disorder of *qi*. When *qi* flows adversely which is induced accidentally by fury, sputum will ascend with *qi* and block the seven orifices, resulting in syncope.

4. Syncope due to indigestion   Intemperance in eating will cause indigestion and the disorder in transport, which will hinder *qi* in its function, resulting in syncope.

Key Points: Sudden reversed flow of *qi* and disturbance in its ascending and descending——Irregular circulation of *qi* and blood——Syncope

Diagnosis and Discrimination

Syncope is a morbid condition characterized by sudden fainting and loss of consciousness accompanied with cold limbs, which may happen at all times and places.

Discrimination should be made firstly between this disease and apoplexy as well as epilepsy, all of which have the same symptom of sudden fainting, and secondly between this disease and colic by ascaris, both of which share the similar symptom of cold limbs.

Disease / Discrimination	Syncope	Apoplexy	Epilepsy	Colic by ascaris
Senses	Obnubilation	Unconsciousness	Obnubilation	Imputability
Accompanied symptoms	Sudden fainting; cold limbs	Distortion of the face; hemiplegia	Frothy salivation; superduction of eyes; spasm of limbs; or bleating or pig-howling	Severe abdominal pain; masses can be felt; cold limbs or vomiting ascariases
Appearances after reviving	No symptoms of distortion of the face or hemiplegia	Often with sequelae	As a healthy person	As a healthy person after the ascariases driven out

Selecting Treatment by Differentiating Syndromes

There are obvious and respective causes for syncopes to take place.

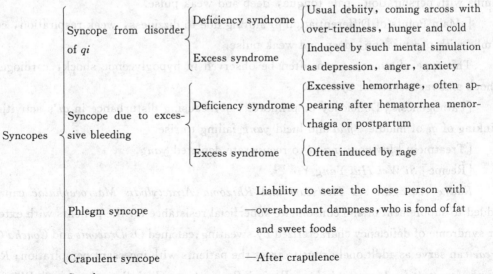

Common Syndromes:

1. Syncope from disorder of *qi*

(1) Excess syndrome

[Symptoms] Sudden fainting, comma, trismus, clenched fists, rude respiration or cold limbs; thin and whitish fur, indistinct pulse or deep and wiry pulse.

[Main Points of Differentiation] Sudden fainting after mental irritation, trismus, cold limbs, rude respiration, wiry pulse.

This type of syncopes is commonly seen in hysterical syncope, vasodepressor syncope (vosovagol syncope).

[Pathogenesis] Disorder of the liver - *qi* causing reversed flow of *qi* to accumulate in the chest and block the seven orifices.

[Treatment] Checking upward adverse flow of *qi* and relieving stagnation.

[Recipe] *Wu Mo Yin Zi*[43].

Semen Amomi Cardamomi, *Liqnum Santali*, *Flos Caryophylli* and *Herba Agastachis* can be added accordingly to regulate the flow of *qi* and relieve the chest stuffiness; in case of hyperactivity of the liver - *yang* manifested as dizziness, headache and flushed face, add *Ramulus Uncariae cum Uncis*, *Concha Haliotidis* and *Magnetitum* to calm the liver and suppress the excessive *yang*; *Poria cum Ligno Hospite*, *Radix Polygalae* and *Semen Ziziphi Spinosae* can be used as additional drugs to tranquilize the patients with the symptom of irregular laugh or cry after reviving, or uneasy sleeping.

Mental stimulation will bring on repeated attacks of the disease, *Xiao Yao San*[222] can be taken in normal times for regulating the flow of *qi* to alleviate mental depression.

[Nursing Points] Pay attention to the regulation and stillness of emotions to avoid anger.

(2) Deficiency syndrome

[Symptoms] Fainting due to dizziness, pale complexion, weak respiration, cold limbs with perspiration, pale tongue, deep and weak pulse.

[Main Points of Differentiation] Fainting due to dizziness, weak respiration, cold limbs with perspiration, deep and weak pulse.

This type of syncopes can often be observed in hypoglycemic shock, cardiogenic shock and vasodepressor syncope.

[Pathogenesis] Deficiency of primordial *qi*, causing disturbance in *qi*'s activities, sinking of *qi* of middle - *jiao* and lucid *yang* failing to rise.

[Treatment] Invigorating *qi* to recuperate depleted *yang*.

[Recipe] *Si Wei Hui Yang Yin*[78].

Radix Astragali seu Hedysari and *Rhizoma Atractylodis Macrocephalae* can be added to supplement *qi* and consolidate superficial resistance for the patients with exterior syndrome of deficiency characterized by sweating; calcined *Os Draconis* and *Concha Ostreae* can serve as additional drugs to treat the patients with incessant perspiration; *Rhizoma Atractylodis Macrocephalae*, *Poria*, *Pericarpium Citri Reticulatae* and *Rhizoma*

Pinelliae may be added to strengthen the spleen and reduce phlegm for those patients who have a poor appetite and cough with polysputum; And with *Radix Polygalae* and *Semen Ziziphi Spinosae* as additional drugs for nourishing the heart to calm the mind, patients with palpitation and unsteadiness can be treated.

[Nursing Points] Strike a proper balance between work and rest; keep away from cold and wind pathogen; keep emotional balance and avoid uncooked or cold food.

2. Syncope due to excessive bleeding

(1) Excess syndrome

[Symptoms] Sudden fainting, coma, lockjaw, cyanotic complexion, purplish lips; red tongue, usually deep and wiry pulse.

[Main Points of Differentiation] Occurrence after fury, sudden fainting, lockjaw, cyanotic complexion and purplish lips.

This type of syncopes can be observed in cases of cerebrovascular spasm, hypertensive cerebral diseases and cardiogenic shock.

[Pathogenesis] Violent rage brings on ascending blood along with the upward invasion of the hyperactive liver - *qi* which obstruct mental activities.

[Treatment] Promoting blood circulation and checking upward adverse flow of the *qi*.

[Recipe] *Tong Yu Jian* [224].

In case of irritation, dizziness, headache, add *Ramulus Uncariae cum Uncis*, *Concha Haliotidis*, *Radix Gentianae*, *Radix Polygalae* and *Rhizoma Acori Graminei*, *Flos Chrysanthemi*, *Concha Margaritifera Usta* to calm the liver and tranquilize mind.

[Nursing Points] Keep emotional balance to navoid fury; avoid pungent food, tobacco and alcohol; and patients should be closely observed of the conditon.

(2) Deficiency syndrome

[Symptoms] Sudden fainting, pale complexion, pallor of the lips, shivering limbs, sinking eyes, opening mouth, cold skin with perspiration, shallow breath, pale tongue, hollow pulse or thready rapid and weak pulse.

[Main Points of Differentiation] Onset often after excessive bleeding, sudden fainting, pale complexion, pallor of the lips, shivering limbs and cold skin, opening mouth, pale tongue.

This type of syncopes is commonly seen in hemorrhagic shock, cardiogenic shock and hypoglycemic shock.

[Pathogenesis] Excessive blood loss leading to its failure in supplying nourishment upward.

[Treatment] Replenishing and restoring *qi* and blood.

[Recipe] *Du Shen Tang*[194] or *Ren Shen Yang Ying Tang*[11].

For emergency case, firstly get *Du Shen Tang*[194] taken in order to supplement *qi* and restore depleted *yang*, then ask the patient to take *Ren Shen Yang Ying Tang*[11]. In case of incessant bleeding, add *Herba Agrimoniae*, *Nodus Nelumbinis Rhizomatis* and *Cacumen Biotae* to stop bleeding; *Radix Aconiti* and *Rhizoma Zingiberis* can serve as additional drugs to warm *yang* for patients with shallow breath and cold skin and perspiration; Add *Arillus Longan*, *Radix Polygalae* and *Semen Ziziphi Spinosae* for patients with palpitation and insomnia to ease the mind and relieve mental strain.

[Nursing Points] Keep the patient under close observation; be sure to have enough rest and supplement nutriment.

3. Syncope due to phlegm stagnation

[Symptoms] Sudden fainting, laryngeal rales or salivating, rude respiration, whitish and greasy fur, deep and slippery pulse.

[Main Points of Differentiation] Sudden fainting, laryngeal rales, whitish and greasy fur.

This type of syncopes can be commonly observed in pulmonary encephalopathy and hypertensive encephalopathy.

[Pathogenesis] Phlegm-dampness at ordinary times encountered with fury resulting in reversed flow of *qi* and causing accumulation of phlegm to check the functional activities of *qi* and block the seven orifices.

[Treatment] Promoting the circulation of *qi* and eliminating phlegm.

[Recipe] *Dao Tan Tang*[121].

In case of serious accumulation of phlegm and *qi*, add *Semen Coicis* and *Semen Sinapis Albae* to resolve phlegm and send down abnormally ascending *qi*; for patients with phlegm-dampness resulting in heat-transmission marked by dry mouth, constipation, yellowish and greasy fur and rapid slippery pulse, add *Radix Scutellariae*, *Fructus Gardeniae*, *Caulis Bambusae in Taemiam* and *Semen Trichosanthis* to reduce heat and purge fire.

[Nursing Points] Avoid fat, sweet, oily and greasy food.

4. Syncope due to indigestion

[Symptoms] After crapulence appearing, sudden fainting, oppressed breath, abdominal distention, thick and greasy fur, slippery and forceful pulse.

[Main Points of Differentiation] Syncope often occurring after crapulence, thick greasy fur, slippery and foreful pulse.

[Pathogenesis] Crapulence making stagnation in the stomach and upward reversed flow of *qi* resulting in the blocked mentality.

[Treatment] Regulating the middle-*jiao* and removing food retention and promoting digestion.

[Recipe] *Shen Zhu San*[186] with *Bao He Wan*[193]

Soon after crapulence, firstly give the patient salt water for inducing vomiting to expell pathogenic factor of excess type, then prescribe *Shen Zhu San*[186] and *Bao He*

$Wan^{[193]}$. In case of abdominal distention and constipation, use *Xiao Cheng Qi Tang*[29] to remove stagnancy downwards.

[Nursing Points] Be abstemious in eating and drinking and avoid crapulence. Have light diet.

Summary

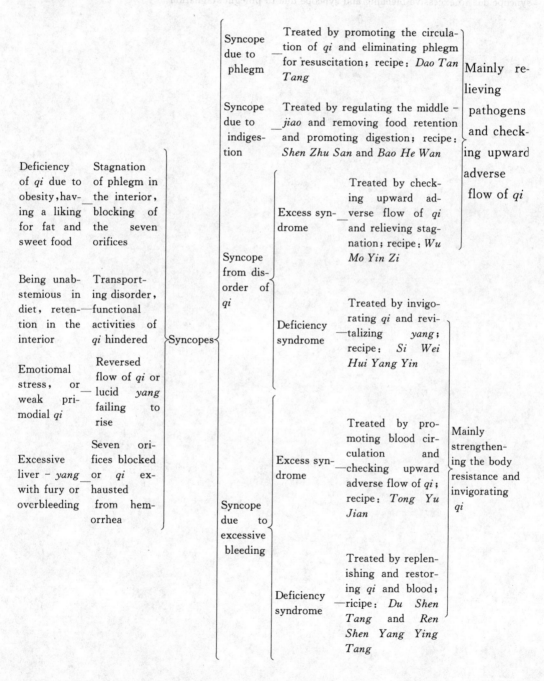

Discussions

1. What are the clinical characteristics of syncope and what are the differences between syncope and apoplexy and epilepsy?

2. What are the differences of the pathogeneses and treatments of syncope from disorder of *qi*, syncope due to excessive bleeding and syncope due to phlegm stagnation?

10 Apoplexy

General

Apoplexy (or apoplectic stroke) is a morbid condition marked by sudden fainting and loss of consciousness with distortion of the face, hemiplegia, dysphasia; or manifested only as a wry face and hemiplegia.

The differentiating treatments for the disease are referential to hypertensive cerebral hemorrhage, cerebral thrombosis, cerebral embolism, subarachnoid hemorrhage, lacunar cerebral infarction, transient cerebral ischemia, as well as the same symptoms caused by peripheral facial paralysis in Western Medicine.

Etiology and Pathogenesis

1. Asthenia of vital - *qi* due to accumulated impairment Senile decay leads to deficiency of the liver - *yin* and kidney - *yin*, and the hyperactivity of liver - *yang*; excessive thinking causes deficiency of *qi* and blood leading to *yin* deficiency in the lower - *jiao*, hyperactivity of *yang* and stirring of wind, upward movement of *qi* and blood to hinder mental activity, hence fainting occurs followed by apoplexy.

2. Intemperance in eating Intemperance in alcohol, greasy and sweet food, or false appearance of strong constitution but actual *qi* deficiency will cause dysfunction of the spleen and accumulation of dampness to turn into phlegm - fire. Consequently the liver - wind complicated with phlegm - fire will invade the channels and collaterals, hindering the mental activity and further rsulting in apoplexy.

3. Emotional injury Overacting of five emotions will cause excessive heart - fire; usual deficiency of *yin*, if complicated with emotional injury, will cause hyperactivity of liver - *yang*, the upward adverse flow of *qi* and blood, and mental disorder, further resulting in fainting and apoplexy.

4. Attacked by pathogenic factors due to *qi* deficiency When *qi* and blood are insufficient, wind pathogen will attack the channels and collaterals, causing obstruction of *qi* and blood; if usual excess of phlegm - dampness is induced by exopathic wind, it will obstruct the channels and collaterals, leading to apoplexy.

Key Points:

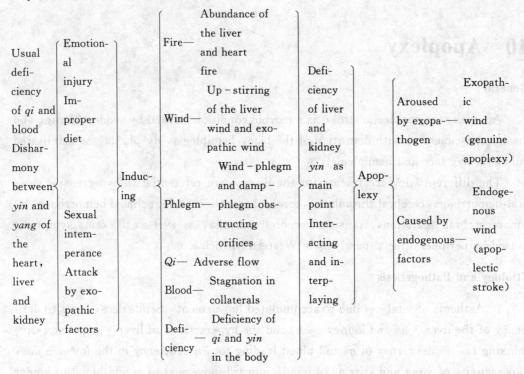

Diagnosis and Discrimination

The disease is manifested by acute onset, various causes and changeable conditions with clinical symptoms of sudden fainting accompanied by distortion of the face, hemiplegia and dysphasia, or only with a wry face and hemiplegia as its clinical symptoms. Among clinical cases most of which are caused by endogenous factors, but, of course, there are some cases which are aroused by exopathogens. Considering its sudden onset and changeable conditions, which are charcteristic of wind in the nature, it is named "*Zhong Feng*" (apoplexy). This is different in meaning from the "*Zhong Feng*" syndrome mentioned in Treatise on Febrile Diseases, which is the result of *Taiyang* channel being invaded by pathogenic wind and cold.

The same symptom of sudden fainting is shared by this disease, syncope and epilepsy, so discrimination should be made. Refer to chapter on Syncope. There are also some similar symptoms shared by this disease and convulsive disease. Here are the discriminations:

Discrimination \ Disease	Apoplexy	Convulsive disease
Distortion of the face, hemiplegia	Yes	No
Convulsion of limbs, even opisthotonus	No	Yes

Selecting Treatment by Differentiating Syndromes

There are differences in its degree and urgency.

A mild case - only blood vessels, channels and collaterals affected without pathological changes in *zang* and *fu* organs and mental symptoms——apoplexy involving the channels and collaterals;

A serious case - affection extending to viscera accompanied by mental variations——apoplexy involving the *zang* and *fu* organs.

1. Apoplexy involving the channels and collaterals

(1) Deficiency of channels and collaterals, and the invasion of pathogenic wind

[Symptoms] Numbness of skin, tingle limbs, sudden distortion of the face, dysphasia, salivation, even hemiplegia, sometimes accompanied with aversion to cold, fever, rigidity of the trunk and arthralgia; thin and whitish fur, and rapid and floating pulse.

[Main Points of Differentiation] Numbness of the skin, tingle limbs, sudden distortion of the face, dysphasia, sometimes accompanied with symptoms of pathogenic factor attacking the exterior of the body. In a clear state of mind.

This type of apoplexy is common with facial paralysis, transient cerebral ischemia and lacunar cerebral infarction.

[Pathogenesis] Deficiency of vital - *qi*, deficidncy of the collaterals and failure of superficial - *qi* to protect the body against diseases leading to the invasion of channels and collaterals by pathogenic wind to obstruct *qi* and blood.

[Treatment] Expelling the wind, nourishing the blood and clearing collaterals.

[Recipe] *Da Qin Jiu Tang*[22].

If without interior heat, *Gypsum Fibrosum* and *Radix Scutellariae* may be subtracted, while *Rhizoma Typhonii* and *Scorpio* may be added to expell the wind, remove the phlegm and clear collaterals; if wind - heat syndrome is encountered, subtract pungent and warm - property drugs such as *Rhizoma seu Radix Notopterygii*, *Radix Ledebouriellae* and *Radix Angelicae Sinensis*, and add *Folium Mori*, *Flos Chrysanthemi* and *Herba Menthae* to dispell wind and remove heat; in case of vomiting due to abundance of phlegm, greasy fur and slippery pulse, subtract *Radix Rehmanniae*, and add *Rhizoma Pinelliae*, *Rhizoma Arisaematis*, *Exocarpium Citri Reticulatae* and *Poria* to remove the phlegm and dampness. For senile patients, add *Radix Astragali seu Hedysari* to supplement *qi* and strengthen the body resistance.

[Nursing Points] Regulate daily life; be on guard against wind pathogen; keep the affected side warm and prevent fatigue. Avoid cold and uncooked food.

(2) Deficiency of liver - *yin* and kidney *yin* and upward invasion of liver - *yang*

[Symptoms] Usual dizziness and headache, tinnitus and giddiness, hyposleeping with polydream, sudden distortion of the face, rigidity of the tongue and dysphasia, or heavily sluggish limbs, even hemiplegia; red tongue with greasy fur, wiry, thready and rapid pulse or wiry and slippery pulse.

[Main Points of Differentiation] Usual dizziness and headache, tinnitus and giddiness suddenly attacked by distortion of the face, rigidity of the tongue and dysphasia in a clear state of mind.

This type of apoplexy is observable in cerebral thrombosis, lacunar cerebral infarction and transient cerebral ischemia.

[Pathogenesis] Usual deficiency of the kidney - yin and hyperactivity of the liver - yang cause up - stirring of wind - yang which coerce phlegm into running about in channels and collaterals, resulting in the impeded vessels and collaterals.

[Treatment] Nourishing yin and suppressing hyperactive yang, and calming the wind and clearing collaterals.

[Recipe] *Zhen Gan Xi Feng Tang*[291].

Rhizoma Gastrodieae, *Ramulus Uncariae cum Uncis* and *Flos Chrysanthemi* can be added to heighten the effect in calming the liver to stop the wind. In case of heavier accumulation of phlegm, add *Arisaema cum Bile*, *Succus Bambusae* and *Bulbus Fritillariae Cirrhosae* to resolve phlegm and clear heat;In case of serious headache,add *Cornu Saigae Tataricae*, *Concha Haliotidis* and *Spica Prunellae* to subdue the endopathic wind and yang.

[Nursing Points] Keep the affected side warm; have light and low - fat diet in normal times; and regulate emotions to keep away from anger and excitement. Avoid sexual intemperance.

2. Apoplexy involving the zang and fu organs

This is a case of apoplexy manifested by sudden fainting and loss of consciousness. There are some differences in clinical symptoms between excess syndrome of stroke and prostration syndrome.

Excess syndrome of stroke—dominating of pathogen and loss of consciousness as its main symptoms—excess syndrome—eliminating the pathogenic factor for urgent case;

Prostration syndrome—yang - qi about to collapse as its characteristic—deficiency syndrome—strengthening the body resistance for urgent case.

(1) Excess syndrome of stroke

The case is marked by sudden fainting, loss of consciousness, trismus, clenched fists, constipation and dysuria,and spasm of limbs. It can be divided into excessive -syndrome of coma with heat syndrome and excessive syndrome of coma with cold manifestations.

①Excessive - syndrome of coma accompanied by heat syndrome

[Symptoms] Besides the above symptoms of excess syndrome of stroke, there are others as flushed face, fever, rude respiration, saburra and fidgets, yellowish and greasy fur, wiry, slippery and rapid pulse.

[Main Points of Differentiation] Sudden fainting, flushed face, fever, trismus, constipation and dysuria, yellowish and greasy fur, wiry, slippery and rapid pulse.

This type is commonly seen in cerebral embolism, hypertensive cerebral hemorrhage and subarachnoid hemorrhage.

[Pathogenesis] Hyperactivity of the liver - *yang* causes wind stirring inside and *yang* ascending and the upward adverse flow of *qi* and blood complicated with phlegm and fire to block the seven orifices.

[Treatment] Removing heat from the liver and calming the endopathic wind; and inducing resuscitation with drugs pungent in flavor and cool in property.

[Recipe] *Zhi Bao Dan*[109] or *An Gong Niu Huang Wan*[111].

Adopt *Ling Yang Jiao Tang*[246] as a continuation to remove heat from the liver and calm the endopathic wind, and to nourish *yin* and suppress the excessive *yang*. In case of convulsion, add *Scorpio*, *Subspinipes Mutilans*, *Bombyx Batryticatus*; for patient with polyphlegm, add *Succus Bambusae*, *Bambusa Textilis*, *Arisaema cum Bile*; in case of polyphlegm and lethargy, add *Radix Curcumae* and *Radix Calami Aromatici* to strengthen the effect of eliminating phlegm for resuscitation.

[Nursing Points] Make less movements of the patients; avoid stimulation and keep close observation.

②Excessive syndrome of coma with cold manifestations

[Symptoms] Besides the above symptoms of excess syndrome of stroke, there are others as pale complexion with dark lips, lying motionless without dysphoria, warmless limbs and profuse sputum and saliva, whitish and greasy fur, and deep, slippery and moderate pulse.

[Main Points of Differentiation] Sudden fainting, trismus, pale complexion with dark lips, warmless limbs, whitish and greasy fur, and deep, slippery and moderate pulse.

This type is often seen in hypertensive cerebral hemorrhage and subarachnoid hemorrhage.

[Pathogenesis] Excessive phlegm - dampness being taken upwards by wind to block the seven orifices, and internally to obstruct channels and collaterals.

[Treatment] Eliminating phlegm and calming the endopathic wind; and inducing resuscitation with drugs pungent in flavor and warm in property.

[Recipe] *Su He Xiang Wan*[128].

Di Tan Tang[215] serves as a continuation to eliminate phlegm and calm the endopathic wind; and *Rhizoma Gastrodiae* and *Ramulus Uncariae cum Uncis* can be added to calm the liver to stop the wind.

[Nursing Points] During coma, take care to eliminate phlegm; prevent infection and keep stool unobstructed.

(2) Prostration syndrome

[Symptoms] Sudden fainting, unconsciousness, closed eyes with open mouth, snores, feeble breath, cold limbs with relaxed hands, polyhidrosis, incontinence of urine and faeces, paralysed body, flaccid tongue, and thready weak pulse or feeble pulse.

[Main Points of Differentiation] Sudden fainting, closed eyes with open mouth, cold limbs with relaxed hands, polyhidrosis, paralysed body, incotinence of urine and faeces, feeble pulse.

This type is common with hypertensive cerebral hemorrhage and subarachnoid hemorrhage.

[Pathogenesis] Upward floating of *yang* with *yin* fluid consumed below making severe exhaustion of vital-*qi* and cardiac neurasthenia.

[Treatment] Supplementing *qi* and restoring *yang*; and using emergency treatment to rescue patient from perishing of *yang* and *yin*.

[Recipe] *Shen Fu Tang*[167] plus *Sheng Mai San*[84].

In case of continual polyhidrosis, add *Radix Astragali seu Hedysari*, calcined *Os Draconis*, calcined *Concha Ostreae* and *Fructus Corni* to arrest sweating and stop prostration syndrome.

[Nursing Points] Take care to keep warm; avoid stimulation; and keep close observation of the patients.

(3) Sequelae

When a patient of apoplexy has been rescued from coma, various sequelae will be left with him, such as hemiplegia, dysphasia or distortion of the face, so timely treatment should be given including synthetical methods as acupuncture and moxibustion, massage therapy and massotherapy accompanied with suitable excercises to promote curative effect.

①Hemiplegia

Hemiplegia, weak-feeling in the limbs accompanied with, on affected side, edema in the hand and foot, distortion of the face, sallow complexion, pale tongue and fine and weak pulse, belonging to the morbid condition of deficiency of *qi* and stagnation of blood, and stasis in vessels and collaterals. The treatments for the disease are invigorating *qi* and promoting blood circulation; and clearing and activating the channels and collaterals with the recipe *Bu Yang Huan Wu Tang*[141].

②Dysphasia

The symptoms of rigidity of the tongue with stammer, numbness of limbs, and wiry and slippery pulse show a morbid state of stagnation in collaterals due to phlegm by wind. The recipe for it is *Jie Yu Dan*[279] to induce resuscitation, promote *qi* circulation and remove obstruction in the collaterals.

In case of dysphasia, palpitation, shortness of breath, soreness of the loins and knees, which are the symptoms of deficiency of the kidney essence, use *Di Huang Yin Zi*[104] with substraction of *Cortex Cinnamomi* and *Radix Aconiti praeparata*, and addition of *Semen Armeniacae Amarum*, *Radix Platycodi* and *Semen Oroxyli* to recover voice and induce resuscitation.

③Distortion of the face

The state is caused by accumulation of phlegm and wind in collaterals. The treatment for it is expelling the wind, removing phlegm and clearing obstruction in the collaterals with the recipe of *Qian Zheng San*[181].

Summary

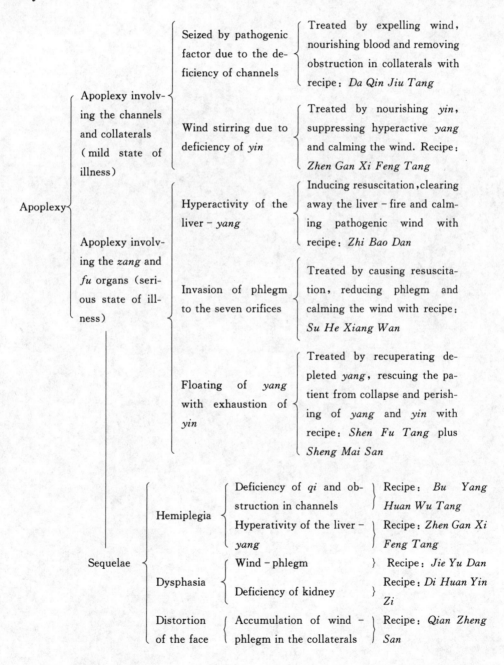

Discussions

1. What are the similatities and differences between apoplexy involving the channels and collaterals and that involving the *zang* and *fu* organs in their symptoms and pathogeneses?

2. What is excess syndrome of stroke, and what is prostration syndrome? And the differences between them?

3. What are the treatments for apoplexy in its convalecent stage?

11　Convulsive Disease

General

Convulsive disease is a morbid state manifested as stifffness of the neck and back, spasm of limbs, even opisthotonus.

The differentiating treatments for the disease are referential to epidemic cerebrospinal meningitis, epidemic encephalitis and tubercular meningitis as well as hyperpyretic convulsion, tetany and cerebroma named by Western Medicine, marked by stiffness of the neck and back and spasm of limbs.

Etiology and Pathogenesis

1. Accumulation of pathogen in channels and collaterals   Wind-cold-dampness accumulating in channels and collaterals causes the impaction of *qi* and blood in circulation and contracture of tendons from want of nourishment resulting in convulsion.

2. Convulsion due to intense heat   Excessive heat in the body will consume the body fluid, whose impairment further results in convulsive state due to the tendons from want of nourishment.

3. Deficiency of *yin* and blood   A convulsive condition due to impaired nourishment of tendons because of the consumption of *yin* and blood by hemorrhage or by polyhidrosis, or by purgation, or owing to the usual state of deficiency of both *yin* and blood.

Key Points:

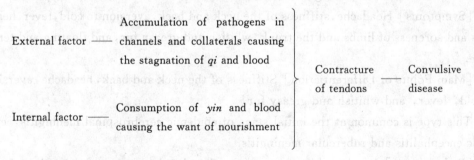

Diagnosis and Discrimination

Convulsive disease is a morbid condition showing stiffness of the neck and back, spasm of limbs, even opisthotonus, without clear seasonal feature.

Apoplexy, epilepsy and convulsive disease have the symptom of spasm in common, so it is necessary to make a distinction. About the distinction between apoplexy and convulsive disease, consult chapter10 Apoplexy; as to the distinction between epilepsy and convulsive diseaes, see the following:

Disease Distinction	Convulsive disease	Epilepsy
Symptoms of muscles, tendons and vessels	Stiffness of the neck and back, spasm of limbs, even opisthotonos	In coma, contracture of tendons and spasm of limbs
Accompanied symptoms	Commonly seen in the courses of various diseases, probably accompanied with symptoms of other diseases	Frothy salivating if onset, or making abnormal crying; as a normal person after regaining consciousness

Selecting Treatment by Differentiating Syndromes

It is better to differentiate in detail the syndrome as caused by external factors or internal injury, and of deficiency or excess type.

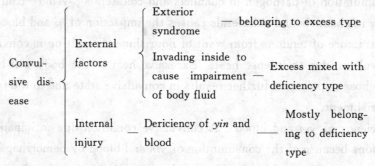

Common Syndromes:

1. Accumulation of pothogens in channels and collaterals

[Symptoms] Headache, stiffness of the neck and back, aversion to cold, fever, heaviness and soreness of limbs and the trunk, whitish and greasy fur, and floating and tense pulse.

[Main Points of Differentiation] Stiffness of the neck and back, headache, aversion to cold, fever, and whitish and greasy fur.

This type is common at the initial stage of epidemic cerebrospinal meningitis, epidemic encephalitis and tubercular meningitis.

[Pathogenesis] Wind-cold-dampness causing the obstruction of channels and collaterals and resulting in the disharmony between *ying* and *wei* in superficies.

[Treatment] Expelling wind and cold; and regulating the *ying* and removing dampness.

[Recipe] *Qiang Huo Sheng Shi Tang*[155].

In case of severe cold which belongs to stiff spastic disease, choose *Ge Gen Tang*[259]. In case of dominant wind pathogen with headache, sweating, and deep and thready pulse, which belongs to soft spastic disease, use *Gua Lou Gui Zhi Tang*[207];

when damp heat pathogens invade collaterals causing contracture of muscles, thirst but no desire for drinking, scanty dark urine, yellowish and greasy fur, and rapid and slippery pulse, adopt *San Ren Tang*[15] to clear away heat, eliminate dampness and dredge the channels and collaterals.

[Nursing Points] Keep away from cold and damp condition; and avoid cold and uncooked food.

2. Convulsion due to intense heat

[Symptoms] Fever, distension in the chest, trismus, teeth grinding, stiff neck and back, even opisthotonos, rigidity and spasm of the extremities, abdominal distention, constipation, dry throat and thirst, fidgets, and even coma with delirium, yellowish and greasy fur, and wiry and rapid pulse.

[Main Points of Differentiation] Stiff neck and back, trismus, even opisthotonos, fever, fidgets, yellowish and greasy fur, and wiry and rapid pulse.

This type is often seen in epidemic encephalitis, epidemic encephalitis and tuberculous meningitis as well as other convulsions with high fever.

[Pathogenesis] Excessive heat invades *Yangming* and stagnates in middle-*jiao* causing the obstruction of *qi* in *fu*-organs; and the impairment of body fluid by intense heat will cause heat-pathogen to disturb mental activity.

[Treatment] Purging intense heat to store body fluid; and nourishing *yin* to increase body fluid.

[Recipe] *Zeng Ye Cheng Qi Tang*[284].

In case of the impairment of body fluid by excessive heat without fullness of *fu*-organs, use *Bai Hu Jia Ren Shen Tang*[89] to remove heat in order to store body fluid; in case of serious spasm, *Lumbricus*, *Scorpio*, *Flos Chrysanthemi* and *Ramulus Uncariae Cum Uncis* may be added to calm the endopathic wind and remove obstruction of the collaterals; for severe fidgets, add *Herba Lophatheri* and *Fructus Gardeniae* to clear away the heat in the heart and relieve fidgets.

[Nursing Points] Be careful to observe the changes of consciousness, sweating, stool and urine in order to give proper treatments; and special nursing is needed in case of spasm to avoid the development of complications as asphyxia and fracture.

3. Deficiency of *yin* and blood

[Symptoms] Usually in the state of deficiency of *yin* and blood, or after bleeding or over-sweating or purging, stiffness of the neck and back, spasm of limbs, dizziness, blurred vision, sweating, listlessness, short breath, pink tongue, and wiry and thready pulse.

[Main Points of Differentiation] Stiffness of the neck and back, spasm of limbs, dizziness, blurred vision, pink tongue with little fur, and thready pulse.

This type is common in various cephalitidis, meningitides, tetanies and cerebroma.

[Pathogenesis] Deficiency of both *yin* and blood resulting in the disability to nourish tendons and the brain; and the failure of superficial-qi to protect the body against diseases due to the exhausted consumption of vital qi.

[Treatment] Nourishing yin and blood.

[Recipe] *Si Wu Tang*[79] and *Da Ding Feng Zhu*[19].

In case of dizziness, fidgets and insomnia, add *Fructus Gardeniae*, *Herba Lophather*, *Flos Chrysanthemi* and *Caulis Polygoni Muliflori* to remove heat and relieve mental stress; for the state of poor appetite with fullness of abdomen, add *Fructus Amoni*, *Endothelium corneum Gigeriae Galli* and *Pericarpium Citri Reticulatae* to regulate the flow of qi in the stomach. In case of diarrhea and pale complexion, add *Radix Codonopsis Pilosulae* and *Rhizoma Atractylosis Macrocephalae* to reinforce qi and the spleen.

[Nursing Points] Have a diet rich in fresh fruit and nutrients; and avoid pungent food.

Summary

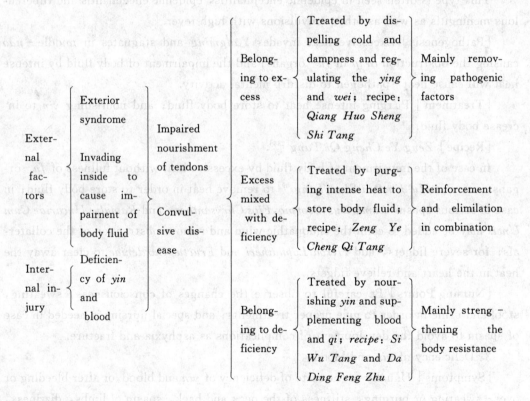

Discussions

1. What are the major pathogeneses of convulsive disease?

2. What are the respective treatments and recipes for convulsion due to accumulation of pathogen in channels and collaterals, convulsion due to intense heat and that due to deficiency of yin and blood?

12 Headache

General

Headache discussed here refers to the morbid condition with headache as its main symptom of internal diseases.

The differentiating treatments given in this chapter are referential to headache caused by influenza, paranasosinusitis, glaucona, prosopalgia, occipital neuralgia, hypertension, anemia, neuroses, vascular headache, postconcussional syndrone, meningitides and cerebroma by Western Medicine.

Etiology and Pathogenesis

1. Headache due to exopathogen Because of carelessness in daily life, or sitting or sleeping in the wind, one is likely to be attacked by wind, cold, dampness or heat pathogens, which go from the superficies to the channels and collaterals and further upward to the top of the head. Thus obstruction of the luccid *yang* follows, and the unsmooth flow of *qi* and blood will block the collaterals, resulting in headache.

2. Headache due to internal injury The brain gets nutrients from the food essence transformed by the spleen and stomach and essence - blood supplied by the liver and kidney. When the liver dysfunction occurs from impairment by emotional disorder, heat is generated which ascends to the head causing headache; deficiency of kidney - water causes its failure in nourishing wood, leading to deficiency of the liver - *yin* and kidney - *yin* and hyperactivity of the liver - *yang*, which ascends and disturbs the head resulting in headache; deficiency of the spleen and stomach causes that of *ying* - blood which fails to nourish the brain and gives rise to headache.

Key Points:

Exopathic cause	Pathogen invading top of the head causing the obstruction of *qi* and blood	Stagnation or inadequate supply of nutrients	— Headache
Endopathic cause	Stagnated fire ascending, hyperactivity of the liver - *yang*, deficiency of nutrients in brains, and deficiency of *qi* and blood		

Diagnosis and Discrimination

Headache, in Traditional Chinese Internal Medicine, refers to a morbid condition with headache as its main symptom, which will come on all the year round.

Headache and dizziness may happen at the same time; or they may appear separately. Here is the comparision:

Disease Discrimination	Headache	Dizziness
Cause	Affection by exopathogen; internal injury	Mostly internal injury
Differentiation of the disease	Mostly deficiency complicated with excess	Mainly deficiency

Selecting Treatment by Differentiating Syndromes

In differentiating the syndromes of headache, attention should be paid to its pathogeneses, as well as its nature, lasting period, peculiarity and location.

Headache
- Acute onset, sharp pain and fever manifested as cramping pain, jumping pain, buring pain, swollen pain and lasting pain — Affection by exopathogen, mostly of excess syndrome
- Slow onset, slight pain and fever marked by vague pain, void pain, dizzy pain, long-lasting, aggravated with overstrain, onset by fits and starts — Caused by internal injury, mostly of deficiency syndrome

Probably deficiency complicated with excess

Common Syndromes:

Affection by exopathogen

1. Headache due to wind-cold pathogen

[Symptoms] Headache by fits and starts, extending to the neck and back, aversion to cold and wind, being more fierce in wind, without thirst, thin and whitish tongue fur and floating pulse.

[Main Points of Differentiation] Headache, aversion to cold and wind, thin and whitish tongue fur.

This type is commonly seen in influenza.

[Pathogenesis] Wind-cold invading the superficies to obstruct lucid *yang* in spreading.

[Treatment] Expelling wind and cold pathogens.

[Recipe] *Chuan Xiong Cha Tiao San*[23].

In case of wind-cold invading the *Jueyin* channel causing the pain on top of the head, retching, vomiting frothy saliva, even cold limbs, adopt *Wu Zhu Yu Tang*[135] minus *Radix Ginseng* and *Fructus Ziziphi Jujubae*; and add *Rhizoma Pinelliae*, *Rhizoma et Radix Ligustici* and *Rhizoma Ligustici Chuan Xinong* to expell cold and lower the adverse flow of *qi*.

[Nursing Points] Keep away from wind-cold; avoid cold and uncooked food.

2. Headache due to pathogenic wind-heat

[Symptoms] Distending pain in the head, splitting sensation if serious, fever, aversion to wind, flushed face, blood-shot eyes, thirst with desire to drink, constipation, yellowish urine, red tongue with yellowish fur, and rapid and floating pule.

[Main Points of Differentiation] Distending pain in the head, fever, yellowish urine and constipation; yellowish fur, and rapid and floating pulse.

This type can be seen in influenza, meningitis and vascular headache.

[Pathogenesis] Pathogenic wind-heat invading the *seven orifices*, resulting in the consumption of body fluid by excessive heat.

[Treatment] Dispelling wind and removing heat.

[Recipe] *Xiong Zhi Shi Gao Tang*[106].

To relieve fever, drugs of pungent and cool property as *Radix Scutellariae*, *Herba Menthae* and *Fructus Gardeniae* should be adopted to take the place of *Rhizoma seu Radix Notopterygii* and *Rhizoma et Radix Ligustici* in the recipe, for they two are drugs pungent in flavor and warm in property. If the state of consumption of body fluid by excessive heat is serious, *Rhizoma Asphodeloidei*, *Herba Dendrobii* and *Radix Trichosanthis* can be added to promote the production of body fluid to quench thirst.

[Nursing Points] Avoiding pungent food.

3. Headache due to pathogenic wind-dampness

[Symptoms] Headache as if wrapped by something, heavy trunk and limbs, poor appetite, sense of suppression in the chest, difficulty in micturition, loose stool, whitish and greasy fur, and soft and floating pulse.

[Main Points of Differentiation] Headache as if wrapped by something, heavy trunk and limbs, sense of suppression in the chest, poor appetite, and whitish and greasy fur.

This type is observable in neuroses, paranasosinusitis and influenza.

[Pathogenesis] Pathogenic wind-dampness invading top of the head to disturb the mentality; retention of dampness in middle-*jiao* obstructing lucid *yang* in dispersing.

[Treatment] Dispelling pathogenic wind and removing dampness.

[Recipe] *Qiang Huo Sheng Shi Tang*[155].

In case of retention of dampness pathagen with symptoms of sense of suppression in the chest, poor appetite and loose stool, add *Rhizoma Atractylodis*, *Cortex Magnoliae Officinalis*, *Pericarpium Citri Reticulatae* and *Fructus Aurantii* to eliminate dampness and relieve epigastric distention.

[Nursing Points] Taking light food; and avoiding fat and sweet food.

Internal injury

1. Headache due to the liver-*yang*

[Symptoms] Headache with dizziness, restlessness, irritability, insomnia sometimes with hypochondiac pain, flushed face, bitter taste; thin and yellowish fur, and wiry and strong pulse.

[Main Points of Differentiation] Headache with dizziness, restlessness, irritability, hypochondriac pain, bitter taste, and wiry pulse.

This type is commonly seen in hypertension and involutional hypertension.

[Pathogenesis] Hyperactivity of the liver - yang invading the seven orifices; hyperactivity of the liver - fire disturbing mental activity.

[Treatment] Calming the liver and suppressing hyperactivity of yang.

[Recipe] *Tian Ma Gou Teng Yin*[33].

Concha Ostreae and *Os Draconis* may be added to promote the effect of calming hyperactivity of the liver - yang. In case of severe headache accompanied with hypochondriac pain, bitter taste, constipation, deep - colored urine, and hyperactivity of the liver - fire, add *Radix Curcumae*, *Radix Gentianae* and *Spica Prunelae* to purge the liver of pathogenic fire; in case of deficiency of the liver - and - kidney - yin marked by headache mild in the morning and severe in the evening, or more serious with tiredness, and wiry and thready pulse, *Radix Rehmanniae*, *Radix Polygoni Multiflori*, *Fructus Ligustri Lucidi* and *Fructus Lycii* may be added to nourish the liver and kidney.

[Nursing Points] Regulate emotions; avoid pungent food and food apt to induce fire.

2. Headache due to the kidney deficiency

[Symptoms] Headache with empty sensation often accompanied with dizziness and aggravated with overstrain, weakness and soreness of the loins and knees, listlessness, nocturnal emission, leukorrhea, tinnitus, insomnia, reddened tongue with little fur, weak and thready pulse.

[Main Points of Differentiation] Headache with dizziness, weakness and soreness of the loins and knees, tinnitus, insomnia, weak pulse.

This type is often seen in neurasthenic headache.

[Pathogenesis] The brain is in want of marrow because of deficiency of the kidney; and loins are the residence of the kidney, so if the kidney is in deficient state, the bones in loins are short of nutrients.

[Treatment] Nourishing yin and supplementing the kidney.

[Recipe] *Da Bu Yuan Jian*[17].

If the patient is on the mend, *Qi Ju Di Huang Wan*[129] may be adopted to nourish the kidney - yin to make a synergism; in case of headache and aversion to cold, warmlessness of limbs, pale tongue and deep, thready and moderate pulse, *You Gui Wan*[68] may be taken to warm and recuperate the kidney - yang and essence and blood.

[Nursing Points] Taking better care of oneself; having animal diet; being cautious to daily life; and avoiding excessive sexual intercourse.

3. Headache due to deficiency of blood

[Symptoms] Headache with dizziness, palpitation and restlessness, listlessness, pale complexion, pale tongue with thin and whitish fur, and thready and weak pulse.

[Main Points of Differentiation] Headache with dizziness, pale complexion, palpitation, pale tongue and weak pulse.

This type is often seen in headaches caused by various anemiae.

[Pathogenesis] Deficiency of *qi* and blood unable to nourish the brain resulting in the want of nourishment of heart.

[Treatment] Nourishing *qi* and blood.

[Recipe] *Jia Wei Si Wu Tang*[98].

In case of obvious deficiency of *qi*, heavy listlessness which will be more serious with over-working, sweating and short breath, add *Radix Astragali seu Hedysari*, and *Radix Ginseng*.

[Nursing Points] Supplement nutrition; take a good rest.

4. Headache due to stagnation of phlegm

[Symptoms] Headache with dizziness, stuffiness and fullness in the chest and epigastriun, vomiting of sputum and saliva, whitish and greasy fur and slippery pulse.

[Main Points of Differentiation] Headache with dizziness, vomiting of sputum and saliva, whitish greasy fur, slippery pulse.

This type is often seen in hypertension, vascular headache and neurosis.

[Pathogenesis] Dysfunction of the spleen in transport causing stagnation of phlegm in the middle-*jiao* to disturb the mentality and lucid *yang* to fail to ascend.

[Treatment] Resolving phlegm and lowering the adverse flow of *qi*.

[Recipe] *Ban Xia Bai Zhu Tian Ma Tang*[92].

Cortex Magnoliae Officinalis and *Fructus Tribuli* may be added to strengthen the effect; in case of heat by stagnation of phlegm with symptoms of bitter taste, dyschezia, yellowish and greasy fur, and slippery and rapid pulse, add *Radix Scutellariae*, *Caulis Bambusae in Taeniam* and *Fructus Aurantii Immaturus* to promote circulation of *qi*, clear away heat and dry dampness.

[Nursing Points] Avoid fat, sweet and greasy food.

5. Headache due to blood stasis

[Symptoms] Lasting headache with fixed aching spot as pain as being drilled, some with a history of head wound, purplish tongue, whitish and thin fur, and thready and weak pulse.

[Main Points of Differentiation] Lasting headache with fixed aching-spot as pain as being drilled, purplish tongue or with ecchymosis.

This type is common in postconcussional syndrome and cerebroma.

[Pathogenesis] Accumulation of blood stasis and stagnation of channels and collaterals.

[Treatment] Promoting blood circulation to remove blood stasis.

[Recipe] *Tong Qiao Huo Xue Tang*[223].

Radix Curcumae, *Rhizoma Acori Graminei*, *Herba Asari* and *Radix Angelicae Dahuricae* may be added to regulate the flow of *qi*, induce resuscitation and alleviate pain. In case of severe headache, add *Scorpio*, and *Scolopendra*, *Eupolyphoge Sinensis*; in case of lasting headache accompanied with deficiency of *qi* and blood, add *Radix Astragali seu Hedysari* and *Radix Angelicae Sinensis* to replenish and restore *qi* and blood.

[Nursing Points] Regulate life and strike a proper balance between work and rest; keep away from wind and cold, and avoid greasy and sweet food.

Summary

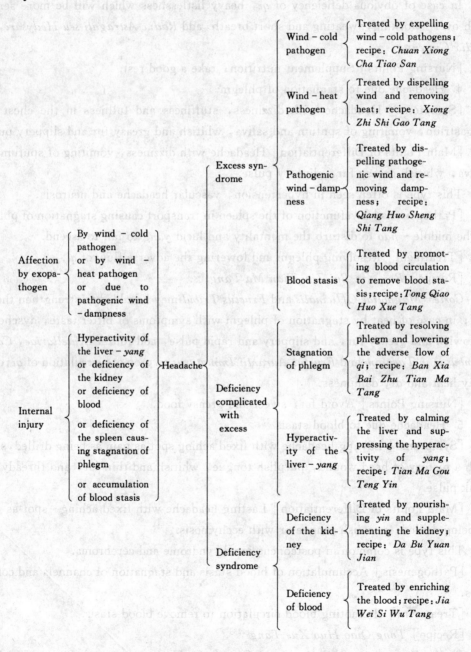

Discussions

1. What are the symptomatic differences between the headache due to exopathy and the headache due to internal injury?

2. Tell respectively the symptomatic features, treatments and recipes of headaches due to hyperactivity of the liver - *yang*, deficiency of blood, stagnation of phlegm and accumulation of blood stasis.

13 Vertigo (*Xuan Yun*)

General

Xuan means blurred vision, and *Yun* dizziness. *Xuan Yun* (vertigo) is a morbid state with symptoms of dizziness and dim eyesight, in severe case, the patient will feel as if boarding a vehicle or boat, feel whirling and is unable to stand long, which sometimes is even complicated with nausea, vomiting and sweating.

The differentiating treatments for the disease are referential to Ménière's disease, senile vertigo, hypertension, hypotension, neurosis and anemia as well as other encephalopathia with the symptom of distinct vertigo by Western Medicine.

Etiology and Pathogenesis

1. Hyperactivity of the liver - *yang*   A kind of vertigo resulting from the usual constitution of *yang* - excess, hyperactvity of the liver - *yang*; or from the usual constitution of deficiency of the kidney - *yin*, lack of nourishment in the liver, hyperactivity of the liver - *yang*; or from melancholy, anger, stagnation of *qi* turning to fire - syndromes, wind - *yang* stirrig to disturb the head.

2. Deficiency of *qi* and blood   Vertigo caused by lasting illness which leads to the consumption of *qi* and blood; or by blood loss without replenishing; or by deficiency of the spleen and stomach which fail in transporting food stuff and transforming it into *qi* and blood and further bring on the deficiency of *qi* and blood, deficiency of the former will make lucid *yang* fail to rise, while deficiency of the latter will cause the lack of nourishment in the brain.

3. Deficiency of the kidney - essence   Vertigo due to congenitial deficiency of the kidndy - essence and the kidndy - *yin*, for the kidney stores vital essence which forms marrow; or due to deficiency of the kidney because of old age, or lasting illness; or due to excessive sexual intercourse which consumes the kidney - essence and causes its failure in forming marrow. As the brain is the sea of marrow, its lack of marrow will result in vertigo.

4. Stagnation of phlegm in middle - *jiao*   Vertigo caused by being addicted to drink and fat and sweet food which are harmful to the spleen and stomach causing their failure in transport and leading to the accumulation of dampness to turn into phlegm which stagnates in the middle - *jiao* and makes lucid *yang* fail to rise and turbid *yin* to descend.

Key Points:

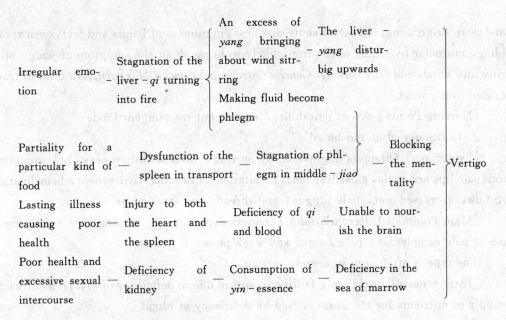

Diagnosis and Discrimination

Vertigo is characterized by dizziness and blurred vision without distinct attack season.

Vertigo sometimes is accompanied with headache and vice versa. For details, refer to chapter 12 Headache.

Selecting Treatment by Differentiating Syndromes

When a disease is diagnosed as vertigo, the next step is to differentiate syndromes. Clinically there are cases of deficiency syndrome and those of deficiency complicated with excess among which most common cases are hyperactivity of the liver - yang and deficiency of qi and blood.

1. Hyperactivity of the liver - yang

[Symptoms] Dizziness, tinnitus, headache with distension, aggravated by vexation, intermittent flushed face, restlessness, irritability, insomnia, dreamful sleep, bitter taste, red tongue with yellowish fur and wiry pulse.

[Main Points of Differentiation] Dizziness, tinnitus, headache with distension and often aggravated by anger.

This type is common in hypertension.

[Pathogenesis] Hyperactivity of the liver - yang invading the seven orifices.

[Treatment] Calming the liver; and nourishing the liver and kidney.

[Recipe] *Tian Ma Gou Teng Yin*[33].

In case of overabundance of the liver - fire, add *Radix Genntianae*, *Flos Chrysanthemi* and *Cortex Moutan Radicis* as synergists to purge the liver of pathogenic fire; in case of constipation, add *Dang Gui Long Hui Wan*[114] to purge the liver of pathogenic fire and clear *fu*-organs; in case of acute dizziness, numbness of hands and feet, even trembling, muscular twitching and cramp, likely to bring about the symptom of *yang*-stirring into wind, add *Os Draconis*, *Concha Ostreae* and *Concha Margaritifera Usta* to tranquilize liver-wind.

[Nursing Points] Avoid irritability; and do not eat pungent food.

2. Deficiency of *qi* and blood

[Symptoms] Dizziness aggravated by moving, onset with tiredness, pale complexion, pale lips and nails, glossiless hair, palpitation, insomnia, listlessness, disinclination to talk, decreased diet, pale tongue, and thready and weak pulse.

[Main Points of Differentiation] Dizziness aggravated by moving, onset with tiredness, pale complexion, pale tongue and weak pulse.

The type is often seen in anemic vertigo.

[Pathogenesis] Lucid *yang* failling to spread due to deficiency of *qi*, and insufficient supply of nutrients for the brain caused by deficiency of blood.

[Treatment] Tonifying *qi* and blood, and strengthening the spleen and stomach.

[Recipe] *Gui Pi Tang*[95].

In case of anorexia, loose stool, insufficiency of the spleen and stomach, it is better to get *Radix Angelicae Sinensis* fried, *Radix Aucklandiae* stewed, and add *Poria*, *Semen Coiccis*, *Rhizoma Alismatis*, *Fructus Amoni* and *Massa Fermentata Medicinalis* as synergists to strengthen the spleen and stomach. In case of serious deficiency of blood, add *Radix Rehmanniae Praeparata*, *Colla Corii Asini* and *Radix Astragali Seu Hedysari* (with larger amount) to invigorate *qi* and enrich the blood; in case of cold limbs and dull pain in the abdomen, add *Ramulus Cinnamoni* and *Rhizoma Zingiberis* to warm the middle-*jiao* and assist *yang*.

[Nursing Points] Take nourishing food; and avoid over-working.

3. Insufficiency of the kidney-essence

[Symptoms] Dizziness with listlessness, insomnia and dreamful sleep, amnesia, soreness and weakness of the loins and knees, nocturnal emission and tinnitus. When it shows dominant deficiency of *yin*, one can see the symptoms of dysphoria with feverish sensation in chest, palms and soles, red tongue, wiry, thready and rapid pulse; and when it shows dominant deficiency of *yang*, the symptoms will be cold limbs, pale tongue, thready, deep and weak pulse.

[Main Points of Differentiation] Dizziness, soreness and weakness of the loins and knees, nocturnal emission and tinnitus; patients of dominant deficiency of *yin*, showing heat of deficiency type; of deficiency of *yang*, displaying aversion to cold.

This type is observable in senile vertigo, anemic vertigo and Ménière's disease.

[Pathogenesis] Insufficient kidney-essence unable to supply the brain and the loins; the kidney's failure in arresting spontaneous emission due to deficiency; patients with deficiency of *yin* having internal heat while with deficiency of *yang* having external cold.

[Treatment] Replenishing *yin* to tonify the kidney for deficiency of *yin*; reinforcing the kidney and supporting *yang* for deficiency of *yang*.

[Recipe] *Zuo Gui Wan*[65] for deficiency of *yin*.

In case of severe heat in the body, add *Carapax Trionycis* fried, *Rhizoma Anemarrhenae*, *Cortex Phellodendri* and *Cortex Lycii Radicis* to nourish *yin* and remove heat.

You Gui Wan[68] for deficiency of *yang*.

. In case of serious dizziness, floating of *yang* due to *yin* deficiency, *Os Draconis*, *Concha Ostreae* and *Concha Margaritifera Usta* may be added to the above two recipes to check exuberant *yang*.

[Nursing Points] Take more animal food; and avoid excessive sexual intercourse.

4. Stagnation of phlegm

[Symptoms] Dizziness with feeling of heaviness in the head as if covered by something, suppression and fullness of the chest, nausea, poor appetite and somnolence, whitish and greasy fur, slippery and soft-floating pulse.

[Main Points of Differentiation] Dizziness, heaviness in the head as if covered by something, suppression and fullness of the chest, nausea, whitish and greasy fur, slippery and soft-floating pulse.

This type is common in hypertension, Ménière's disease and senile vertigo.

[Pathogenesis] Stagnation of phlegm in middle-*jiao* covering the lucid *yang*, making the turbid *yin* fail to descend and resulting in disorder of *qi*.

[Treatment] Eliminating dampness and removing phlegm; and strengthening the spleen and stomach.

[Recipe] *Ban Xia Bai Zhu Tian Ma Tang*[92].

In case of serious dizziness, frequent vomiting, add *Ochra Haematitum*, *Caulis Bambusae in Taeniam* and *Rhizima Zingiberis* to prevent vomiting by checking the adverse flow of *qi* with heavy material; in case of fullness in the stomach, anorexia, add *Semen Amoni Cardamomi* and *Fructus Amomi* to regulate the stomach with fragrance; in case of tinnitus, repeated viberating sound in the ear, add *Bulbus Allii Fistulosi*, *Radix Curcumae* and *Rhizoma Calami* to activate *yang* and induce resuscitation; in case of phlegm obstructing functional activities of *qi* with symptoms of expanding pain in the head and eyes, vexation, bitter taste, thirst but drinking little, yellowish and greasy fur, slippery and wiry pulse, adopt *Wen Dan Tang*[270] plus *Rhizima Coptidis* and *Radix Scutellariae* which are bitter in taste and cold in property and able to dry dampness, to remove heat and phlegm.

[Nursing Points] Take light food and avoid greasy and sweet stuffs.

Summary

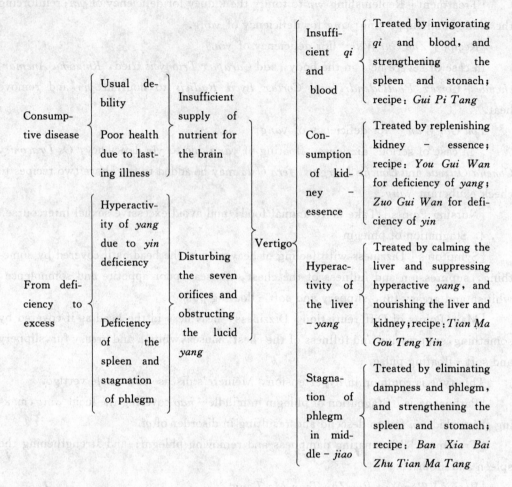

Discussions

1. What are the pathogeneses of vertigo?
2. Describe the main symptoms, treatments and recipes of hyperactivity of the liver – *yang*, deficiency of *qi* and blood, deficiency of the kidney – essence and stagnation of phlegm in middle – *jiao*.

14 Insomnia

General

Insomnia is a morbid condition marked by being unable to get regular sleep.

The differentiating treatments for this disease are referential to neurosis and some chronic diseases with insomnia as their main symptom (e. g. hypertensive insomnia, dyspeptic insomnia and anemic insomnia) by Western Medicine.

Etiology and Pathogenesis

1. Over-anxiety and over-tiredness hurting the heart and the spleen The injury of the heart leads to the consumption of *yin* blood resulting in mental derangement; while the injury of the spleen causes the state of poor appetite leading to the shortage of nutrients to become *ying* blood to supply the heart resulting in irritability.

2. *Yang* and *yin* failling in coordination and the same case being with the heart and the kidney Usual debility or lasting illness consumes the kidney-*yin* and causes its failure in supplying nutrients for the heart and discordance between water and fire, resulting in exuberance of the heart-*yang*; or overacting of five emotions and flaming of the heart-fire make the heart and kidney fail in coordination; exuberance of the heart-fire leads to mental disorder and irritability resulting in insomnia.

3. Hyperactivity of fire due to *yin* deficiency, up-stirring of the liver-*yang* Injury by emotions leads to the irregularity of the liver and convertion of the stagnated *qi* into fire flaring up; or hyperactivity of *yang* due to deficiency of *yin* disturbs the heart and causes irritability resulting in insomnia.

4. Insuff iciency of the heart and gallbladder qi, mental upset Insufficiency of the heart and gallbladder *qi* will cause one's hesitation in making a decision, and his susceptbility to being frightened, leading to mental upset. Thus occurs insomnia.

5. Disorder of the stomach-*qi* and restless sleep Enterogastric impairment due to improper diet causes the undigested food to become phlegm-heat to block the middle-*jiao* and its upward stirring leads to disorder of the stomach-*qi* resulting in insomnia.

Key Points:

Over-anxiety
Imbalance between labor and rest } Impairment of spleen and heart } Insufficiency of *qi* and blood

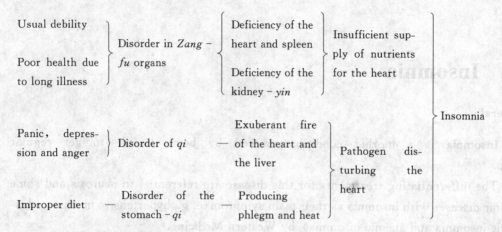

Diagnosis and Discrimination

Insomnia is a morbid state marked by being unable to get regular sleep, often accompanied with poor apptite and listlessness. If there is only sign of decreasing sleep without other symptoms, the case should not be regarded as insomnia. It is normal for a senile to keep waking after a period of sleep at night. And occasional sleeplessness due to emotional influence or the change of life surroundings should not be considered as insomnia.

Selecting Treatment by Differentiating Syndromes

To make clinical differentiating, firstly it is important to know that insomnia is manifested as having difficulty in going to sleep or sleeping but not deeply; secondly one shoule distinguish deficiency syndrome from excess syndrome.

Deficiency syndromes: Mostly due to deficiency of *yin* − blood caused by dysfunction of the heart, spleen, liver and kidney.

Excess syndrome: Mostly due to fire − syndrome caused by stagnation of the liver − *qi*, dyspepsia, stagnation of phlegm and disorder of the stomach.

Common Syndromes :

Excess syndromes

1. Fire due to stagnation of the liver − *qi*

[Symptoms] Insomnia, irritability, anorexia, thirst with preference for drink, red eyes, bitter taste, dark urine, constipation, red tongue with yellowish fur, and wiry and rapid pulse.

[Main Points of Differentiation] Insomnia, irritability, red eyes, bitter taste, wiry and rapid pulse.

This type is often seen in neurasthenic insomnia.

[Pathogenesis] Impairment of the liver by anger making the disorder of the liver − *qi* and fire generated, fire disturbing the heart resulting in insomnia.

[Treatment] Relieving the depressed liver, and removing heat assisted with tranquilliaing the mind.

[Recipe] *Long Dan Xie Gan Tang*[64].

Add *Poria cum Ligno Hospite*, *Os Draconis* and *Concha Ostreae* to ease mental stress. In case of fullness and oppressed feeling in the chest and susceptibility to sighing, add *Radix Curcumae* and *Rhizoma Cyperi* to soothe the liver and relieve stagnation.

[Nursing Points] Regulate emotions to avoid anger and anxiety; and do not eat pungent food.

2. Internal up-stirring by accumulation of phlegm-heat

[Symptoms] Insomnia, heavy feeling in the head, oppressed feeling in the chest, polyphlegm, aversion to food, eructation, acid regurgitation, nausea, vexation, bitter taste, blurred vision, greasy and yellowish fur, and slippery and rapid pulse.

[Main Points of Differentiation] Insomnia, excessive sputum, chest distress, aversion to food, regurgitation of sour saliva, yellowish greasy fur, slippery and rapid pulse.

This type is common in dyspeptic insomnia.

[Pathogenesis] Dyspepsia causing accumulation of dampness to become phlegm which turns into heat to invade the upper-*jiao* leading to vexation and insomnia.

[Treatment] Resclving phlegm and removing heat; regulating the stomach to ease the mind.

[Recipe] *Wen Dan Tang*[270].

Rhiaoma Coptidis and *Radix Pittospori* may be added to clear away the heart-fire. In case of palpitation, add *Concha Margaritifera Usta* and *Cinnabaris* to tranquilize and relieve palpitation. In case of severe phlegm-heat and constipation, *Meng Shi Gun Tan Wan*[289] may be adopted to remove the heat and phlegm to ease the mind.

[Nursing Points] Have light food and take less fat and sweet food.

Deficiency syndromes

1. Excessive fire due to deficiency of *yin*

[Symptoms] Vexation, insomnia, palpitation, dizziness, tinnitus, amnesia, soreness in the loins, oneirogmus, dysphoria with feverish sensation in chest, palms and soles, dry mouth with little fluid, red tongue with little fur, and thready and rapid pulse.

[Main Points of Differentiation] Vexation, insomnia, soreness in the loins, oneirogmus, dysphoria with feverish sensation in chest, palms and soles, red tongue with little fur.

This type is observable in hypertensive insomnia.

[Pathogenesis] Deficiency of the kidney-*yin* failing in coordination with the heart causing hyperactivity of fire of the heart and liver, deficiency-fire flaring up to disturb mental activities.

[Treatment] Nourishing *yin* to reduce pathogenic fire and tranquilizing the mind by nourishing the heart.

[Recipe] *Huang Lian E Jiao Tang*[231].

In case of flushed face, serious dizziness and tinnitus, add *Concha Ostreae*, *Plastrum Testudinis* and *Magnetium* to check exuberant *yang* and ease mental strain.

[Nursing Points] Do not have pungent diet; and avoid sexual intercourse and overstrain.

2. Deficiency of both the heart and spleen

[Symptoms] Excessive dreaming and aptness to wake during sleep, palpitation, amnesia, dizziness, tiredness in limbs, listlessness, poor appetite, dim complexion, pale tongue with thin fur, and thready and weak pulse.

[Main Points of Differentiation] Excessive dreaming and aptness to wake during sleep, palpitataion, amnesia, poor appetite, tiredness in limbs, pale tongue and weak pulse.

This type is observable in anemic insomnia.

[Pathogenesis] Deficiency of both the heart and spleen making blood fail to nourish the heart, resulting in mental derangement.

[Treatment] Invigorating the heart and spleen to promote production of *qi* and blood.

[Recipe] *Gui Pi Tang*[95].

In severe case of deficiency of heart - blood, add *Redix Rdhmanniae Praeparata*, *Radix Paeoniae Alba* and *Colla Corii Asini* to nourish heart blood; in severe case of insomnia, add *Fructus Schisandrae* and *Semen Biotae* to nourish the heart and tranquilize the mind; or add *Flos Abliziae*, *Caulis Polygoni Multiflori*, *Os Draconis* and *Concha Ostreae* to tranquilize the mind; if accompanied with oppressed feeling in eigastrium, poor appetite and slippery and greasy fur, add *Rhizoma Pinelliae*, *Pericarpium Citri Reticulatae*, *Poria* and *Cortex Magnoliae Officinalis* to strengthen the spleen, regulate the flow of *qi* and remove phlegm.

[Nursing Points] Have good rest and nutritive food.

3. Deficiency of *qi* of the heart and gallbladder

[Symptoms] Insomnia or excessive dreaming and aptness to be waken, timidness, palpitation, aptness to be frightened, short breath, fatigue, dribbling urination, pale tonge, and wiry and thready pulse.

[Main Points of Differentiation] Insomnia, or excessive dreaming, aptness to be waken, timidness, palpitation and aptness to be frightened.

This type is common in neurasthenic insomnia.

[Pathogenesis] Deficiency of the heart - *qi* causing irritability while deficiency of gallbladder - *qi* leading to the symptom of being susceptible to fright.

[Treatment] Supplementing *qi* to relieve fright and ease the mind.

[Recipe] *An Shen Ding Zhi Wan*[112].

In case of floating-yang due to deficiency of blood and insomnia due to vexation, *Suan Zao Ren Tang*[280] is suitable.

[Nursing Points] Take regular exercise; adjust emotions; do not have strong tea or coffee before sleep; and smoke less.

Summary

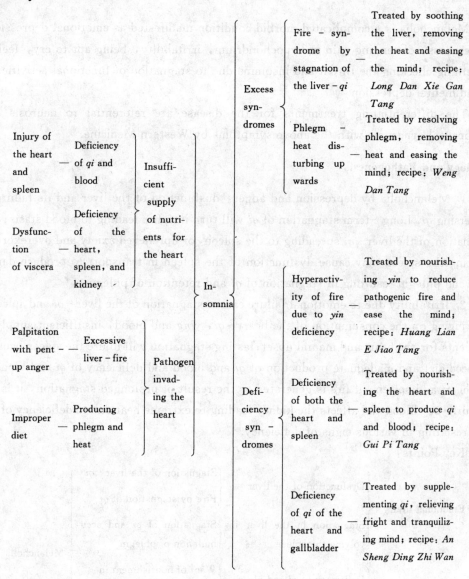

Discussions

1. What are the pathogenic factors of insomnia?
2. Make a description of main points of defferentiation, therapeutic methods and recipes of fire by stagnation of the liver-qi and deficiency of both the heart and spleen.

15 Melancholia

General

Melancholia is a complicated morbid condition manifested as emotional depression, restlessness, distending pain in hypochondrium, irritability, being apt to cry, feeling something checking the throat and insomnia due to stagnation of functional activities of qi and mental depression.

The differentiating treatments for the disease are referential to neurosis and menopausal syndrome with the above symptoms by Western Medicine.

Etiology and Pathogenesis

1. Melancholia by depression and anger, dusfunction of the liver and its failure in dispersing qi. Long-term stagnation of qi will turn into fire leading to blood stasis; and stagnation of the liver-qi spreading to the spleen, or uprelieved axiety and overexertion injuring the spleen may cause dysfunction of the spleen in transport to produce dampness and phlegm resulting in stagnation of qi and retention of phlegm.

2. Irritability due to emotional failure causes stagnation of the liver-qi and spleen-qi bringing on the consumption of the heart-qi, ying and blood, insufficient supply of nutrients for the heart and mental upset; lasting stagnation will injure the spleen causing reduced diet and inadequate production of qi and blood and deficiency of qi and blood in the heart and spleen; if fire is generated as the result of prolonged stagnation, it is apt to hurt yin-blood and affects the kidney leading to extreme heat due to deficiency of yin and resulting in various signs of deficiency.

Key Points:

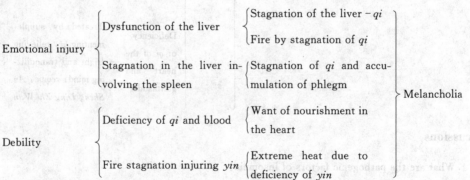

Diagnosis and Discrimination

This disease is a morbid state characteriaed by emotional depression and the stagnation of functional activities of *qi*.

It is necessary to make a discrimination between the disease and epilepsy both of which are concerned with emotions.

Disease Discrimination	Melancholia	Epilepsy
Symptomatic features	Gloomy mind, restlessness, listlessness, suspicion, axiety, insomnia	Delusion, paraphasia, insaneness
State of consciousness	Generally in normal state	Cold expression, being lost in reverie, or dementia

Selecting Treatment by Differentiating Syndromes

After melancholia is diagnosed, differentiation should be made between excess syndrome and deficiency syndrome before selecting a treatment. Excess syndrome is treated by relieving the depressed liver and regulating the circulation of *qi* while deficiency syndrome by invigorating *qi* and blood to strengthen the body resistance.

Excess syndrome

1. Stagnation of the liver - *qi*

[Symptoms] Gloomy mind, restlessness, susceptibility to signing, distending pain in chest and hypochondrium with unfixed paining - spot, eructation, fullness in stomach, abdominal distention, poor appetite, or vomiting, without menses in women, greasy and thin fur, and wiry pulse.

[Main Points of Differentiation] Gloomy mind, susceptible to signing, distending pain in chest and hypochondrium, wiry pulse.

This type is observable in neurosis and menopausal syndrome.

[Pathogenesis] Emotional injury making dysfunction of the liver and leading to stagnation of the liver - *qi* and that of functional activities of *qi*.

[Treatment] Soothing the liver and regulating the circulation of *qi*. Relieving mental depression.

[Recipe] *Chai Hu Shu Gan San*[211].

Radix Curcumae and *Pericarpium Citri Reticulatae Viride* are adopted to strengthen the effect of regulating the circulation of *qi*. *Yue Ju Wan*[264] may be taken as a synergist. In case of frequent eructation, depression feeling in chest and epigastrium, add *Flos Inulae*, *Ochra Haematitum* and *Pericarpium Citri Reticulatae* to calm the liver and lower the adverse flow of *qi*; in case of abdominal distention caused by food stagnation, add *Fructus Crataegi*, *Massa Fermentata Madicinalis* and *Endothelium Corneum Gigeriae Galli* to remove food stagnation.

[Nursing Points] Keep opitimistic mood; medical personnel and the relatives of the patient should take good care of the patients.

2. Fire due to stagnation of *qi*

[Symptoms] Irritability, fullness in the chest and hypochondrium, gastric upset, acid regurgitation, dry mouth, bitter taste, constipation, or headache, red eyes, tinnitus, red tongue with yellowish fur, and wiry and rapid pule.

[Main Points of Differentiation] Irritability, dry mouth, bitter taste, red tongue with yellowish fur, wiry and rapid pulse.

This type is common in neurosis.

[Pathogenesis] Fire by stagnation of *qi* tending to flare up and causing the liver-fire to disturb the stomach and impair body-fluid.

[Treatment] Purging the liver of pathogenic fire; relieving depression and regulating the stomach.

[Recipe] *Dan Zhi Xiao Yao San*[52] with *Zuo Jin Wan*[67].

In case of severe constipation, add *Radix Gentianae* and *Radix et Rhizoma Rhei* to relieve constipation by purgation.

[Nursing Points] Keep opitimistic mood and have less pungent food; medical personnels should take good care of the patients.

3. Stagnation of *qi* and phlegm

[Symptoms] Feeling something checking the throat that cannot be coughed up nor swallowed down, stuffiness in chest or accompanied with pain in hypochondrium, whitish and greasy fur, and slippery and wiry pulse.

[Main Points of Differentiation] Feeling something checking the throat, stuffiness in chest.

This type is often seen in neurosis.

[Pathogenesis] Stagnation of the liver-*qi* involving the spleen causes dysfunction of the spleen in transport and the production of dampness and phlegm resulting in disorder of *qi*.

[Treatment] Resolving phlegm, promoting circulation of *qi* and relieving the stagnation.

[Recipe] *Ban Xia Hou Pu Tang*[93].

Rhizoma cyperi Praeparata, *Fructus Aurantii Immaturus*, *Fructus Citri Sarcoda ctyli*, *Flos Inulae* and *Ochra Haematitum* may be added to strengthen the effect of regulating the flow of *qi* to alleviate mental depression and resolving phlegm to check the adverse flow of *qi*. If accompanied with the symptoms of vomiting, bitter taste, yellowish and greasy fur which are the signs of phlegm-heat, *Wen Dan Tang*[270] may be used with *Radix Scutellariae*, *Bulbus Fritillariae* and *Fructus Trichosandthis* as additional drugs to reduce phlegm and clear away heat for promoting functional activities of *qi*.

[Nursing Points] Have ease of mind; and take light food.

Deficiency syndrome

1. Mental injury by melancholy

[Symptoms] Being lost in reverie, restlessness, anxiety apt to cry, intermittent yawn, pale tongue with whitish and thin fur, and thready and wiry pulse.

[Main Points of Differentiation] Being lost in reverie, anxiety apt to cry, intermittent yawn.

This type is common in hysteria.

[Pathogenesis] Pent-up melancholy consuming the heart-*qi* leading to the consumption of *ying*-blood and insufficient supply of nutrients for the heart.

[Treatment] Nourishing the heart to calm the mind.

[Recipe] *Gan Mai Da Zao Tang*[71].

To strengthen the function of nourishing the heart and tranquilizing the mind, add *Semen Biotae*, *Semen Zizyphi Jujubae*, *Poria Cum Ligno Hospite* and *Flos Albiziae*.

[Nursing Points] Medical personnel should be kind and do painstaking ideological work to divert the patient's attention.

2. Deficiency of both the heart and spleen

[Symptoms] Over-anxiety, palpitation, timidness, insomnia, amnesia, pale complexion, dizziness, listlessness, poor appetite, pale tongue, and thready and weak pulse.

[Main Points of Differentiation] Over-anxiety, palpiataion, insomnia, pale complexion, listlessness, poor appetite.

This type is observable in neurosis.

[Pathogenesis] Over-anxiety causing dysfunction of the spleen in transport bringing about insufficient supply of nutrients for the heart and deficiency of both the heart and spleen.

[Treatment] Invigorating the spleen, nourishing the heart and replenishing *qi* and blood.

[Recipe] *Gui Pi Tang*[95].

Radix Curcumae and *Flos Albiziae* may be added to relieve stagnation and ease the mind.

[Nursing Points] Develop peace of mind; keep opitimistic mood; and adjust diet.

3. Excessive fire due to deficiency of *yin*

[Symptoms] Vexation, irritability, palpitation, insomnia, dizziness or emission, soreness in loins, menstrual disorder in women, red tongue, wiry, thready and rapid pulse.

[Main Points of Differentiation] Insomnia, vexation, dizziness, palpiation, red tongue with little fur, wiry, thready and rapid pulse.

This type is common in menopausal syndrome.

[Pathogenesis] Deficiency of liver-*yin* and kidney-*yin* and consumption of *ying*-blood causing insufficient supply of nutrients for the heart and flaring-up of deficiency-fire.

[Treatment] Nourishing *yin*, removing heat, and tranquilizing the mind.

[Recipe] *Zi Shui Qing Gan Ying* [271].

Concha Margaritifera Usta, *Magnetitum* and *Pig Iron Cinder* may by added for tranquilizing the mind with heavy materals. In case of soreness in loins, emission and acratia, add *Plastrum Testudinis*, *Rhizona Anemarrhenae*, *Cortex Eucommiae* and *Concha Ostreae* to tonify the kidney and reinforce essence. For irregular menstruation, add *Rhizona Cyperi* and *Herba Leonuri* to regulate the flow of *qi* for alleviating mental depression and normalize menstruation.

[Nursing Points] Develop a peaceful and opitimistic mood; and avoid pungent food and alcohol.

Summary

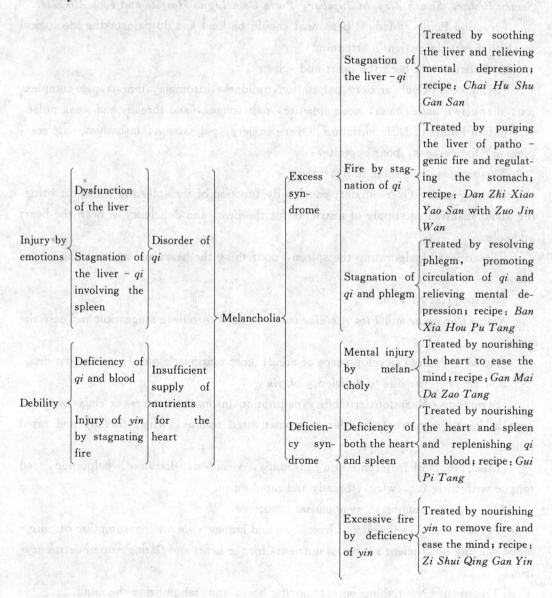

Discussions

1. What is the general of melancholia?
2. What are the respective etiologies and pathogeneses, symptoms, treatments and recipes of stagnation of the liver-*qi* and deficiency of both the heart and spleen?

— 355 —

16 Mania – Depressive Psychosis

General

Mania – depressive psychosis shows two morbid states marked by abalienation and abnormal mentality. Depressive psychosis is manifested as silence, dementia, paraphasis, quietness and hyperpleasure, while mania as tumult, restlessness, beating and scolding and polyanger.

The differentiating treatments for the diseases are referential to schizophrenia, manic – depressive psychosis, involutional psychosis, psychotenic reaction as well as some kinds of neuroses by Western Medicine.

Etiology and Pathogenesis

1. **Imbalance between *yin* and *yang*** A breakdown of *yin – yang* equilibrium leads to hyperactivity of *yang* upward due to *yin* deficient downward causing the disturbance of the mentality resulting in disorder of mental activities.

2. **Emotional depression** Anger and panic impair the liver and kidney, or being subject to changing moods will consume the heart – *yin* and cause insufficiency of *yin* – fluid in the liver and kidney, insufficient supply of nutrients for the liver and its dysfunction leading to symptoms such as silence, dementia, paraphasis; or deficiency of the heart – *yin* will bring on flaring heart – fire and adverse flow of *qi* in the liver and gallbladder resulting in a vesanic condition of ravings and scolding.

3. **Phlegm *qi* disturbing upward** A vesanic state due to phlegm *qi* disturbing upward the seven orifices and blocking the heart making a confused mind displaying signs of mania, restlessness, singing, laughing, scolding, climbing walls and getting on roofs.

4. **Stagnation of *qi* and blood** A vesanic condition by stagnation of *qi* and blood obstructing channels and collaterals and further resulting in the disconnection between the brain – *qi* and *qi* of the *zang* and *fu* organs.

Key Points:

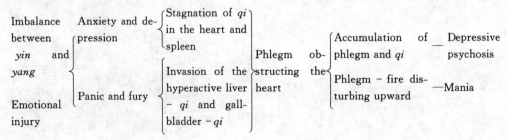

Diagnosis and Discrimination

Mania – depressive psychosis belongs to amentia. Depressive psychosis is characterized by silence and hyperpleasure, while mania marked by move – liking and polyanger. They share the same sign of abnormal mental state with epilepsy, but patients of epilepsy are as normal as healthy persons at ordinary times, when the disease comes on, symptoms of sudden fainting and loss of consciousness will appear, while patients of vesanic diseases are usually in the state of abnormal mentality of various degrees. Whether there is a goat – bleat with frothy saliva or not before on – coming is one of the distinguishing signs between epilepsy and amentia.

Selecting Treatment by Differentiating Syndromes

The pathogeneses of vesanic disease are stagnation of *qi* and phlegm – fire, imbalance between *yin* and *yang* resulting from the pathogenic changes in the liver, gallbladder, heart and spleen. Clinical differentiation should be made between vesanic diseases and mania.

Vesanic diseases
- Depression, silence, dementia, self – murmuring → Depressed psychosis : Treated by soothing the liver and regulating *qi*, eliminating phlegm for resuscitation
- Tumult, beating, scolding, restlessness → Mania : Treated by tranquilizing the mind, removing the phlegm and purging the liver of pathogenic fire

Common syndromes:

Depressive psychosis

1. Stagnation of phlegm and *qi*

[Symptoms] Depression, cold complexion, dementia, paraphasia or self – murmuring, being subject to changing moods, no desire for eating, greasy fur, and wiry and slippery pulse.

[Main Points of Differentiation] Depression, dementia, paraphasia, greasy fur and slippery pulse.

This type is seen in depression, involutional melancholia and neurosis.

[Pathogenesis] Over- anxiety stagnating the liver – *qi* and checking the spleen – *qi* to send up nutrients, leading to the stagnation of *qi* and phlegm to obstruct mental activities.

[Treatment] Regulating the flow of *qi* to alleviate mental depression, and eliminating phlegm for resuscitation.

[Recipe] *Shun Qi Dao Tan Tang* [191].

Kong Xian Dan[238] may be used for severe cases in order to remove phlegm stagnation in chest. In case of mental confusion, being lost in a reverie, dull expression, paraphasia, staring-eyes, and whitish and greasy fur due to phlegm, firstly use *Su He Xiang Wan*[128] to induce resuscitation with aromatics, and secondly adopt *Si Qi Tang*[75] plus *Arisaema cun Bile*, *Radix Curcumae*, *Rhizoma Calami* and *Radix Polygalae* to reduce phlegm and promote the circulation of *qi*.

[Nursing Points] Pay attention to psychotherapy. Avoid greasy, sweet and phlegm-producing food.

2. Deficiency of both the heart and spleen

[Symptoms] Trauce, palpitation apt to panic, susceptible to sorrow and crying, tiredness, reduced diet, pale tongue, weak and thready pulse.

[Main Points of Differentiation] Trauce, palpitation apt to panic, reduced diet, tiredness, pale tongue and thready pulse.

This type is common in involutional psychosis and neurosis.

[Pathogenesis] Insufficient blood in the heart causing the lack of nutrients for the heart, deficiency of *qi* and blood resulting in dysfunction of the spleen in transport.

[Treatment] Invigorating the spleen, nourishing the heart, replenishing *qi* and easing the mind.

[Recipe] *Yang Xin Tang*[185].

It is better to adopt *Gan Mai Da Zao Tang*[71] at the same time to nourish the heart and moisten dryness for the cure of madness, and sorrow with aptness to cry and trauce.

[Nursing Points] Paying attention to psychotherapy; and regulating the diet.

Mania

1. Phlegm-fire disturbing upward

[Symptoms] Sudden onset, at the beginning displaying the signs of choleric mood, headache, insomnia, angry-staring eyes, flushed face and eyes, and then suddenly becoming mad, climbing walls, getting on roofs, scolding, shouting, regardless of close or distant relationship, or damaging things and injuring persons, having excessive strength, not eating nor sleeping, deep-red tongue, yellowish and greasy fur, wiry large, slippery and rapid pulse.

[Main Points of Differentiation] Sudden onset, flushed face and eyes, madness, not eating and sleeping, deep-red tongue, yellowish and greasy fur, wiry, large, slippery and rapid pulse.

This type is observable in mania and schizophrenia.

[Pathogenesis] Fury impairing the liver bringing on the flaming-up of the liver-fire and arousing phlegm-heat to disturb mental activities.

[Treatment] Tranquilizing the mind, removing phlegm and purging the liver of pathogenic fire.

[Recipe] *Sheng Tie Luo Yin*[85].

In case of abundant phlegm-fire with yellowish and greasy fur, use *Meng Shi Gun Tan Wan*[289] at the same time to purge intense heat and remove phlegm; and then adopt *An Gong Niu Huang Wan*[111] to remove heat from the heart and restore consciousness. In case of excessive heat in *Yangmin* with symptoms of replete constipation, yellowish and rough fur, replete and large pulse, use modified *Cheng Qi Tang*[100] to clear away pathogenic factors and purge the excess-fire from the stomach and intestines.

[Nursing Points] Take safety measures to avoid accidents. And do not eat pungent, fat and sweet food.

2. Impairment of *yin* by excessive fire

[Symptoms] Lasting madness showing decreasing, inclination with tiredness, talkative, being apt to panic, intermittent dysphoria, thin physique, flushed face, red tongue with little fur, thready and rapid pulse.

[Main Points of Differentiation] Lasting madness, tiredness, dysphoria, red tongue with little fur.

This type is seen at the later stage of mania.

[Pathogenesis] Lasting madness consuming *qi* and impairing *yin*; insufficiency of *qi* making the degree of madness decrease while deficiency of *yin* causing the flaring-up of the heart-fire.

[Treatment] Nourishing *yin* to reduce pathogenic fire, and tranquilizing the mind.

[Recipe] *Er Yin Jian*[3]

Ding Zhi Wan[156] may be used as an adjustment.

[Nursing Points] Regulate daily life; avoid smoking, drinking and pungent food.

Summary

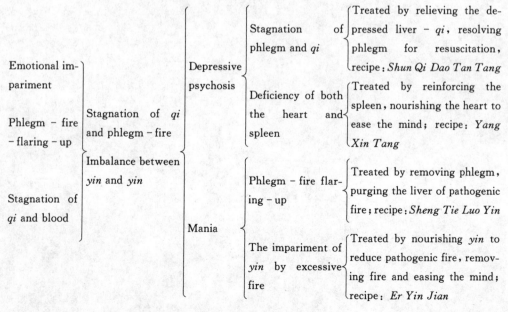

Discussions

1. What are the pathogenetic and clinical differences between depressed psychosis and mania?

2. What are the respective symptoms, treatments and recipes of stagnation of phlegm – *qi* in depressed psychosis, and those of phlegm – fire flaring – up in mania?

17 Epilepsy

General

Epilepsy is a kind of paroxysmal mental disorder characterized by episodic mental confusion (trauce), even sudden fainting and loss of consciousness, frothy salivation, upward turning of eyeballs, convulsion of limbs, or crying like a pig or sheep, being mentally normal as usual after regaining consciousness.

The differentiating treatment for this disease is referential to the epilepsy in Western Medicine.

Etiology and Pathogenesis

1. Emotional disorder Epilepsy caused by the generation of wind and heat due to *yin* unable to keep *yang* well, resulting from the disorder of functional activities of *qi*, and the impairment of kidney and liver after sudden onset of convulsion.

2. Congenital factors The diseases that occur in childhood, are related to congenital factors. If the mother was suddenly frightened during the period of pregnancy, the consumption of mother's essence and the deficiency of kidney will cause the growth of unnormal fetal. The baby will suffer from epilepsy after birth.

3. Brain trauma Epilepsy caused by falling down, or being striken or difficulty in birth leading to the impairment of brain, stagnation of *qi*, stasis of blood and the obstruction of collaterals.

Key Points:

Emotional disorder	The stagnation of liver-*qi* and heart-*qi*	Obstruction of wind-phlegm caused by the accumulation of phlegm and the adverse rising of *qi*
Occurrence after illness (trauma)	Functional disorder of *zang*-organs	Disorder of functional activites of *qi* and obstruction of phlegm
Congenital factors		

→ Epilepsy

Diagnosis and Discrimination

Epilepsy is characterized by episodic mental confusion, or sudden fainting and loss of consciousness, frothy salivation and crying like a pig or sheep. It may occur anywhere at any time.

Epilepsy, apoplexy and *jue*-syndrome, each of them presents sudden loss of con-

— 361 —

sciousness. So they should be distinguished. The detailed contents can be seen in the chapters of Apoplexy and *Jue* - Syndrome.

Selecting Treating by Differentiating Syndromes

In clinic, epilepsy should be treated in a clear knowledge of *Biao*, *Ben*, deficiency and excess. In case of frequent occurrence, the treatment should be aimed at treating Biao (symptoms), i.e, emphatically keeping the adverse rising *qi* downwards and eliminating phlegm, waking up patient from unconsciousness and arresting epilepsy by calming wind - syndrome. In normal time, the treatment should be emphatically aimed at treating *Ben* (root cause), i.e, invigorating the spleen to remove phlegm, tonifying the liver and kidney, and tranquilizing the mind by nourishing heart - blood.

Common Types:

1. Obstruction of wind - phlegm

[Symptoms] Before the onset of epilepsy, there are some aural symptoms of dizziness, feeling of oppression over the chest, and lassitude; during the attack, it is manifested as sudden loss of consciousness, convulsion, frothy salivation, some accompanied with crying, urinary and fecal incontinence; and some with just a transient loss of consciousness or mental confusion but without convulsion; whitish and greasy fur, wiry and rapid pulse.

[Main Points of Differentiation] At usual times, the patient remains fully conscious; during the attack, it is manifested as sudden loss of consciousness, convulsion, frothy salivation, crying, or just transient mental confusion.

[Pathogenesis] Obstruction of wind - phlegm and the mind being disturbed caused by stirring up of the liver - wind and phlegm; or phlegm generating inside and going upward with wind.

[Treatment] Eliminating phlegm and calming liver - wind, regaining consciousness and arresting epilepsy.

[Recipe] *Ding Xian Wan*[157].

[Nursing Points] Live a regular life and eat light food. Avoid eating mutton and drinking alcohol, etc. which can generate fire and induce epilepsy. Don't go to the dangerous part and do dangerous work in order to avoid accidents.

2. Excessive phlegm - fire inside

[Symptoms] During the attack, manifested as loss of consciousness, convulsion, frothy salivation, or roaring; at usual times, manifested as irritability, upset, insomnia, difficult expectoration, bitter taste and dry feeling in the mouth, constipation, red tongue with yellowish and greasy fur, wiry and slippery, rapid pulse.

[Main Points of Differentiation] During the attack, manifested as loss of consciousness, roaring; during the silent stage, manifested as irritability, bitter taste in the mouth, constipation, which are caused by phlegm - heat, red tongue with yellowish and greasy fur, slippery and rapid pulse.

[Pathogenesis] Predominating liver - fire causes the generation of wind and consumes body fluid resulting in the generation of phlegm, which goes upward and disturbs the mentality.

[Treatment] Clearing away liver - fire, eliminating phlegm, waking up patients from unconsciousness.

[Recipe] *Long Dan Xie Gan Tang*[64] with *Di Tan Tang*[215].

On the basis of the above recipe, *Concha Haliotidis*, *Ramulus Uncariae cum Uncis*, *Succus Bambosae*, *Lumbricus*, etc. may be added to strengthen the action of calming liver to relieve wind - syndrome (such as convulsion, dizziness), eliminating phlegm and arresting epilepsy. In case of costipation caused by phlegm - fire obstruction, *Zhu Li Da Tan Wan*[117] should be used to eliminate phlegm and purge fire.

[Nursing Points] Eat less pungent, greasy and sweet food in order to avoid producing fire and phlegm. Avoid going to dangerouse parts alone or doing dangerous work; when epilepsy occurs, unbutton the patient's dress and make his head turn to one side to prevent the phlegm from getting into trachea.

3. Deficiency of the heart and the kidney

[Symptoms] Prolonged epilepsy, amnesia, palpitation, dizziness, blurred vision, soreness in the loins and knees, lassitude, thin and greasy fur, thready and weak pulse.

[Main Points of Differentiation] Repeated attack for a long time, amnesia, palpitation, soreness in the loins, lassitude.

[Pathogenesis] Repeated occurrence of epilepsy consumes *qi* and impairs *yin*, resulting in the deficiency of heart - blood and kidney - *qi*.

[Treatment] Tonifying heart and kidney, invigorating spleen and removing phlegm.

[Recipe] *Da Bu Yuan Jian*[17] with *Liu Jun Zi Tang* [45].

In case of deficiency of the kidney, use *He Che Da Zao Wan*[152]. In case of prolonged epilepsy, manifested as mental confusion, fear, depression, anxiety, *Gan Mai Da Zao Tang*[71] is used in combination to nourish heart and moisturize dryness.

[Nursing Points] Have some proper physical training. Avoid excessive mental irritation and sexual intercourse.

Summary

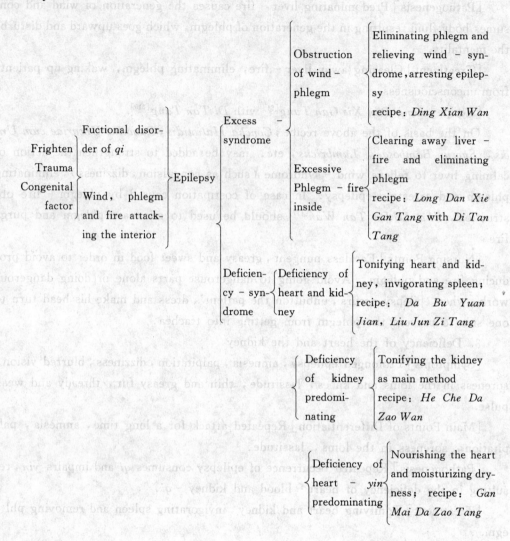

Discussions

1. What is the pathogenesis of epilepsy?
2. What are the respective symptoms, therapeutic principles and recipes of obstruction of wind-phlegm and excessive phlegm-fire inside?

18 Stomachache

General

Stomachache refers to a disease with frequent pain in the epigastrium as the main symptom.

The treatment by differentiating syndromes of the disease is referential to gastro-duodenal ulcer, acute or chronic gastritis, gastroptosia, gastroneurosis, prolapse of gastric mucosa and gastric cancer, etc. with the same symptom as the above in Western Medicine.

Etiology and Pathogenesis

1. **Stomach being attacked by exogenous pathogen** The attack of exogenous cold or overeating of uncooked and cold food will lead to accumulation of cold in middle-*jiao*, which hinders the stomach-*yang*, and obstructs the functional activities of *qi*, resulting in stomachache.

2. **Stagnation of liver-*qi*** Stomachache due to the stagnation of the functional activities of *qi* and the failure of stomach-*qi* in descending resulting from anxiety, worry and anger impairing the liver and causing stagnated liver-*qi* to attack the stomach.

3. **Deficiency-cold of the spleen and stomach** Stomachache resulting from the deficiency-cold in the middle-*jiao* and the impairment of spleen and stomach by overstrain or abnormal ingestion.

Key Points

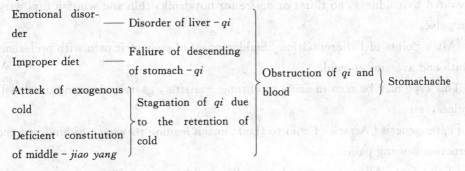

Diagnosis and Discrimination

Regular or sudden pain appearing between the pit of stomach and the umbilicus, including distending pain, pinching pain, dull pain and severe pain, is the main symptom of stomachache. It is often accompanied with some symptoms of the functional disorder of spleen and stomach such as feeling of fullness and distension over the epigastrium and abdomen, acid regurgitation and eructation with fetid odour, nausea, vomiting, no desire for eating, dry stool or loose stool as well as some general symptoms such as lassitude, sallow complexion, emaciation and edema.

Stomachache should be distinguished from angina pectoris, abdominal pain and hypochondriac pain. Angina pectoris, which is characterized by sudden onset of severe or pinching or suffocative pain, is a serious case of chest pain and appears in the left chest. The symptoms and prognosis of it are completlely different from those of stomachache. The position of abdominal pain is somewhat different from that of stomachache. It involves the whole part between epigastrium and the pubic bone. Since stomach lies in abdomen and connects with intestines, therefore, stomachache may involve abdomen and abdominal pain may also involve stomach in very few specific cases. So, they should be distinguished from each other. Distending pain lying in one or two sides of hypochondriac region is the main symptom of hypochondriac pain, which is helpful to differentiation.

Selecting Treatment by Differentiating Syndromes

In clinic, stomachache can be classified into deficiency syndrome and excess syndrome.

Deficiency syndrome —— Slow onset, prolonged course, mild pain, preference for pressing

Excess syndrome—— Acute onset, short course, severe pain, refusal of pressing

Common Types:

1. Attack of cold pathogen to the stomach

[Symptoms] Sudden onset of epigastric pain which can be alleviated by warmth and aggravated by coldness, no thirst or desire for hot drink, thin and whitish fur, wiry and tense pulse.

[Main Points of Differentiation] Sudden onset of epigastric pain with preference for warmth and aversion to cold.

This type may be seen in acute or chronic gastritis, gastric ulcer and duodenal bulbar ulcer, etc.

[Pathogenesis] Attack of cold to the stomach leading to *yang-qi* hindered and the obstruction causing pain.

[Treatment] Alleviating pain by expelling cold.

[Recipe] Warm local area or take decocted ginger water infused with brown sugar for mild cases; use modified *Liang Fu Wan*[139] for severe cases; if ineffective, use *Ban Xia Hou Pu Tang*[93]; in case of being accompanied with food stagnation, add *Fructus Aurantii Immaturus*, *Massa Fermentata Medicinals* and *Endothelium Corneum Gigeriae*

Galli to relieve dyspepsia.

[Nursing Points] Avoid raw and cold food. Eat ginger and brown sugar, etc. which can warm the stomach.

2. Stagnation of food

[Symptoms] Distention feeling over the the epigastrium, even epigastric pain, eructation with fetid odour and acid regurgitation, vomiting of indigested food, pain alleviated after vomiting, or unsmooth defecation, thick and greasy fur, slippery pulse.

[Main Points of Differentiation] Feeling of fullness and distention over the epigastrium, no appetite, eructation with fetid odour and acid regurgitation.

This type is commonly seen in acute gastritis, gastroduodenal ulcer.

[Pathogenesis] Retention of undigested food in stomach and intestines leading to the functional disorder of *qi* and blocking transportation.

[Treatment] Relieving dyspepsia.

[Recipe] *Bao He Wan*[193] with *Fructus Aurantii Immaturus*, *Semen Arecae*, etc.

If ineffective, use *Xiao Cheng Qi Tang*[29] with *Radix Aucklandiae*, *Rhizoma Cyperi*, etc; in case of the generation of fire caused by the stagnation of food after the attack of cold, manifested as acute onset of epigastric pain, accompanied with yellowish fur, constipation, or fever, add *Natrii Sulfas* to pruge heat and indigestion.

[Nursing Points] Eating less and light food.

3. Deficiency-cold of spleen and stomach

[Symptoms] Dull pain over the epigastrium, vomiting of watery fluid, preference for warmth and pressure, cold hands and feet, loose stool, pale tongue with whitish fur, weak or deep and thready pulse.

[Main Points of Differentiation] Dull pain with preference for warmth and pressure.

This type may be seen in gastroduodenal ulcer, etc.

[Pathogenesis] Deficiency-cold of the spleen and stomach leading to the retention of fluid.

[Treatment] Expelling cold by warming middle-*jiao*.

[Recipe] *Huang Qi Jian Zhong Tang*[235].

In case of acid regurgitation, add *Fructus Euodiae* to warm liver and stomach, and relieve gastric hyperacidity, besides, *Concha Arcae* may be added; in case of vomiting of much thin fluid, add *Rhizoma Zingiberis*, *Pericarpium Citri Reticulatae*, *Rhizoma Pinelliae*, *Poria*, etc. to warm stomach and relieve the fluid-retention; in case of severe pain with vomiting and cold limbs caused by excessive cold, use *Da Jian Zhong Tang*[20] to warm and invigorate middle-*jiao qi*, or use *Li Zhong Wan*[229] to expell cold by warming middle - *jiao*. Therefore, middle - *jiao yang* functions normal, cold and all the symptoms disappear.

[Nursing Points] Avoid raw and cold food, and cold - dampness.

4. Hyperactive liver - *qi* attacking stomach

[Symptoms] Feeling of distention and oppression over the epigastrium, wandering pain radiating to the hypochondriac region, frequent belching, unsoomth defecation, which is usually induced by emotional upset, thin and whitish tongue fur, deep and wiry pulse.

[Main Points of Differentiation] Distending and wandering pain over the epigastrium radiating to the hypochondriac region, and related to emotional changes.

This type is commonly seen in gastroneurosis, and chronic gastritis.

[Pathogenesis] Stagnated liver - *qi* caused by emotional upset attacking the stomach.

[Treatment] Dispersing the stagnated liver - *qi*.

[Recipe] *Chai Hu Shu Gan San*[211].

Radix Curcumae, *Pericarpium Citri Reticulatae Viride* and *Radix Aucklandiae*, etc. may be chosen to strengthen the effect of regulating the functional activities of *qi* and relieving mental depression.

In case of severe pain, add *Fructus Meliae Toosendan*, *Rhizoma Corydalis* to strengthen the effect of promoting the circulation of *qi* and relieving pain; in case of frequent belching, add *Lignum Aquilariae Resinatum*, *Flos Inulae* to keep the adverse - rising *qi* downwards or use *Chen Xiang Jiang Qi San*[136].

[Nursing Points] Regulate emotions and avoid irritation.

5. Accumulation of heat in the liver and stomach

[Symptoms] Acute burning pain over the epigastrium, irritability, acid regurgitation, gastric upset, dryness and bitter taste in the mouth, red tongue with yellowish fur, wiry or rapid pulse.

[Main Points of Differentiation] Burning pain over the epigastrium, gastric upset, irritability, dryness and bitter taste in the mouth.

This type is commonly seen in gastritis, gastroduodenal ulcer and prolapse of gastric mucosa.

[Pathogenesis] Heat attacking the stomach and rushing up, caused by prolonged stagnation of liver - *qi*.

[Treatment] Clearing away heat in the liver and stomach, regulating the stomach and relieving pain.

[Recipe] *Hua Gan Jian*[49].

Zuo Jin Wan[67] may be added to disperse the stagnation with drugs of acrid taste and clear away fire with drugs of bitter taste. Endogenous heat is most likely to consume *yin* fluid, so, those drugs which can relieve pain by eliminating stagnation of *qi* and regulate the functional activities of *qi* but not impair *yin* - fluid, such as *Fructus Citri*, *Fructus Citri Sarcodactylis* and *Flos Mume Albus*, etc. may be added.

[Nursing Points] Avoid pungent and greasy food.

6. Retention of blood stasis

[Symptoms] Localized stabbing pain and tenderness over the epigastrium which is more severe after eating, or vomiting of blood, defecating of dark feces, dark purplish tongue, uneven pulse.

[Main Points of Differentiation] Localized or stabbing pain over the epigastrium.

This type may be seen in carcinoma of stomach, gastric ulcer, prolapse of gastric mucosa.

[Pathogenesis] Prolonged stagnation of functional activities of *qi* leading to the retention of blood stasis, further resulting in the impairment of stomach collaterals and pain.

[Treatment] Dredging the collaterals by dissipating blood stasis, regulating *qi* and stomach.

[Recipe] *Shi Xiao San*[86] with *Dan Shen Yin*[51].

In case of vomiting of blood, dark stools caused by bleeding, exclude *Lignum Santali*, *Fructus Amomi* and add charred *Radix Rubiae*, *Radix Notoginseng* and *Lignum Dalbergiae Odoriferae*, etc. to stop bleeding by eliminating the blood stasis.

[Nursing Points] Take easily digested food. Avoid raw and cold food or overeating.

7. Stomach *yin* - deficiency

[Symptoms] Dull pain over the epigastrium, dry mouth and throat, dry stools, red tongue with little saliva, thready and rapid pulse.

[Main Points of Differentiation] Dull pain, dry mouth and throat, red tongue with little saliva.

This type may be seen in chronic atrophic gastritis.

[Pathogenesis] Prolonged stomachache will cause *yin* - deficiency and *qi* stagnation, and lack of nutrients in the stomach - collaterals and the disturbance of deficiency heat internally.

[Treatment] Benefiting stomach by nourishing stomach - *yin*.

[Recipe] *Yi Guan Jian*[1] with *Shao Yao Gan Cao Tang*[108].

Fructus Citri, *Fructus Citri Sarcodactylis* and *Flos Mume Albus* may be chosen to regulate *qi* and relieve pain. In case of gastric upset or acid regurgitation, add *Zuo Jin Wan*[67] to relieve gastric hyperacidity and regulate stomach; in case of gastric acidity obviously reduced, add *Fructus Mume*, *Fructus Chebulae* accordingly to strengthen the effect of nourishing *yin* with sour and sweet drugs; for the case with constipation, add *Fructus Cannabis*, *Semen Trichosanthis* to moisturize the intestine and ralex the bowels.

[Nursing Points] Eat easily digested food. Avoid pungent, greasy, raw and cold, coarse and hard food. Have more meals a day but less food at each.

Summary

Stomachache	Cold syndrome — Attack of cold to stomach	Expelling cold and alleviating pain	*Liang Fu Wan*
	Heat syndrome — Accumulation of heat in liver and stomach	Clearing away the heat in liver and stomach, regulating stomach and relieving pain	*Hua Gan Jian*
	Deficiency syndrome — Deficiency cold of spleen and stomach	Warming middle-*jiao* to expel cold	*Huang Qi Jian Zhong Tang*
	Deficiency syndrome — Deficiency of stomach-*yin*	Nourishing stomach-*yin* and regulating *qi*	*Yi Guan Jian* with *Shao Yao Gan Cao Tang*
	Excess syndrome — Stagnation of food	Relieving dyspepsia	*Bao He Wan*
	Excess syndrome — Hyperactivity of liver-*qi* attacking stomach	Dispersing the stagnated liver-*qi*	*Chai Hu Shu Gan San*
	Excess syndrome — Retention of blood stasis	Dredging the collaterals by dissipating blood stasis, regulating *qi* and stomach	*Shi Xiao San* with *Dan Shen Yin*

Discussions

1. What is the difference between stomachache and angina pectoris?

2. What are the main etiology and pathogenesis of stomachache?

3. How do you differentiate and treat the syndromes of liver-*qi* attacking stomach and asthenia-cold of spleen and stomach?

19 Vomiting

General

Vomiting is a morbid condition with symptom of forcible expulsion of the contents of the stomach through the mouth caused by the adverse rising of stomach - qi.

Vomiting may appear separately and may also be seen in many kinds of acute or chronic diseases.

The treatment by differentiating syndromes of the disease is referential to acute or chronic gastritis, peptic ulcer, neurogenic vomiting, otogenic vomiting, psychogenic vomiting and other disease with the symptom of vomiting in Western Medicine.

Etiology and Pathogenesis

1. **Attack of exogenous evils** Vomiting resulting from food going up along with the adverse - rising stomach - qi due to wind, cold, summer - heat, dampness and filthy evils attacking stomach.

2. **Improper diet** Vomiting caused by the failure of stomach - qi in descending due to overeating or the retention of undigested greasy, raw and cold food; or by the adverse rising of phlegm and fluid in the epigastrium due to the failure of transformation of food into refined materials, resulting from the dysfunction of the spleen and stomach in transportation and transformation.

3. **Emotional disorder** Anxiety, worry and anger often causes the dysfunction of the liver. When the stomach is affected, vomiting occurs as the result of the rising of food along with the adversed stomach - qi.

4. **Deficiency of spleen and stomach** Vomiting caused by the retention of cold turbid evil in middle - *jiao* due to the deficiency of middle - *jiao yang* and deficiency of the spleen and the stomach after illness; or by the deficiency of stomach - *yin* which fails to nourish the stomach and the failure of stomach - qi in descending.

Key Points:

Attack of exopathogens
Internal damage caused by seven emotions
Improper diet
Overstrain
} Stomach - qi adversely rising instead of descending } Vomiting

Diagnosis and Discrimination

Any disease chiefly manifested as vomiting may refer to the differentiation and treatment herein.

Vomiting, regurgitation and hiccup all belong to the pathological changes of the adverse rising of stomach *qi*. So, they should be distinguished. Vomiting is the morbid condition of something cast out of the mouth with sound; regurgitation refers to the morbid condition of something eaten in the morning and vomited at night or vice versa, or indigested food vomited after being taken for a long time. Hiccup is the condition of repeated, frequent and short characteristic sound coming from the throat which can not be controlled.

Selecting Treatment by Differentiating Syndromes

Excess and deficiency syndromes of vomiting should be differentiated. Excess syndrome is mostly caused by exogenous evils and improper diet, and marked by acute onset and short course. Deficiency syndrome is commonly caused by the dysfunction of spleen and stomach, and marked by chronic onset and long course. Now they will be discussed separately as follows.

Excess - syndrome

1. Invasion of exogenous evils to stomach

[Symptoms] Sudden onset of vomiting accompanied with chilliness, fever, headache, general aching, feeling of oppression in the chest, feeling of distress and burning, epigastric pain and diarrhea, ropy and greasy mouth, whitish and greasy fur, soft - floating and moderate pu-lse.

[Main Points of Differentiation] Sudden onset of vomiting, headache and general aching or accompanied with chillness and fever.

This type is commonly seen in gastrointestinal type influenza, acute gastritis, cholecystitis and pancreatitis.

[Pathogenesis] Attack of exogenous evils to the stomach leading to the functional disorder of *qi*, and the adverse rising of turbid *qi*.

[Treatment] Expelling superficial evils and relieving exterior syndrome, eliminating turbid - evil with drugs of fragrant flavour.

[Recipe] *Huo Xiang Zheng Qi San*[288].

In case of being accompanied with retention of indigested food, manifested as feeling of oppression over the chest and abdominal distension, exclude *Rhizoma Atractylodis Macrocephalae*, *Radix Glycyrrhizae* and *Fructus Ziziphi Jujubae*, add *Endothelium Corneum Gigeriae Galli* and *Massa Fermentata Medicinals* to relieve dyspepsia; in case of predomination by superficial evil, manifested as chillness, fever, anhidrosis, add *Radix*

Ledebouriellae and *Herba Schizonepetae*, etc. to relieve exterior syndrome by expelling wind; in case of vomiting accompanied with restlessness and thirst caused by the affection of summer-heat dampness, exclude sweet taste and warm natured drugs and add *Rhizoma Coptidis*, *Herba Eupatorii* and *Folium Nelumbinis*, etc. to clear away summer-heat evil; in case of being affected by filthy evil, take *Yu Shu Dan*[60] first to stop vomiting by removing filthy evil.

[Nursing Points] Avoid raw and cold, fat and sweet food and the attack of wind-cold evil.

2. Retention of food

[Symptoms] Vomiting of sour and putrid content, feeling of fullness and distension over the epigastrium and abdomen, pain with aversion to pressure, belching and anorexia, which become severe after taking food and get relieved after vomiting, loose stool or dry stool, thick and greasy fur, slippery and replete pulse.

[Main Points of Differentiation] Vomiting of sour and putrid content, belching and anorexia.

This type is commonly seen in acute gastritis and pylorochesis.

[Pathogenesis] Retention of food leading to the disorder of transportation and transformation, and the obstruction of the functional activities of *qi* resulting in the adverse rising of turbid *qi*.

[Treatment] Relieving dyspepsia, regulating stomach and lowering the adverse-rising *qi*.

[Recipe] *Bao He Wan*[193].

In case of much indigested food, manifested as fullness of abdomen and constipation, add *Radix et Rhizoma Rhei* and *Fructus Aurantii Immaturus* to relieve dyspepsia, and make *fu* unobstructed enabling the turbid *qi* to go down to stop vomiting. In case of vomiting immediately after eating, halitosis and thirst, yellowish fur, rapid pulse caused by the rushing up of heat accumulation in stomach, use *Zhu Ru Tang*[118] to clear away the heat in stomach and lower the adverse-rising *qi*.

[Nursing Points] Eat less and vegetable food.

3. Retention of phlegm and fluid

[Symptoms] Vomiting of thin and mucous fluid, fullness of epigastrium, loos of appetite, dizziness, palpitation, whitish and greasy fur, slippery pulse.

[Main Points of Differentiation] Vomiting of thin and mucous fluid, dizziness and palpitation.

This type is commonly seen in chronic gastritis, pylorochesis and auditory vertigo.

[Pathogenesis] Dysfunction of the spleen in transportation and transformation leading to the retention of phlegm and fluid, resulting in the failure of stomach-*qi* in descending and the adverse rising of turbid fluid.

[Treatment] Invigorating spleen and warming middle – *jiao*; eliminating fluid retention, lowering adverse – rising *qi*.

[Recipe] *Xiao Ban Xia Tang*[26].

In case of vomiting of much fluid and mucous, add *Semen Pharbitidis*, and *Semen Sinapis Albae* 2g which are grained into powder and filled into capsules, and taken in three separate doses a day to strengthen the effect of resolving phlegm and fluid retention. In case of stomach – *qi* unable to descend caused by the accumulation of phlegm – heat in the stomach, manifested as dizziness, upset, insomnia, nausea and vomiting, etc., use *Wen Dan Tang*[270] to clear away gallbladder heat and regulate stomach, eliminate phlegm and relieve vomiting.

[Nursing Points] Eat light food. Avoid fat and sweet, raw and cold food. Stop smoking and drinking alcohol. Keep proper balance between work and rest to avoid recurrence.

4. Attack of liver – *qi* to stomach

[Symptoms] Vomiting, acid regurgitation, frequent belching, feeling of oppression and pain in the chest and hypochondrium which can be aggravated by depression and anger, redness of tongue margin, thin and greasy fur, wiry pulse.

[Main Points of Differentiation] Vomiting and acid regurgitation, belching, hypochondric pain which is often related to the emotional changes.

This type may be seen in acute or chronic gastritis, gastro – duodenal bulbar ulcer and psychogenic vomiting, etc.

[Pathogenesis] The stagnated liver – *qi* attacking the stomach resulting in the failure of stomach – *qi* in descending.

[Treatment] Dispersing the stagnated liver – *qi* and regulating stomach, lowering adverse – rising *qi* and relieving vomiting.

[Recipe] *Ban Xia Hou Pu Tang*[93] and *Zuo Jin Wan*[67] with modification.

In case of being accompanied with bitter taste in the mouth, gastric upset and constipation, add slight *Radix et Rhizoma Rhei* and *Fructus Aurantii Immaturus* to relax bowels and lower turbid *qi*; in case of severe heat – syndrome, add *Caulis Bambusae in Taeniam* and *Fructus Aurantii Immaturus* to clear away the liver – fire.

[Nursing Points] Keep a good mood and avoid emotional irritation.

Deficiency – syndrome

1. Deficiency – cold of spleen and stomach

[Symptoms] Epigastric distension after eating a little bit more, even nausea and vomiting, lassitude, dry mouth but no desire for drinking, preference for warmth and intolerance to cold, pale complexion, even cold extremities, loose stool, pale tongue with whitish and greasy fur, soft – floating and weak pulse.

[Main Points of Differentiation] Vomiting induced immediately after eating little unsuitable food, cold extremities, loose stool.

This type is commonly seen in chronic gastritis and peptic ulcer.

[Pathogenesis] Dysfunction of the spleen and stomach leading to deficiency of middle - *jiao yang* and the functional disorder of transportation and transformation.

[Treatment] Invigorating spleen by warming middle - *jiao* and lowering adverse rising *qi* by regulating stomach.

[Recipe] *Li Zhong Wan*[229].

Fructus Amomi, *Rhizoma Pinelliae* and *Pericarpium Citri Reticulatae*, etc. may be added to regulate the circulation of *qi* and lower adverse - rising *qi*. In case of incessant vomiting, add *Fructus Euodiae* to relieve vomiting by warming middle - *jiao*, and lowering adverse - rising *qi*.

[Nursing Points] Have more meals a day but less food at each, and avoid raw and cold food.

2. Deficiency of stomach - *yin*

[Symptoms] Recurrence of vomiting and sometimes retching, dry mouth and throat, seeming hunger but no desire for eating, reddish tongue with little saliva, thready and rapid pulse.

[Main Points of Differentiation] Retching, dry mouth and throat, reddish tongue with little saliva.

This type may be seen in chronic atrophic gastritis, pylorochesis and psychogenic vomiting, etc.

[Pathogenesis] The lack of nourishment in the stomach and the failure of stomach - *qi* in descending caused by stomach - *yin* being consumed by heat evil uncleared away in the stomach.

[Treatment] Nourishing stomach - *yin*, relieving vomiting by lowering adverse - rising *qi*.

[Recipe] *Mai Men Dong Tang*[124].

In case of severe impairment of body fluid, reduce the amount of *Hizoma Pinelliae*, use *Radix Adenophorae Strictae* to replace *Radix Ginseng*, and add *Herba Dendrobii*, *Radix Trichosanthis*, *Caulis Bambusae in Taeniam* and *Rhizoma Anemarrhenae*, etc. to promote the production of body fluid and nourish stomach - *yin*; in case of dry and hard stool, add *Fructus Cannabis* and *Semen Trichosanthis*, etc. to moisten the intestines and relax bowels.

[Nursing Points] Avoid eating sweet, greasy, pungent and dry - natured food and avoid smoking, and drinking alcohol.

Summary

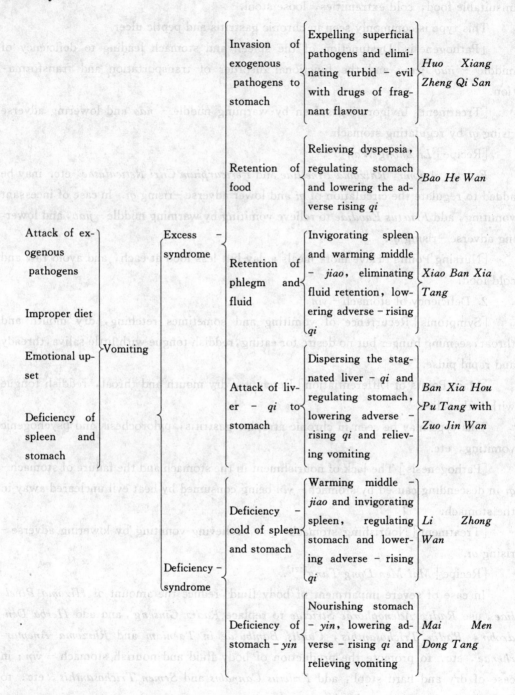

Discussions

1. Please relate the etiology and pathogenesis of vomiting.
2. What are the common types of vomiting? Try to relate the main symptoms, therapeutic principles, recipes of each type.

20 Hiccup

General

Hiccup is a morbid state characterized by uncontrolled, frequent and short sound coming from throat caused by the adverse rising *qi*.

It is usually seen in gastrointestinal neurosis by Western Medicine. The treatment by differentiating syndromes of the disease may serve as a reference to the hiccup caused by some diseases located in esophagus, stomach, intestines, peritoneum, mediastinum and brain.

Etiology and Pathogenesis

1. Improper diet   Hiccup caused by cold staying in middle - *jiao* and stomach - *yang* hindered due to overeating of cold and raw food or overtaking of cool and cold - natured drugs; or by internal exuberance of dryness and heat resulting from overeating of pungent food or overtaking of warm and dry - natured drugs.

2. Emotional upset   Hiccup resulting from mental irritation or emotional upset which leads to stagnation of *qi* and its convertion into fire which, in turn, attacks the stomach; or from prolonged retention of phlegm and undigested food which turn to heat, and result in stomach - *qi* unable to descend.

3. Insufficiency of vital energy   Hiccup resulting from consumption of middle - *jiao qi* or impairment of stomach - *yin* after severe or prolonged illness or caused by misuse of emetic or purgatives. In case of pathologic changes involving the kidney, the hiccup is often caused by the adverse rising *qi* of the *Chong* Channel with stomach - *qi* irritating the diaphrogm, which results from the dysfunction of kidney in receptivity.

Key Points:

Improper diet
Emotinal depression } Pathogens attacking stomach
Deficiency of vital *qi* —— Deficiency - *qi* rising adversely
} The adverse rising of stomach - *qi* —— Hiccup

Diagnosis and Discrimination

The cases with uncontrolled, frequent sound from the throat caused by the adverse - rising *qi* can be diagnosed as hiccup. Hiccup, retch and belch are all caused by the adverse rising of stomach - *qi*, but their characteristics are different. Retch is characterized by only sound of vomiting without anything but saliva. Its long, deep and thick sound is different from the frequent, uncontrolled and short sound of hiccup. Belch refers to the condition with fullness and distension in the chest and epigastrium which is caused by the stagnation of *qi* in middle – *jiao* and alleviated after belching, sometimes accompanied with food or acid and putrid odour.

Selecting Treatment by Differentiating Syndromes

In differentiating hiccup, deficiency syndrome, excess syndrome, cold syndrome and heat syndrome should be distinguished. Continuous, loud and strong sound of hiccup at the beginning of a disease usually belongs to excess syndrome. Intermittent, low and weak sound of hiccup mostly belongs to deficiency syndrome. The condition of hiccup aggravated by coldness and alleviated by warmth, manifested as cold feeling over the epigastrium and whitish fur on the tongue, usually belongs to cold syndrome. The case with symptoms of halitosis, polydispia, costipation, red tongue with yellowish fur usually belongs to heat syndrome.

Common Types:

Excess syndrome

1. Retention of cold in the stomach

[Symptoms] Deep, slow and strong sound of hiccup, uncomfortable sensation over the epigastrium which can be alleviated by warmth and aggravated by coldness, poor appetite, no thirst, whitish and moist fur on the tongue, slow, moderate pulse.

[Main Points of Differentiation] Deep, slow and strong sound of hiccup which can be alleviated by warmth and aggravated by coldness.

This type is commonly seen in gastrointestinal neurosis, esophagitis, gastritis.

[Pathogenesis] Retention of cold leads to the adverse rising of stomach – *qi*.

[Treatment] Expelling cold by warming middle – *jiao*, smoothing hiccup by lowering the adverse – rising *qi*.

[Recipe] *Ding Xiang San*[7].

In case of cold predomination, *Cortex Cinnamomi*, *Fructus Euodiae* may be added to lower the adverse – rising *qi* by warming *yang* and expelling cold. In case of fullness sensation over the epigastrium and eructation with foul odour caused by the retention of phlegm and indigested food, add *Cortex Magnoliae Officinalis*, *Fructus Aurantii Immaturus*, *Pericarpium Citi Reticulatae* to promote the circulation of *qi*, eliminate phlegm and stagnated food.

[Nursing Points] Don't eat raw and cold food or drink cold beverage. Avoid attack of wind – cold.

2. Rising up of stomach – fire

[Symptoms] Continuous, strong and sonorous sound of hiccup which rushes out of the mouth, halitosis, polydispia, deep – coloured urine, constipation, yellowish fur, slippery and rapid pulse.

[Main Points of Differentiation] Sonorous sound of hiccup, halitosis, polydispia, deep-coloured urine, costipation.

This type is commonly seen in gastritis and gastrectasia.

[Pathogenesis] The retention of phlegm and undigested food in stomach for a long time leading to the generation and rising up of stomach-fire.

[Treatment] Clearing away stomach-fire, lowering adverse-rising qi to stop hiccup.

[Recipe] *Zhu Ye Shi Gao Tang*[116] with *Calyx Kaki*, *Caulis Bambusae in Taeniam*.

In case of constipation, feeling of fullness and oppression in the epigastrium and abdomen, *Xiao Cheng Qi Tang*[29] is used in combination to eliminate heat by making *fu-qi* normal. After *fu-qi* gets unblocked, stomach-qi can desend normally. As a result, hiccup stops naturally.

[Nursing Points] Avoid pungent or fried food.

3. Stagnation of *qi*

[Symptoms] Continuous sound of hiccup which is often induced or aggravated by emotional upset, accompanied with oppression feeling in the chest, poor appetite, feeling of distention and oppression over the epigastrium and the hypochondrium, increased borborygmus, wind from bowels, thin and whitish fur, wiry pulse.

[Main Points of Differentiation] Continuous sound of hiccup which is often induced and aggravated by emotional upset.

This type is commonly seen in hysteria, gastritis.

[Pathogenesis] Emotional depression causing liver-qi to attack stomach, thus resulting in the adverse rising of stomach-qi.

[Treatment] Lowering the adverse-rising qi, regulating the stomach to stop hiccup.

[Recipe] *Wu Mo Yin Zi*[43].

On the basis of the above recipe, add *Flos Syzygii Aromatici*, *Ochra* to stop hiccup by lowering the adverse-rising qi and add *Fructus Meliae Toosendan*, *Radix Curcumae* to alleviate mental depression by dispersing the stagnated liver-qi. In case of fire-syndrome caused by the stagnation of qi, manifested as upset, constipation, bitter taste in the mouth, red tongue, wiry and rapid pulse, add *Fructus Gardeniae*, *Rhizoma Coptidis*, etc. to clear away liver-fire and regulate stomach-qi. In case of the adverse rising of qi and the retention of phlegm, manifested as dizziness, blurring vision, sometimes nausea, thin and greasy fur, wiry and slipery pulse, use *Xuan Fu Dai Zhe Tang*[244] or *Er Chen Tang*[2] modified to lower the adverse-rising qi, eliminate phlegm and regulate the stomach.

[Nursing Points] Avoid mental irritation. Keep a good mood.

Deficiency - syndrome

1. *Yang* deficiency of spleen and stomach

[Symptoms] Uncontinuous, low and week sound of hiccup, pale complexion, cold hands and feet, poor appetite, feeling of distention over the epigastrium, lassitude, pale tongue with whitish fur, deep and thready pulse.

[Main Points of Differentiation] Low and weak sound of hiccup, cold hands and feet, poor appetite, distending feeling in the epigastrium.

This type may be seen in urinaemia, advanced carcinoma of stomach, etc.

[Pathogenesis] Dysfunction of the spleen and stomach leading to the disorder of ascending and descending and the adverse rising of deficiency - *qi*.

[Treatment] Invigorating and warming spleen and stomach, regulating middle - *jiao* and lowering adverse - rising *qi*.

[Recipe] *Li Zhong Tang*[229] with *Fructus Euodiae* and *Flos Syzygii Aromatici*.

In case of incessant hiccup, epigastric fullness and rigidity, *Xuan Fu Dai Zhe Tang*[244] is used in combination to regulate middle - *jiao* and lower adverse - rising *qi* with sedatives with heavy material (such as minerals, shells); in case of being accompanied with the deficiency of kidney - *yang*, manifested as chilliness, cold extremities, soreness and weakness in the loins and knees, swollen and tender tongue, sunken and slow pulse, add *Radix Aconiti Praeparata*, and *Cortex Cinnamomi* to warm the kidney and support *yang*; in case of being accompanied with food stagnation, add small amount of *Pericarpium Citri Reticulatae*, *Fructus Hordei Germinatus* to promote the circulation of *qi* and remove food stagnation; in case of severe deficiency of middle - *jiao qi*, manifested as uncontinuous, low and weak sound of hiccup, poor appetite, loose stool, lassitude, feeble pulse, use *Bu Zhong Yi Qi Tang*[140] suitably.

[Nursing Points] Avoid greasy, raw and cold food. Take decocted ginger water infused with brown sugar or have some pieces of ginger in the mouth usually. Keep warm.

2. Deficiency of stomach - *yin*

[Symptoms] Uncontinuous, short and hasty sound of hiccup, dry mouth and tongue, restlessness, red and dry tongue or with fissure, thready and rapid pulse.

[Main Points of Differentiation] Short and hasty sound of hiccup, dry mouth and tongue, red and dry tongue.

This type may be seen in cerebritis, cerebroma, cerebral hemorrhage, gastrointestinal neurosis, urinaemia, intestinal obstruction, etc.

[Pathogenesis] Febrile disease or overusing diaphoresis and emetic therapy leading to the deficiency of body fluid, the lack of nourishment in the stomach and the failure of stomach - *qi* in descending.

[Treatment] Nourishing the stomach and promoting the production of body fluid, regulating stomach and stopping hiccup.

[Recipe] *Yi Wei Tang*[217].

Folium Eriobotryae, *Herba Dendrobii*, *Calyx Kaki* may be added to the above recipe to lower the adverse-rising *qi* and stop hiccup. In case of severe deficiency of stomach -*qi*, manifested as no desire for eating, *Ju Pi Zhu Ru Tang*[286] is used in combination to benifit *qi* and regulate middle - *jiao*.

[Nursing Points] Eat light, sweet and cold-natured food such as mung bean tea, lotus root powder, pear juice; avoid drinking alcohol, smoking cigarettes and eating pungent food such as onion, garlic, (Chinese) chives, hot pepper, etc.

Summary

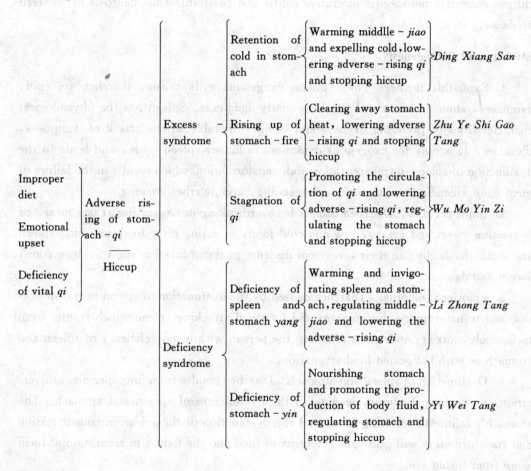

Discussions

1. What are the characteristics of deficiency, excess, cold, heat syndromes of hiccup?

2. How many types are the pathogenesis of hiccup divided into?

3. How many common types are there in the excess-syndrome of hiccup? How do you differentiate and treat them?

21 Diarrhea

General

Diarrhea refers to the morbid state marked by increased frequency and liquidity, even watery fecal discharge.

The treatment by differentiating syndromes of the disease is applicable to acute or chronic enteritis, nonspecific ulcerative colitis and gastrointestinal neurosis in Western Medicine.

Etiology and Pathogenesis

1. Exopathic factors The common exogenous evils causing diarrhea are cold, dampness, summer – heat and fire, especially dampness. Spleen has the physiological characterisitics of prefering dryness and being vulnerable to the attack of dampness, therefore, it is easy for exogenous dampness to impair spleen – yang and leads to the dysfunction of spleen in transportation and transformation, which results in the failure of lucid yang ascending and turbid yin descending, and diarrhea ensuing.

2. Improper diet Diarrhea caused by overdrinking or overeating at one meal, or overeating sweet and greasy, raw and cold food, or eating dirty food impairing spleen and stomach, leading to their functional disorder in transportation and transformation, ascent and descent.

3. Emotional disorder Diarrhea caused by the dysfunction of spleen in transportation and transformation due to stagnated liver – qi attacking spleen which results from melancholy, anxiety and terror affecting the person with usual deficiency of spleen and stomach or with indigested food stagnation.

4. Dysfunction of spleen and stomach Diarrhea results from improper diet or overstrain, or prolonged illness, leading to the dysfunction of spleen and stomach. The stomach's failure in receiving food, and the dysfunction of the spleen in transportation and transformation will cause the retention of food and the failure in separation of lucid yang from turbid yin.

5. Deficiency of kidney – yang Diarrhea resulting from the disorder of transportation and transformation due to the failure in warming the spleen, which is caused by the deficiency of kidney – yang after prolonged illness or because of old age.

Key Points:

```
Exogenous cause  { Impairment of the spleen caused by excessive dampness }  } Functional disorder
                                                                              of spleen in trans-  } Diarrhea
Endogenous cause { Retention of dampness caused by the dysfunction of spleen } portation and trans-
                                                                              fomation
```

Diagnosis and Discrimination

Diarrhea is characterized by increased frequency and liquidity of fecal discharge, which can occur in any season of a year, especially in summer and autumn.

The pathology of both diarrhea and dysentery occur in the instestines. Either of them has abdominal pain and abnormal defecation. So, they should be distinguished from each other.

Discrimination \ Disease	Diarrhea	Dysentery
Stool	Loose stool, even watery stool, smooth defecating	Unsmooth defecating of bloody and purulent stool
Abdominal pain	Having or not having; accompanied with distending feeling over the epigastrium, borborygmus, paroxysmal, disappearing after diarrhea	Definitely having; accompanied with tenesmus, persistent, still being or reduced after defecating
Feces examination	Usually no obviously abnormal, or a small amount of red blood cells, white blood cells and pus cells may be seen	A great amount of red blood cells and pus cells can be seen

Selecting Treatment by Differentiating Syndromes

After establishing diagnosis, differentiation should be carried out. Cold, heat, deficiency and excess type should be distinguished from one another at first.

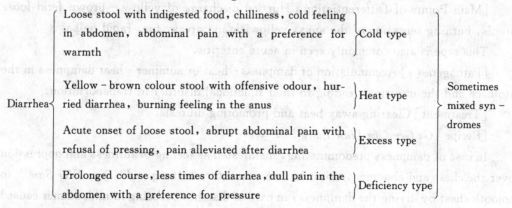

```
         { Loose stool with indigested food, chilliness, cold feeling
         { in abdomen, abdominal pain with a preference for   } Cold type
         { warmth
         { Yellow-brown colour stool with offensive odour, hur-                  } Sometimes
Diarrhea { ried diarrhea, burning feeling in the anus         } Heat type       } mixed syn-
         { Acute onset of loose stool, abrupt abdominal pain with                 dromes
         { refusal of pressing, pain alleviated after diarrhea } Excess type
         { Prolonged course, less times of diarrhea, dull pain in the
         { abdomen with a preference for pressure              } Deficiency type
```

Common Types

1. Attack of exogenous evils

(1) Cold-dampness blocking the spleen

[Symptoms] Thin stool, even watery stool, abdominal pain, borborygmus, fullness sensation over the epigastrium, poor appetite, sometimes accompanied with chilliness, fever, stuffy nose, headache, aching pain of limbs, pale tongue, thin and whitish or whitish and greasy fur, soft and floating, and moderate pulse.

[Main Points of Differentiation] Thin and loose stool, abdominal pain with borborygmus.

This type is commonly seen in acute enteritis.

[Pathogenesis] Cold-dampness stagnating in superficies and attacking the stomach and the intestines leading to functional disorder of the spleen in transportation and transformation, ascent and descent.

[Treatment] Eliminating dampness with drugs of fragrant flavour, expelling cold evil to relieve superficies-syndrome.

[Recipe] *Huo Xiang Zheng Qi San*[288].

In case of superficies-syndrome predominating caused by cold-dampness, add *Herba Schizonepetae*, *Radix Ledebouriellae*, *Rhizoma Seu Radix Notopterygil*, *Radix Angelicae Pubescentis* and *Fructus Viticis*; for the case of distention and fullness of chest and abdomen, lassitude, whitish and greasy fur caused by dampness predominating, increase the amount of *Rhizoma Atractylodis*, *Cortex Magnoliae Officinalis* and *Poria*, or use *Wei Ling Tang*[182]; in case of watery stool, add *Semen Plantaginis* and *Rhizoma Alismatis* to remove wetness.

[Nursing Points] Avoid eating raw and cold food and being attacked by wind-cold.

(2) Accumulation of dampness-heat

[Symptoms] Diarrhea with abdominal pain, hurried discharge of yellow-brown and fetid stool, or difficulty in defecating, burning sensation of the anus, dysphoria with thirst, oliguria with yellow urine; red tongue with yellowish and greasy fur, soft and floating and rapid pulse or slippery and rapid pulse.

[Main Points of Differentiation] Hurried discharge of yellow-brown fetid loose stools, burning sensation of the anus, yellowish and greasy fur, rapid pulse.

This type is also commonly seen in acute enteritis.

[Pathogenesis] Accumulation of dampness-heat or summer-heat dampness in the stomach and the intestines leading to their functional disorder in transportation.

[Treatment] Clearing away heat and promoting diuresis.

[Recipe] *Ge Gen Qin Lian Tang*[260].

In case of dampness predominating, manifested as feeling of fullness and oppression over the chest and abdomen, thirst but no desire for drinking, add *Ping Wei San*[70] to smooth chest by drying the dampness; in case of diarrhea occuring in midsummer caused by summer-heat dampness predominating, manifested as watery diarrhea, spontaneous presiration, dim complexion, add *Herba Agastachis*, *Herba Elsholtziae Seu Moslae*, *Testa Dolichoris*, *Folium Nelumbinis*, etc. to clear away summer-heat and eliminate dampness; in case of being accompanied with food retention, manifested as poor appetite or anorexia, add *Massa Fermentata*, *Medicinals*, *Fructus Hordei Germinatus* and *Fructus Crataegi* to relieve dyspepsia by promoting digestion.

[Nursing Points] Avoid greasy and sweet food.

(3) Retention of food in stomach and intestines

[Symptoms] Loose stools with the odour of rotten eggs accompanied with indigested food, abdominal pain relieved after diarrhea, borborygmus, feeling of fullness and oppression over the epigastrium and abdomen, eructation with acid and fetid odour, loss of appetite, dirty or thick and greasy fur, slippery pulse.

[Main Points of Differentiation] Stool with the smell of rotten eggs, eructation with acid and fetid odour, loss of appetite, thick and greasy fur, slippery pulse.

This type is commonly seen in acute enteritis.

[Pathogenesis] Retention of indigested food in the stomach and the intestines leading to the functional disorder of *qi* and transportation.

[Treatment] Promoting digestion to relieve dyspepsia.

[Recipe] *Bao He Wan*[193].

For the case of unsmooth diarrhea caused by severe food retention, use *Zhi Shi Dao Zhi Wan*[172] to relieve dyspepsia and remove dampness – heat in accordance with the principle of treating diarrhetic diseases with cathartics. This type is mostly seen in children, so, use relieving dyspepsia herbs combined with raw *Radix et Rhizoma Rhei* and *Fructus Aurantii Immaturus*, which have dredging effect, to calm and assist healthy energy by eliminating evils. Do not let evils remain and make patient's condition worse because of the delay for the fear of using purgation.

[Nursing Points] Eat less and have a vegetarian diet.

(4) Hyperactive liver – *qi* attacking the spleen

[Symptoms] Abdominal pain and diarrhea usually occur after emotional changes (depression, anger, emotional tension). Feeling of distension and oppression in the chest and hypochondria usually, eructation, poor appetite, reddish tongue, wiry pulse.

[Main Points of Differentiation] The occurrence of diarrhea is related to emotional changes, especially depression and anger. Feeling of distension in the hypochondria, wiry pulse.

This type is commonly seen in gastrointestinal neurosis and may also be seen in chronic nonspecific colitis.

[Pathogenesis] Functional disorder of the spleen in transportation and transformation caused by stagnated liver – *qi* attacking it.

[Treatment] Checking hyperfunction of the liver and strengthening the spleen.

[Recipe] *Tong Xie Yao Fang*[269].

In case of obvious stagnation of liver – *qi*, manifested as fullness and distension over the hypochondria, sighing, bitter taste in the mouth, add *Radix Bupleuri*, *Rhizoma Cyperi*, *Radix Curcumae* and *Pericarpium Citri Reticulatae Viride*, etc. accordingly to strengthen the effect of dispersing the stagnated liver – *qi* and alleviating mental depression; in case of being accompanied with eructation with fetid odour, distension in the epigastrium caused by food retention, add *Endothelium Corneum Gigeriae Galli*, *Fructus Hordei Germinatus* and *Fructus Crataegi* to relieve dyspepsia by promoting digestion.

[Nursing Points] Avoid anxiety, worry, anger and depression.

(5) Insufficiency of the spleen and stomach

[Symptoms] Sometimes loose stool and sometimes diarrhea with indigested food, increased frequency of defecating after taking little greasy food, poor appetite, feeling of uncomfort and fullness in the epigastrium and abdomen, sallow complexion, lassitude, pale tongue with whitish fur, thready and weak pulse.

[Main Points of Differentiation] Sometimes loose stool and sometimes diarrhea, sallow complexion, lassitude, prolonged course.

This type may be seen in chronic enteritis and chronic nonspecific ulcerative colitis, etc.

[Pathogenesis] Insufficiency of the spleen and stomach leading to food stagnation and the failure in separation of lucid – *yang* from turbid – *yin*.

[Treatment] Invigorating the spleen and benefiting the stomach.

[Recipe] *Shen Ling Bai Zhu San*[169].

In case of excessive *yin* – cold inside caused by the hypofunction of the spleen – *yang*, manifested as cold pain in the abdomen, cold hands and feet, use *Li Zhong Tang*[229] with *Fructus Euodiae* and *Cortex Cinnamomi* to expell cold by warming the middle – *jiao*. For the case with prolapse of rectum caused by descending of middle – *jiao qi* resulting from chronic diarrhea, *Bu Zhong Yi Qi Tang*[140] is used to benefit and lift up middle – *jiao qi* (spleen – *qi*).

[Nursing Points] Have more meals a day but less food at each. Avoid greasy, cold and raw food, and overeating.

(6) Deficiency of kidney – *yang*

[Symptoms] Diarrhea following borborygmus, commonly occurring before dawn (morning diarrhea), accompanied with abdominal pain, and relieved after diarrhea, chilliness, soreness and weakness of loins and knees, pale tongue with whitish fur, deep and thready pulse.

[Main Points of Differentiation] Morning diarrhea (cock – crowing diarrhea), intolerance of cold, soreness of loins, deep and thready pulse.

This type may be seen in chronic enteritis and chronic nonspecific colitis, etc.

[Pathogenesis] Functional disorder of the spleen in transportation and transformation caused by deficient kidney – *yang* failing to warm it.

[Treatment] Warming the kidney and invigorating the spleen, stopping diarrhea with astringent method.

[Recipe] *Si Shen Wan*[82].

Deficiency of kidney – *yang* is usually accompanied with deficiency of spleen – *yang*, so, *Si Shen Wan* with *Li Zhong Wan*[229] is often used. In case of lingering diarrhea due to the descending of middle – *jiao qi* caused by old age, suitably add *Radix Astragali Seu Hedysari*, *Radix Codonopsis Pilosulae* and *Rhizoma Atractylodis Macrocephalate* to benefit *qi* and invigorate the spleen or use *Tao Hua Tang*[205] in combination to stop diarrhea by astringent method.

[Nursing Points] Eat some warm – natured food such as parched flour and millet gruel, etc. Avoid raw and cold food.

Summary

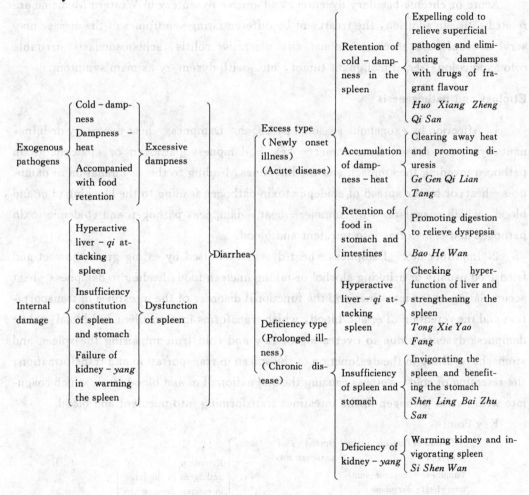

Discussions

1. How should you distinguish the cold, heat, excess and deficiency types of diarrhea in clinic?

2. How many types is diarrhea classified into? What are the key points of differentiation, therapeutic principles and recipes of each type?

3. How do you differentiate diarrhea from dysentery?

22 Dysentery

General

Dysentery is a intestinal infectious disease with frequent discharge of mucous and bloody stool, abdominal pain, tenesmus as main symptoms and commonly seen in summer and autumn.

Acute or chronic bacillary dysentery and amebic dysentery in Western Medicine are related to it. In addition, the treatment by differentiating syndromes of the disease may serve as a reference to chronic nonspecific ulcerative colitis, schistosomiasis, irritable colon and colon-rectal malignant tumor, etc. with dysentery as main symptom.

Etiology and pathogenesis

1. **Affection by exogenous seasonal pathogen** Dampness-heat dysentery or fulminant dysentery caused by summer-heat-dampness pathogen or epidemic toxin pathogen invading the stomach and the intestines, leading to the accumulation of dampness-heat; or by the spread of epidemic toxin pathogen leading to the blocking of *qi* and blood, which coagulates with summer-heat-dampness pathogen and epidemic toxin pathogen and transforms into purulent and blood.

2. **Improper diet** Dampness-heat dysentery caused by eating greasy, sweet and fried food usually or drinking alochol or taking unclean food, leading to dampness-heat accumulating in the intestines and the functional disorder of the intestines in transportation and the retention of *qi* and blood, which transforms into purulent and blood; cold-dampness dysentery due to overeating of raw and cold fruit impairing the spleen and stomach, resulting in the dysfunction of the spleen in transportation and transformation; the retention of cold-wetness causing the stagnation of *qi* and blood stasis which coagulate with putrid pathogen in the intestines transforming into purulent and blood.

Key Points:

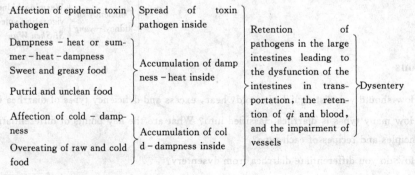

Diagnosis and Discrimination

All the conditions with increased frenquency of defecating little bloody and mucous stool, abdominal pain and tenesmus can be diagnosed as dysentery. Acute dysentery mostly occurs in summer and autumn, but chronic one can be seen in any season of a year.

The clinical manifestions of dysentery are simmilar to those of diarrhea. Both occur in the stomach and intestines. The etiology of both is difficult to be distinguished. Both of them commonly occur in summer and autumn, so, they should be distinguished from each other (the detailed content can be found in the section of Diarrhea.)

Selecting Treatment by Differentiating Syndromes

After establishing diagnosis, the differentiation should be carried on. At first, cold, heat, deficiency and excess syndromes should be distinguished.

The condition with symptoms of thin mucous and bloody stool without foul odour, pale complexion and chilliness, or dull pain in the abdomen which can be relieved by warmth and pressure, belongs to cold syndrome; the condition marked by the symptoms of obvious tenesmus, red tongue with yellowish and greasy fur, slippery and rapid pulse or soft and floating and rapid pulse, sometimes accompanied with fever and even lingering high fever, belongs to heat syndrome; the case with symptoms of tenesmus which can not be alleviated by defecating, dull pain in the abdomen which can be reduced after pressure, mostly belongs to deficiency type; the condition with symptoms of tenesmus which can get alleviated after defecating, fullness and distension of abdomen, abdominal pain with tenderness often followed by strong desire for defecating which can get temporarily reduced after defecation, mostly belongs to excess type.

Common types:

1. Dampness – heat dysentery

[Symptoms] Abdominal pain, tenesmus, discharge of purulent and bloody stool, burning sensation in the anus, oliguria with deep – coloured urine, yellowish and greasy fur, slippery and rapid pulse.

[Main Points of Differentiation] Burning sensation in the anus, oliguria with deep – coloured urine.

This type is commonly seen in acute bacillary dysentery.

[Pathogenesis] Accumulation of dampness – heat in intestines leading to the impairment of vessels, stagnation of *qi* and blood stasis, and the functional disorder of intestines in transportation.

[Treatment] Clearing away heat and relieving accumulation, regulating *qi* and promoting the circulation of blood.

[Recipe] *Shao Yao Tang*[107].

In case of being accompanied with superficies - syndrome such as chilliness, fever and headache, add *Radix Puerariae*, *Fructus*, *Forsythiae* and *Herba Schizonepetae*, etc; in case of being accompanied with food stagnation, add *Massa Fermentata Medicinals* and *Fructus Crataegi*; in case of heat predominating, manifested as discharge of little purulent and much bloody stool, or only bloody stool, serious fever, thirst with strong desire for drinking, red tongue with yellowish fur, slippery and rapid pulse, use *Bai Tou Weng Tang*[88] to clear away heat and toxic materials. Besides, *Flos Lonicerae*, *Radix Paeoniae*, *Fructus Aurantii Immaturus* and *Radix Glycyrrhizae* can also be added accordingly.

[Nursing Points] Have a good rest. Eat liquid or semiliquid diet which is light and easily digested and avoid pungent, sweet and fat food.

2. Fulminant dysentery

[Symptoms] Sudden onset, high fever, thirst, headache, irritability, intense abdominal pain, even coma and convulsion, frequent discharge of bright, purplish, bloody and purulent stool, tenesmus which is more severe than that in dampness - heat type, crimson tongue with yellowish and dry fur, slippery and rapid pulse.

[Main Points of Differentiation] Sudden onset, high fever, irritability, even presence of symptoms of mental disorder, intense abdominal pain and tenesmus.

This type is commonly seen in toxic dysentery and acute schistosomiasis.

[Pathogenesis] Accumulation of epidemic toxic pathogen in intestines leading to the consumption of *qi* and blood and the blockage of orifices.

[Treatment] Clearing away heat pathogen and cooling blood, removing toxic material and eliminating stagnation.

[Recipe] *Bai Tou Wong Tang*[88] with other drugs

Radix scutellariae, *Flos Lonicerae*, *Radix Paeoniae Rubra*, *Cortex Moutan Radicis*, *Radix Sanguisorbae* and *Rhizoma Dryopteris Crassirhizomae*, etc. may be added accordingly to strengthen the effect of clearing away heat in *Xuefen* and removing toxic material. In case of critical condition caused by heat and toxic pathogens disturbing cardiac atrophy, manifested as coma and delirium, even convulsion, wiry and thready pulse, crimson tongue, yellowish and dry fur, add *Cornu Antelopis* and fresh *Radix Rehmanniae*, etc. Besides, use *Shen Xi Dan*[187] or *Zhi Xue Dan*[267] in combination to clear away heat pathogen and remove toxic material, wake up patients from unconsciousness and relieve muscular spasm.

[Nursing Points] Observing the patient's condition closely. Rescuing patient with combined Chinese and Western Medicine if necessary. Eat less and have a vegetarian diet

3. Cold - dampness dysentery

[Symptoms] Diarrhea with mucous and bloody stool in which mucous is predominating, or with only mucous stool, accompanied with abdominal pain, tenesmus, loss of appetite, feeling of fullness and oppression over epigastrium, heavy feeling of the head and body, pale tongue, whitish and greasy fur, soft and floating and slow pulse.

[Main Points of Differentiation] Diarrhea with much mucous and little bloody stool, or only mucous stool, epigastric oppression, heavy feeling of head and body.

This type is commonly seen in chronic bacillary dysentery, chronic nonspecific ulcerative colitis and irritable colon.

[Pathogenesis] Retention of cold-dampness pathogen in intestines leading to the stagnation of functional activities of *qi* and the disorder of transportation.

[Treatment] Warming middle-*jiao* and dispeling cold, eliminating dampness and relieving stagnation.

[Recipe] *Wei Ling Tang*[182] with modification.

For the case with dysentery, the method of promoting urination excessively is unsuitable, so, *Rhizoma Alismatis* and *Polyporus Vmbellatus* are not applicable. In case of cold predominating, add *Rhizoma Zingiberis Praeparatae* and *Cortex Cinnamomi* to dispel cold and regulate the functional activities of *qi*.

[Nursing Points] Avoid raw and cold fruits to prevent cold from impairing the *yang* of spleen and stomach. Eat light diet such as vegetable, millet gruel, etc.

4. *Yin*-deficiency dysentery:

[Symptoms] Diarrhea with purulent and bloody stool or with sticky bright red blood, burning pain in the abdomen, long straining at stool but in vain, poor appetite, restlessness, dry mouth, crimson tongue with little fur or red tongue without fur and lack of saliva, thready and rapid pulse.

[Main Points of Differentiation] Diarrhea with purulent and bloody stool or with sticky bright red blood, long straining at stool but in vain, crimson tongue or red tongue without fur.

This type is commonly seen in chronic bacillary dysentery, chronic nonspecific ulcerative colitis, carcinoma of colon and rectal carcinoma.

[Pathogenesis] Prolonged dysentery and remaining dampness-heat resulting in the consumption of *yin*-fluid and the retention of dampness-heat in intestines.

[Treatment] Nourishing *yin* and regulating *yingfen*, clearing away dampness-heat in the intestines and relieving dysentery.

[Recipe] *Zhu Che Wan*[166] with modification.

Radix Paeoniae Albe and *Radix Glycyrrhizae* can be added to regulate *yingfen* and relieve pain by nourishing *yin* with sour and sweet drugs; *Fructus Trichosanthis* may also be added to smooth the flow of *qi*; in case of the consumption of body fluid by deficiency-heat, manifested as thirst, oliguria and dry tongue, use *Radix Adenophorae Strictae* and *Herba Dendrobii* to promote the production of body fluid by nourishing *yin*; in case of diarrhea with much blood, add *Cortex Moutan Radicis*, *Radix Paeoniae Rubra*, *Herba Ecliptae* and the charcoal of *Radix Sanguisorbae* to stop bleeding by cooling blood; in case of dampness-heat uncleared away completely, manifestied as bitter taste in the mouth and burning sensation in the anus, add *Cortex Phellodendri* and *Cortex Fraxini* to clear away dampness - heat.

[Nursing Points] Avoid pungent and fried food as well as overstrain.

5. Deficiency - cold dysentery

[Symptoms] Diarrhea with mucous or thin stool, even incontinence of feces, or dull pain in the abdomen, poor appetite, listlessness, cold limbs, soreness of loins, chilliness, pale tongue with thin and whitish fur, deep, thready and weak pulse.

[Main Points of Differentiation] Diarrhea with thin or mucous stool, even incontinence of feces, cold limbs and soreness of loins.

This type is commonly seen in chronic bacilliary dysentery, chronic nonspecific ulcerative colitis and irritable colon.

[Pathogenesis] Retention of cold - dampness in the intestines after prolonged dysentery leading to the deficiency of spleen - *yang* and kidney - *yang*, resulting in the descent of middle - *jiao qi* and its failure to control.

[Treatment] Warming and invigorating spleen and kidney, arresting the incontinence of feces by using astringent therapy.

[Recipe] *Zhen Ren Yang Zang Tang*[198] with modification.

In case of severe deficiency - cold syndrome, use *Fu Zi Li Zhong Tang*[146] in combination to dispel cold by warming the middle - *jiao*; in case of food stagnation remaining, use small amount of drugs which can relieve despepasia such as *Fructus Aurantii*, *Fructus Crataegi* and *Massa Fermantata Medicinals*, or add *Semen Raphani*; in case of proctoptosis (prolapse of rectum) caused by the deficiency of spleen - *qi* and the collapse of vital *qi* after prolonged dysentery, use *Bu Zhong Yi Qi Tang*[140] instead of the above recipe to benefit middle - *jiao qi*, lift up prolapsing *zang* - *fu* organs by lifting up lucid *yang*.

[Nursing Points] Eat nutritious but not greasy food. Avoid overstrain and wind - cold.

6. Recurrent dysentery

[Symptoms] Lingering and intermittent dysentery with mucous or bloody stool, abdominal pain with tenesmus, poor appetite, lassitude and aversion to cold, somnolence, pale tongue with greasy fur, soft - floating or feeble and rapid pulse.

[Main Points of Differentiation] Dysentery with a chronic course and a tendency of relapse.

This type is commonly seen in chronic bacilliary dysentery, chronic amebic dysentery, chronic nonspecific ulcerative colitis and chronic schistosomiasis.

[Pathogenesis] The remaining of pathogens and the deficiency of vital *qi* after prolonged dysentery leading to the cold - syndrome associated with heat - syndrome, and the functional disorder of stomach and intestines in transportation.

[Treatment] Warming the middle - *jiao* and clearing away the pathogens in the intestines, regulating *qi* and relieving stagnation.

[Recipe] *Lian Li Tang*[134] with modification.

Semen Arecae, *Radix Aucklandiae* and *Fructus Aurantii Immaturus*, etc. may be added to regulate *qi* and relieve stagnation.

[Nursing Points] Having Light and easily digested food. Eating raw garlic and purslane regularly in summer and autumn as a means of prevention. Taking exercise and alternating work and rest to strengthen the constitution.

Summary

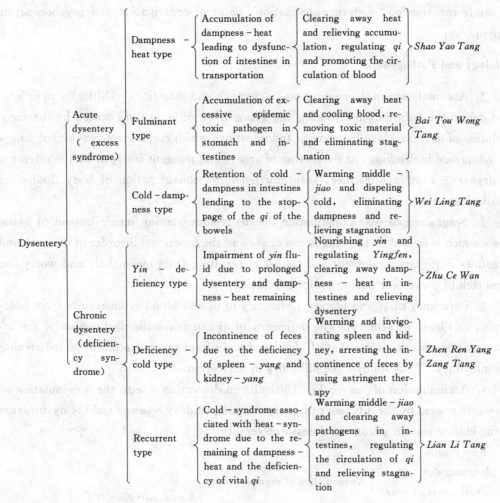

Discussions

1. What is dysentery? How many types is it classified into?

2. How do you differentiate and treat dampness - heat dysentery and recurrent dysentery?

3. Please relate the pathogenic characteristics, clinical manifestations and therapeutic method of fulminant dysentery.

23 Constipation

General

Constipation refers to a morbid condition with symptom of difficult and prolonged fecal discharge.

The treatment by differentiating syndromes of the disease may serve as a reference to senile constipation, dietetic constipation, habitual constipation and psychoneurotic constipation.

Etiology and Pathogenesis

1. Accumulation of dryness – heat in stomach and intestines   Difficulty in defecation due to the failure of distributing and going down of body fluid caused by the accumulation of dryness – heat in stomach and intestines which results from exuberant *yang*, or indulgence in drinking, or overeating of greasy and pungent food; or by the retention of dryness – heat in intestines, resulting from the consumption of body fluid after febrile diseases.

2. Stagnation of *qi*   Constipation due to residue staying inside instead of going down which is caused by the stagnation of *qi*, and the functional disorder of stomach and intestines in digestion, descent and transport resulting from melancholy and worry, or from lack of movement during prolonged sitting.

3. Deficiency of *qi* and blood   Deficiency of *qi* and blood often results from overstrain, or illness or senility. The deficiency of *qi* can cause the dysfunction of the intestines in transport, while that of blood and body fluid can cause failure in moistening the intestines. Thus follows the difficulty in defacation.

4. Accumulation of *yin* – cold   Difficulty in defecation due to the accumulation of *yin* – cold caused by the dificiency of genuine – *yang* (kidney – *yang*) and the dysfunction of the kidney resulting from weakness, or senility.

Key Points:

Improper diet / Usual excess of *yang*	Accumulation of dryness – heat	
Anxiety or less movement	Stagnation of functional activities of *qi*	Functional disorder of the large intestines in transportation → Constipation
Debility after illness	Deficiency of *qi* and blood / Retention of *yin* – cold	

Diagnosis and Discrimination

In diagnosis, doctors must get some idea of the patient's habits of life, diet and defecation in order to identify the reasons causing constipation.

The common manifestations of constipation are dry and impacted feces, difficulty in defecation, the bowel movement occurring once every 3 to 5 or 7 to 8 days, sometimes even longer. Prolonged constipation usually causes other symptoms such as hemorrhoid, hematochezia and anal fissure, etc. The obstructed *qi* of the bowels due to constipation often causes fullness and distention of abdomen, even abdominal pain, poor appetite, dizziness and distending feeling of head, restless sleep, etc. in some cases.

Some cord-like masses varying in size, which are formed by stool, can be touched over the left lower abdomen after prolonged constipation. Those should be distinguished from *Zheng Jia* and *Ji Ju* (both manifested as abdominal mass). If the mass is caused by constipation, it will disappear or become smaller after purgation. The mass caused by *Zheng Ji* can not be moved by pushing or pressing and will not disappear after purgation, while that by *Jia Ju* is movable and appears intermittently.

Selecting Treatment by Differentiating Syndromes

Constipation may be classified into heat-type, *qi*-stagnated type, deficiency-type and cold-type, or into two kinds i.e. deficiency-syndrome and excess-syndrome. Excess-syndrome includes heat-type constipation and *qi*-stagnated type constipation; deficiency syndrome incluses *qi*-deficiency, blood-deficiency, and *yang*-deficiency (cold-type).

Purgation should be used as the main method for treating constipation, but purgatives can not be used singly. It should be used together with orther drugs which are chosen according to the pathogenesis. The treatment of excess-syndrome should be aimed at clearing away heat and nourishing the intestines, promoting the circulation of *qi* and dispersing stagnation; the treatment of deficiency-syndrome should be aimed at tonifying *qi* and nourishing blood, eliminating constipation by using some warm-natured purgatives.

Common Types:

1. Heat-type

[Symptoms] Dry stool, oliguria with deep-coloured urine, flushed face, fever, sometimes accompanied with abodominal distention and pain, dry mouth, halitosis, red tongue with yellowish or yellowish and dry fur, slippery and rapid pulse.

[Main Points of Differentiation] Dry stool, fever, deep-coloured urine, distending pain in the abdomen.

This type may be seen in the constipation caused by diet or febrile disease.

[Pathogenesis] Accumulation of heat in the stomach and the intestines consuming body fluid and leading to the retention of dry stool and the obstructed *qi* of the bowels.

[Treatment] Clearing away heat and moisturizing intestines.

[Recipe] *Ma Zi Ren Wan*[240].

In case of severe dry stools hard to be defecated for many days, add *Natii Sulfas Exsiccatus* to soften the dry feces and dissipate the mass, clear away heat and relax bowels; in case of stagnation of fire in liver channel, manifested as reddish eyes, irritablity, red tongue and wiry pulse, add *Radix Gentianae*, *Radix Scutellariae*, *Fructus Gardeniae* to clear away heat and purgate fire, or in combination with *Geng Yi Wan*[131] to remove pathogenic heat from liver and relax bowels; in case of the patient's suffering from hemorrhoid, constipation, defecating with much blood caused by accumulation of dryness-heat in the stomach and the intestines, add *Flos Sophorae*, *Radix Sanguisorbae* to cool blood and stop bleeding. In case of slight dryness-syndrome, manifested as only constipation, take *Qing Lin Wan*[148] to clear away heat in *fu* organs with mild purgation in order to avoid the recurrence of constipation.

[Nursing Points] Avoid eating fried, greasy, sweet and pungent food, and drinking alcohol. Have light food.

2. Stagnation of *qi*

[Symptoms] Dry and hard stool, desire for defecation but nothing defecated, frequent belching, feeling of fullness and oppression over the chest and hypochondria, even distending pain in the abdomen, poor appetite, thin and greasy fur, wiry pulse.

[Main Points of Differentiation] Dry and hard stool, desire for defecation but nothing defecated, frequent belching, feeling of fullness and oppression over the chest and hypochondria.

This type is commonly seen in gastrointestinal neurosis.

[Pathogenesis] Emotional upset leading to the obstruction of the *qi* of the bowels and functional disorder of the intestines in transportation.

[Treatment] Promoting the circulation of *qi* and dispersing stagnation.

[Recipe] *Liu Mo Tang*[47].

In case of the generation of fire evil resulting from prolonged stagnation of *qi*, manifested as bitter taste in the mouth, dry throat, yellowish fur, wiry and rapid pulse, add *Radix Scutellariae*, *Fructus Gardeniae* to clear away heat and purge fire.

[Nursing Points] Regulate emotional activities. Avoid depression and anger.

3. Deficiency syndrome

(1) *Qi*-deficiency

[Symptoms] Defecating with great efforts accompanied with sweating and shortness of breath, not so hard and dry feces, lassitude after defecation, pale complexion, fatigue, timidness, pale tongue, thin and whitish fur, feeble pulse.

[Main Points of Differentiation] Defecating with great efforts, sweating, shortness of breath, fatigue, timidness, feeble pulse.

This type may be seen in senile constipation, habitual constipation and dietetic constipation, etc.

[Pathogenesis] Deficiency of lung-qi and spleen-qi leading to the dysfunction of the large intestines in transportation.

[Treatment] Tonifying qi and moisturizing the intestines.

[Recipe] *Huang Qi Tang*[234].

In case of obvious qi-deficiency, add *Radix Condonopsis Dilosulae*, *Rhizoma Atractylodis Macrocephalae* to strengthen the effect of benefiting qi; in case of dragging and distending feeling of the anus caused by qi collapse due to the deficiency of qi, *Bu Zhong Yi Qi Tang*[140] is used in combination to lift up the collapse by benefiting qi and make spleen-qi and lung-qi sufficient. Then, the transporting function of the intestines will become normal, which will result in normal defecation.

[Nursing Points] Avoid eating fried and pungent food; take often vegetables, fruits and honeys; cultivate the good habit of defecating at fixed time.

(2) Blood-deficiency

[Symptoms] Dry and hard stool, pale complexion, palpitation, dizziness, blurring vision, pale tongue and lips, thready pulse.

[Main Points of Differentiation] Dry and hard stool, pale complexion, pale tongue and lips, thready pulse.

This type may be seen in senile people, puerpera and those people in poor condition who are at the restoration stage of a disease.

[Pathogenesis] Deficiency of blood and body fluid leading to the failure in moisturizing the intestines.

[Treatment] Moisturizing dryness by nourishing blood.

[Recipe] *Run Chang Wan*[214].

In case of endogenous heat pathogen caused by the deficiency of blood and yin, manifested as feverish sensation accompanied with restlessness, dry mouth, red tongue with little saliva, add *Radix Scrophulariae*, raw *Radix Polygoni Multiflori*, *Rhizoma Anemarrhenae* to clear away heat and promote the production of body fluid. In case that the body fluid has been recovered but the stool is still dry, *Wu Ren Wan*[39] is used to moisturize the intestines and relax bowels.

[Nursing Points] Adjust daily life. Avoid overstrain. Medicated diet and dietetic treatment can be used in coordination. For example, grind black sesame, walnut kernel and pine nut kernel into fine powder to be taken with honey after infusion.

4. Cold type (yang-deficiency)

[Symptoms] Difficulty in defecation, clear and profuse urine, pale complexion, cold extremities, preference for warmth and avorsion to cold, cold pain of the abdomen, or soreness and cold sensation of loins, pale tongue with whitish fur, deep and slow pulse.

[Main Points of Differentiation] Difficulty in defecation, cold pain of abdomen, cold extremities.

[Pathogenesis] The stagnation of functional activities of *qi* and dysfunction of the intestines in transportation caused by the generation of cold interior resulting from the deficiency of *yang*.

[Treatment] Warming *yang* and relaxing bowels.

[Recipe] *Ji Chuan Jian*[183].

In case of excessive *yin*-cold interior, use *Ban Liu Wan*[94].

[Nursing Points] Avoid raw, cold food and wind-cold.

Besides, for the cases with constipation, being in a good mood, taking exercises, having rational diet and defecating at fixed time, etc. will do good to the treatment. As for the cases with no feces due to not taking food after febrile diseases or prolonged illness, the purgative therapy should not be used immediately, instead, benefiting stomach-*qi* is needed. After the amount of diet is increased, the defecation will become normal.

Summary

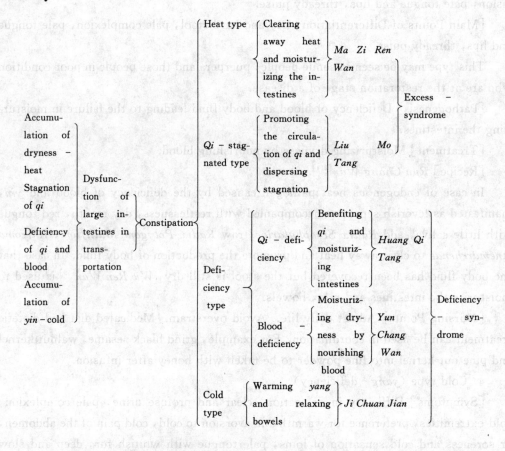

Discussions

1. Please relate the etiology and pathogenesis of constipation.

2. How do you use purgative therapy correctly for treating constipation?

3. How many types is the constipation commonly classified into? What are the key points of differentiation, therapeutic principles and recipes for each type?

24 Parasitic Syndrome (*Chong Zheng*)

General

Parasitic syndrome refers to the disorder caused by worms which parasitize in the intestines of human body.

The treatment by differentiating syndromes of the disease is referential to the symptoms caused by ascariasis, taeniasis, ancylostomiasis, oxyursis, fasciolopsiasis.

Etiology and Pathogenesis

1. **Dietetic factors** Dietetic factors, which include improper diet and dirty diet, are the main factors that bring on parasitic syndrome. Improper diet is inclusive of overeating of raw and cold or greasy and sweet food, while dirty diet eating of uncleaned food sticked with worm eggs, unprepared fish or meat. Worm eggs in nails, clothes or bedding eatten along with food also can cause this disease.

2. **Entering through skin** The ancylostomiasis often results from hookworm larva getting into human body through skin when people touch the soil in doing farmwork as well as from dirty diet.

3. **Accumulation of dampness – heat** On the one hand, accumulation of dampness –heat pathogen does good to the parasitizing of worms; on the other hand, worms may disturb the activities of *qi* and lead to the functional disorder of *zang – fu*, which results in generation of dampness – heat.

4. **Worms disturbing inside while vital *qi* is deficient** In case of the functional disorder of *zang – fu* caused by *qi* –deficiency, especially the dysfunction of the spleen and stomach, the disturbance of worms can lead to various kinds of diseases.

Key Points:

Improper diet → Generation of dampness – heat → Accumulation of dampness – heat

Dirty diet → Eggs being eatten

Attack of toxin pathogen in stool → Worms getting into human body from skin

→ Worms parasitizing in the intestines → Disturbing the function of the spleen and stomach and consuming *qi* and blood → Parasitic syndrome

Diagnosis and Discrimination

At the beginning of parasitic diseases, no symptoms or occasionally some symptoms appear. After prolonged illness, with the consumption of refined essence, poor appetite, recurrence of abdominal pain and restless sleep will occur, and the patients often become thin. In addition to making diagnosis based on feces examination, those special symptoms caused by various worms may serve as a reference for clinical diagnosis.

Ascariasis: Irregular occurrence of abdominal pain around the anvel with visible mass which moves up and down.

Taeniasis: Distending pain in the abdomen, diarrhea or defecating of white proglottids (the bodies of worms).

Ancylostomiasis: Sallow complexion with edema face, emaciation, lassitude, polyphagia and easy hunger or heterorexia.

Oxyursis: Itching on the anus at night, some small white wriggling worms can be seen around the anus, and make sleep restless.

Fasciolopsiasis: Generally, no obvious symptoms; at the late stage, slight abdominal pain and diarrhea start appearing.

In clinic, yellowness and edema caused by ancylostomiasis should be distinguished from those caused by jaundice. The patients suffering from jaundice present yellow coloration of general skin and sclera without edema, accompanied with hypochondriac pain, tea-coloured urine, poor appetite, etc. which result from dampness-heat predominating inside. The patients suffering from ancylostomiasis present sallow complexion with edema face, without icteric sclera, accompanied with lassitude, etc.

Selecting Treatment by Differentiating Syndromes

Deficiency syndrome and excess syndrome must be distinguished at first and then the treatment is applicated. Generally, the treatment for parasitic syndrome is expelling worms before regulating spleen and stomach.

1. Ascariasis

[Symptoms] Intermittent abdominal pain around the anvel, gastric upset, even vomiting or defecating of roundworms, abdominal mass caused by roundworms; in severe case, manifested as poor appetite, sallow complexion, emaciation, itching in the nostril, teeth grinding and salivation during sleep.

[Main Points of Differentiation] Intermittent abdominal pain around the anvel, itching in the nostril, teeth grinding and salivation during sleep.

[Pathogenesis] Roundworms staying inside leading to the generation of dampness-heat and the functional disorder of *qi*.

[Treatment] Expelling or calming roundworms, invigorating spleen and regulating stomach.

[Recipe] *Hua Chong Wan*[48], *Wu Mei Wan*[56].

Hua Chong Wan is suitably applicated for the case of slight abdominal pain or no abdominal pain to dispel roundworms. *Wu Mei Wan* is used for the case of severe abdominal pain, vomiting and nausea to alleviate pain by calming roundworms.

[Nursing Points] Pay attention to the hygiene of diet.

2. Taeniasis

[Symptoms] Dull pain or feeling of fullness and distention in the abdomen, or diarrhea, itching on the anus, emaciation and lassitude after prolonged illness; sometimes some white proglottides can be found in stool or on the underpunts.

[Main Points of Differentiation] Distending pain in the abdomen, defecating of white proglottids.

[Pathogenesis] Taenia in the intestines obstructing the functional activities of *qi* and disturbing the function of the spleen and stomach, resulting in the disorder of transportation and transformation and the consumpation of refined materials.

[Treatment] Expelling taenia, regulating the spleen and stomach.

[Recipe] Some simple recipes listed below can be used.

(1) Take *Semen Arecae* with *Semen Cucurbitae Moschatae*, two hours later, dissolve *Natii Sulfas Exsiccatus* 9~18g in warm boiled water and take it at a draught. Two or three hours later, some proglottids will be defecated out.

(2) Take *Omphalia* powder 20g each time, once a day, continuously for three days.

(3) *Pericarpium Granati* 25g is decocted in water for oral dose. The drug is unsuitable for patients suffering from stomach disease.

[Nursing Points] Only when taenia and scolex (cephalomere) completely defecated out can the patient get completely cured. After taenia being expelled, the patient should take some Chinese drugs which can invigorate the spleen and stomach. Pay attention to the hygiene of diet. Do not eat uncooked pork or beef.

3. Ancylostomiasis

(1). Retention of dampness due to the dysfunction of the spleen

[Symptoms] Sallow complexion or yellowish complexion with a puffy face, polyphagia and easy to be hungery, distending feeling in the abdomen after eating, or preference for eating raw rice, tea and charcoal, etc. lassitude, weakness of limbs, pale tongue with thin fur, soft and floating pulse.

[Main Points of Differentation] Sallow complexion with a puffy face, polyphagia and easy to be hungry, or preference for eating special things.

[Pathogenesis] Deficiency of *qi* and blood, and retention of wetness caused by the dysfunction of the spleen and stomach in transportation and transformation resulting from hookworm disturbing the functional activities of *qi* .

[Treatment] Invigorating spleen and drying the wetness, regulating middle - *jiao* and nourishing blood.

[Recipe] *Huang Bing Jiang Fan Wan*[236].

(2) Deficiency of *qi* and blood

[Symptoms] Pale or sallow complexion and skin, edema of face and feet, even general edema, feeling of fullness and discomfort in the stomach, lassitude, dizziness, tinnitus, palpitation, shortness of breath, pale and enlarged tongue, weak pulse.

[Main Points of Diferentiation] Pale or sallow skin, edema of face and feet, palpitation, shortness of breath.

[Pathogenesis] Hookworm in the intestines sucking the essential substance and consuming qi and blood resulting in the deficiency of qi and blood.

[Treatment] Tonifying qi and blood.

[Recipe] *Ba Zhen Tang*[13].

In case of feeling of oppression over the epigastrium, poor appetite, add *Radix Aucklandiae*, *Fructus Amomi* to regulate the functional activities of qi and the stomach. For two types of ancylostomiasis (hookworm disease), the treatment of expelling hookworm is needed. *Semen Torreyae*, *Omphalia*, *Semen Arecae*, *Radix Stemonae*, *Fructus Carpesii*, *Rhizoma Dryopteris Crassirhizomae* etc. can be used according to the patient's condition.

[Nursing Points] Pay attention to protecting partial skin. Do not touch the ground (soil) with bear feet and body. Suitably take the food nutritious and easily digested. The patient in severe condition should have a good rest.

4. Oxyursis

[Symptoms] Unusually itching on the anus, especially at night, restless sleep. When itching occurs, some small white wriggling worms can be found around the anus. Severe case is marked by irritability, poor sleep, dizziness, poor appetite, sallow complexion, emaciation, or nausea and vomiting, abdominal pain, diarrhea.

[Main Points of Differentiation] Itching on the anus at night, some smallwhite wriggling worms can be seen around the anus.

[Pathogenesis] Pinworms wriggling around the anus causing itching, and their staying in the intestines leading to the functional disorder of the spleen in transportation, and transformation and the stagnation of functional activities of qi.

[Treatment] Expelling oxyurid (pinworm) and relieving itching.

[Recipe] *Zhui Chong Wan*[196].

Fructus Quisqualis, *Fructus Carpesii*, *Semen Torreyae*, *Semen Arecae* etc., which can expel worms, may be selected. Besides internal remedy, *Radi Stemonae* may be decocted in water for clyster.

[Nursing Points] Pay attention to personal hygiene. Clothes and bedclothes should be washed and changed regularly.

5. Fasciolopsasis

[Symptoms] Generally, no obvious clinical manifestation; some cases manifested as slight abdominal pain and diarrhea, or nausea and vomiting, lassitude or distending feeling in the abdomen, edema after prolonged illness.

[Main Points of Differentiation] Slight abdominal pain and diarrhea, or lassitude, edema.

[Pathogenesis] Stagnation of functional activities of *qi*, the disorder of reception, and transportation caused by fasciolopsises staying in the intestines; the dysfunction of the spleen and stomach after prolonged illness causes the deficiency of *qi* and blood, the retention of wetness.

[Treatment] Expelling fasciolopsises as the main method, and invigorating spleen in coordination.

[Recipe] For expelling fasciolopsises, make *Semen Arecae* 50g into small pieces and soak it in water overnight, after that, decoct it for one hour and take it at a draught before meal, continuously take it for two or three days.

For invigorating spleen and regulating stomach, use *Xiang Sha Liu Jun Zi Tang*[189]; For the case with abdominal distention and edema, add *Herba Plantaginis*, *Cortex Acanthopanacis Radicis*, dried *Pericarpium Lagenariae Sicerariae* to eliminate wetness by promoting diuresis.

[Nursing Points] Pay attention to the hygiene of diet. Eat washed vegetable and cooked food. Raw *Trapanatans* should be washed with boiled water before eating.

Summary

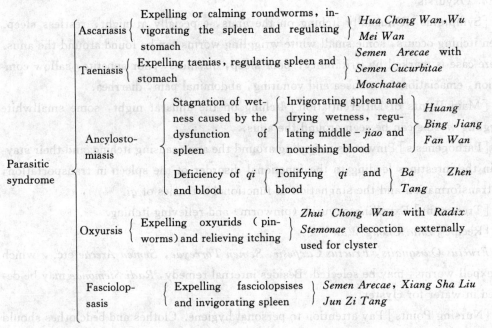

Discussions

1. How does the parasitic syndrome happen?

2. What are the clinical manifestations when roundworms stay in intestines? How should you treat it?

3. What are the effective recipes and drugs to be used for taeniasis?

25 Abdominal Pain

General

Abdominal pain refers to a morbid condition manifested as pain which takes place below the stomach and above the suprapubic hair margin.

The syndrome of abdominal pain involves a wide scope. When we deal with the syndromes chiefly characterized by abdominal pain such as enterospasm, acute pancreatitis, gastrointestinal neurosis, adhesive ileus, mesenteriopathy and peritoneopathy, partial enteritis and colitis in Western Medicine, we can consult the selecting treatment by differentiating syndrome of this illness.

Etiology and Pathogenesis

1. Exopathic factor Abdominal pain results from dysfunction of the spleen in transporting, distributing and transforming nutrients, which is caused by pathogens of cold, heat, summer-heat and dampness invading the abdomen, and which causes in turn, stagnation of *qi* due to a lingering pathogenic factor in the body.

2. Improper diet Abdominal pain may result from crapulence or uncontrolled intake of unhygienic food; it may also be caused by retention of food and generation of heat-dampness as the result of taking too much enriched fatty diet and acrid food; or it could be the result of stagnation of *qi* in *fu*-organs due to the accumulation of heat in the stomach and intestines.

3. Emotional disorder The injury of the liver by melancholy and anger can lead to dysfunction of the liver (wood) to spread out freely and stagnation of *qi* and blood; or lead to transverse invasion of the hyperactive liver-*qi*, which results in incoordination between the stomach and the spleen, and obstruction of *qi*. All the reasons as mentioned above will give rise to abdominal pain.

4. Insufficiency of *yang* Dysfunction of the spleen in transporting, distributing and transforming the nutrients is due to insufficiency of the spleen-*yang*; insufficiency of the spleen-*yang*, deficiency of *qi* and blood are caused by retention of cold-dampness and unable to warm and reinforce viscera and bowels (*zang* and *fu*). As a result, abdominal pain occurs.

Moreover, stagnation of *qi* and blood stasis and obstruction of channels and collaterals caused by abdominal operation or traumatic injury can give rise to abdominal pain.

Key Points:

```
Exopathogenic factor ⎫   Qi of fu-organs being  ⎫
Improper diet        ⎬   unable     to    descend⎬
Emotional disorder   ⎭   smoothly                ⎪    Disorder of qi leading⎫
                                                 ⎬    to   obstruction   of ⎬ Abdominal pain
                         ⎧ Insufficiency cold in ⎪    channels              ⎭
Insufficiency of yang ⎨  zang and fu not warmed  ⎪
                         ⎩ and reinforced        ⎭
```

Diagnosis and Discrimination

Clinically, a syndrome manifested as pain which is located below the stomach and above the suprapubic hair margin belongs to the field of abdominal pain.

Abdominal pain due to internal diseases should be differentiated from those induced by acute appendicitis or periappendicular abscess, hernia, cholera, dysentery and *Ji Ju*. Abdominal pain due to acute appendicitis or periappendicular abscess is often characterized by a serious pain which apperas in the right lower abdomen with aversion to pressure and gets relieved by genuflexion and aggravated by extension on the right foot; abdominal pain caused by hernia may often be accompanied by a cramping sensation of the lower abdomen with radiation to the part of medial femora; abdominal pain induced by cholera is often characterized by a continued colic with vomiting and diarrhea, cold clammy extremities and spasm; in dysentery, the abdominal pain is often accompanied by tenesmus with pus and blood in the stool; while the visible abdominal mass may be always shown in *Ji Ju*. As for the abdominal pain due to women's diseases, it is often accompanied by abnormalities in menstruation, leukorrhea, pregnancy and labor.

Selecting Treatment by Differentiation Syndromes

As concerns differentiating syndrome of abdominal pain, we should differentiate the character of pain carefully. All kinds of the pain manifested as sudden onset and tenderness during the attack belong mainly to the excess type; while the dull pain with prelief by pressing belongs to the deficiency type; the acute pain with abdominal distension, constipation and inability to get relieved by warming mainly belongs to the heat type; while the pain aggravated by cold and relieved by hot compress or eating hot food mainly belongs to the cold type; abdominal distention with wandering pain is mainly due to the stagnation of *qi*; while a fixed and stabbing pain is caused by the stasis of blood.

Common Syndromes:

1. Accumulation of cold

[Symptoms] Sudden abdominal pain, relievied by warming and aggravated by cold, normal sense of mouth and no thirst, copious clear urine, normal or loose stool, whitish and greasy fur, deep and tense pulse.

[Main Points of Differentiation] Aggravated by cold and relievied by warmth. This type may be seen in enterospasm and enteritis.

[Pathogenesis] Obstruction of *qi* and blood due to *yang - qi* being unable to transport caused by invasion of pathogenic cold.

[Treatment] Warming the middle - *jiao* to dispel cold.

[Recipe] *Liang Fu Wan*[139] with *Zheng Qi Tian Xiang San*[62].

In case of dominant pathogenic cold with violent pain and cold extremities, deep and thready pulse, add *Radix Aconiti praeparata*, and *Cortex Cinnamomi* to activate *yang* with drugs pungent in flavor and heat in property, and to disperse cold and relieve pain; in case of cramping sensation and cold pain belonging to stagnancy of *qi* of the liver channel, add *Evodia rutaecarpa* (Juss.) Benth, *Fructus Foenicuii*, and *Lignum Aquilariae Resinatum* to warm the liver channel and dispel the pathogenic cold; in case of abdominal cold pain with constipation, add *Radix Aconiti Praeparata*, *Radix et Rhizoma Rhei* to warm and promote the circulation of *qi* of the *fu* - organs.

[Nursing Points] Cold, uncooked, greasy food, and pathogens of wind - cold should be avoided.

2. Stagnation of dampness - heat

[Symptoms] Abdominal pain with tenderness, chest distress, constipation or loose stool with difficult defecation, extreme thirst and desire for drinking, spontaneous perspiration, scanty dark urine, greasy yellowish fur, slippery and rapid pulse.

[Main Points of Differentiation] Abdominal pain with tenderness, chest distress, constipation with dark urine, greasy yellowish fur, rapid pulse.

This type can be seen in acute enteritis, acute pancreatitis, intestinal obstruction and so on.

[Pathogenesis] Obstruction of *qi* of the *fu* - organs due to disturbance of visceral function caused by accumulation of dampness - heat in the interior.

[Treatment] Remove obstruction of *qi* of the *fu* - organs to expel the pathogenic heat.

[Recipe] *Da Cheng Qi Tang*[21].

In case of constipation being not severe while the damp - heat pathogen dominant, remove *Natrii Sulphas* and add *Radix Scutellariae*, *Radix Pittospori*, etc. ; if abdominal pain radiates to the hypochondrium, add *Radix Bupleuri* and *Radix Curcumae*.

[Nursing Points] The greasy and pungent food should be avoided and a bit of vegitarian diet may be recommended.

3. Deficiency of middle - *jiao* and interior cold

[Symptoms] A paroxysmal continuous abdominal pain with preference for warmth and aversion to cold, and preference for pressing when aching which is aggrravated after starvation and tiredness and slightly relieved after taking food or rest; loose stool, accompanied with listlessness and fatigue, shortness of breath, and aversion to cold; pale tongue with whitish fur, deep and thready pulse.

[Main Points of Differentiation] Abdominal pain with preference for pressing, relieved by eating, loose stool, aversion to cold.

This type can be seen in chronic enteritis, and chronic inflamation of mesentery and peritoneum.

[Pathogenesis] Cold originating from the interior and the channels being unable to be nourished properly caused by the insufficiency of the spleen - *yang*.

[Treatment] Warming the middle - *jiao* and invigorate the spleen - *yang* to relieve spasm and pain.

[Recipe] *Xiao Jian Zhong Tang*[28].

In case of listlessness and shortness of breath, or soft stool with difficulty in defecation resulting from deficiency of *qi* and weakness, add *Radix Astragali seu Hedysari* to invigorate *qi*. Marked by cold of insufficiency type of abdominal pain accompanied by vomiting and cold extremities with indistinctive pulse, take *Da Jian Zhong Tang*[20] to warm the middle - *jiao* to dispel cold. In case of abdominal pain with frequent defecation, cold limbs, deep and slow pulse belonging to insufficiency of the spleen and kidney -*yang*, take *Fu Zi Li Zhong Tang*[146] to warm and invigorate the spleen and kidney.

[Nursing Points] The cold and uncooked or greasy food should be avoided and light diet may be recommended.

4. Retention of food

[Symptoms] Abdominal pain with distension and tenderness, poor appetite, eructation with fetid odor, acid regurgitation, diarrhea caused by abdominal pain or the pain relieved after diarrhea, or constipation, greasy fur with slippery and replete pulse.

[Main Points of Differentiation] Abdominal pain with distension and tenderness, poor appetite, eructation with fetid odor.

This type is often seen in acute gastroenteritis, incomplete intestinal obstruction, etc.

[Pathogenesis] Retention of food in the stomach and intestines resulting in disturbance in ascending and descending and dysfunction of the spleen in transporting, distributing and transforming the nutrients, which leads to obstruction of *qi* of *fu* - organs and adverse rising of turbid *qi*.

[Treatment] Promoting digestion and removing stagnancy.

[Recipe] *Bao He Wan*[193] or *Zhi Shi Dao Zhi Wan*[172].

[Nursing Points] Being moderate in eating and drinking, avoiding overeating, frequent small meals, fasting treatment for a short time if necessary.

5. Stagnation of *qi* and blood stasis

[Symptoms] In case of dominant stagnation of *qi*, the symptom is marked by abdominal distension or wandering pain with radiation to the lower abdomen which is relieved by eructation or wind from bowels, while aggravated by anger, thin fur with wiry pulse; the type of dominant blood stasis is marked by fixed and severe pain, blueish-purple tongue with wiry or uneven pulse.

[Main Points of Differentiation] Stagnation of *qi* characterized by a dominant distending pain and wandering pain, while blood stasis, by a dominant stabbing and fixed pain.

This type is seen in acute pancreatitis, intestinal adhesion, chronic nonspecific ulcerative colitis, gastrointestinal neurosis, etc.

[Pathogenesis] Abdominal pain caused by obstruction of the channels or stagnation of *qi* due to disorder of the liver-*qi*; or by accumulation of blood stasis resulting from persistent pain injuring the collaterals.

[Treatment] Promote the flow of *qi* and blood circulation. In case of stagnation of *qi* in dominance, relieve the depressed liver, soothe the liver and regulate the circulation of *qi*; if blood stasis in dominance, remove it by promoting blood circulation.

[Recipe] *Chai Hu Shu Gan San*[211], or *Shao Fu Zhu Yu Tang*[57].

Concerning stagnation of *qi* and blood stasis, the former is always considered a light state of the illness while the latter a serious one; in order of the time, onset of the stagnation of *qi* is earlier than the blood stasis, and the latter is often accompanied with the former. Therefore, in the treatment of blood stasis, we often add drugs for regulating the flow of *qi* to promote *qi* in motion to render blood circulating normally while in the treatment of stagnation of *qi*, add drugs for promoting blood flow such as *Radix Curcumae*, *Rhizoma Corydalis*, etc. to promote the blood circulation to render the flow of *qi* in motion normally.

[Nursing Points] Keeping to proper diet and avoiding crapulence; regulating mental activities and avoiding melancholy, anxiety and anger.

Summary

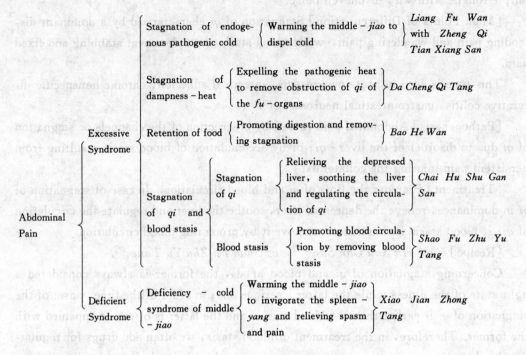

Discussions

1. How do you understand the etiology and pathogenesis of abdominal pain?

2. Retell the main points of differentiation and discrimination in each of syndromes.

3. Retell the symptoms, treatment and recipe of the abdominal pain in the types respectively of accumulation of cold, of stagnation of *qi* and blood stasis, and of deficiency of middle – *jiao* with cold of *zang* – organs.

26 Hypochondriac Pain

General

Hypochondriac pain is chiefly manifested as pain of hypochondriac regions by one side or two sides. It is a common kind of subjective symptom in clinic.

This illness may be seen in many kinds of diseases in Western Medicine such as acute hepatitis, chronic hepatitis, hepatic parasitosis, hepatic abscess, liver cirrhosis, liver cancer, acute or chronic cholecystitis, gallstones, ascariasis of biliary tract and intercostal neuralgia. The selecting treatment by differentiating syndromes herein is referential to the diseases whose main symptom is characterized by hypochondriac pain.

Etiology and Pathogenesis

1. Stagation of the liver - qi Emotional depression or rage injuring the liver can cause dysfunction of the liver to spread out freely, and disorder in governing the flow of qi as well. Thus, hypochondric pain occurs due to obstruction of the liver - qi and blockage of the collaterals.

2. Blocking of blood circulation by blood stasis If the stagnation of the liver qi continues for a long period, blood circulation will be blocked and blood stasis accumulated. So hypochondriac pain appears due to the obstruction of hypochondriac collaterals. The injury of hypochondriac collaterals caused by overload leading to blood stasis, which may obstruct the hypochojndriac collaterals and cause hypochondriac pain.

3. Deficiency of the liver - yin The morbid condition is caused by chronic illness, overstrain or hypererosia. The deficiency of essence and blood can lead to deficiency of the liver - yin, so that the liver and its channels can not be nourished by blood. This condition will result in hypochondriac pain in the end.

4. Dampness - heat in the liver and the gallbladder Under the circumstances of invasion by exopathogens or improper diet, dysfunction of the spleen in transporting, distributing and transforming the nutrients can lead to stagnation of phlegm - dampness and generation of heat induced by stagnancy of the liver - qi, which results in disorder of the liver and gallbladder to spread out freely, so that the hypochondriac pain appears.

Key Points:

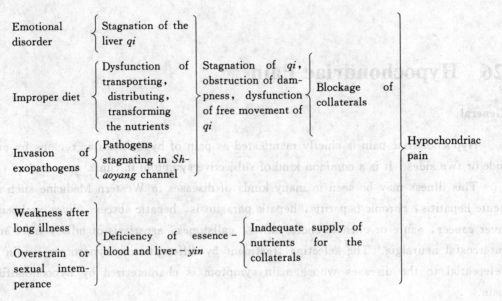

Diagnosis and Discrimination

A syndrome chiefly manifested as pain of costal regions by one side or two sides clinically can be diagnosed as hypochondriac pain.

Clinical diagnosis of hypochondriac pain should be differentiated from chest pain or stomachache carefully because all the three kinds of pains have the same symptom of stagnation of the liver – qi, the same pathogenesis basically and the same clinical manifestation and consequent obscurity in diagnosis.

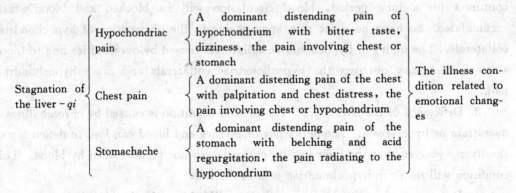

Selecting Treatment by Differentiating Syndromes

As regard to differentiating syndrome of hypochondriac pain, differentiating the state of qi, and blood is the first concern. Generally speaking, distention belongs to stagnation of qi and it manifests as wandering pain; stabbing pain belongs to blood stasis chiefly and it manifests as fixed pain; vague pain belongs to deficiency of yin and its pain is continuous. As for the hypochondriac pain caused by dampness – heat, it often manifests as a severe pain with bitter taste and yellowish tongue coating.

Common Syndromes:

1. Stagnation of the liver-qi

[Symptoms] Hypochondriac distention by left side, by right side or by two sides is characterized by wandering pain. It varys along with emotional changes and is accompanied with chest distress, dyspnea, poor appetite and frequent belching. Thin whitish fur with wiry pulse or wiry-thready pulse is common manifestations.

[Main Points of Differentiation] Hypochondriac distention with wandering pain and its onset relating to emotional factors.

This type is commonly seen in acute and chronic hepatitis, cholecystitis.

[Pathogenesis] Stagnation of the liver-qi, and dysfunction of free movement of qi leading to blockage of collaterals in the hypochondriac regions.

[Treatment] Soothing the liver and regulating the circulation of qi.

[Recipe] *Chai Hu Shu Gan San*[211].

Add *Rhizoma Cyperi praeparata*, *Pericarpium Citri Reticulatae Viride*, *Pericarpium Citri Reticulatae*, *Radix Curcumae*, *Rhizoma Corydalis*, *Fructus Meliae Toosendan* to regulate the flow of qi to alleviate mental depression and pain. In case of a severe stagnation of qi and a permanent hypochondriac pain, add discretionally *Flos Mume Albus*, *Retinervus Luffae Fructus*, *Fructus Citri Sarcodactylis*, *Fructus Tribuli*, *Flos Rosae Rugosae*, *Flos Albiziae* to regulate the flow of qi to alleviate mental depression; in case of fire induced by stagnation of the liver-qi and the pain manifested as burning pain accompanied with dry mouth and bitter taste, aptness to vex and anger, dysuria and constipation, red tongue with yellowish fur and wiry-rapid pulse, *Dan Zhi Xiao Yao San*[52] may be chosen. Add *Rhizoma Coptidis*, *Radix Curcumae* to dispel heat of the liver and alleviate mental depression.

[Nursing Points] Normalizing emotions, avoiding emotional depression and anger, avoiding pungent or greasy food.

2. Blood stasis

[Symptoms] A permanant hypochondriac pain as if stabbed and with a fixed location, and aggravation especially at night, or palpable mass under the hypochondrium, purple tongue with thin whitish fur, deep-uneven pulse.

[Main Points of Differentiation] Stabbing pain in the hypochondrium with a fixed position and its aggravation especially at night.

This type may be seen in chronic hepatitis, cirrhosis and liver cancer.

[Pathogenesis] Stagnation of qi and stasis of blood leading to obstruction of hypochondriac collaterals.

[Treatment] Regulating the flow of qi to remove obstruction in the collaterals and promoting blood circulation to remove blood stasis.

[Recipe] *Xuan Fu Hua Tang*[245].

Add *Radix Curcumae*, *Semen Persicae*, *Rhizoma Corydalis*, *Radix Angelicae Sinensis* to enhance effectiveness of regulating the flow of qi and promoting blood circulation as physician thinks fit. In case of a severe stasis of blood, *Fu Yuan Huo Xue Tang*[190] can be chosen to promote blood circulation and remove blood stasis, and clear and activate the channels and collaterals. In case of mass of hypochondrium and the vital -*qi* being not weak so much, add *Rhizoma Sparganii*, *Rhizoma Zedoariae*, *Eupolyphaga seu Steleophaga*, etc. to strengthen the effectiveness of removing blood stasis and lumps.

[Nursing Points] Keeping a reasonable life style and a regularity of work and rest, easing mental anxiety and not being greedy for gain, eating light food.

3. Deficiency of the liver - *yin*

[Symptoms] Vague pain of the hypochondrium manifested as a continuous pain and its aggravation during overwork, dry mouth and throat, vexation, dizziness, tiredness, red tongue with a little fur, thready - wiry pulse or thready - rapid pulse.

[Main Points of Differentiation] Vague pain in hypochondrium, dry throat and vexation, red tongue with a little fur.

This type is often seen in chronic hepatitis or cirrhosis.

[Pathogenesis] Deficiency of the liver - *yin* caused by deficiency of essence and blood, giving rise to malnutrition of hypochondriac collaterals.

[Treatment] Nourishing *yin* and blood, nourishing the liver to regulate the collaterals.

[Recipe] *Yi Guan Jian*[1].

In case of dysphoria and feverish sensation in the chest, add *Gardenia Jasminoides Ellis* (parched), *Semen Ziziphi Spinosae* to clear away heat and tranquilize the mind; as for dizziness, add *Rhizoma Polygonati*, *Fructus Ligustri Lucidi*, *Flos Chrysanthemi* to tonify the kidney and remove heat from the liver.

[Nursing Points] Fresh vegetables and fruits, bean products, and enriched animal protein food could be chosen. Avoid pungent, greasy food, and abstain from indulgence in sexual activities and overstrain.

4. Dampness and heat in the liver and gallbladder

[Symptoms] Hypochondriac pain, chest distress, bitter taste and poor appetite, nausea and vomiting, conjunctival congestion, icteric sclera, dark urine, yellowish greasy fur with rapid and slippery pulse.

[Main Points of Differentiation] Hypochondriac pain, bitter taste, yellowish eyes, body and urine, yellowish greasy fur and rapid and slippery pulse.

This type is mainly seen in icteric viral hepatitis, acute cholecystitis, ascariasis biliary tract, etc.

[Pathogenesis] Blockage of hypochondriac collaterals resulting from dysfunction of the liver and gallbladder caused by dampness - heat.

[Treatment] Clearing away heat and promoting diuresis.

[Recipe] *Long Dan Xie Gan Tang*[64].

In case of fever with jaundice, add *Herba Artemisiae Capillaris*, *Cortex Phellodendri* to clear away heat and promote diuresis to eliminate jaundice; in case of a severe pain in the hypochondrium with vomiting of ascaris, take *Wu Mei Wan*[56] firstly to relieve colic caused by ascaris, and then, the vermifuge; in case of lithogenesis due to dampness-heat scorching the fluid, resulting in blockage of biliary tract and marked by a severe pain in the hypochondrium radiating to the shoulder and back, add *Herba Lysimachiae*, *Spora Lygodii*, *Radix Curcumae*, etc. to normalize the function of the gallbladder and remove gallbladder stone; if constipation and abdominal distention, caused by consumption of the body fluid due to excessive heat, occur, add *Radix et Rhizoma Rhei*, *Natrii Sulphas* to expel the pathogenic heat to loosen the bowels.

[Nursing Points] Abstain from indulgence in sexual activities and avoid greasy and pungent food. Fresh vegetables and fruits, bean products or light food could be chosen.

Summary

Hypochondriac pain	Excessive Syndrome	Stagnation of the liver *qi*	Soothing the liver and regulating the circulation of *qi*	*Chai Hu Shu Gan San*
		Blocking of blood circulation by stagnancy	Regulating the flow of *qi* to remove obstruction in the collaterals and promoting blood circulation and removing blood stasis	*Xuan Fu Hua Tang*
		Dampness-heat in the liver and gallbladder	Clearing away heat and promoting diuresis	*Long Dan Xie Gan Tang*
	Deficiency Syndrome	Deficiency of the liver-*yin*	Nourishing *yin* and blood, nourishing the liver to regulate the collaterals	*Yi Guan Jian*

Discussions

1. Retell the etiology and pathogenesis of the hypochondriac pain.
2. How many common syndromes does the hypochondriac pain cover? What are the main points of differentiation in each?
3. What are the clinical characters of the stagnation of the liver-*qi* in the hypochondriac pain? How to treat it?

27 Jaundice

General

Jaundice is the morbid condition chiefly manifested as icteric sclera, xanthochromia and dark brownish urine. Among them, the icteric sclera is an important character of this illness.

There is the same exposition about the implication of jaundice either in Traditional Chinese Medicine or Western Medicine. This covers approximately the hepatocellular jaundice, obstructive jaundice and hemolytic jaundice. All the diseases manifested as jaundice including icteric viral hepatitis, icteric infectious mononucleosis, cholestatic hepatitis, cholecystitis, cholelithiasis, leptospirosis and medicamentous liver lesion, etc. can consult the selecting treatment by differentiating syndrome herein.

Etiology and Pathogenesis

1. **Exopathic factor** This type of jaundice occurs as a result of exogenous affection of seasonal pathogens or pathogenic damp–heat so that exopathogens accumulate in the body, stagnate in the middle–*jiao* and result in dysfunction of the stomach and the spleen in transporting, distributing and transforming the nutrients which will cause endogenous damp–heat. In this circumstances, intertwinement of exogenous dampness with endogenous heat affect the liver and gallbladder so that bile overflow to muscle, skin and the urinary bladder, which is manifested as icteric sclera, yellowish skin and brownish urine.

2. **Improper diet** The stomach and spleen can be impaired by unhygienic food, too much eating or hunger, or too much drinking so that dysfunction of the stomach and spleen causes pathogenic dampness being generated internally. Moreover, stagnation of pathogenic dampness leads to damp–heat occurrence which affects the liver and gallbladder resulting in circulation of bile abnormally and overflow to muscle and skin, so that jaundice occurs.

3. **Insufficiency–cold of the the spleen and stomach** The impaired spleen and stomach *yang* due to insufficiency in natural endowment or after illness will cause pathogenic dampness obstructing internally and dampness–cold being generated. When dampness–cold accumulates in the middle–*jiao*, bile circulation is obstructed, and bile overflows to muscle and skin leading to jaundice in the end.

4. **Transforming from *Ji Ju* Syndrome** When biliary tract is obstructed by stagnation of blood stasis due to syndrome of *Ji Ju* for a long duration, bile overflows leading to jaundice; while pathogenic dampness obstructing circulation of *qi*, stagnation

of *qi* and blood stasis may generate many kinds of symptoms of blood stasis.

Under the circumstances of exopathogenic factor or improper diet, the pathogenesis refers to tranformation from pathogenic dampness into pathogenic heat so that *yang* jaundice occurs; in terms of insufficiency – cold of the spleen and stomach *yang* or transforming from *Ji Ju* syndrome, it refers to transformation from pathogenic dampness into pathogenic cold, so *yin* jaundice occurs.

Key Points:

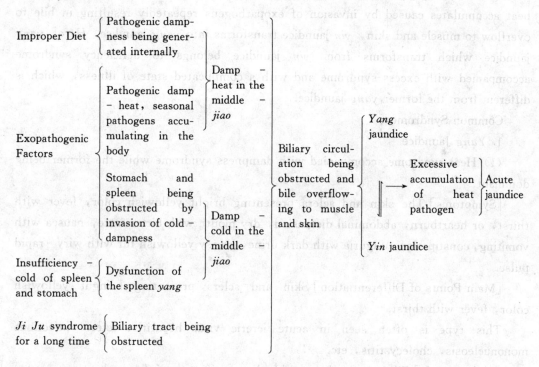

Diagnosis and Discrimination

According to icteric sclera, xanthochromia and dark urine, the diagnosis of jaundice can be established. Especially icteric sclera is the most significant diagnostic basis, because it is an indication which appears earlier and disappears latest.

Clinically, we should differentiate jaundice from sallow complexion of insufficiency type. The pathogenesis of jaundice refers to retention of dampness in the liver and spleen leading to bile overflowing outwardly, and its cardinal symptoms include icteric sclera, xanthochromia and dark brownish urine. While the sallow complexion of insufficiency type is due to malnutrition of the muscle and skin caused by deficiency of *qi* and blood, and its cardinal symptom is sallow complexion including general skin but sclera.

Selecting Treatment by Differentiating Syndromes

As concerns differentiating syndrome of jaundice, we should differentiate *yang* jaundice from *yin* jaundice. In *yang* jaundice, the illness course is shorter, its skin presents bright yellowish color, and belongs to heat syndrome or excess syndrome; while in *yin* jaundice, the course is longer, its skin presents dark and gloomy yellowish color, and belongs to cold syndrome or deficiency syndrome. TCM believes that in a certain condition, transfoming of *yang* jaundice into *yin* jaundice and vice versa may take place. When dysfunction of the spleen - *yang* caused by a delayed treatment or protracted course of *yang* jaundice leads to transformation from pathogenic dampness into pathogenic cold, *yang* jaundice transforms into *yin* jaundice; while pathogenic damp - heat accumulates caused by invasion of exopathogens repeatedly resulting in bile to overflow to muscle and skin, *yin* jaundice transforms into *yang* jaundice. Here, *yang* jaundice which transforms from *yin* jaundice belongs to deficiency syndrome accompanied with excess syndrome and with a complicated state of illness, which is different from the former *yang* jaundice.

Common Syndromes:

1. *Yang* Jaundice

(1) Heat syndrome accompanied with dampness syndrome while the former being dominant.

[Symptoms] The skin and sclera presenting bright yellowish color, fever with thirst, or heartburn, abdominal distension, dry mouth with bitter taste, nausea with vomiting, constipation, oliguria with dark urine, greasy yellowish fur with wiry - rapid pulse.

[Main Points of Differentiation] Skin and sclera presenting bringht yellowish color, fever with thirst.

This type is often seen in acute icteric viral hepatitis, icteric infectious mononucleosis, cholecystitis, etc.

[Pathogenesis] Bile overflowing outside due to affection of damp - heat.

[Treatment] Clearing away heat and promoting diuresis, detoxicating and resolving mass.

[Recipe] *Yin Chen Hao Tang*[177].

Add drugs capable of excreting dampness such as *Poria*, *Polyporus*, *Talcum Pulveratum*, etc. to dispel dampness through urination; in case of abdominal distention, add *Radix Curcumae*, *Fructus Melia Toosendan*, *Pericarpium Citri reticulate Viride* to sooth the liver and regulate the circulation of *qi*; of nausea and vomiting, add *Pericarpium Citri Reticulatae*, *Caulis Bambusae in Taeniam* to check upward adverse flow of *qi* to stop vomiting; in case of vexation with heartburn, add *Rhizoma Coptidis*, *Radix Gentianae*; of vexation with insomnia, epistaxis, add *Radix Paeoniae Rubra*, *Corex Moutan Radicis* to remove heat from the blood to stop bleeding; during remission of constipation and fever, and the fur changing from yellowish one to whitish one, add the drugs of invigorating the spleen for eliminating dampness such as *Rhizoma Atractylodis Macrocephalae*, *Poria*, etc, and remove the drugs bitter in taste and cold in nature which can clear away internal heat at the same time in order to avoid the impairement of the spleen - *yang* and avoid transforming from *yang* jaundice into *yin* jaundice.

[Nursing Points] An enriched soft diet or semiliquid diet is recommended, while the pungent, greasy food and wine should be avoided. Take bed rest and having ease of mind.

(2) Damp syndrome accompanied with heat syndrome while the former being dominant

[Symptoms] The skin and sclera presenting yellowish color but not bright, recessive fever, heavyness in the head and limbs, feeling of fullness in the chest and upper abdomen, poor appetite, thirst but not to drink too much, nausea with vomiting, abdominal distension, loose difficult stool, scanty dark urine, greasy, thick, light, yellowish fur, wiry, slippery pulse or soft and floating, moderate pulse.

[Main Points of Differentiation] The skin and sclera presenting yellowish color but not bright, fever with heavyness in the limbs, nausea and vomiting and abdominal distention.

This type of syndrome is often seen in icteric viral hepatitis, cholecystitis, etc.

[Pathogenesis] Disorder of the flow of the liver *qi* and bile overflowing outside caused by retained heat due to blockage of dampness.

[Treatment] Removing dampness by diuresis to eliminate turbid pathogens, removing heat to expel jaundice.

[Recipe] *Yin Chen Wu Ling San*[175] with *Gan Lu Xiao Du Dan*[74] with modification. In case of obstructed flow of *qi* due to accumulation of dampness, manifested as chest or abdominal rigidity or distention, nausea, and poor appetite, add *Rhizoma Atractylodis*, *Cortex Magnoliae Officinalis*, *Rhizoma Pinelliae* to invigorate the spleen for eliminating dampness, to promote circulation of *qi* and regulate the stomach.

[Nursing Points] Have proper diet, abstain from pungent, greasy or sweet food, and drinking.

2. Acute Jaundice

[Symptoms] Jaundice presenting golden color with sudden onset, characterized by a rapid aggravating brown yellowish pigmentation of the skin and sclera, high fever, polydipsia, hypochondriac pain with feeling of fullness in the abdomen, coma, delibrium, epistaxis, bloody urine, skin ecchymosis, dark -red tongue with dry yellowish fur, wiry - slippery, rapid pulse or thready rapid pulse.

[Main Points of Differentiation] Sudden onset, jaundice presenting golden color, high fever, polydipsia, coma, delibrium and blood troubles.

This illness can be seen in acute or subacute fatal hepatitis.

[Pathogenesis] Bile overflowing outwardly caused by invasion of a violent toxic heat affecting the liver and gallbladder.

[Treatment] Clearing away heat and toxic material, removing heat from *yingfen* to induce resuscitation.

[Recipe] *Xi Jiao San*[274].

Add *Radix Rehmanniae*, *Cortex Moutan Radicis*, *Radix Scrophulariae*, *Herba Dendrobii*, etc. to increase effectiveness of removing pathogenic heat from blood. In case of coma, delibrium, take compatible with *An Gong Niu Huang Wan*[111] or *Zhi Bao Dan*[109] in compatibility with the above recipe to remove heat pathogen from the blood to induce resuscitation; in case of a dominant blood trouble such as epistaxis, bloody urine or skin ecchymosis, add *Radix Sanguisorbae*, *Cacumen Biotae*, etc. to remove heat pathogen from the body to stop bleeding; in case of oliguria or difficulty in passing water, or ascites, add *Caulis Aristolochiae Manshuriensis*, *Rhizoma Imperatae*, *Herba Plantaginis*, *Pericarpium Arecae*, etc. to clear away heat pathogen by diuresis.

[Nursing Points] Take bed rest under close observation of the state of illness. Liquid food is recommended while pungent, greasy and fried food should be avoided.

3. *Yin* Jaundice

[Symptoms] The skin and sclera presenting dark gloomy yellowish color, fullness sensation in the epigastrium with poor appetite, abdominal distention, loose stool, mental fatigue, aversion to cold, tastelessness but not thirst, pale tongue with greasy fur, soft-floating and moderate or deep-slow pulse.

[Main Points of Differentiation] The skin and sclera presenting dark gloomy yellowish color, fullness sensation in the epigastrium, loose stool, mental fatigue, moderate pulse.

This type can be seen in cholestatic hepatitis, chronic icteric viral hepatitis.

[Pathogenesis] Bile overflowing outwardly due to dysfunction of *yang-qi* and dysfunction of the liver and spleen caused by cold-dampness pathogens stagnating.

[Treatment] Strengthening the spleen and stomach, warming and expelling pathogenic cold-dampness.

[Recipe] *Yin Chen Zhu Fu Tang*[176].

Add *Radix Curcumae*, *Cortex Magnoliae Officinalis*, *Poria*, *Alisma Plantago Acuatica*, etc. to promote the circulation of *qi* to induce diuresis. In case of stagnation of the liver *qi* and deficiency of the spleen leading to dysfunction of the liver and spleen, marked by feeling of fullness in the epigastrium and abdomen, dull pain in the hypochondriac regions, poor appetite, fatigue, constipation alternating with loose stool, wiry and thready pulse, add *Xiao Yao San*[222] to sooth the liver and to strengthen the spleen; if accompanied by hypochondriac distention due to fixed mass, gloomy yellowish skin, purple tongue with wiry-thready pulse, it belongs to the syndrome of deficiency of both *qi* and blood and obstruction of the collaterals and channels by turbid pathogens, take *Xiao Shi Fan Shi San*[266] to remove turbid pathogens and phlegm and to soften hard mass. In case of jaundice for a long duration, stagnation of *qi* and blood stasis accompanied by mass, stabbing pain on the chest and hypochondriac regions, tenderness, take *Bie Jia Jian Wan*[290] to remove blood stasis by promoting blood circulation; in case of insufficiency cold of the spleen and stomach with poor appetite, abdominal distention, and lassitude, add *Xiang Sha Liu Jun Zi Tang*[189] to strengthen the function of spleen and stomach.

[Nursing Points] An enriched digestible food should be recommended while the uncooked, greasy and pungent food should be avoided; internal injury caused by overstrain and sexual activity should be avoided.

Summary

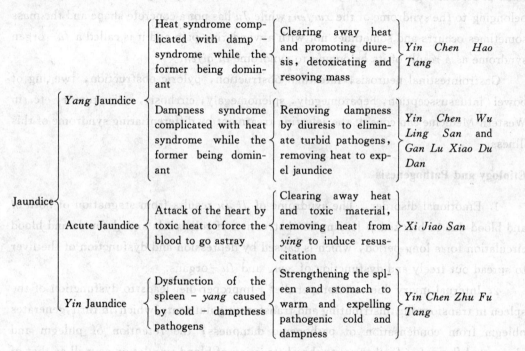

Discussions

1. What is jaundice? Retell its etiology and pathogenesis.
2. Retell the differentiation among *yang* jaundice, *yin* jaundice and acute jaundice.
3. Retell the main symptoms treatment and recipe of the *yang* jaundice.

28 The Syndrome of *Ji Ju* (Abdominal Mass)

General

Ji Ju refers to the morbid condition manifested as mass in the abdomen with pain or distention. TCM believes that *Ji* has a specific shape and a fixed position presenting pain fixed at certain region, and physicians call *Ji* a *zang* - organ syndrome in virtue of its belonging to the syndrome of the *xuefen*; while *Ju* has not a concrete shape and the mass sometimes occurrs and sometimes not with a wandering pain and it is called a *fu* - organ syndrome as a result of its belonging to syndrome of *qifen*.

Gastrointestinal neurosis, intestinal obstruction, pyloric obstruction, twisting of bowel, intussussception, hepatomegaly, splenomegaly, cirrhosis, celiac tumor, etc. in Western Medicine can consult the selecting treatment by differentiating syndrome of this illness.

Etiology and Pathogenesis

1. Emotional disorder   The syndrome of *Ji Ju* results from stagnation of both *qi* and blood due to blocked *qi* leading to obstruction of collaterals and channels and blood circulation for a long period, which is caused by depression and dysfunction of the liver to spread out freely and dysfunction of *zang* and *fu* - organs.

2. Internal injury due to improper diet   Improper diet leads to dysfunction of the spleen in transforming, distributing and transforming nutrients, which, in turn, generates phlegm from condensation of pathogenic dampness; the retention of phlegm and obstructed flow of *qi* further cause the obstruction of blood circulation as well as that of the channels and collaterals.

3. Invasion by cold - dampness   Abdominal mass is formed by stagnation of *qi* and blood as the result of dysfunction of spleen and dampness phlegm accumulated in the body, which is caused by invasion of cold - dampness.

4. Shifting to abdominal mass from other diseases   Stagnation of *qi* and blood caused by retention of pathogenic dampness after jaundice or due to a permanent jaundice; the dampness - phlegm retention resulting in obstruction of collaterals and channels during chronic malaria; stagnation of *qi* and blood due to disharmony between the liver and spleen caused by infection of schistosome; deficiency of spleen - *qi* and blockage of blood circulation after chronic diarrhea or dysentery. All the above conditions can give rise to the syndrome of *Ji Ju*.

Key Points:

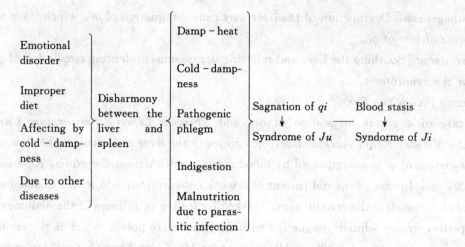

Diagnosis and Discrimination

Mass in the abdomen is characteristic of both *Ji* and *Ju* syndromes. Of a longer course, *Ji* syndrome has gradually formed palpatle masses of different sizes, harder quality and fixed position, which is serious and difficult to deal with; of shorter course, *Ju* symdrome has indefinite paroxysmal intervals and is characteriaed by visible peristalsis with wandering pain or distention and by its relief followed by the diappearance of distention and masses. *Ju* syndrome is easy to deal with because of its mild nature.

Ji Ju should be differentiated from the symptom of fullness sensation. Fullness sensation is a kind of subjective symptom caused by abdominal distention or obstructed flow of *qi*, and no mass can be palpated; while *Ji Ju* refers to mass in the abdomen with pain or distention and it not only has subjective symptom but has mass to be palpated.

Selecting Treatment by Differentiating Syndromes

Although there is difference between *Ji* and *Ju*, clinically we often call *Ji* and *Ju* the same syndrome simultaneously, namely, syndrome of *Ji Ju*, because stagnation of *qi* transforms into *Ju* whose generation is earlier, and syndrome of *Ju* for a long period may lead to occurrence of blood stasis and gives rise to the syndrome of *Ji*.

Common syndromes are as follows:

1. Syndrome of *Ju*

(1) Stagnation of the liver *qi*

[Symptoms] Retention of *qi* in the abdomen with an intermittent attack of distention or wandering pain accompanied by abdominal discomfort or hypochondriac distention, thin fur with wiry pulse.

[Main Points of Differentiation] A wandering pain in the abdomen due to retention of *qi* presenting paroxysmal attack.

This syndrome can be seen in gastrointestinal neurosis.

[Pathogenesis] Dysfunction of the liver may cause stagnation of *qi*, which leads to the disorder of fow of *qi*.

[Treatment] Soothing the liver and relieving depression, promoting circulation of *qi* to relieve the syndrome of *Ju*.

[Recipe] *Xiao Yao San*[222].

In case of a severe stagnation of *qi*, add *Rhizoma Ciperi*, *Pericarpium Citri Reticulatae Viride*, *Radix Aucklandiae*, etc. to sooth the liver and regulate the flow of *qi*; if stagnation of *qi* is accompanied by blood stasis, add *Rhizoma Corydalis*, *Rhizoma Zedoariae*, etc. In case of the old patient or a weak constitution, add *Radix Codonopsis Pilosulae* to consolidate the constitution. Marked by feeling of fullness in the abdomen, poor appetite, greasy whitish tongue fur with wiry moderate pulse, which is the result of cold-dampness obstructing the middle-*jiao*, take *Mu Xiang Shun Qi San*[36] to warm the middle-*jiao* to dispel cold, to promote circulation of *qi* to remove dampness.

[Nursing Points] Keeping equilibrium in emotional activities and refraining from depression and agner.

(2) Retention of indigested food and obstruction of phlegm

[Symptoms] Abdominal pain or distention, constipation, poor appetite, stripe-like mass in the abdomen sometimes. Aggravation of distending pain due to great pressure, greasy fur with wiry, slippery pulse.

[Main Points of Differentiation] Stripe-like mass in the abdomen with tenderness, constipation, poor appetite.

This type can be seen in incomplete intestinal obstruction, intussusception.

[Pathogenesis] Retention of food in the intestinal tract leading to dysfunction of the spleen giving rise to the generation of dampness-phlegm and obstruction of food and phlegm resulting in stagnation of *qi*.

[Treatment] Removing stagnancy and relaxing the bowels, regulating the flow of *qi* and resolving the phlegm.

[Recipe] *Liu Mo Tang*[47].

In case of a dominant phlegm-dampness, add *Pericarpium Citri Reticulatae*, *Rhizoma Pinelliae*, *Poria* to enhance the effectiveness of resolving phlegm and normalizing function of the stomch and spleen. In case of a dominant phlegm-dampness with indigestion and greasy fur in spite of normal circulation of *fu*-organs *qi*, take *Ping Wei San*[70] plus *Fructus Crataegi*, *Massa Fermentata Medicinalis* to reinforce the spleen and promote digestion and to dry dampness and eliminate phlegm. The syndrome of *Ju* is often seen in the excess type, but its repeated attack is likely to injure the spleen. In this circumstance, take *Xiang Sha Liu Jun Zi Tang*[189] frequently to reinforce the spleen and normalize the function of the stomach and spleen so that the body resistance is strengthened.

[Nursing Points] Refrain from greasy or pungent food, and light and vegetarian food is recommended.

2. Syndrome of *Ji*

(1) Stagnation of *qi* and obstructed flow of blood

[Symptoms] The mass of *Ji* is soft in quality and has a fixed position with distending pain, thin fur and wiry pulse.

[Main Points of Differentiation] The mass of *Ji* is soft in quality and has a fixed position with distending pain.

This syndrome may be seen in hepatomegaly, splenomegaly, intestinal obstruction and intussusception.

[Pathogenesis] Stagnation of *qi* and obstructed flow of blood leads to the disharmony of channels and collaterals, whose accumulation transforms into mass.

[Treatment] Regulating the flow of *qi* to promote circulation of blood, removing obstruction in the collaterals and eliminating *Ji*.

[Recipe] *Jin Ling Zi San*[162] with *Shi Xiao San*[86].

In case of a dominant stagnation of *qi* and blood stasis accompanied by manifestation of cold syndrome, take *Da Qi Qi Tang*[16]. If marked by alternating attacks of chills and fever with pantalgia, greasy whitish fur with floating – wiry – full pulse, being accompanied with wind – cold type of exterior syndrome, take *Wu Ji San*[42] to disperse wind – cold syndrome to regulate the flow of *qi* and to remove *Ji*.

[Nursing Points] Keeping equilibrium in emotional activities and striking a proper balance between work and rest, and avoiding wind – cold.

(2) Accumulation of blood stasis in the body

[Symptoms] Dominant abdominal mass with fixed pain, darkish complexion, emaciation, fatigue, poor appetite, alternating spells of fever and chill, amenorrhea in women's cases, dark purple tongue or with ecchymoses and petechiae, thready and uneven pulse.

[Main Points of Differentiation] Obvious abdominal mass with a fixed pain, dark purple tongue.

This syndrome is commonly seen in hepatosplenomegaly, cirrhosis and tumor in the abdominal cavity.

[Pathogenesis] Stagnation of *qi* and blood due to abdominal mass for a long duration resulting in obstruction of collaterals and channels.

[Treatment] Removing blood stasis and softening hard masses, regulating the function of spleen and stomach.

[Recipe] *Ge Xia Zhu Yu Tang*[282].

Add *Fructus Meliae Toosendan*, *Rhizoma Sparganii*, *Rhizoma Zedoariae*, etc. to enhance the effectiveness of removing blood stasis and softening hard masses. In case of a hard and large mass with pain, add *Bie Jia Jian Wan*[290] to remove blood stasis and soften the hard masses.

[Nursing Points] Avoid melancholy, anger, and hard work.

(3) Weakened body resistance with accumulation of blood stasis

[Symptoms] Weakness due to a long period of illness, hard mass, aggravating pain gradually, sallow or darkish complexion, obvious emaciation, poor appetite, pale purple tongue without any fur, thready, rapid or wiry thready pulse.

[Main Points of Differentiation] Hard masses, obvious emaciation, sallow or darkish complexion.

This syndrome can be seen in cirrhosis, liver cancer, carcinoma of stomach, etc.

[Treatment] Invigorating primodial *qi* and blood, removing blood stasis by promoting blood circulation.

[Recipe] *Ba Zhen Tang*[13] with *Hua Ji Wan*[50].

In case of evident impairment of *yin*, dizziness, uncoated and smooth tongue with thready rapid pulse, add *Radix Rhihmaniae*, *Radix Glehnia*, *Fructus Lycii*, *Herba Dendrobii*, etc to nourish *yin* and promote the production of body fluid; in case of gingival bleeding, nosebleed, add discretionaly *Capejasmine*, *Cortex Moutan Radicis*, *Rhizoma Imperatae*, *Radix Rubiae*, *Radix Notoginseng*, etc to remove heat from the blood and remove blood stasis to stop bleeding; in case of deficiency of *yang*, aversion to cold and cold limbs, pale tongue with deep thready pulse, add *Radix Astragali seu Hedydari*, *Radix Aconiti Praeparata*, *Cortex Cinnamomi*, *Rhizoma Alisma Plantago Aquatica*, etc. to warm *yang* and invigorate *qi* to induce diuresis and alleviate edema.

[Nursing Points] Take proper diet, lead a regular life, keep optimistic and avoid overwork.

Summary

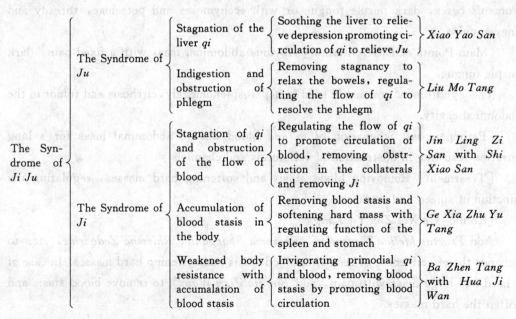

Discusstions

1. Retell the key points of etiology and pathogenesis in the syndrome of *Ji Ju*.
2. What are the differences and connections between the syndrome of *Ji* and *Ju*?
3. Retell the main symptoms, pathogenesis, treatment and recipe of the syndrome of *Ju* due to stagnation of liver-*qi*.

29 Tympanites

General

Tympanites is a morbid state manifested as abdominal distention like a drum, sallow complexion and visible blood vessels.

The disease is commonly seen in ascites due to cirrhosis. Besides, the differentiating treatments for the disease are referential to tuberculous peritonitis, abdominal neoplasm, chronic constrictive pericarditis and nephrotic syndrome in Western Medicine.

Etiology and Pathogenesis

1. Improper diet   Addiction to alcohol or fat, sweet and greasy food generates dampness and heat, whose accumulation in the middle – *jiao* causes a mixture of clear and turbid *qi* and the failure of food essence to be transported, leading to the transformation from internally accumulated turbid dampness into tympanites.

2. Emotional impairment   Anxiety, depression and anger impairs the liver and spleen, leading to dysfunction of the liver in purgation and stagnation of *qi*. If this continues for a period of time, blood stasis and obstruction of channels and collaterals occur. The dysfunction of the liver in promoting the free flow of *qi* invades the spleen and stomach and makes the spleen fail in transport. This, in turn, generates retention of water within the body, and tympanites is converted from the stagnation of *qi*, blood and water.

3. Infected by poison of schistome   Infection of schisosome – poison without timely treatment impairs the liver and spleen causing obstruction of the channels and collaterals to hold up functional activites of *qi* and making disturbance in ascending and descending, and mixing clear – *qi* up with turbid – *qi*. Tympanites is thus gradually formed.

4. Deuteropathy   Tympanites is likely to occur after other diseases impair the liver and spleen, leading to dysfunction of the liver in purgation and dysfunction of the spleen in transport, e. g. lasting jaundice imparis the liver and spleen and blocks the circulation of *qi* and blood causing stagnation in channels and collaterals which results in tympanites that will get larger and larger to worsen the state of obstructed functional activities of *qi* and may well bring about the stagnation of dampness.

Key Points:

Improper diet
Emotional impairment
Infected by schistosome poison
Deuteropathy
} → { Impairment of the liver, spleen and kidney / Stagnation of *qi*, blood stasis and retention of water } → Tympanites

Diagnosis and Discrimination

The major clinical mark of tympanites is abdominal distention. At the initial stage, flatulence is its characteristic. Although the patient feels distent in the abdomen, the abdomen is soft when pressed and will give out drumbeats - sound when knocked. Only when turning is made, can a vibrato of water be heard. At the later stage, ascitic fluid increases, and the abdomen distends to stretch tight with a full and hard feeling accompanied with symptoms of protruding acromphalus, standing - out veins, and blood stasis in vessels. Besides, the symptoms of sallow complexion, icteric sclera and red lines on the skin are referential for diagnosing the disease.

Tympanites should be distinguished from hydrops. Tympanites is marked by abdominal distention with unclear extremital tumefaction. It is at the later stage that extremital tumefaction appears accompanied with dark green complexion, red lines on the face and neck, hardness under the ribs and standing - out veins on the abdominal skin; And hydrops begins from eyelids spreading to the head, face and limbs. Or it starts from lower limbs extending to the whole body with symptoms of white complexion, soreness of loins, tiredness, or complicated with ascites.

Selecting Treatment by Differentiating syndromes

To make a differentiation of tympanites, firstly excess syndrome should be differentiated from deficiency syndrome. Generally speaking, heat belongs to excess syndrome, while coldness to deficiency one; slippery and forceful pulse belongs to excess syndrome, while floating and thready pulse to deficiency one; rough and forceful breath to excess syndrome, while haggard complexion and shortness of breath to deficiency one; young people with stagnation of *qi* and blood to excess syndrome while senile people with listlessness and timidness to deficiency one.

Common Syndromes:

1. Stagnation of *qi* and dampness

[Symptoms] Abdominal distention being soft if pressed, distention or pain under the ribs, reduced diet, distent - feeling after eating, eructation, oliguria, whitish and greasy fur, and wiry pulse.

[Main Points of Differentiation] Abdominal distention being soft if pressed, distention or pain under the ribs, distent - feeling becoming worse after eating.

This type is often seen in ascites due to cirrhosis.

[Pathogenesis] Stagnation of the liver - *qi* and deficiency of the spleen causing retention of dampness in the middle - *jiao* and the fullness of turbid *qi*.

[Treatment] Relieving the depressed liver and regulating the flow of *qi*, and removing fullness by eliminating dampness.

[Recipe] *Chai Hu Shu Gan San*[211] or *Wei Ling Tang*[182].

In case of stuffiness in chest and epigastrium, abdominal distention, desire for eructation which are the symptoms of stagnation of *qi*, add *Fructus Citri Sarcodactyli*, *Lignum Aquilariae Resinatum* and *Radix Aucklandiae* to regulate functional activities of *qi*; in case of retention of dampness in the middle – *jiao*, oliguria, abdominal distention and greasy fur, add *Fructus Amomi*, *pericarpium Arecae*, *Rhizoma Alismatis* and *Semen Plantaginis* to promote the effect of invigorating the spleen for eliminating dampness; in case of deficiency of the spleen – *yang*, listlessness, loose stool, pale tongue, add *Radix Codonopsis Pilosulae*, *Radix Aconiti*, *Rhizoma Zingiberis* and *Pericarpium Zanthoxyli* to warm *yang* and replenish *qi* and to invigorate the spleen for eliminating dampness; if accompanied with stabbing pain under the ribs, purplish tongue, uneven pulse and stagnation of *qi* and blood, add *Rhizona Corydalis*, *Rhizoma Zedoariae* and *Radix Salviae Miltiorrhizae* to promote blood circulation for removing blood stasis.

[Nursing Points] Keep ease of mind; Avoid harmful stimulation; Regulate daily life and have light food.

2. Cold – dampness blocking the spleen

[Symptoms] Abdominal distention as if a water bladder if pressed, in severe case, the face showing slight general edema, the lower limbs having general edema, stuffiness in epigastrium relieved when heated, listlessness, aversion to cold, being disinclined to move about, oliguria, loose stool, whitish and greasy fur, and moderate pulse.

[Main Points of Differentiation] Abdominal distention as if a water bladder if pressed, aversion to cold, listlessness, general edema and loose stool.

This type is common in ascites due to cirrhosis and nephrotic syndrome.

[Pathogenesis] Deficiency of the spleen – *yang* causing stagnation of cold – dampness and fluid.

[Treatment] Warming the middle – *jiao* to strengthen the spleen, and promoting the circulation of *qi* to induce diuresis.

[Recipe] *Shi Pi Yin* [159].

In severe case of dampness, add *Cortex Cinnamomi*, *Umbellate Pore* and *Rhizoma Alismatis* to promote functional activity of *qi* in bladder for diuresis; in case of deficiency and shortness of breath, add *Radix Astragali Seu Hedysari* and *Radix Codonopsis Pilosulae* to invigorate the spleen – *qi* and the lung – *qi*; in case of distending pain in ribs and abdomen, add *Radix Curcumae*, *Pericar Pium Citri Reticulatae Virid* and *Fructus Amomin* to regulate the flow of *qi* and regulate the spleen and stomach.

[Nursing Points] Do not have uncooked, cold, fat and sweet food; and keep away form cold and dampness.

3. Accumulation of damp – heat pathogen

[Symptoms] Hard, full and distending abdomen, dysphoria with smothery sensation, bitter taste, thirst with no desire for drinking, sallow complexion and skin, difficult and dark urine, constipation or loose stool, redness on the tip and margin of the tongue, yellowish and greasy fur or mixed with gray and black color, and wiry and rapid pulse.

[Main Points of Differentiation] Hard, full and distending abdomen, dysphoria with smothery sensation, bitter taste, sallow complexion and dark urine.

This type is often seen in ascites due to cirrhosis and abdominal oncoma.

[Pathogenesis] Accumulation of damp-heat and stagnation of turbid fluid causing disorder of *qi*.

[Treatment] Clearing away heat, eliminating dampness, and purging the turbid fluid.

[Recipe] *Zhong Man Fen Xiao Wan*[38] with *Yin Chen Hao Tang*[177].

In case of severe heat, add *Fructus Forsythiae*, *Radix Gentianae* and *Herba Lobeliae Radicantis* to clear away heat and toxic material; In case of difficult and dark urine, add *Pericarpium Lagenariae* and powder of *Crichet* (separately swallowed) to promote diuresis for inducing resuscitation. If sudden change of the disease takes place in urgent state with symptoms of massively spitting blood and hematorrhea, use *Xi Jiao Di Huang Tang*[273] plus *Radix Notogingseng*, *Herba Agrimoniae* and *Radix Sanguisorbae* to remove pathogenic heat from blood and stop bleeding. In case of severe damp-heat covering pericardium with symptoms of unconsciousness, dysphoria, even howling with glaring eyes, convulsion in limbs, constipation, dark urine, yellowish fur and rapid pulse, adopt *An Gong Niu Huang Wan* [111] or *Zhi Bao Dan*[109] to remove heat for inducing resuscitation; In case of severe phlegm-stagnation with symptoms of lethargy, paraphasia, unconscious state becoming deeper gradually, thick and greasy fur, thready, soft and floating pulse, use *Su He Xiang Wan*[128] to induce resuscitation with aromatics.

[Nursing Points] Lie on bed, have light food and avoid fried, pungent and hard food.

4. Blood stasis in the liver and spleen

[Symptoms] Hard, full and distending abdomen, explosive vessels, stabbing pain in hypochondrium and abdomen, darkish complexion, netlike echymoses on the face, neck, chest and arms, red scars on the palms, dark-purple lips, thirst but inability to swallow water, dark stool, purplish red tongue or with purple spots, uneven and hollow pulse.

[Main Points of Differentiation] Hard, full and distending abdomen, explosive vessels, stabbing pain in hypochondrium and abdomen, dark-purple tongue.

This type is seen in ascites due to cirrhosis and abdominal oncoma.

[Pathogenesis] Retention of wetness within the body and stagnated blood circulation.

[Treatment] Removing blood stasis by promoting blood circulation and promoting the circulation of *qi* to induce diuresis.

[Recipe] *Tiao Ying Yin* [219].

If the mass under the hypochondrium gets larger, add *Squama Manitis*, *Eupolyphoge Sinensis Hirudo*, *Tabanus* and *Concha Ostreae* or take *Bie Jia Jian Wan*[290] to remove blood stasis and resolve the mass. In case of debility due to lasting illness, deficiency *qi* and blood, or impairment of vital *qi* by elimination of extravasated blood, adopt *Ba Zhen Tang*[13] to enrich *qi* and blood; in case of dark stool, add *Radix Notoginseng*, *Radix Rubiae* and *Cacumen Biotae* to remove the blood stasis for stopping bleeding.

[Nursing Points] Take light food. Avoid fried, pungent and hard food.

5. Insufficiency of the spleen – *yang* and the kidney – *yang*

[Symptoms] Abdominal distention relieved in the morning and aggravated at night, sallow or white complexion, stuffiness in epigastrium, poor appetite, palpitation, listlessness, aversion to cold, cold limbs or general edema in legs, oliguria with difficulty, enlarged purplish tongue, and deep, wiry and weak pulse.

[Main Points of Differentiation] Abdominal distention worsening at night, listlessness, aversion to cold, general edema in legs, pale tongue.

This type is observable in nephrotic syndrome, ascites due to cirrhosis and chronic constrictive pericarditis.

[Treatment] Warming and invigorating the spleen and kidney, and promoting the circulation of *qi* and diuresis.

[Recipe] *Fu Zi Li Zhong Tang*[146] with *Wu Lin San*[41].

In case of general edema in legs and oliguria, *Ji Sheng Shen Qi Wan*[184] may be added to nourish *yin*, assist *yang* and promote the circulation of *qi* and diuresis. If complicated with blood stasis such as blue veins standing – out on the abdominal wall, add *Radix Paeoniae Rubra*, *Semen Persicae*, *Rhizoma Sparganii* and *Rhizoma Zedoariae* to promote circulation of blood and remove blood stasis.

[Nursing Points] Lie on bed, with semiprone position. Have light food and avoid fat, sweet and greasy diet.

6. Deficiency of the liver – *yin* and kidney – *yin*

[Symptoms] Full, hard and distending abdomen, in severe case even with blue veins standing – out, thin physique, darkish complexion, purple lips, dry mouth, irritability, nosebleed, gingival hemorrhage, scanty dark urine, deep – red tongue with little fluid, wiry, thready and rapid pulse.

[Main Points of Differentiation] Full, hard and distending abdomen with blue veins standing – out, dry mouth, irritability, nosebleed, gingival hemorrhage, deep – red tongue with little fluid.

This type is common in ascites due to cirrhosis, ascites due to tubercular peritonitis and abdominal oncoma.

[Pathogenesis] Deficiency of the liver – *yin* and kidney – *yin* and stagnation of functional activities of *qi* causing the accumulation of wetness in the body and unsmooth circulation of blood.

[Treatment] Nourishing the liver and kidney, removing heat from the blood and eliminating blood stasis.

[Recipe] *Yi Guan Jian*[1] with *Ge Xia Zhu Yu Tang*[282].

In case of internal heat, dry mouth, deep-red tongue with little fluid, add *Radix Scrophulariae* and *Herba Dendrobii*; if accompanied with hectic fever, add *Radix Stellariae* and *Cortes Lycii Radicis*; for oliguria, add *Poluporus Umbelltus* and *Talcum*; in case of nosebleed and gingival hemorrhage, add *Herba Agrimoniae* and *Rhizoma Imperatae*; in case of coma, use *Zi Xue Dan*[267] for emergency case, or use *An Gong Niu Huang Wan*[111] to wake up the patient from unconsciousness by clearing away heat from the *yinfen*.

[Nursing Points] Have light, nutritious and digestible food. Adjust emotions. Avoid excessive sexual intercourse. And guard against exopathogen.

Summary

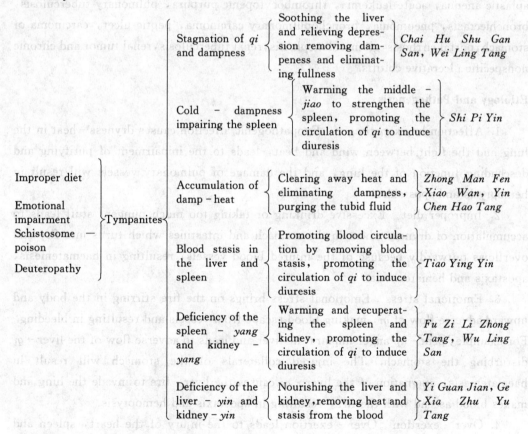

Improper diet Emotional impairment Schistosome poison Deuteropathy	Tympanites	Stagnation of *qi* and dampness	Soothing the liver and relieving depression removing dampeness and eliminating fullness	*Chai Hu Shu Gan San, Wei Ling Tang*
		Cold-dampness impairing the spleen	Warming the middle-*jiao* to strengthen the spleen, promoting the circulation of *qi* to induce diuresis	*Shi Pi Yin*
		Accumulation of damp-heat	Clearing away heat and eliminating dampness, purging the tubid fluid	*Zhong Man Fen Xiao Wan, Yin Chen Hao Tang*
		Blood stasis in the liver and spleen	Promoting blood circulation by removing blood stasis, promoting the circulation of *qi* to induce diuresis	*Tiao Ying Yin*
		Deficiency of the spleen-*yang* and kidney-*yang*	Warming and recuperating the spleen and kidney, promoting the circulation of *qi* to induce diuresis	*Fu Zi Li Zhong Tang, Wu Ling San*
		Deficiency of the liver-*yin* and kidney-*yin*	Nourishing the liver and kidney, removing heat and stasis from the blood	*Yi Guan Jian, Ge Xia Zhu Yu Tang*

Discussions

1. What is tympanises?
2. Retell the pathogeneses and common types of tympanites.
3. Describe the main symptoms, treatments and recipes of cold-dampness impairing spleen, accumulation of damp-heat and deficiency of the liver-*yin* and kidney-*yin*.

30 Bleeding Syndrome

General

Bleeding syndrome refers to the diseases caused by failure of blood to circulate in the vessels, or bleeding through nine orifices or through the skin. In internal medicine, the common types of bleeding are nosebleed, gingival hemorrhage, hemoptysis, haematemesis, henatochezia, urohematin and purpura.

The differentiating treatments for bleeding syndrome here are referential to hemorrhagia caused by various acute and chronic diseases in Western Medicine, such as aplastic anemia, acute leukemia, thrombocytopenic purpura, pulmonary tuberculosis, bronchiectasis, pneumonia, bronchopulmonary carcinoma, peptic ulcer, carcinoma of stomach, portal cirrhosis, glomerulonephritis, renal tuberculosis, renal tumor and chronic nonspecific ulcerative coltitis.

Etiology and Pathogenesis

1. Affection by exopathogen   Exopathogenic affection causes dryness – heat in the lung and the fight between wind and heat, leads to the impairment of purifying and descending function of the lung, and the damage of pulmonary vessels will result in hemoptysis and apostaxis.

2. Improper diet   Excessive drinking or taking too much pungent stuff leads to accumulation of dryness – heat in the stomach and intestines which turns into fire and overflows outwardly because of the injured blood vessels, resulting in haematemesis, apostaxis and hematochezia.

3. Emotional stress   Emotional stress brings on the fire stirring in the body and upward adverse flow of *qi*, making blood escape from vessels and resulting in bleeding. For example, pent – up anger impairs the liver and leads to adverse flow of the liver – *qi* disturbing the stomach. The injured collaterals of the stomach will result in haematemesis; stagnation of the liver – *qi* causes the liver – fire to invade the lung and makes blood ascend with the fire, resulting in apostaxis and hemoptysis.

4. Over – exertion   Over – exertion leads to the injury of the heart, spleen and kidney. When *qi* is impaired it will fail to command blood; and when essence – *qi* is impaired, hyperactivity of fire due to *yin* deficiency will arise and further generate bleeding.

5. After febrile disease or lasting illness   Either condition consumes excessively the body fluid, and causes hyperactivity of fire due to *yin* – deficiency; it may result in

the lack of vital *qi* and make *qi* fail to control blood; it may also bring about stagnation of blood vessels, leading to the failure of blood to circulate in the vessels. All the above mentioned conditions may give rise to bleeding.

Diagnosis and Discrimination

Bleeding syndrome is marked by blood failing to flow along its vessels, in which case, it will bleed through the mouth or nose (such as nosebleed, hemoptysis or haematemesis), or via two lower orifices (as urohematin or hematochezia), or out of the skin (i. e. purpura).

Discrimination should be made among coughing of blood, hemoptysis and haematemesis in clinic. Bleeding with cough is coughing of blood in which blood comes from the lung; hemoptysis refers to blood brought up immediately after coughing; while bleeding with vomiting is haematemesis in which blood comes from the stomach. Coughing of blood is scarlet mixed with phlegm in frothy form, small blood mass or mouthful of blood are often in hemoptysis which are brought up by coughing, while haematimesis is dark purple or deep – red blood mixed with food – residue or blood mass and is often accompanied with hematochezia.

As to hematochezia, there is a distinction in its sources, that is far – source or near – source. Far source bleeding comes from the stomach and small intestines mixed with stool, pitch – dark or dull purple color. And near – source bleeding originates from sigmoid colon, rectum or anus, separate from stool, or wrapping the stool, in scarlet color.

Blood in urine is divided into hematuria and stranguria complicated by hematuria. Bleeding with urine without pain is hematuria, while painful and dribbling urination with blood is stranguria complicated by hematuria. In this chapter, only hematuria is discussed, and the latter will be included in stranguria.

Selecting Treatment by Differentiating Syndromes

In differentiating syndromes of bleeding, firstly bleeding – spots and connected foci in viscera should be diagnosed. Secondly deficiency syndrome and excess syndrome should be distinguished, including heat of excess type, deficiency of *yin* and deficiency of *qi*. Generally speaking, heat of excess type is marked by acute condition, short course, bright purple blood in thick quality and large amount, and the patients mostly have a strong constitution in combination with some symptoms of heat of excess type; deficiency of *yin* is characterized by chronic condition, long course, scarlet or pink blood intermittently and with small amount, and the patients have a thin figure in combination with some symptoms of internally – accumulated heat due to deficiency of *yin*; deficiency of *qi* is manifested as protracted course, dull – colored blood in thin quality and small amount, but sometimes acute onset and large amount may occur, and the patients have a poor constitution and often are accompanied with some symptoms of *yang*-deficiency.

The treatments for bleeding syndrome can be summarized as treating pathogenic fire, syndrome of *qi* and bleeding; treating pathogenic fire means purging fire for patients with heat of excess type and nourishing *yin* to reduce fire for patients with heat of deficiency type; treating syndrome of *qi* refers to clearing up the *qifen* and descending *qi* for excess syndrome and invigorating *qi* for deficiency syndrome; by treating bleeding is meant removing heat from the blood to stop bleeding, astringing to arrest bleeding and promoting blood flow to stop bleeding.

Common syndromes:

1. Nosebleed

①Invasion of the lung by pathogenic heat

[Symptoms] Nosebleed, dry mouth, painful throat or accompanied with fever, cough with little phlegm, red tongue with thin fur, and rapid pulse.

[Main Points of Differentiation] Nosebleed, dry mouth and nose, fever.

This type is common in nosebleed by infective diseases and paroxysmal diseases.

[Pathogenesis] Accmulation of heat in the lung consumes the lung - *yin* causing bleeding due to blood - heat.

[Treatment] Clearing away heat from the lung and removing heat from the blood to stop bleeding.

[Recipe] *Sang Ju Yin* [227].

Cortex Moutan Radicis, *Rhizoma Imperatae*, *Herba Ecliptae* and *Cacumen Biotae* may be added to remove heat from the blood for stopping bleeding. In case of excessive lung - heat without exterior syndrome, subtract *Herba Menthae* and *Radix Platycodi*, and add *Radix Scutellariae* and *Fructus Gardeniae* to purge intense heat from the lung; in case of severe *yin* impairment, dry mouth, nose and throat, add *Radix Scrophulariae*, *Radix Ophiopogonis* and *Radix Rehmanniae* to nourish *yin* for moistening the lung.

[Nursing Points] Pay attention to climatic changes to avoid exopathogenic factors. Do not eat pungent and fried food.

②Excessive stomach - heat

[Symptoms] Nosebleed, sometimes accompanied with gingival hemorrhage in scarlet color, thirst with desire for drink, dry nose and mouth, ozostomia, dysphoria, constipation, red tongue with yellowish fur and rapid pulse.

[Main Points of Defferentiation] Nose bleed in scarlet color with large amount, thirst, constipation, red tongue with yellowish fur, rapid pulse.

This type is seen in nosebleed caused by febrile diseases and primary thrombocytopenic purpura.

[Pathogenesis] Flaring up of the stomach - fire causing bleeding.

[Treatment] Purging stomach - fire and removing heat from the blood to stop bleeding.

[Recipe] *Yu Nu Jian*[59].

Rhizoma Imperatae, *Herba Seu Radix Cirsii Japonici*, *Herba Cephalanoploris* and *Nodus Nelambinis Rhizomatis* may be added to remove heat from the blood for stopping bleeding. In case of serious heat, add *Radix Pittospori*, *Cortex Moutan Radicis* and *Radix Scutellariae* to clear heat and fire; in case of constipation, add *Radix et Rhizoma Rhei* to remove heat from *fu* - organs; in case of serious *yin* impairment with symptoms of thirst, red tongue with little fur, thready and rapid pulse, add *Radix Trichosanthis*, *Herba Dendrobii* and *Rhizoma Polygonati Odorati* to nourish the stomach for promoting the production of body fluid.

[Nursing Points] Restrain from smokes and alcohol, and pungent food.

③Flaming - up of the liver - fire

[Symptoms] Nosebleed, headache, dizziness, tinnitus, irritability, red eyes, bitter taste, red tongue, wiry and rapid pulse.

[Main Points of Differentiation] Nosebleed, headache, red eyes, bitter taste.

The type is observable in hypertension and febrile diseases.

[Pathogenesis] Fire due to stagnation of *qi* causing flaring - up of the liver - fire, resulting in bleeding.

[Treatment] Purging the liver of pathogenic fire and removing heat from the blood to stop bleeding.

[Recipe] *Long Dan Xie Gan Tang*[63].

Rhizona Imperatae, *Pollen Typhae*, *Herba seu Radix Cirsii Japonici*, *Herba Cephalanoploris* and *Nodus Nelumbinis Rhizomatisi* may be added to remove heat from the blood for stopping bleeding. In case of consumption of *yin* fluid, dry mouth and nose, red tongue with little fluid and thready and rapid pulse, subtract *Herba Plantaginis*, *Rhizoma Alismatis* and *Radix Angelicae Sinensis*, and add *Radix Scrophulariae*, *Radix Ophiopogonis*, *Fructus Ligustri Lucidi* and *Herba Ecliptae* to nourish *yin* and eliminate heat.

[Nursing Points] Regulate emotions to avoid anger; do not eat pugent food.

④Deficiency of *qi* and blood

[Symptoms] Nosebleed, sometimes complicated with gingival hemorrhage, hemato hidrosis, listlessness, pale complexion, dizziness, tinnitus, palpitation, restless, pale tongue, and thready and weak pulse.

[Main Points of Differentiation] Nosebleed, pale complexion, dizziness, palpitation, listlessness.

This type is seen in aplastic anemia and leukemia.

[Pathogenesis] Deficiency of *qi* and blood makes *qi* fail to command blood, leading to bleeding.

[Treatment] Invigorating *qi* to control blood.

[Recipe] *Gui Pi Tang*[95].

Herba agrimoniae, *colla corii asini* and *Radix Rubiae* may be used to increase the effectiveness in stopping beeding.

[Nursing Points] Take nutrient food; avoid tiredness.

2. Gingival hemorrhage

① Excessive stomach-fire

[Symptoms] Gingival hemorrhage in scarlet color, red, swollen and painful gums, headache, ozostomia, constipation, red tongue with yellowish fur, full and rapid pulse.

[Main Points of Differentiation] Gingival hemorrhage in scarlet color, painful gums, ozostomia and constipation.

This type is observable in thrombocytopenic purpura and aplastic anemia.

[Pathogenesis] Stomach-fire flaming up to impair vessels.

[Treatment] Purging fire from the stomach, and removing heat from the blood to stop bleeding.

[Recipe] *Jia Wei Qing Wei San*[99] with *Xie Xin Tang*[153].

Rhizoma Imperatae, *Herba Seu Radix Cirsii Japonici* and *Nodus Nelumbinis Rhizomatis* may be added to remove heat from the blood and stop bleeding.

[Nursing Points] Give up smoking and drinking alcohol; and do not take pungent, greasy and dry food.

② Excessive fire due to deficiency of *yin*

[Symptoms] Gingival hemorrhage in pink color, often induced by heat, dysphoria, and tiredness, unfixed teeth, red tongue with little fur, thready and rapid pulse.

[Main Points of Differentiation] Gingival hemorrhage, unfixed teeth, red tongue with little fur.

This type is common in thrombocytopenic purpura and aplastic anemia.

[Pathogenesis] Deficiency of the liver-*yin* and kidney-*yin* making the fire flare up, causing bleeding.

[Treatment] Nourishing *yin* to reduce pathogenic fire and removing heat from the blood to stop bleeding.

[Recipe] *Zi Shui Qing Gan Yin*[271] with *Qian Gen San*[178].

In case of severe deficiency-fire with symptoms of low fever, feverish sensation in the palms and soles, add *Cortex lycii Radicis*, *Radix Cynanchi Atrati* and *Rhizoma Anemarrhenae* to remove deficiency fire.

[Nursing Points] Refrain from smokes, alcohol and pungent food.

3. Hemoptysis

① Impairment of the lung by dryness-heat

[Symptoms] Itching throat, cough, phlegm with blood streaks, dry mouth and nose or with fever, red tongue with little fluid and thin and yellowish fur, and rapid pulse.

[Main Points of Differentiation] Itching throat, cough, phlegm with blood streads.

This type is seen in acute tracheobronchitis and bacterial pneumonia.

[Pathogenesis] Pathogenic wind-heat and dryness make the lung fail to purify and descend *qi* causing damage of pulmonary collaterals.

[Treatment] Removing heat, nourishing the lung and relieving vessels to stop bleeding.

[Recipe] *Sang Xing Tang* [226].

Rhizoma Imperatae and *Radix Rubiae* may be added to remove heat from the blood and stop bleeding; in case of serious impairment of fluid, add *Radix Scrophulariae* and *Radix Ophiopogonis* to nourish *yin* and moisturize dryness.

[Nursing Points] Avoid tiredness. Have nutritious and digestible food. And do not take pungent food.

②The liver-fire invading the lung

[Symptoms] Intermittent cough, phlegm with blood streaks, or scarlet blood only distending pain in the chest and hypochondrium, irritability, bitter taste, red tongue with thin and yellowish fur wiry and rapid pulse.

[Main Points of Differentiation] Cough, phlegm with blood streaks, distending pain in the chest and hypochondrium.

The type is common in bronchiectasis and pulmonary tuberculosis.

[Pathogenesis] Flaring-up of the liver-fire causing impairment of purifying and descending function of the lung and damage of pulmonary collaterals.

[Treatment] Purging the pathogenic fire in liver and lung, and removing heat from the blood to stop bleeding.

[Recipe] *Xie Bai San* [154] with *Dai Ge San* [287].

Radix Rehmanniae, *Herba Ecliptae*, *Rhizoma Imperatae*, *Herba Seu Radix Cirsii Japonici* and *Herba Cephalanoploris* may be added to clear away heat from the blood and stop bleeding. In case of dominant liver-fire with dizziness, red eyes and irritability, add *Cortex Moutan Radicis*, *Fructus Gardeniae* and *Radix Scu tellariae* to purge the pathogenic fire in the liver; if coughing brings up blood with large amount in scarlet color, *Xi Jiao Di Huang Tang* [273] may be used plus *Radix Notoginseng* powder (infused in boiling water) to remove heat and fire, and stop bleeding.

[Nursing Points] Adjust emotions to avoid anger. Refrain from smokes or alcohol, and pungent food.

③The lung-heat syndrome due to *yin* deficiency

[Symptoms] Cough with a little phlegm, phlegm with blood streaks or repeated coughing with blood in scarlet color, dry mouth and throat, flushing of zygomatic region, hectic fever, night sweating, red tongue with little fur, and thready and rapid pulse.

[Main Points of Differentiation] Cough, dry throat, phlegm with blood streaks, hectic fever and night sweating.

This type is often seen in pulmonary tuberculosis and cancer of lung.

[Pathogenesis] The lung-heat due to deficiency of *yin* causing impairment of purifying and descending function of the lung and damage of pulmonary collaterals.

[Treatment] Nourishing *yin*, moisturizing the lung and relieving pulmonary collatrals to stop bleeding.

[Recipe] *Bai He Gu Jin Wan*[103].

Rhizoma Bletillae, *Nodus Nelumbinis Rhizomatis*, *Rhizoma Imperatae* and *Radix Rubiae* may be added to stop bleeding. In case of repeated coughing with blood, or coughing with blood in large amount, add *Colla Corii Asini* and *Radix Notoginseng* to nourish blood and stop bleeding; in case of hectic fever and flushing of zygomatic region, add *Herba Artemisiae*, *Carapax Trionycis*, *Cortex Lycii Radicis* and *Radix Cynanchi Atrati* to remove deficiency heat; for night sweating, add *Radix Oryzae Glutinosae*, *Fructus Tritici Levis*, *Fructus Schisandrae* and *Concha Ostreae* to induce astringency.

[Nursing Points] Do not take pungent food; avoid smoking and drinking alcohol.

4. Hematemesis

①Excessive heat in stomach

[Symptoms] Fullness, even pain in the stomach, red or deep purple blood when vomiting, and often mixed up with food residue, ozostomia, constipation or dark stool, red tongue with yellowish and greasy fur, and slippery and rapid pulse.

[Main Points of Differentiation] Red blood when vomiting, fullness in the stomach, ozostomia, constipation, and slippery and rapid pulse.

This type is common in acute and chronic gastritis and peptic ulcer.

[Pathogenesis] Accumulation of heat in the stomach impairing stomach collaterals, causing failure of descending of the stomach - *qi*.

[Treatment] Clearing away heat in the stomach and removing the blood stasis for hemostasis.

[Recipe] *Xie Xin Tang*[153] with *Shi Hui San*[5].

In case of vomiting caused by adverse flow of the stomach - *qi*, add *Ochra Haematitum*, *Caulis Bambusae in Taeniam* and *Flos Inulae* to regulate the stomach - *qi* and relieve the adverse flow of *qi*.

[Nursing Points] Be abstemious in eating and drinking. And avoid pungent food, smoking and drinking alcohol.

②The liver - fire invading the stomach

[Symptoms] Red or deep - purple blood when vomiting, bitter taste, painful hypochondrium, irritability, insomnia and dreamful sleep, deep - red tongue, wiry and rapid pulse.

[Main points of Differentiation] Vomiting with red blood, bitter taste and painful hypochondrium.

This type is observable in acute and chronic gastritis and peptic ulcer.

[Pathogenesis] Flaring - up of the liver - fire invading the stomach, causing impairment of stomach collaterals.

[Treatment] Purging the liver-fire and stomach heat and removing heat from the blood to stop bleeding.

[Recipe] *Long Dan Xie Gan Tang*[64].

Rhizona Imperatae, *Nodus Nelunbinis Rhizomatis*, *Herba Ecloptae* and *Radix Rubiae* may be added to elimiate heat from the blood and arrest bleeding.

[Nursing Points] Keep a cheerful mood. Do not have pungent or indigestible food.

③Bleeding due to deficiency of *qi*

[Symptoms] Continual vomiting with blood of alternate mildness and severity and in dull color, listlessness, palpitation, shortness of breath, pale face, pale tongue, thready and weak pulse.

[Main Points of Differentiation] Continual Vomiting with blood, palpitation, shortness of breath, listlessness, weak pulse.

This type can be observed in bleeding due to gastroduodenal bulbar ulcer.

[Pathogenesis] Deficiency of *qi* in middle-*jiao* impeding its ability to command blood, resulting in bleeding.

[Treatment] Strengthening the spleen, nourishing the heart and replenishing *qi* for commanding blood.

[Recipe] *Gui Pi Tang*[95].

Herba Agimoniae, *Rhizoma Bletillae*, *Os Sepiella seu Sepiae* and baked ginger may be added to warm the channels and arrest bleeding.

[Nursing Points] Avoid smoking, drinking alcohol and pungent food; adujst moods and daily life; and have nutrient but light diet.

5. Hematochezia

①Dampness-heat in intestinal tract

[Symptoms] Scarlet blood in stool, constipation, or loose stool, sometimes accompanied with abdominal pain, bitter taste, yellowish and greasy fur, soft and floating, and rapid pulse.

[Main Points of Differentiation] Scarlet blood in stool, bitter taste, yellowish and greasy fur.

This type is common in chronic nonspecific ulcerative colitis.

[Pathogenesis] Accumulation of dampness-heat impairing intestinal collaterals, and thus impeding the transporting ability of intestines and obstructing functional activities of *qi*.

[Treatment] Eliminating dampness-heat and removing heat from the blood to stop bleeding.

[Recipe] *Di Yu San*[105].

[Nursing Points] Refrain from smoking, drinking alochol and avoid pungent, greasy and sweet food.

②Insufficiency – cold of the spleen and stomach

[Symptoms] Deep – purple or dark blood in stool, listlessness, loose stool and pale tongue.

This type is seen in chronic nonspecific ulcertive colitis and gastroduodenal bulbar ulcer.

[Pathogenesis] Insufficiency – cold of the spleen and stomach causing deficiency of *qi* in middle – *jiao*, thus impeding the ability of *qi* to command blood and resulting in bleeding in the stomach and intestines.

[Treatment] Inigorating the spleen, warming the middle – *jiao* and nourishing blood to stop bleeding.

[Recipe] *Huang Tu Tang* [230].

Rhizoma Bletillae and *Os Sepiella seu Sepiae* may be added as hemostyptics; *Radix Notoginseng* and *Ophicalcitum* can be used to promote the circulation of blood and arrest bleeding. In case of serious deficiency *yang* with aversion to cold and cold limbs, add *Cornu Cervi Degelatinatum*, Baked Ginger and *Folium Artemisiae Argyi* to warm *yang* and arrest bleeding.

[Nursing Points] Regulate daily life; avoid wind – cold; do not eat uncooked or cold food; and prevent over – working.

6. Hematuria

①Excessive heat in lower – *jiao*

[Symptoms] Dark urine with burning sensation during urination, scarlet urohematin, vexation, thirst, flushed face, aphthae, restless sleep, red tongue and rapid pulse.

[Main Points of Diffentiation] Dark urine with burning sensation during urination, scarlet urohematin.

This type is seen in acute nephritis, renal tuberculosis and renal tumor.

[Pathogenesis] Excessive heat in lower – *jiao* impairing vessels, causing bleeding from bladder.

[Treatment] Clearing away heat and purging fire, removing heat from the blood to stop bleeding.

[Recipe] *Xiao Ji Yin Zi* [31].

[Nursing Points] Avoid pungent and greasy food.

②Excessive fire due to deficency of the kidney

[Symptoms] Scanty dark urine with blood, dizziness, tinnitus, flushing of zygomatic region, hectic fever, lassitude in loins and knees, red tongue, thready and rapid pulse.

[Main Points of Differentiation] Scannty dark urine with blood, tinnitus, hectic fever, lassitude in loins and knees.

This type can be observed in renal tuberculosis and renal tumor.

[Pathogenesis] Deficiency of the kidney – *yin* causing deficiency fire to flare up in the body and impair vessels.

[Treatment] Nourishing *yin* to reduce pathogeic fire, and removing fire from the blood to arrest bleeding.

[Recipe] *Zhi Bai Di Huang Wan* [160].

Herba Ecliptae, *Herba Seu Radix Cirsii Japonici*, *Herba Cephalanoploris*, *Nodus Nelumbinis Rhizomatis* and *Pollen Typhae* may be added to remove heat from the blood, and arrest bleeding.

[Nursing Points] Regulate daily life and refrain from excessive sexual intercourse, avoid smoking, drinking and pungent food.

③Failure of the spleen in governing blood

[Symptoms] Hematuria for a long period, dim complexion, tiredness, short breath, low voice, sometimes accompanied with gingival hemorrhage, hematohidrosis, pale tongue, thready and weak pulse.

[Main Points of Differentiation] Urohemation for a long period, dim complexion, short breath, tiredness, pale tongue and weak pulse.

This type is common in urohematin caused by hematopathy.

[Pathogenesis] Insufficiency of the spleen – *qi* makes the spleen fail in governing blood, thus resulting in irregular blood circulation.

[Treatment] Invigorating the spleen for controlling blood.

[Recipe] *Gui Pi Tang*[95].

[Nursing Points] Have nutritious but not greasy food and avoid over – eating.

④unconsolidation of the kidney – *qi*

[Symptoms] Lasting urohematin in pink color, dizziness, tinnitus, listlessness, soreness in loins, pale tongue, and deep and weak pulse.

[Main Points of Differentiation] Lasting urohematin in pink color, tinnitus, soreness in loins.

This type is observable in renal tumor and renal tuberculosis.

[Pathogenesis] Unconsolidation of the kidney – *qi* with decline of its reserving function causing bleeding with urine.

[Treatment] Invigorating the kidney – *qi* to stop bleeding.

[Recipe] *Wu Bi Shan Yao Wan*[34].

[Nursing Points] Be moderate in sexual intercourse. Avoid Smoking, drinking alcohol and pungent food.

7. Purpura

①Bleeding due to blood – heat

[Symptoms] Dark – purple dots or mass on the skin, accompanied with nosebleed, gingival hemorrhage, hematochezia and urohematin, or fever, thirst, constipation, red tongue with yellowish fur, wiry and rapid pulse.

[Main Points of Differentiation] Dark – purple dots or mass on the skin, fever, thirst, constipation, red tongue with yellowish fur and rapid pulse.

This type is often seen in thrombocytopenic purpura, aplastic anemia and acute leukemia.

[Pathogenesis] Accumulation of heat in vessels causing bleeding.

[Treatment] Clearing away heat and toxic material, and removing heat from the blood to stop bleeding.

[Recipe] *Xi Jiao Di Huang Tang* [273].

In case of severe toxic heat, fever, wide spots of blood, add *Gypsum Fibrosum*, *Radix Gentianae* and *Radix Arnebiae seu Lithospermi*, plus *Zi Xue Dan*[267] (infused in boiling water).

[Nursing Points] Avoid tiredness. Pay attention to climatic changes to guard against exopathogen. Have nourishing and digestible food. Avoid pungent food and smoking and drinking alcohol.

②Hyperactivity of fire due to *yin* deficiency

[Symptoms] Intermittent occurrence of dark – purple blood dots or mass accompanied with nosebleed, gingival hemorrhage or menorrhagia, flushed cheeks, irritability, thirst, feverish sensation of the palms and soles, and sometimes with hectic fever, night sweat, red tongue with little fur, thready and rapid pulse.

[Main points of Differentiation] Ecchymosis and dots in scarlet or purple color, hectic fever, night sweat, red tongue with little fur.

This type can be observed in thrombocytopenic purpura, allergic purpura and aplastic anemia.

[Pathogenesis] Hyperactivity of fire due to *yin* deficiency impairing vessels, causing bleeding marked on the skin.

[Treatment] Nourishing *yin* to reduce pathogenic fire and relieving vessels to arrest bleeding.

[Recipe] *Qian Gen San*[178].

In case of severe *yin* deficiency, add *Radix Scrophulariae*, *Plastrum Testudinis* and *Herba Ecliptae* to nourish *yin* and eliminate heat.

[Nursing Points] Have nutrient and digestible food. Avoid pungent food and fish, shrimp, crab and milk.

③Failure of *qi* in commanding blood

[Symptoms] Lasting illness with repeating hematohidrosis, listlessness, dizziness, pale or sallow complexion, poor appetite, pale tongue, and thready and weak pulse.

[Main points of Differentiation] Dull purple blood dots on the skin appearing repeatedly and aggravated after over–working.

This type is common in thrombocytopenic purpura and chronic aplastic anemia.

[Pathogenesis] Consumption of *qi* and blood, and failure of *qi* in commanding blood leading to bleeding marked on the skin.

[Treatment] Tonifying *qi* to make it able to command blood.

[Recipe] *Gui Pi Tang*[95].

Herba Agrimoniae, palm charcoal, *Radix Sanguisorbae*, *Pollen Typhae*, *Radix Rubiae* and *Radix Arnebiae seu Lithospermi* may be added to strengthen the effect of arresting bleeding and removig blood stasis. If accompanied with deficiency of the kidney-*qi* with soreness of loins and knees, add *Fructys Corni*, *Semen Cuscutae* and *Radix Dipsacy* to tonify the kidney and invigorate *qi*.

[Nursing Points] Build up the body to guard against exopathogen. Avoid smoking, drinking, pungent food and over-working. Take nutrient and digestible food.

Summary

Bleeding syndrome	Nosebleed	Pathogenic heat invading the lung	Removing heat from the lung and blood to stop bleeding	*Sang Ju Yin*
		Excessive heat in the stomach	Removing heat from the stomach and blood to arrest bleeding	*Yu Nu Jian*
		Flaming-up of the liver-fire	Removing fire from the liver and blood to stop bleeding	*Long Dan Xie Gan Tang*
		Deficiency of *qi* and blood	Tonifying *qi* to command blood	*Gui Pi Tang*
	Gingival hemorrhage	Excessive fire in the stomach	Eliminating fire and heat from the stomach and blood to arrest bleeding	*Jia Wei Qing Wei San* with *Xie Xin Tang*
		Hyperactivity of fire due to *yin* deficiency	Nourishing *yin* to reduce fire and removing heat from blood to stop bleeding	*Zi Shui Qing Gan Yin* with *Qian Gen San*
	Hemopysis	Dryness-heat impairing the lung	Removing heat and moisturizing the lung, relieving vessels to stop bleeding	*Sang Xing Tang*
		The liver-fire invading the lung	Removing heat from the liver, lung and blood to stop bleeding	*Xie Bai San* with *Dai Ge San*
		The lung-heat caused by *yin* deficiency	Nourishing *yin*, moisturizing the lung and relieving vessels to arrest bleeding	*Bai He Gu Jin Tang*
	Hematemesis	Accumulation of heat in the stomach	Removing heat from the stomach and eliminating blood stasis to stop bleeding	*Xie Xin Tang* and *Shi Hui San*
		The liver-fire invading the stomach	Removing heat from the liver, stomach and blood to arrest bleeding	*Long Dan Xie Gan Tang*
		Bleeding due to *qi* deficiency	Strengthening the spleen, nourishing the heart and invigorating *qi* to command blood	*Gui Pi Tang*
	Hematochezia	Damp-heat in the intestinal tract	Removing the damp-heat, cooling the blood to arrest bleeding	*Di Yu San*
		Deficiency cold in the spleen and stomach	Strengthening the spleen, warming the middle-*jiao* and nourishing blood to stop bleeding	*Huang Tu Tang*
	Urohematin	Excessive heat in lower-*jiao*	Removing heat from lower-*jiao* and cooling blood to stop bleeding	*Xiao Ji Yin Zi*
		Excessive fire due to deficiency of the kidney	Nourishing *yin* to reduce fire and removing heat from blood to stop bleeding	*Zhi Bai Di Huang Wan*
		Failure of the spleen in commanding blood	Tonifying the spleen for commanding blood	*Gui Pi Tang*
		Unconsolidation of the kidney-*qi*	Tonifying the kidney-*qi* for stopping bleeding	*Wu Bi Shan Yao Wan*
	Purpura	Bleeding due to heat in blood	Clearing away heat and toxic material and removing heat from the blood to arrest bleeding	*Xi Jiao Di Huang Tang*
		Excessive heat due to *yin* deficiency	Nourishing *yin*, removing heat and relieving vessels to stop bleeding	*Qian Gen San*
		Failure of *qi* in commanding blood	Tonifying *qi* to command blood	*Gui Pi Tang*

Discussions

1. What is bleeding syndrome? And how many common types are there?
2. What are the treatments for bleeding syndrome?
3. How do you distinguish hemoptysis from hematemesis? What are their respective common types? And what are the main points of differentiation, respective treatments and recipes for them?

31 Edema

General

Edema is a morbid condition marked by retention of water in the body making the skin swell such as palpebebral edema, cephaledema, facial edema, edema of limbs, even general edema. If serious, it may well be accompanied with hydrothorax and ascites.

The differentiating treatments for the disease are referential to acute and chronic nephritis, nephrotic syndrome, cardiac edema, idiopathic edema, premenstrual tensional syndrome, myxedema and dystrophic edema in Western Medicine.

Etiology and Pathogenesis

Edema is the clinical reflection of dysfunction of the *zang* and *fu* organs and irregular activities of *qi*. The root cause is dysfunction of the kidney, with the lung, spleen and *san-jiao* involved in.

1. Wind-cold pathogen leading to failure of the lung in maintaining normal water metabolism The lung is the upper resource of water, and its function is to ascend vital *qi* and descend turbid *qi*. When the lung is affected by pathogens, its functional activities will be disturbed, which will cause retention of water, and counteraction between wind and water pathogens, resulting in the swelling of the skin.

2. Disturbance of the spleen-*qi* by toxin and dampness Toxin of carbuncle, furuncle and pyogenic infections or pathogenic dampness gathering in the spleen causes dysfunction of the spleen in transport, leading to disorder of water metabolism and resulting in swelling of the skin.

3. Accumulation of dampness-heat obstructing the *san-jiao* Dampness-heat accumulating for a long time in the *san-jiao* causes disorder of *qi* and impaired water metabolism resulting in edema.

4. Edema due to insufficiency of *yang* and the kidney-*qi* Insufficiency of *yang-qi*, the kidney-*qi* and the kidney-essence leads to dysfunction of the spleen and lung and that of the urinary bladder, giving rise to edema.

Key Points:

Pathogenic wind invading the body	{ Dysfunction of the lung in ascending and descending, irregular water metabolism
Pathogenic dampness invading the body	{ Disturbance of the spleen – *qi* causing failure of the spleen in transport
Accumulation of dampness – heat	{ Dysfunction of the *san – jiao* making stagnation of *qi* and retention of water
Weakness due to overstrain	{ Consumption of the kidney – essence leading to edema due to *yang* insufficiency

} Accumulation of pathogenic water in the body giving rise to swelling of the skin } Edema

Diagnosis and Discrimination

Edema is characterized by swelling of the skin and muscles. Discrimination should be made between edema and fluid – retention syndrome as well as tympanites.

Discrimination \ Disease	Edema	Tympanites	Fluid – retention Syndrome
Etiology and pathogenesis	Abnormal water metabolism due to dysfunction of the lung, spleen and kidney	Dysfunction of the liver, spleen and kidney	Dysfunction of the lung, spleen and kidney
Characteristics	Having case history of nephroses, pale complexion, swelling of the flabby skin in the face and limbs; hydrothorax or ascites appearing only in serious cases, without outstanding veins on the abdominal surface	Having case history of hepatopathy, dimmish and bluish complexion, ascites without edema of limbs, slight swelling of the lower limbs seen in severe case, outstanding veins on the abdominal surface	Fluid – retention in some part of the body

Selecting Treatment by Differentiating Syndromes

In differentiating syndromes of edema, the major point is to distinguish *yin* syndrome from *yang* syndrome, and the next is to differentiate exterior syndrome from interior syndrome, cold syndrome form heat syndrome and deficiency syndrome from excess syndrome. At the same time, attention should be paid to changes of pathogeneses, superficiality and origin as well as acute and chronic cases.

Common Types:
1. *Yang Shui* (edema of *yang* syndrome)
① *Feng Shui* (edema of wind syndrome)

[Symptoms] Palpebral edema followed rapidly by that of the limbs and the whole body, accompanied with fever, aversion to cold, soreness in limb joints, difficulty in urination, or cough with dyspnea, painful throat, reddish or whitish tongue, floating and slippery pulse, or deep and tight pulse.

[Main Points of Differentiation] Palpebral edema rapidly spreading to the whole body, complicated with exterior syndrome of wind-cold or wind-heat.

This type is seen at the initial stage of acute nephritis.

[Pathogenesis] Pathogenic wind invades the lung and impairs the ascending and descending function of the lung causing abnormality in water metabolism and resulting in swelling.

[Treatment] Expelling wind, removing heat and promoting water metabolism by activating dispersing function of the lung.

[Recipe] *Yue Bi Jia Zhu Tang* [262].

In case of dominant wind-heat, add *Rhizoma Imperatae*, *Fructus Forsythiae* and *Radix Isatidis* to remove heat and activate dispersing function of the lung; in case of wind-cold, add *Folium Perillae Acutae*, *Radix Lede Bouriellae* and *Ramulus Cinnalmomi*, and subtract accordingly *Gypsum Fibrosum*; in case of deficiency of *wei-yang* with sweating and aversion to wind, use *Fang Ji Huang Qi Tang*[122] to invigorate the lung and *wei* for promoting water metabolism.

[Nursing points] Have light food; avoid wind-cold; and avoid overstrain.

②Pathogenic dampness invading the body

[Symptoms] Palpebral edema spreading to the whole body, difficulty in urination, carbuncle and sore, even ulcer accompanied with fever, aversion to cold, red tongue with thin and yellowish fur, floating, slippery and rapid pulse.

[Main Points of Differentiation] Palpebral edema spreading to the whole body, exterior syndrome of wind-heat, sore and carbuncle, floating, slippery and rapid pulse.

This type is common in acute nephritis.

[Pathogenesis] Pathogenic dampness accumulates in the lung and *wei* and affects the *zang-fu* organs, and the dysfunction of the spleen and lung will make dampness turn into heat, resulting in swelling.

[Treatment] Ventilating the lung, removing pathogen and promoting water metabolism to alleviate edema.

[Recipe] *Ma Huang Lian Qiao Chi Xiao Dou Tang*[243].

In case of excessive heat caused by the retention of pathogenic dampness, add *Flos Lonicerae*, *Herba Taraxaci*, *Radix Isatidis* and *Viola Yedoensis*; in case of ulceration with pus, add *Radix Sophorae Flavescentis* and *Rhizoma Smilacis Glabrae*; in case of serious swelling due to heat in the blood, add *Cortex Moutan Radicis*, *Radix Paeoniae Rubra* and *Radix et Rhizoma Rhei*.

[Nursing Points] Avoid pungent and fried food. Regulate daily life.

③Retention of wetness within the body

[Symptoms] General edema, sunken surface when pressed with finger, lassitude, oliguria, chest tightness and nausea, poor appetite, whitish and greasy fur, deep and moderate pulse, slow onset with long period.

[Main Points of Differentiation] General edema, sunken surface when pressed with finger, long course of illness, lassitude, chest tightness and nausea.

This type may be observed in chronic nephritis, nephrotic syndrome, right heart failure and alimentary edema.

[Pathogenesis] Disturbance of the spleen - yang by internally accumulated dampness causes dysfunction of the spleen and retention of wetness within the body, resulting in edema.

[Treatment] Strengthening the spleen to eliminate wetness, activating yang to promote diuresis.

[Recipe] *Wei Ling Tang*[182] with *Wu Pi Yin*[40].

In case of serious edema with asthma, add *Herba Ephedrae*, *Semen Lepidii Seu Descurainiae* and *Semen Armeniacae Amarum* to facilitate the flow of the lung - qi for relieving asthma.

[Nursing Points] Have nutrient, digestible and low salt diet.

④Excessive dampness - heat

[Symptoms] General edema, bound and glossy skin, feeling stuffy in epigastrium, excessive thirst, dark urine, constipation, yellowish and greasy fur, slippery and rapid pulse, or deep and rapid pulse.

[Main Points of Differentiation] General edema, bound and glossy skin, feeling stuffy in epigastrium, excessive thirst, dark urine, constipation, yellowish and greasy fur.

This type is observable in acute nephritis

[Treatment] Removing dampness - heat by promoting water metabolism.

[Recipe] *Shu Zao Yin Zi* [275].

In case of serious edema, adopt *Wu Ling San*[41]; if accompanied with dyspnea, use *Ting Li Da Zao Xie Fei Tang*[261]; if yin - fluid is consumed with dominant heat syndrome due to lasting accumulation of dampness - heat, choose *Zhu Ling Tang*[257]; for serious case of constipation and abdominal distention, *Ji Jiao Li Huang Wan*[24] may be used.

[Nursing Points] Have light and low salt diet. Avoid smoking, drinking alcohol and pungent food.

2. *Yin Shui* (edema of yin syndrome)

①Insufficiency of the spleen - yang

[Symptoms] General edema, specially the part below the loins, sunken surface with difficulty in recovery if pressed, stuffiness in epigastrium, abdominal distention, poor appetite, loose stool, sallow complexion, listlessness, cold limbs, oliguria, pale tongue, whitish and greasy fur, deep and moderate pulse.

[Main Points of Differentiation] Pitting edema specially below the loins, listlessness, cold limbs, poor appetite, loose stool, deep and moderate pulse.

This type is seen in chronic nephritis, nephrotic syndrome, cardiac edema, alimentary edema and the late stage of myxedema.

[Pathogenesis] Insufficiency of the spleen-*yang* leads to dysfunction of the spleen in transport and makes *yang* fail in transforming *qi*, resulting in edema.

[Treatment] Warming the spleen-*yang* to promote water metabolism.

[Recipe] *Shi Pi Yin*[159].

In case of obvious *qi* deficiency, add *Radix Ginseng* and *Radix Astragali seu Hedusari* to warm the middle-*jiao* and tonify the spleen; in case of serious edema and oliguria, add *Ramulus Cinnamomi* and *Rhizoma Alismatis* to promote the function of the urinary bladder.

[Nursing Points] Keep away from wind-cold. Have nutrient and low salt diet.

②Deficiency of the kidney-*qi*

[Symptoms] Edema of the head, face and the whole body, specially the part below the loins, sunken surface with difficulty in recovery if pressed, palpitation, short breath, heaviness, soreness and coldness of the loins, oliguria or polyuria, listlessness, cold limbs, pale or grey complexion, pale and emlarged tongue, whitish fur, deep, slow, thready and weak pulse.

[Main Points of Differentiation] General pitting edema, specially below the loins, heaviness, soreness and coldness of the loins, listlessness, cold limbs, deep, slow, thready and weak pulse.

This type can be seen in chronic nephritis, neurosis, cardiogenic pulmonary edema, alimentary edema and the late stage of mucoid edema.

[Treatment] Warming the kidney to reinforce *yang-qi* and promoting water metabolism.

[Recipe] *Ji Sheng Shen Qi Wan*[184] with *Zhen Wu Tang*[199].

In case of hyperdiuresis, subtract *Rhizoma Alismatos* and *Semen Plantaginis*, and add *Oetheca Mantidis* and *Fructus Psoraleae*; in case of palpitation and cyanotic lips, use larger amount of *Radix Aconiti*, and add *Ramulus Cinnamomi*, *Radix Salviae Miltiorrhizae* and *Rhizoma Zingiberis* to warm *yang* and remove stasis; in case of dyspnea and shortness of breath, add *Gecko* and *Fructus Schisandrae*, or take *Hei Xi Dan*[268]; in case of listlessness, nausea and uric taste in the mouth, add *Radix Aconiti*, *Rhizoma Coptidis* and *Radix et Rhizoma Rhei*.

[Nursing Points] Have low salt diet. Avoid wind-cold.

Summary

Edema is commonly seen in clinic, the differentiation of which should be conducted with a close observation of the functional changes of the *zang-fu* organs (the kidney, the spleen, and the lung). It is important to distinguish *yin* syndrome from *yang* one, and the primary cause from the secondary one, paying special attention to the interchanges between the excess and deficiency syndrome as well as the cold and heat syndromes. The common treatments for this disease include ventilating the lung to benefit sweating, reinforcing the spleen and warming the kidney, removing stasis and purging turbid *qi*, promoting water metabolism, which should be selected on the basis of careful and accurate differentiation.

Edema	Yang Shui	*Feng Shui* — The lung failing to ascend and descend *qi* and water	Expelling wind, removing heat and promoting water metabolism by activating dispersing function of the lung; recipe: *Yue Bi Jia Zhu Tang*
		Pathogenic dampness invading the body — Dysfunction of the spleen and lung	Ventilating the lung, removing pathogenic dampness and promoting water metabolism to alleviate edema; recipe: *Ma Huang Lian Qiao Chi Xiao Dou Tang*
		Retention of wetness within the body — Disturbance of the spleen-*yang* by dampness	Strengthening the spleen, activating *yang* and promoting water metabolism; recipe: *Wei Ling Tang* with *Wu Pi Yin*
		Excessive dampness-heat — Accumulation of dampness-heat in the *san-jiao*	Removing dampness-heat by promoting water metabolism; recipe: *Shu Zao Yin Zi*
	Yin Shui	Insufficiency of the spleen-*yang* — Abnormal water metabolism	Warming the spleen-*yang* to promote water metabolism; recipe: *Shi Pi Yin*
		Deficiency of the kidney-*qi* — Failure of *yang* in transforming *qi*	Warming the kidney to reinforce *yang-qi* and promoting water metabolism; recipe: *Ji Sheng Shen Qi Wan* with *Zhen Wu Tang*

Discussions

1. Retell the etiology and pathogenesis of edema.
2. How is edema distinguished from tympanites?
3. Retell the symptoms, main points of differentiation, treatments and recipes of various types of *Yang shui*.

32 Stranguria

General

Stranguria is a syndrome characterized by frequent, painful and dripping urination, contracture of lower abdomen, and pain involving waist and abdomen.

The differentiating treatments for the disease are referential to the above symptoms seen in urinary infection, urinary calculus, tuberculosis of urinary system, prostatitis, chyluria and urinary tumor in Western Medicine.

Etiology and Pathogenesis

1. Dampness–heat in the urinary bladder   Excessive intake of pungent, greasy or sweet food, or excessive alcohol generate dampness–heat which spreads downward to the urinary bladder, resulting in stanguria. The symptom manifested as burning pain with urine is known as heat–stranguria; if the impurity in the urine turns into stone as the result of lasting accumulation of dampness–heat, it is called stone–stranguria; if the dampness–heat gathers in the urinary bladder and causes disturbance in *qi* transformation which impedes the decomposition of essence and excretion so that the essence is excreted along with the urine, giving rise to greasy urine, it is called grease–stranguria; if excessive heat impairs the vessels and causes irregular blood circulation manifested as difficult and painful urination with blood, it is known as blood–stranguria.

2. Insufficiency of the spleen and kidney   Insufficiency of the spleen and kidney may result from comsumption of vital *qi* by dampness–heat as the result of protracted stranguria, or from one of the following factors such as senile decay, long illness, debility, over–working or improper sexual intercourse. Insufficiency of the spleen will cause sinking of *qi* in middle–*jiao*, while insufficiency of the kidney will lead to unconsolidation of vital *qi* in lower–*jiao*, which will result in stranguria. If the stranguria comes on with over–working, it is named overstrain–stranguria; if the stranguria is caused by deficiency and sinking of *qi* in middle–*jiao*, it is *qi*–stranguria of deficiency type; when the urine is like fat and grease due to insufficiency of the kidney *qi* and unconsolidation of *qi* in lower–*jiao*, it is grease–stranguria. When the urine is accompanied with blood because deficiency of the kidney–*yin* causes deficiency–fire to impair vessels resulting in stranguria, the stranguria is called blood–stranguria.

3. Stagnation of the liver–*qi*   *Qi*–stranguria of excess type is caused by impairment of the liver due to fury which will cause stagnation of *qi* to become fire and the accumulation in lower–*jiao* will impede the function of the urinary bladder with the symptoms of distention of lower abdomen, difficult, painful and dribbling urination.

Diagnosis and Discrimination

The discrimination of stranguria from other disceses is as follows:

1. *Long Bi* *Long Bi* is marked by difficulty in urination and oliguria, even no urine if serious, among the symptoms of which difficulty in urination is similar to that of stranguria. The discrimination between the two is that stranguria has the symptom of frequent and painful sensation during urination, which will not appear in *Long Bi*.

2. Hematuria Blood-stranguria and hematuria have in common the symptoms of bleeding with urination, dark urine, and even pure blood excreted sometimes. Discrimination should focus on whether there is painful sensation during urination. If there is, it belongs to the former; if not, the latter.

3. Turbid urine Discrimination should be made between turbid urine and stranguria. Although the urine is turbid in both cases, difficult and painful sensation during urination is accompanied with stranguria, while there is no such sensation in turbid urine.

Selecting Treatment by Differentiating Syndromes

1. Heat-stranguria

[Symptoms] Frequent urination, oliguria, hot and painful discharge of reddish urine, distention, pain and cramping sensation of the lower abdomen, sometimes with chills and fever, bitter taste, nausea, lumbago aversion to press, or constipation, yellowish and greasy fur, soft and floating and rapid pulse.

[Main Points of Differentiation] Frequent urination, oliguria, hot and painful discharge of reddish urine, constipation, yellowish and greasy fur.

This type is seen in urethritis, cystitis, pyelonephritis, cystomhthisis and renal tuberculosis.

[Pathogenesis] Accumulation of dampness-heat in lower-*jiao* causing dysfunction of the urinary bladder.

[Treatment] Clearing away heat, promoting diuresis and urination.

[Recipe] *Ba Zheng San*[12].

In case of constipation and distention of abdomen, take a larger amount of *Radix et Rhizoma Rhei*, and add *Fructus Aurantii Imaturus* to remove heat from *fu*-organs; if accompanied with chills and fever, bitter taste and nausea, *Xiao Chai Hu Tang*[30] may be added to treat *Shaoyang* disease by mediation; in case of impairment of *yin* by dampness-heat, subtract *Radix et Rhizoma Rhei*, and add *Radix Rchmanniae*, *Rhizoma Anemarrhenae* and *Rhizoma Imperatae* to replenish *yin* and remove heat.

[Nursing Points] Avoid pungent, greasy and sweet food; have light food and drink much boiled water.

2. Stone-stranguria

[Symptoms] Urine often complicated with stones, difficulty in urination, interruption of urination, urethralgia, cramping senstaion of the lower abdomen, or colic of the loins and abdomen, urine with blood, red tongue, thin and yellowish fur, or wiry and rapid pulse. If the case of urine with stones have lasted a long time, such symptoms will occur as dim complexion, listlessness, lassitude, pale tongue with teeth marks, thready and weak pulse; or dull pain in the loins and abdomen, feverish sensation in the palms and soles, red tongue with little fur, thready and rapid pulse.

[Main Points of Differentiation] Interruption of urination, urethralgia, cramping sensation of the lower abdomen, or urine with blood.

This type is common in urinary tract calculi.

[Pathogenesis] Excessive in take of greasy, sweet and pungent food leads to accumulation of dampness - heat in the lower - *jiao* which affects the urine and gradually turns into stones. As a result, the urinary tract is obstructed and the vessels impaired.

[Treatment] Clearing away heat, promoting diuresis, promoting urination and removing stones.

[Recipe] *Shi Wei San*[63].

In case of colic of the loins and abdomen, *Radix paeoniae Alba* and *Radix Glycyrrhizae* may be added to relieve spasm and pain; in case of urine with blood, add *Herba Cephalanoploris*, *Rasix Rehmanniae* and *Nodus Nelumbinis* to remove heat from blood and stop bleeding; if accompanied with fever, add *Herba Tara Xaci*, *Cortex Phellodendri* and *Radix et Rhizoma Rhei* to remove heat; in case of lasting stone - stranguria showing deficiency syndrome complicated with excess syndrome, its symptoms and causes should be dealt with at the same time; in case of deficiency of *qi* and blood, adopt *Er Shen San*[4] and *Ba Zhen Tang*[13]. While *Liu Wei Di Huang Wan* [46] and *Shi Wei San* [63] should be used for cases of consumption of *yin* - fluid.

[Nursing Points] Take light food; avoid pungent, fat and sweet food.

3. *Qi* - stranguria

[Symptoms] Excess syndrome: Difficult and dribbling urination, fullness and pain of the lower abdomen, whitish and thin fur, deep and wiry pulse.

Deficiency syndrome: Distending sensation in the lower abdomen, dribbling urination, pale complexion, pale tongue, weak, thready and feeble pulse.

[Main Points of Differentiation] Excess syndrome: Difficult in urination, fullness and pain of the lower abdomen, wiry pulse; deficiency syndrome: distending sensation in the lower abdomen, dribbling urination, feeble pulse.

This type is seen in urinary tuberculosis, tumor of urinary bladder and prostatitis.

[Treatment] Promoting the circulation of *qi* to promote water metabolism for excess syndrome; invigorating the spleen and replenishing *qi* for deficiency syndrome.

[Recipe] *Chen Xiang San*[137] with other herbs for excess syndrome.

In case of oppressed feeling in chest and fullness in the hypochondrium, add *Peri-*

carpium Citri Reticulatae Viride, *Radix Linderae* and *Fructus Foenicuii* to normalize the flow of the liver - *qi*; in case of long course with stagnation of *qi* and blood stasis, add *Flos Carthami*, *Radix Paeoniae Rubia* and *Radix Achyranthis Bidentatae* to activate blood flow and remove blood stasis.

Bu Zhong Yi Qi Tang[140] for deficiency syndrome.

If complicated with deficiency of blood and the kidney, *Ba Zhen Tang*[13] may be adopted with double amount of *Poria* plus *Cortex Eucommiae*, *Fructus Lycii* and *Radix Achyranthis Bidentatae* to tonify *qi*, nourish blood and replenish the spleen and the kidney.

[Nursing points] Adjust emotions; avoid depression and anger; regulate daily life and avoid overstrain.

4. Blood - stranguria

[Symptoms] Excess Syndrome: Hot urine, difficulty and stabbing sensation in urination, dark - red urine sometimes complicated with blood mass, or vexation, yellowish fur, and slippery and rapid pulse.

Deficiency syndrome: Pink urine, dull pain and difficulty in urination, lassitude and soreness in loins and knees, pink tongue, thready and rapid pulse.

[Main points of Differentiation] Excess syndrome: Dark - red urine, stabbing pain with fullness sensation; deficiency syndrome: pink urine without marked feeling of pain.

The type can be observed in acute pyelonephritis, cystitis, urinary tract infection, urinary calculus, tuberculosis of urinary system, urinary benign tumor and malignant tumor.

[Pathogenesis] Dempness-heat accumulating in the urinary bladder impairs vessels causing bleeding; or lasting illness leads to deficiency of the kidney - *yin*, and deficiency - fire burns the vessels resulting in bleeding.

[Treatment] Clearing away heat to promote urination and removing heat from blood to stop bleeding for excess syndrome; nourishing *yin* to remove heat and restoring *qi* to arrest bleeding for deficiency syndrome.

[Recipe] *Xiao Ji Yin Zi*[31] with *Dao Chi San*[120] for excess syndrome; *Zhi Bai Di Huang Wan*[160] for deficiency syndrome to nourish *yin* and remove heat, and *Herba Ecliptae*, *Colla Corii Asini* and *Herba Cephalanoploris* may be added to restore *qi* and stop bleeding.

[Nursing Points] Have light food with cool property; avoid pungent, fat, sweet and fried diet.

5. Grease - stranguria

[Symptoms] Excess syndrome: swill - like urine, cotton - like sediment with oily floating surface, or compalicated with coagulate of blood, painful, difficult and burning sensation in the urinary tract, red tongue with yellowish and greasy fur, soft and floating and rapid pulse.

Deficiency syndrome: lasting illness with repeated attack, oily urine with lessened difficulty and pain in urination, thin physique, dizziness, lacking strength, soreness in loins and knees, pale tongue with greasy fur, thready and weak pulse.

[Main Points of Differentiation] Excess syndrome: swill-like urine, pain in urination; deficiency syndrome: lasting illness, repeated attack, oily urine, lessened pain in urinary tract.

This type is seen in Filatia bancrofti and chyluria caused by tuberculous infection and oncoma.

[Pathogenesis] Dampness-heat descending to bring on disturbance in *qi* transformation; or deficiency of the kidney causing unconsolidation of primordial *qi* and its inability to control oily fluid, bringing about oily urine.

[Treatment] For excess syndrome: removing heat to promote water metabolism and separating essence from turbid substance; for deficiency syndrome: tonifying the kidney.

[Recipe] *Cheng's Bi Xie Fen Qing Yin*[272] with modification for excess syndrome; *Gao Lin Tang*[281] for deficiency syndrome.

In case of insufficiency of the spleen and kidney, sinking of *qi* in middle-*jiao* and unconsolidation of the kidney-*qi*, use *Bu Zhong Yi Qi Tang*[140] and *Qi Wei Du Qi Wan*[8] to supplement *qi*, make the descending *qi* ascend, and nourish the kidney.

[Nursing Points] Avoiding pungent, greasy and sweet food in case of excess syndrome; having nutrient and digestible diet in case of deficiency syndrome.

6. Overstrain-stranguria

[Symptoms] Dribbling urination by fits and starts, coming on with over-working, soreness in loins and knees, listlessness, pale tongue, and weak pulse.

[Main Points of Differentiation] Dribbling urination, coming on with over-working.

The type is commonly seen in chronic pyelonephritis and chronic prostatitis.

[Pathogenesis] Over-working causing deficiency of the spleen and kidney, and retention of dampness.

[Treatment] Invigorating the spleen and tonifying the kidney.

[Recipe] *Wu Bi Shan Yao Wan*[34] with modification.

In case of insufficiency of the spleen and *qi* descent, manifested as distention and tenesmus in the lower abdomen, and dribbling urination, use *Bu Zhong Yi Qi Tang*[140] as a synergist in order to replenish *qi* and make the descending *qi* ascend; in case of deficiency of the kidney-*yin*, manifested as flushed complexion, and dysphoria with feverish sensation in chest, palms and soles, *Zhi Bai Di Huang Wan*[160] may be used to nourish *yin* for reducing pathogenic fire.

[Nursing Points] Have nutrient, ungreasy and digestible food; avoid overstrain caused by sexual intercourse.

Summary

Stranguria refers to the morbid condition manifested as frequent, brief, difficult and dribbling urination with stabbing pain and cramping sensation in the lower abdomen, sometimes involving the loin and abdomen.

It is classified into six types, the differentiation of which should focus on their different characteristics and the excess or deficiency syndrome they are of. However, there is a certain relationship between them, marked by the interchanges of excess syndrome to deficiency syndrome as well as one type to the other. A sound knowledge of this relationship is helpful in clinical practices.

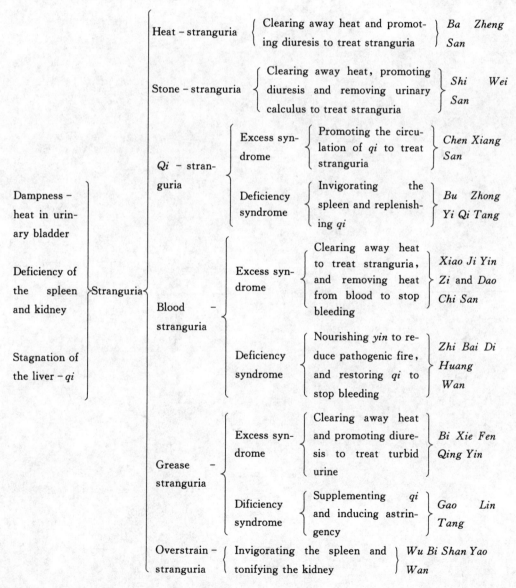

Discussions

1. How is blood-stranguria distinguished from urohematin?
2. How are the six types of stranguria distinguished?
3. Retell the main symptoms, treatments and recipes of the heat-stranguria and stone-stranguria.

33 Long Bi

General

Long Bi (Retention of Urine) refers to the disease chiefly characterized by oliguria or dribbling urination, or anuria in severe cases. *Long* is the term for slow onset of the disease with dysuria, and scanty dribbling urination; *Bi* is the term for an acute attack of the disease with anuria.

This disease includes dysuria or anuria due to obstruction of urinary system as well as oliguria and anuria because of renal dysfunction, etc. in the Western Medicine.

Etiology and Pathogenesis

Though the diseased sites are at the urinary bladder, *Long Bi* is closely related to *san-jiao*, the lung, the spleen, the kidney and the liver. The detailed descriptions are as follows:

1. Accumulation of dampness-heat   *Long Bi* occurs as a result of dysfunction of *qi* of the urinary bladder due to the stagnation of dampness-heat in the urinary bladder or the mixed accumulation of dampness and heat caused by the kidney-heat invading the bladder.

2. Excessive accumulation of the lung-heat   It is known that the lung serves as the upper source of water. *Long Bi* forms because of heat accumulation in the upper-*jiao* and failure in distributing body fluid resulting in urine retention; or because of a downward flow of heat from the upper-*jiao* to the bladder, which gives rise to accumulation of heat in both upper-*jiao* and lower-*jiao*.

3. Failure of the spleen-*qi* in ascending   The spleen is in charge of transporting and transforming nutrients. If the spleen-*qi* is insufficient, there may appear dysfunction of ascending the clear and descending the turbid, which leads to *Long Bi*.

4. Stagnation of the liver-*qi*   *Long Bi* is caused by endogenous impairment by seven emotions leading to stagnation of the liver-*qi* and dysfunction of *qi*, which results in urine retention.

5. Obstruction of urethra   *Long Bi* is also the result of agglutination of blood stasis or uretheral claculi obstructing urethra and the bladder.

6. Deficiency of the kidney-*qi*   *Long Bi* forms because of deficiency of the kidney-*yang* and decline of the vital *qi*, which brings about dysfunction of the bladder.

Diagnosis and Discrimination

Discrimination of *Long Bi* and Stranguria (*Lin* Syndrome)

Diseases \ Discrimination	*Long Bi*	Stranguria
Pain sensation with urination	No	Dribbling urination with stabbing pain
Amount of urine	Oliguria or anuria	Frequent urination, brief and difficult with total amount being generally normal
Difficult urination	Yes	Yes

Selecting Treatment by Differentiating Syndromes

First of all the differentiation of *Long Bi* lies in a clear distinction between deficiency and excess. Excess syndrome is characterized by an acute attack of the disease, dark yellow urine, burning sensation during urination, wiry and rapid pulse; while deficiency syndrome is mostly marked by slow onset of the disease, difficult urination, and weak pulse.

The treatment of *Long Bi* should follow the principle that "*Fu* is functioning well by being clear", with "being clear" as a focus. But considering the different causes of this disease the treatment should be planned accordingly, and the medicines for promoting urination can not be abused. The detailed descriptions are in the following:

1. Dampness - heat in the urinary bladder

[Symptoms] Urine retention or oliguria, scanty dark yellow urination with burning sensation, lower abdominal distention or constipation, bitter taste with sticky mouth, red tongue with yellowish sticky fur, and rapid pulse.

[Main Points of Differentiation] Anuria or oliguria, scanty dark yellow urination with burning sensation, red tongue with yellowish fur and rapid pulse.

[Pathogenesis] Excessive liquor or fatty and sweet food will lead to the stagnation of damp - heat in the spleen and the stomach, whose descending to the urinary bladder will result in dysfunction of *qi*.

[Treatment] Eliminating dampness and heat and promoting urination.

[Recipe] *Ba Zheng San*[12] with modification.

In case of impairment of *yin* due to excessive heat, dry mouth with red tongue and little salive, add *Radix Rehmannia* and *Radix Ophiopogonis*; in case of restlessness, add *Rhizoma Coptidis*, *Lophatherum*, etc.

[Nursing Points] Preferring a light diet and avoiding pungent, fatty and sweet food.

2. Excessive accumulation of the lung-heat

[Symptoms] Urine retention or dribbling urination, dry throat with a desire for drinking, short and rapid breathing, thin and yellowish fur, and rapid pulse.

[Main Points of Differentiation] Obstructed urination or anuria, short breathing with excessive thirst, and rapid pulse.

[Pathogenesis] Obstruction of *qi* due to heat in the lung, which gives rise to impairment of purifying and descending function of the lung, thus resulting in the failure in the downward transportation of body fluid to the urinary bladder.

[Treatment] Clearing away heat in the lung to promote urination.

[Recipe] *Qing Fei Yin*[249] with modification.

In case of the impairment of *yin* due to excessive heat, add *Rhizom Coptidis*, *Radix Adenophorae Strictae*, *Rhizoma Phragmitis*, etc.

[Nursing Points] Avoiding pungent and greasy food, preferring a light diet.

3. Stagnation of the liver-*qi*

[Symptoms] Mental depression or restlessness and irritability, urine rebtention or hesitant urination, hypochondriac and abdominal distention, red tongue with thin and yellowish fur, wiry pulse.

[Main Points of Differentiation] Urine retention or hesitant urination, accompanied by mental depression, chest and abdominal distention.

[Pathogenesis] Internal injury by seven emotions causes stagnation of the liver-*qi* resulting in obstructed urination.

[Treatment] Relieving the depressed liver-*qi*, and promoting urination.

[Recipe] *Chen Xiang San*[137] with modification.

Add *Rhizoma Cyperi*, *Radix Curcumae*, *Pericarpium Citri Reticulatae Viride* for the sake of strengthening regulation of the flow of *qi*.

In case of stagnation of *qi* turning into fire, add *Cortex Moutan Radicis*, *Radix Pittospori* for clearing away heat, and soothing the liver and regulating the flow of *qi*.

[Nursing Points] Avoid mental depression, anxiety and irritability, refrain from pungent food that induces fire-syndrome.

4. Urethral obstruction

[Symptoms] Dribbling or thready urine, or retention of urine, lower abdominal distention and pain, dark purplish tongue or ecchymosis on the tongue, and uneven pulse.

[Main Points of Differentiation] Retention of urine, or dribbling or thready urine, lower abdominal distention and pain.

[Pathogenesis] Blood stasis or obstructed discharge of sperm, or lump or calculus leads to the obstruction of urinary tract.

[Treatment] Promoting urination by removing stasis and obstruction.

[Recipe] *Dai Di Dang Wan*[87] with modification.

5. Insufficiency of *qi* in middle - *jiao*

[Symptoms] Straining distention of the lower abdomen, feeling for urination but without urine discharged, or oliguria with hesitant urination, lassitude, poor appetite, shortness of breath, pale tongue with thin fur, thready and weak pulse.

[Main Points of Differentiation] Feeling for urinating without urine discharged, straining distention of the lower abdomen, poor appetite and lassitude.

[Pathogenesis] Insufficiency of the spleen - *qi*, descent of *qi* in middle - *jiao* and dysfunction of *qi* in ascending the clear and descending the turbid.

[Treatment] Ascending the clear *qi* and descending the turbid *qi*, to promote water metabolism.

[Recipe] *Bu Zhong Yi Qi Tang*[140] and *Chun Ze Tang*[171].

[Nursing Points] Regulate daily life, avoid fatigue, take in nourishing but light food.

6. Declining of the kidney - *yang*

[Symptoms] Retention of urine or dribbling and difficult urination, pale complexion, lassitude, aversion to cold, coldness below the loins, weakness of knees, pale tongue with whitish fur, deep and thready pulse.

[Main Points of Differentiation] Urine retention or difficult urination, soreness and coldness of the loins and knees, deep thready pulse.

[Pathogenesis] Deficiency of the kidney - *yang* and decline of the vital *qi* leading to the dysfunction of the urinary bladder.

[Treatment] Warming *yang* and supplementing *qi*, and invigorating the kidney to promote urination.

[Recipe] *Ji Sheng Shen Qi Wan*[184].

In case of severe deficiency of *yang*, add *Rhizoma Curculiainis*, *Herba Epimedii*, etc.

[Nursing Points] Take in food rich in nutrients and warm in nature, refrain from excessive sexual intercourse.

Summary

Though *Long Bi* is originated from the disorder of the urinary bladder, it is closely related to *san - jiao*, the lung, the spleen, the kidney and the liver. The disease is caused by such factors as a mixed accumulation of dampness and heat, stagnation of *qi* due to the lung - heat, stagnation of the liver - *qi*, obstruction of urinary passage, insufficiency of *qi* in middle - *jiao*, the deficiency of the kidney - *yang*. In differentiating *Long Bi*, a discrimination of deficiency or excess syndrome should be put in the first place, followed by a differentiation of the condition as being mild or severe, chronic or acute.

	Dysfunction of the urinary bladder – *Long Bi*			
Mixed accumulation of dampness and heat		Dampness-heat in the bladder	Clearing away dampness and heat, promoting urination	Ba Zheng San
Excessive accumulation of heat in the lung		Excessive accumulation of heat in the lung	Clearing away heat in the lung to promote urination	Qin Fei Yin
Stagnation of the liver – *qi*		Stagnation of the liver – *qi*	Relieving the depressed liver *qi*, and promoting urination	Chen Xiang San
Urethral obstruction		Urethral obstruction	Promoting urination by removing stasis and obsturction	Dai Di Dang Wan
Failure of the spleen – *qi* in ascending		Insufficiency of *qi* in middle-*jiao*	Ascending the clear *qi* and descending the turbid *qi*, to promote water metabolism	Bu Zhong Yi Qi Tang and Chun Zhe Tang
Deficiency of the kidney – *yang*		Declining of the kidney – *yang*	Warming *yang* and supplementing *qi*, and invigorating the kidney to promote urination	Ji Sheng Shen Qi Wan

Discussions

1. How is *Long Bi* discriminated from stranguria?
2. Retell the chief symptoms, treatments and recipes of *Long Bi* caused respectively by accumulation of dampness – heat in the urinary bladder, urethral obstruction and deficiency of the kidney – *yang*.

— 465 —

34 Lumbago

General

Lumbago is a morbid condition chiefly manifested by pain in the lumbar region, which may appear on one side or on both sides. Lumbago is closely related to the kidneys, as they are located in the lumbar region.

In Western Medicine, the diseases with lumbago as a primary symptom are rheumatism, ankylosing spondylitis, lumbar muscle strain, acute lumbar sprain, prolapse of lumbar intervertebral disc, hyperosteogeny of lumbar vertebra, tuberculosis and tumour of lumbar vertebra, renal diseases, pelvic diseases and so on. The differentiation and treatment herein are referential to the above mentioned diseases.

Etiology and Pathogenesis

1. Invasion of cold - dampness   Lumbago occurs in the patients who are attacked by cold - dampness as they sit or sleep on the damp ground, or live in a cold and damp place, or wade into the water, or walk in the rain, leading to obstruction of channels and collaterals and unsmooth flow of *qi* and blood.

2. Impairment of collaterals due to damp - heat   The patients are attacked by external pathogenic factors of dampness - heat or suffer from internal accumulation of it, or a stagnation of cold - dampness in the body turns into heat, further causing obstruction of channels and collaterals and impairment in lumbar region.

3. Deficiency of the kidney - essence   The patients are usually over fatigued, or weak because of a long sickness course, or insufficient and weak in essence and blood in their old age, or have excessive sexual life, all of which may lead to the deficiency of the kidney - essence and its failure in nourishing channels and collaterals, thus giving rise to lumbago. Lumbago is also due to insufficiency of the kidney - *qi* and the obstrtucted condition of *Du* channel.

4. Blood stasis and stagnation of *qi*   Overstrain, or protracted course of disease, or traumatic injury will cause stagnation of *qi* and blood stasis, which lead to disharmony of the channels and collaterals, resulting in lumbago.

Diagnosis and Discrimination

Lumbago is an independent disease as well as a chief symptom of many diseases. So it is easy to make a diagnosis of lumbago, but it is difficult to discriminate its etiology and pathogenesis, especially difficult to find out its primary cause. In clinic, differentiation and treatment should follow the principle of treating the cause of lumbago with careful consideration of its pathogenesis.

Selecting Treatment by Differentiating Syndromes

First of all in the differentiation of lumbago a clear discrimination should be made of *biao* (the secondary cause) from *ben* (the primary cause), acuteness from chronicity deficiency from excess, and the cold sydrome from the heat syndrome. Lumbago due to invasion of exopathogen belongs to exterior and excess syndrome, manifesting an acute onset of the disease. The treatment of this type is eliminating pathogenic factors and removing obstruction in the collaterals, respectively according to the different causes of colddampness and dampness – heat. Lumbago due to deficiency of the kidney – essence belongs to interior and deficiency syndrome showing repeated chronic attacks. The treatment of this type is tonifying the kidney and supplementing *qi*. Syndrome of excess complicated by deficiency results from the persistent retention of exopathogen leading to an impairment of the kidney – *qi*. Syndrome of deficiency complicated by excess forms because of sudden invasion of excessive pathogenic factors after persistent deficiency of the kidney – *qi* and surface body resistance, for which the principle of treating the secondary as well as the primary should be carried out on the basis of a clear knowledge of pathogenic factors or vital energy being dominant. The cases of lumbago caused by blood stasis due to stagnation of *qi* mostly present the syndrome of excess complicated by deficiency, the treatment of which is chiefly removing the stasis by promoting the circulation of blood, regulating the flow of *qi* to remove obstruction in the collaterals, and after that, it is necessary to regulate and arrest the kidney – *qi* in order to consolidate the therapeutic effect.

1. Lumbago due to cold – dampness

[Symptoms] Sensation of coldness, pains and heaviness in the lumbar region with trouble in turning round and showing increasing seriousness, and not to be relieved in lying position, being aggravated in cloudy and rainy days, whitish and greasy fur, deep and slow pulse.

[Main Points of Differentiation] Coldness, heaviness and pains in the loins, aggravated in cloudy and rainy days.

This syndrome is mostly seen in the patients with rheumatic lumbago, ankylosing spondylitis, hyperosteogeny of lumbar vertebra, etc.

[Pathogenesis] Invasion of pathogenic factors of cold – dampness into the loins resulting in obstruction of the channels and collaterals.

[Treatment] Dispelling cold and dampness, warming the channels and collaterals and promoting the flow of *qi* in them.

[Recipe] *Gan Jiang Ling Zhu Tang*[72].

Add *Ramulus Cinnamomi*, *Radix Achyranthis Bidentatae* to warm channels and remove obstruction in the collaterals, or add *Cortex Eucommiae*, *Ramulus Loranthi*,

Radix Dipsaci to tonify the kidney and stengthen the loins. In case of lumbago on the left or right side by turns involving feet, shoulders or wandering pain of the joints, which shows lumbago accompanied by pathogenic wind, apply *Du Huo Ji Sheng Tang*[195] with modification for eliminating pathogenic wind and activating the collaterals, and tonifying the liver and the kidney.

[Nursing Points] Avoiding wind - cold, applying hot compression on the diseased region.

2. Lumbago due to dampness - heat

[Symptoms] Distending pain in the loins region with hot sensation, aggravated in hot or rainy days, scanty and dark yellow urine, yellowish and greasy fur, soft - floating or wiry rapid pulse.

[Main Points of Differentiation] Lumbago with hot sensation, aggravated by heat, yellowish and greasy fur, and rapid pulse.

This syndrome occurs in the patients of pyelonephritis, chronic pelvic inflammation, etc.

[Pathogenesis] Accumulation of damp - heat leading to the obstruction of *qi* in channels and collaterals.

[Treatment] Clearing away heat to remove dampness, and relaxing muscles and tendons to relieve pain.

[Recipe] *Si Miao Wan*[76] with modification.

Add *Fructus Chaenomelis*, *Caulis Trachelospermi* for strengthening the effect of promoting the normal flow of *qi* and blood in the collaterals to alleviate pain. In case of red tongue with thirst, scanty and dark yellow urine and wiry rapid pulse, which presents dominant heat - syndrome, add *Fructus Gardeniae*, *Rhizoma Alismatis*, *Caulis Akebiae* in favour of clearing away damp - heat.

[Nursing Points] Regulating daily life, avoiding dampness - heat and refraining from acrid, pungent, fatty and sweet food.

3. Lumbago due to blood stasis

[Symptoms] Stabbing pain of loins in a fixed location, with aversion to pressure, mild pain in the day and aggravated at night, difficulty in lying prostrated in mild cases and inability to turn round in severe cases, and most cases with external injury, purplish - dim tongue with ecchymosis and uneven pulse.

[Main Points of Differentiation] Stabbing pain of the loins with a fixed location, purplish dim tongue.

This syndrome is commonly seen in tumour of lumbar vertabra, acute lumbar sprain and contusion, prolapse of lumbar intervertebral, lumbar muscle strain, etc.

[Pathogenesis] Blood stasis due to stagnation of *qi* leading to obstruction of channels and collaterals.

[Treatment] Removing blood stasis to promote blood circulation, and regulating the flow of *qi* to relieve pain.

[Recipe] *Shen Tong Zhu Yu Tang*[145] with modification.

In case of lumbago due to external injury, add *Radix et Rhizoma Rhei*, and take *Radix Notoginseng* powder. In case of hematuria, add *Rhizoma Imperatae*, *Cortex Moutan Radicis*, *Herba Seu Radix Cirsii Japonici* and *Herba Cephalanoploris*.

[Nursing Points] Avoiding bearing a heavy load and overstrain.

4. Lumbago due to deficiency of the kidney

[Symptoms] Lumbago with sore and weak sensation inclined to be pressed and kneaded, weakness of legs and knees aggravated by overwork and relieved in lying position. In case of dominant deficiency of *yang*, the patient will show contracture of the lower abdomen, pale complexion, chilliness of hands and feet, pale tongue and deep thready pulse. In case of dominant deficiency of *yin*, the patient will show restlessness and insomnia, dry mouth and throat, reddish complexion, feverish sensation in palms and soles, red tongue with little fur, thready and rapid pulse.

[Main Points of Differentiation] Soreness of the loins and weakness of the knees aggravated by over-work. In case of dominant deficiency of *yang*, there are manifestations as chilliness of hands and feet, deep and thready pulse. In case of dominant deficiency of *yin*, there appear symptoms of dry throat and insomnia, red tongue with little fur.

This symdrome is usually seen in the patients with tuberculosis of lumbar vertebra, renal diseases and chronic inflammation of pelvic cavity, etc.

[Pathogenesis] The loins is the residence of the kidney. Lumbago occurs when there is deficiency of the kidney-*qi* resulting in the lack of nutrients in the loins and spinal cord.

[Treatment] In case of deficiency of the kidney-*yang*, tonifying the kidney to reinforce *yang*; in case of deficiency of the kidney-*yin*, tonifying the kidney to nourish *yin*.

[Recipe] *You Gui Wan*[68] for the case of deficiency of *yang*, and *Zuo Gui Wan*[65] for the case of deficiency of *yin*.

In case of protracted lumbago without symptoms of deficiency of *yang* or *yin*, take *Qing E Wan*[147] for tonifying the kidney to cure lumbago.

[Nursing Points] Regulate daily life, refrain from excessive sexual life, and take nutritious but ungreasy diet.

Summary

The deficiency of the kidney is the primary cause of lumbago, and invasion by exopathogens, trauma and sprain are the secondary. Therefore, in the treatment of lumbago due to cold-dampness, dampness-heat and blood stasis, herbs to tonify the kidney and reinforce the loins are often adopted for the purpose of strengthening the body resistance to eliminate pathogenic factors.

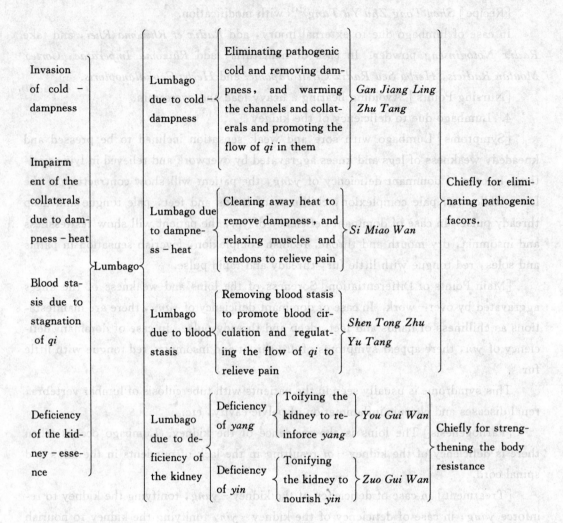

Discussions

1. How is lumbago due to cold-dampness distinguished from that due to dampness-heat?
2. What are the etiology and pathogenesis, main symptoms, therapeutic methods and recipes of lumbago due to deficiency of the kidney?

35 Xiao Ke

General

Xiao Ke is a disease characterized by excessive intake of water, polyphagia, polyuria and emaciation or turbid urine with sweet smell.

In Western Mdicine the treatment of diabetes, diabetes insipidys, hyperthyroidism and psychogenic polydipsia may refer to the differentiation and treatment of this disease.

Etiology and Pathogenesis

1. Intemperance in eating   Excessive intake of fatty and sweet food and alcohol leads to dysfunction of the spleen and stomach and accumulation of pathogenic heat in the body which converts into dryness pathogen and consumes the body fluid, resulting in Xiao Ke.

2. Emotional imbalance   A long period of spirital stimulus may give rise to disturbance of functional activities of qi, which turns further into fire consuming and burning the yin-fluid of the lung and the stomach, thus occurs Xiao Ke.

3. Overstrain and sexual intemperance   Usual deficiency of yin and sexual intemperance will impair yin-essence and cause hyperactivity of fire pathogen induced by deficiency of yin, which goes upward and steams the lung and stomach, thus resulting in Xiao Ke.

Diagnosis and Discrimination

This disease is characterized by excessive intake of water, polyphagia, polyuria and emaciated constitution, which should be discriminated from some other diseases.

1. *Shang Xiao* (Xiao Ke occurring in the upper-jiao) is to be differentiated from polydipsia and excessive intake of water resulting from the consumption of the body fluid by epidemic febrile disease. In both cases the patients show symptoms of excessive intake of water and polydipsia, but the latter has the case history of being affected by exopathic factor of warm pathogen, and there may appear transmission process of the four systems (*wei*, *qi*, *ying* and *blood*) without such symptoms as seen in Shang Xiao marked by polyphagia and polyuria.

2. *Zhong Xiao* (Xiao Ke occurring in the middle-jiao) is to be differentiated from liability to feel hungry and emaciation seen in hyperthyroidism. The former manifested doubled diet, hyperactive digestion and liability to feel hungry, while the latter, involves but does not display as serious condition as the former. The former is often accompanied by symptoms of Shang Xiao and Xia Xiao (Xiao Ke occurring in the lower-

jiao); while the latter by enlargement of the front of neck, trembling fingers, hyperhidrosis, and protruding eyeballs.

3. *Xia Xiao* should be discriminated from overstrain – stranguria and turbid urine. *Xia Xiao* is characterized by much urination with turbid unine; overstrain – stranguria is manifested by frequent and clear urine; and turbid urine is marked by white turbid urine. The volume of urine does not obviously increase in the case of overstrain – stranguria or turbid urine, and in both cases the urine does not have sweet smell.

Selecting Treatment by Differentiating Syndromes

Though the disease is classified into three types: *Shang Xiao*, *Zhong Xiao* and *Xia Xiao*, and differentiated by dryness of the lung, heat in the stomach and deficiency of the kidney, the symptoms of excessive intake of water, polyphagia and polyuria are seen simultaneously in clinic. Whether it is *Shang Xiao* or *Zhong Xiao* or *Xia Xiao*, the treatment should be based on tonifying the kidney and nourishing *yin*. In case of excessive dryness – heat, clearing away heat is a proper way; and in case of impairment of *yin* involving *yang* due to long course of *Xia Xiao*, nourishing both *yin* and *yang* is preferable.

1. *Shang Xiao* Impairment of the body fluid by the lung – heat

[Symptoms] Excessive intake of water and polydipsia, dryness of the mouth and the tongue, frequent and much urination, red tongue tip with slight yellowish fur, rapid and full pulse.

[Main Points of Differentiation] Excessive intake of water and polydipsia and polyuria.

This syndrome is commonly seen in psychogenic polydipsia, diabetes, diabetes insipidus, etc.

[Pathogenesis] Excessive heat in the lung leading to a consumption of lung – *yin*, which gives rise to a failure of distribution of the body fluid.

[Treatment] Clearing away heat and moistening the lung, and promoting the production of the body fluid to quench thirst.

[Recipe] *Xiao Ke Fang*[216] with modification.

If there is the syndrome of consumed *qi* and *yin* due to excessive blazing heat in the lung and the stomach marked by dryness of the tongue with yellowish fur, excessive intake of water and polydipsia, and rapid full pulse, *Bai Hu Jia Ren Shen Tang*[89] may be applied for clearing away heat in the lung and the stomach to promote the production of the body fluid to quench thirst.

[Nursing Points] Take easily digestible food and food likely to promote the production of body fluid instead of pungent food and tabacco and alcohol that are apt to generate heat in the body.

2. *Zhong Xiao* (excessive blazing heat in the stomach)

[Symptoms] Polyphagia with liability to hunger, emaciated constitution, constipation, yellowish fur of the tongue, slippery, full and forceful pulse.

[Main Points of Differentiation] Polyphagia with liability to hunger, emaciated constitution, slippery and full pulse.

This syndrome is usually seen in diabetes, hyperthyroidism, etc.

[Pathogenesis] Hyperactive digestion and consumption of the body fluid due to excessive blazing heat in the stomach.

[Treatment] Clearing away heat in the stomach and nourishing *yin* to promote the production of the body fluid.

[Recipe] *Yu Nu Jian*[59] with *Rhizoma Coptidis* and *Fructus Gardeniae*.

In case of constipation, *Zeng Ye Cheng Qi Tang*[284] may be prescribed for moistening and removing obstruction from the *fu* - organs. When there is a recovery of free movement of the bowels, change to the recipe *Yu Nu Jian*.

[Nursing Points] Refrain from greasy, sweet food and alcohol, and control the intake of cereal; have *Monordica charantia*, *Benineasa Hispida* and legume vegetables

3. Xia Xiao

(1) Deficiency of the kidney - *yin*

[Symptoms] Frequent and much discharge of greasy urine with sweet smell, dry mouth and lips, dysphoria with feverish sensation in chest, palms and soles, red tongue with little fur, deep, thready and rapid pulse.

[Main Points of Differentiation] Frequent and much discharge of greasy urine, dysphoria with feverish sensation in chest, palms and soles, red tongue with little fur.

[Pathogenesis] Internal blazing of deficiency - fire due to deficiency and consumption of the kidney - *yin* gives rise to the failure of the kidney in arresting discharge leading to a loss of refined nutritious substances.

[Treatment] Nourishing *yin* to reinforce the kidney.

[Recipe] *Liu Wei Di Huang Wan*[46].

In case of deficiency of both *qi* and *yin* accompanied by lassitude, shortness of breath, and reddish tongue, add accordingly *Radix Condonopsis Pilosulae*, *Radix Scutellariae* and some other medicines for supplementing *qi*.

[Nursing Points] Refrain from excessive sexual intercourse. Take light and easily digested food to nourish *yin* instead of pungent food.

(2) Deficiency of both *yin* and *yang*

[Symptoms] Frequent discharge of greasy urine, even urination immediately after drinking in serious cases, dark complexion, withered auricle, soreness and weakness of loins and knees, chilliness and cold limbs, impotence, pale tongue with whitish fur, deep, thready and weak pulse.

[Main Points of Differentiation] Frequent discharge of greasy urine, soreness of loins and chilliness, and deep thready pulse.

This syndrome is mostly seen in diabetes insipidus, diabetes, etc.

[Pathogenesis] Consumption of *qi* and *yin*, causes the deficiency and weakness of the renal *qi* resulting in the loss of control of urination.

[Treatment] Warming *yang* and tonifying the kidney to arrest polyuria.

[Recipe] *Jin Gui Shen Qi Wan*[163].

In case of deficiency of *yin* and *yang* as well as *qi* and blood, *Lu Rong Wan*[239] may be used. *Fructus Rubi*, *Oetheca Mantidis*, and *Fructus Rosae Laevigatae* can be added to the two recipes above to tonify the kidney for arresting polyuria.

[Nursing Points] Be moderate in sexual life and regulate daily life, take nutritious food other than greasy one, avoid fatty, sweet and pungent food. Pig pancreas, *Rhizoma Dioscoreae*, and wild rice stem are preferable daily food beneficial to the curing of the disease.

Summary

Xiao Ke is a disease characterized by excessive intake of water, polyphagia, polyuria and emaciation. The disease is chiefly caused by intemperance in eating, emotional imbalance, overstrain and sexual intemperance. The pathogenetic characteristics are deficiency of *yin*, dryness and heat, impairment of both *qi* and *yin*, deficiency of both *yin* ang *yang*, dryness and heat due to deficiency of *yin* showing various symptoms. In addition, dryness and heat due to deficiency of *yin* or deficiency of both *yin* and *yang* will lead to obstructed flow of blood, therefore the onset of *Xiao Ke* is closely related to the blood stasis. Therefore, besides tonifying *yin* and clearing away heat, *Radix Salviae Miltiorrhizae*, *Fructus Crataegi*, *Semen Persicae*, and *Flos Carthami* can be added for promoting blood circulation by removing the blood stasis; at the same time the patients should regulate the daily life and diet to enhance the therapeutic effect.

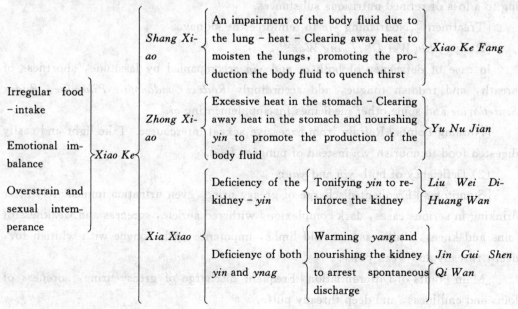

Discussions

1. What are the etiology and pathogenesis of *Xiao Ke*?
2. What are the different types and treatment of *Xiao Ke*? What are the main points of differentiation, pathogenesis outline and recipes?
3. What is the relationship between *Xiao Ke* and blood stasis in their etiology and pathogenesis?

36 Spermatorrhea

General

Spermatorrhea refers to emission not as the result of sexual life. It is physiologically normal for an unmarried male or one married but in separation from the spouse if it occurs one or twice monthly.

The differentiation and treatment herein may serve as a reference to such diseases in Western Medicine as psychoneurosis, chronic prostatitis, vesiculitis, posterior urethritis, epididymitis and the pathologic emission seen in some other chronic diseases.

Etiology and Pathogenesis

1. Hyperactive heart – fire and disharmony between the heart and kidney Weary mind or emotional disorder will consume the heart – *yin* and induce hyperactive heart – *yang* resulting in mental upset and emission with sexual dreams; the hyperactive heart – *yang* will consume the kidney fluid and cause its failure to counteract the heart – fire. Hence the essence house is disturbed and emission follows with dreams.

2. Descent of dampness – heat and disturbance of essence house Liquor and greasy food will impair the spleen and stomach, and generate dampness inside the body, which accumulates and induces heat. When dampness and heat descend and disturb the essence house, spontaneous emission will occur.

3. Spermatorrhea is the result of failure of *qi* to arrest spontaneous discharge of sperm resulting from overstrain and impairment of the heart and the spleen. Patients, who have constant overstrain leading to impairment of *qi*, suffer from insufficiency of *qi* in middle – *jiao* and deficiency of the heart – *qi* and the spleen – *qi*, and more serious deficiency of *qi* whenever they are in the condition of overwork and overanxiety, as a result there appears sinking of lucid *yang* causing the failure of *qi* to control emission.

4. Seminal emission is due to deficiency of the kidney resulting in kidney's failure in arresting spontaneous discharge of sperm because of the early marriage of patients, or intemperance of sexual life or the bad habit of masturbation, or congenital insufficiency and remained persistent deficiency after birth. Nocturnal emission occurs as a result of deficiency – fire to disturb the kidney when there is excess of the kidney – *yang* with deficiency of the kidney – *yin*, while spermatorrhea is due to the deficiency of the kidney – *yang* failing in arresting spontaneous discharge of sperm.

Key Points:

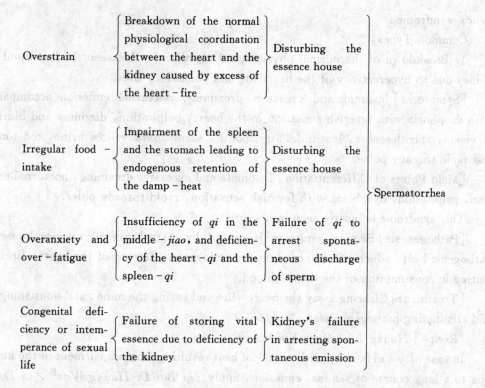

Diagnosis and Discrimination

Spermatorrhea is usually classified into nocturnal emission and involuntary emission. The former refers to emission at night with sexual dreams, while the latter may occur without dreams. In severe cases, because of the kidney's failure in arresting spontaneous emission, there may appear emission with straining motion or at what one sees, hears or touches. Besides, spermatorrhea should also be distinguished from premature ejaculation, the latter refers to extremely short time of intercourse, or emission upon touch, or sex act with emission before intercourse which is immediately followed by flaccid penis and inability to conduct normal intercourse. This differs from emission and involuntary emission manifested as spontaneous discharge of sperms not from sexual intercourse.

Selecting Treatment by Differentiating Syndromes

Spermatorrhea can be classified into nocturnal emission and involuntary emission. The former includes deficiency type or excess type, which initially is caused by heart - fire, stganation of the liver - qi, damp - heat, fire - heat, which disturbs downward the essence house causing the disorder of essence - qi. Furthermore, a long course of emission may lead to deficiency of the kidney. The latter mostly develops from the former, or is due to persisitent deficiency after birth, or sexual strain, and masturbation. Most of the cases display deficiency syndrome.

Common Types:

1. Breakdown of the normal physiological coordination between the heart and the kidney due to hyperactivity of the heart fire and the kidney fire.

[Symptoms] Insomnia and excessive dreaming, nocturnal emission accompanied with dysphoria with feverish sensation in the heart, palpitation, dizziness and blurring of vision, spiritlessness, lassitude, dry mouth, scanty dark yellow urine, red tongue and rapid thready pulse.

[Main Points of Differentiation] Insomnia and excessive dreaming, nocturnal emission, palpitation, dysphoria with feverish sensation, rapid thready pulse.

This syndrome is mostly seen in neurosis.

[Pathogenesis] Seminal emission is caused by disturbance of essence house by pathogenic heat, which is brought about by endogenous flaming of the heart-fire, resulting in consumption of the heart-blood.

[Treatment] Clearing away the heart-fire and easing the mind, and nourishing yin and eliminating pathogenic heat.

[Recipe] *Huang Lian Qing Xin Yin*[232].

In case of yin deficiency with excess of heat resulting from impairment of the kidney due to a long course of seminal emission, apply *Zhi Bai Di Huang Wan*[160] or *Da Bu Yin Wan*[18] to nourish yin and purge intense heat.

[Nursing Points] Keep peaceful mind and exercise moderately, and avoid pungent food and drinking.

2. Disturbance of the essence house due to downward flow of the damp-heat

[Symptoms] Frequent seminal emission, or a little amount of sperm discharged with urination, dark yellow and turbid urination with hot sensatin, or dribbling urination, dysphoria, bitter taste in the mouth, aphtha of the mouth and tongue, loose smelly stool with discharging difficulty, fullness in the stomach and abdomen, yellowish and greasy fur of the tongue, soft-floating and rapid pulse.

[Main Points of Differentiation] Frequent seminal emission, dark yellow and turbid urination with hot sensation, loose smelly stool with discharging difficulty, yellowish and greasy fur of the tongue.

This syndrome usually occurs in prostatitis, vesiculitis and posterior urethritis.

[Pathogenesis] Pathogenic dampness accumulates downward and generates heat, further disturbing the essence house.

[Treatment] Clearing away heat and promoting diureses.

[Recipe] *Cheng's Bi Xie Fen Qing Yin*[272] or *Zhu Du Wan*[256].

In case of downward flow of the spleen-dampness, it is applicable to use *Cang Zhu Er Chen Tang*[126] with *Cortex Phellodendri*, *Radix Bupleuri*, *Rhizoma Cimicifugae*.

3. Failure of *qi* to arrest spontaneous discharge of sperm due to impairment of the heart and the spleen

[Symptoms] Seminal emission after overstrain, palpitation or daze, insomnia and poor memory, sallow complexion, lassitude, poor appetite, loose stool, pale tongue with thin fur, and weak pulse.

[Main Points of Differentiation] Seminal emission after overstrain, palpitation and daze, poor appetite, loose stool, pale tongue and weak pulse.

This syndrome is mostly seen in neurosis.

[Pathogenesis] Seminal emission may be caused by mental distraction resulting from deficiency of *qi*, which is due to deficiency of *qi* and blood in the heart and the spleen, and impairment of *qi* in middle - *jiao* after overstrain.

[Treatment] Regulating the function of the heart and the spleen and nourishing them and supplementing *qi* to arrest spontaneous discharge of sperm.

[Recipe] *Miao Xiang San*[132] or *Bu Zhong Yi Qi Tang*[140].

In case of deficiency of both the heart and spleen resulting from the spleen's being impaired by anxiety, large amount of herbs for supplemeating the heart and spleen to induce ascent of lucid *qi* should be applied instead of those for purgation and astringency.

In case of unsteadiness of the heart -fire resulting from floating of *yang* and insufficiency of *qi*, apply herbs for nourishing *qi* and enriching the blood to ease mental strain, instead of those for clearing away the heart -fire. In clinic *Gui Pi Tang*[95] and *Liu Wei Di Huang Wan*[46] may be adopted with modification.

[Nursing Points] Keep peaceful mind, and alternate work with leisure; nutritious but ungreasy food is preferred, e. g. gruel made with *Radix Astragali seu Hedysari*, or *Semen Nelumbinis* or *Semen Dolichoris*; avoid excessive sexual life.

4. Emission due to deficiency of the kidney and its failure in arresting spontaneous discharge of sperms

[Symptoms] Frequent seminal emission even involuntary emission, soreness and weakness of loins and knees, dizziness and tinnitus, dysphoria with dry throat, insomnia and poor memory, low fever with flushing cheeks, emaciated constitution, night sweat, aplopecia and loose teeth, red tongue with little fur, thready and rapid pulse. Patients with seminal emission for a long course usually show syndromes of chilliness and coldness of the limbs, asynodia and premature ejaculation, oliguria and edema, light -coloured urine or dribbling urination, pale complexion, pale and tender tongue with teeth marks, deep and thready pulse.

[Main Points of Differentiation] Frequent seminal emission or involuntary emission, soreness and weakness of loins and knees, lassitude, poor memory.

This syndrome is mostly seen in neurosis, chronic prostatitis and some other chronic diseases.

[Pathogenesis] Unconsolidation of the essence house resulting from failure of the kidney in storing the essence, and impairment of *yin* involving *yang*.

[Treatment] Nourishing the kidney and tonifying the essence house to control seminal emission.

[Recipe] In case of deficiency of the kidney-*yin*, apply *Liu Wei Di Huang Wan*[46] or *Zuo Gui Wan*[65]. In case of deficiency of *yin* involving *yang*, apply *You Gui Wan*[68].

In the cases of severe seminal emission due to dysfunction of the kidney in storing essence, the above-mentioned recipes should be applied in combination with *Jin Suo Gu Jing Wan*[164], *Shui Lu Er Xian Dan*[58], etc. In case of emission due to deficiency of the kidney resulting from breakdown of the normal hysiological coordination between the heart and the kidney, add *Sang Piao Xiao San*[228], *Ban Long Wan*[258], etc. according to the actual condition to restore the normal coordination between the heart and the kidney and to tranquilize mind to arrest spontaneous emission.

[Nursing Points] Food rich in nutrients are preferable. *Semen Juglandis*, *Fructus Schisandrae*, fresh cowry and soft-shelled turtle are suggested daily food for nourishing *yin* and strengthening *yang*. Lead a regular life, keep in good mood and avoid excessive sexual life.

Summary

Spermatorrhea is mostly caused by disturbance of emotions, irregular food-intake, intemperance of sexual life, etc. The disease is related with the five *zang* organs, especially closely with the heart and the kidney. In the early stage of the disease, it is due to breakdown of the normal physiological coordination between the heart and the kidney resulting from excess of the heart-fire, which mostly belongs to a complicated type of deficiency and excess; the therapeutic principle to treat this type is clearig away the heart-fire and easing mental anxiety, and nourishing *yin* and eliminating pathogenic heat. As the disease is lingering for a long period, it turns into deficiency type characterized by a failure in storing the essence due to deficiency of the kidney and its failure in arresting spontaneous discharge of sperms, and the therapeutic mehtod is nourishing the kidney to arrest spontaneous discharge of sperm. If the disease is caused by sinking of *qi* of middle-*jiao* due to deficiency of *qi*, which results from downward flow of the damp-heat affecting the normal circulation of *qi*, it belongs to a combined type of deficiency and excess mainly resulting from the functional disturbance of the spleen and the stomach, and the treatment of this type should follow the principle of clearing away heat to promote diuresis, and supplementing *qi* and strengthening the spleen. The general therapeutic method is clearing away the heart-fire and easing the mental anxiety for treating pathogenic factors in the upper portion, regulating the function of the spleen and the stomach, and ascending *yang*-*qi* for treating pathogenic factors in the middle portion, and reinforcing the kidney to arrest spontaneous emission for treating pathogenic factors in the lower portion.

Breakdown of the normal physiological coordination between the heart and the kidney due to the hyperactivity of the monarch fire and the ministerial fire	Seminal emission	Breakdown of the normal physiological coordination between the heart and the kidney	Clearing away heart-fire and easing mental anxiety	*Huang Lian Qing Xin Yin*
Disturbance of the essence house due to downward flow of pathogenic damp-heat		Downward flow of pathogenic damp-heat	Clearing away heat and promoting diuresis	*Bi Xie Feng Qing Yin*
Failure of *qi* to arrest spontaneous discharge of sperm due to impairment of the heart and the spleen		Impairment of the heart and the spleen	Regulating the function of the heart and the spleen and nourishing them	*Miao Xiang San* or *Bu Zhong Yi Qi Tang*
Deficiency of the kidney and its failure in arresting spontaneous discharge of sperms		Deficiency of the kidney	Nourishing the kidney to control seminal emission	*Liu Wei Di Huang Wan*, *Zuo Gui Wan* and *You Gui Wan*

Discussions

1. Make brief description of the etiology and pathogenesis of spermatorrhea.
2. What are spermatorrhea, involuntary emission and nocturnal emission?
3. How many types is spermatorrhea classified into? What are the main points of differentiation, therapeutic methods and recipes of each?

37　*Bi* Syndrome

General

Bi Syndrome is marked by soreness and numbness and heaviness of muscles, bones and joints with difficulty in bending and stretching, even arthrocele with burning sensation, which are caused by exopathogens (wind, cold, heat and dampness) invading the body and making *qi* and blood flow unsmoothly.

The differentiating treatments for the disease are referential to rheumatic arthritis, rheumatoid arthritis, gout, scapulohumeral periarthritis and osseous arthritis.

Etiology and pathogenesis

1. Wind, cold and dampness invading the body   Changeable climate and alternate cold and heat, or dwelling in damp places, or wading, or being caught in the rain will cause wind, cold and dampness to attack the body and linger in channels and joints, resulting in *Bi* syndrome as the result of stagnation of *qi* and blood. And clinical manifestations vary with predomination of different pathogens.

2. Affected by exopathogen or heat from other accumulated pathogen. When attack of wind–heat is complicated with dampness, or heat is generated from exopathogens because of usual excess of *yang* or deficiency of *yin*, or from accumulation of wind, cold and dampness, *Bi* syndrome will follow.

Key Points:

Endopathic factors { Usual debility, deficiency of vital *qi*, failure of superficial body resistance to protect the body against diseases }

Exopathic factors { Affected by pathogenic wind, cold, dampness and heat }

→ { Stagnation syndrome in muscles, joints and channels and collaterals } → *Bi* syndrome

Diagnosis and Discrimination

Bi syndrome is caused by wind, cold, dampness and heat manifested as soreness and numbness of muscles, joints and bones, and in severe case, marked by arthrocele with burning sensation.

The affected parts of both *Bi* syndrome and *Wei* syndrome are the limbs and joints, so it is necessary to make a discrimination.

Discrimination \ Disease	Bi syndrome	Wei syndrome
Clinical symptoms	Soreness and heaviness of muscles, bones and joints, difficulty in bending and stretching	Weakness of limbs, emaciated muscles
Pain in limbs and joints	Yes	No

Selecting Treatment by Differentiating Syndromes

To make a differentiation of *Bi* syndrome, one must firstly discriminate *Bi* syndrome due to wind-cold-dampness from that due to heat. The latter is characterized by hematoma of joints with pain and burning sensation, while there is no hematoma of joints with burning sensation, but soreness of joints in the former.

Bi syndrome
- Red and swollen joints with burning pain —— *Re Bi*
- Wandering soreness of joints —— *Xing Bi* (migratory *Bi* syndrome)
- Sharp pain with fixed spot —— *Tong Bi* (*Bi* syndrome aggravated by cold)
- Soreness and heaviness of limbs, numbness of muscles —— *Zhuo Bi*

Common Types:

1. *Bi* caused by wind-cold-dampness

(1) *Xing Bi*

[Symptoms] Wandering soreness of limbs and joints, difficulty in bending and stretching, and sometimes aversion to wind, fever, thin and whitish fur, floating pulse.

[Main Points of Differentiation] Wandering soreness of joints.

This type is seen in rheumatic arthritis.

[Pathogenesis] Wind-cold-damp pathogen accumulating in channels and collaterals to obstruct the flow of *qi* and blood, and exuberant wind pathogen wandering and changing.

[Treatment] Dispelling wind, dredging channels and removing dampness.

[Recipe] *Fang Feng Tang*[123].

If the soreness is mainly in the joints of shoulders and elbows, add *Rhizoma Seu Radix Notopterygii*, *Rhizoma Curcumae Longae*, *Radix Angelicae Dahuricae* and *Rhizoma Ligustici Wallichii* to expell wind, dredge channels and arrest pain; if the soreness is mainly in the joints of knees and ankles, add *Radix Achyranthis Bidentatae*, *Radix Stephaniae Tetrandrae* and *Fructus Chaenomelis* to remove dampness and obstruction in the channels to relieve pain; if the soreness is mainly in loins and knees, add *Cortex Euconniae*, *Ramulus Visci*, *Radix Dipsaci*, *Radix Morindae Officinalis* and *Herba Epimedii* to warm and tonify the kidney, and strengthen muscles and bones; in case of arthrocele, thin and yellowish fur, pathogen turning into heat, use *Gui Zhi Shao Yao Zhi Mu Tang*[203].

[Nursing Points] Keep away from wind-cold; do not expose to wind while sweating; and take warm food.

(2) *Tong Bi*

[Symptoms] Severe pain in joints of limbs with fixed spot, the pain lessened with heat and aggravated with cold, joints unable to bend and stretch, without red color but normal temperature on the painful spot, thin and whitish fur, tense and wiry pulse.

[Main Points of Differentiation] Severe pain of joints with fixed spot and aggravated with cold.

This type is observable in rheumatoid arthritis and the early stage of scapulohumeral periarthritis.

[Pathogenesis] Pathogen of wind-cold-dampness invading the body, and exuberant cold to obstruct channels and collaterals.

[Treatment] Expelling pathogenic cold from-channels and removing wind and dampness.

[Recipe] *Wu Tou Tang*[53].

In case of severe pain, add *Radix Aconiti Praeparate*, *Rhizoma Zingiberis*, *Herba Asari*, *Ramulus Cinnamomi*, etc. to dispel cold and relieve pain; in case of accumulation of cold due to lasting illness accompanied with blood stasis, add *Resina Boswelliae Carterii*, *Resina Commiphorae Myrrha*, *Scolopendra*, *Squama Manitis Praeparata*, *Caulis Spotholobi*, etc. to promote blood circulation, remove obstruction in the collaterals and relieve pain.

[Nursing Points] Guard against cold; have warm food.

(3) *Zhuo Bi*

[Symptoms] Soreness and heaviness of joints with fixed spot, heaviness of hands and feet, difficulty in movement, or numbness of muscles, swelling joints, whitish and greasy fur, soft-floating and moderate pulse.

[Main Points of Differentiation] Soreness and heaviness of joints, numbness of muscles, whitish and greasy fur.

This type is seen in rheumatoid arthritis, scapulohumeral periarthritis and bony arthritis.

[Pathogenesis] Pathogenic wind-cold-dampness stagnating in collaterals, muscles and joints, and exuberant dampness lingering in the body.

[Treatment] Removing dampness and obstruction in the collaterals, expelling wind and clearing away cold.

[Recipe] *Yi Yi Ren Tang*[285].

In case of severe numbness of muscles, add *Cortex Erythrinae* and *Herba siseges-*

beckiae to dispell wind and remove obstruction in the collaterals; in case of swelling of joints, add *Rhizoma Dioscoreae Septemlobae*, *Caulis Aristolochiae Manshuriens is* and *Rhizoma Curcumae Longae umae* to alleviate water retention and remove obstruction in the collaterals.

[Nursing Points] Avoid dwelling in damp and cold places; do not eat uncooked, cold, fat and sweet food.

2. *Bi* syndrome due to wind – heat – dampness

[Symptoms] Painful joints, local swelling with burning sensation, untouchable pain aggravated with heat and lessened with cold, one or several joints involved, accompanied with fever, aversion to wind, sweating, vexation, thirst with desire for cold drinks, yellowish and dry fur, slippery and rapid pulse.

[Main Points of Differentiation] Swelling joints with burning pain aggravated with heat, slippery and rapid pulse.

This type is common in rheumatic arthritis and gout.

[Pathogenesis] Pathogenic fire accumulating in the collaterals and joints causing stagnation of *qi* and blood.

[Treatment] Clearing away heat, expelling wind and dampness, and removing obstruction in the collaterals.

[Recipe] *Bai Hu Jia Gui Zhi Tang*[90].

Flos Lonicerae, *Fructus Forsythiae*, *Cortex Phellodendri*, *Radix Clematidis*, *Radix Stephaniae Tetrandrae* and *Ramulus Mori* may be added to remove wind, heat and obstruction in the collaterals. In case of skin erythema, add *Cortex Moutan Radicis*, *Radix Rehmanniae*, *Radix Raeonie Rubra* and *Caulis Lonicerae* to remove heat from blood and expell wind.

In case of *Re Bi* turning into fire causing impairment of body fluid manifested as swelling of joints, pain as if cut, aggravated at night, high fever, excessive thirst, red tongue with little fluid, wiry and rapid pulse, adopt *Xi Jiao San*[274] plus *Radix Rehmanniae*, *Radix Scro Phulariae* and *Radix Ophiopogonis* to clear away heat and toxic material and remove heat from blood to relieve pain as well as to nourish *yin* for production of fluid.

[Nursing points] Ventilate the house. Avoid pungent, fat and sweet food and alcohol.

Protracted course of *Bi* syndrome will result in body resistance weakened while pathogenic factors prevailing to accumulate in collaterals and turn the body fluid into phlegm. Stagnation of phlegm, in turn, causes alternate dull and severe pain, arthrocele and joint deformity, difficulty in bending and stretching, purplish tongue, whitish and greasy fur, wiry and uneven pulse. In this case, *Tao Hong Yin*[204] should be adopted to resolve and remove phlegm and expell wind to remove obstruction in the collaterals plus *Squama Manitis*, *Lumbricus*, *Scorpio* and *Eupolyphaga seu Steleophaga*, specially for removing obstruction in the collaterals. *Semen Sinapia Albae* and *Arisaema cum Bile* may be added to remove phlegm and disperse accumulation of pathogens.

Long-lasting *Bi* syndrome will also bring on deficiency of *qi* and blood as well as insufficiency of the liver and kidney, in this case, *Du Huo Ji Sheng Tang*[195] with modification may be chosen to eliminate pathogenic factor and support healthy energy, which is a method of reinforcement and elimination in combination, that is, simultaneously using methods of expelling wind, cold and removing dampness together with methods of invigorating *qi* and blood and nourishing the liver and kidney.

In treating *Bi* syndrome, *Radix Aconiti*, *Radix Aconiti Praeparata* and *Herba Asari* are often adopted to expell wind and dampness and relieve pain for cases of *Bi* syndrome due to wind-cold-dampness with sharp pain. At the beginning, take small amount of those drugs, then largen the amount gradually. And their toxicity will be lessened if they have been decocted for a long time, or they are decocted together with *Radix Glycyrrhizae*. Lessen the amount, or stop taking them and adopt remedial measure when intoxication symptoms appear, such as glossolabial numbness, numbness of hands and feet, nausea, palpitation and slow pulse.

Summary

Cause	Syndrome	Type	Treatment
Pathogenic wind-cold-dampness invading the body	*Bi* syndrome due to wind-cold-dampness	Xing Bi	Dispelling wind, cold and dampness and removing obstruction in the collaterals; recipe: *Fang Feng Tang*
		Tong Bi	Expelling pathogenic cold from collaterals and removing wind and dampness; recipe: *Wu Tou Tang*
		Zhuo Bi	Expelling dampness and removing obstruction in the collaterals, and expelling wind and cold; recipe: *Yi Yi Ren Tang*
Affected by pathogenic heat or heat from accumulation of other pathogens	*Bi* syndrome due to wind-heat-dampness		Removing heat and obstruction in the collaterals and expelling wind and dampness; recipe: *Bai Hu Gui Zhi Tang*

Discussions

1. Tell the relationship between *Bi* syndrome and pathogens of wind, cold and dampness.

2. How many types is *Bi* syndrome classified into? Describe their main points of differentiation, treatments and recipes.

38 Flaccidity Syndrome (*Wei Zheng*)

General

Flaccidity syndrome is a morbid condition manifested as flaccidity of tendons and muscles which will result in myoatrophy because it is impossible for tendons and muscles to move freely.

The differentiating treatments for the disease are referential to polyneuritis, acute myelitis, myasthenia gravis, myodystrophy, periodic paralysis, progressive myatrophy and infective sequelae of certral nervous system with the symptom of flaccid paralysis by Western Medicine.

Etiology and Pathogenesis

1. **Impariement of body fluid due to the lung – heat** Affection by pathogenic heat causing high fever to linger a long time, or heat remaining after illness leading to injury of the lung which fails to distribute body fluid to five *zang* organs resulting in malnutrition of tendons, muscles and vessels in limbs and flaccidity.

2. **Invasion of damp – heat** Staying in damp condition for a long time, or being caught in rain or wading across water bringing on invasion of dampness to channels to become heat; or improper diet, or a liking for fat and sweet or pungent food, or over - drink causing impairment of the spleen and stomach and the production of damp – heat, which invades the tendons, muscles and vessels to obstruct the flow of *qi* and blood, resulting in malnurtition of tendons, muscles and vessels and flaccidity syndrome.

3. **Deficiency of the spleen and stomach** The spleen acts as the source of growth and development, so usual weakness of the spleen and stomach or long – lasting illness will impair *qi* of middle – *jiao* causing dysfunction of the spleen and stomach in receiving and transporting essence, deficiency of body fluid, *qi* and blood and malnutrition of five *zang* organs and tendons, resulting in flaccidity showing the symptoms of dysfunction of joints and muscular wasting. Flaccidity syndrome is aggravated if it lasts long and causes deficiency of the spleen and stomach.

4. **Deficiency of the liver and kidney** Inborn debility or excessive sexual intercourse impairs the essence – *qi* and over – strain causes deficiency of *yin* – fluid leading to excess of fire in the kidney and malnutrition of muscles, tendons and vessels resulting in flaccidity. Flaccidity syndrome will also take place in case of syndromes caused by the disorders of five emotions leading to deficiency of the kidney – fluid and excessive heart fire to damage the lung resulting in the failure of the lung in directing the body fluid into five *zang* organs and malnutrition of limbs.

Besides, damp-heat going downwards to impair the liver and kidney will lead to malnutrition of muscles, tendons and vessels.

Key points:

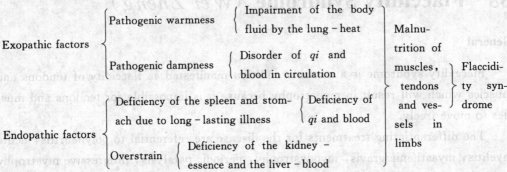

Diagnosis and Discrimination

Flaccidity syndrome is a disease manifested as flaccid limbs unable to move freely as a result of their malnutrition due to the impairment of the *qi* of *zang* organs.

Discrimination should be made between flaccidity syndrome and *Bi* syndrome, for both of them share the same symptom of emaciation and myoatrophy. At the later stage of *Bi* syndrome, the joints are painful and unable to move, therefore emaciation follows from their disease. There is no painful feeling in joints with flaccidity syndrome while there is painful sensation with *Bi* syndrome, and the pathogeneses and treatments of them are different.

Selecting Treatment by Differentiating Syndromes

Myasthenia in legs is a common symptom of flaccidity syndrome, sometimes both hands and feet are involved, in severe case, the patient can not stand up or hold things, when the case lasts a long time, even paralysis will happen.

Clinically flaccidity syndromes can be divided into deficiency syndrome and excess syndrome. Excess syndrome is marked by sudden onset and rapid development due to the impairment of body fluid by the lung-heat or due to the attack of dampness-heat, while deficiency syndrome is characterized by long medical history, slow onset and development due to deficiency of the spleen, stomach, liver and kidney. There are still cases of excess complicated by deficiency or vice versa. The treating principle is regulating the functions of the spleen and stomach, but differentiating syndromes is also important in selecting a treatment.

Common syndromes:

1. The impairment of body fluid by the lung-heat and malnutrition of muscles, tendons and vessels.

[Symptoms] Onset with fever, after abatement of fever appearing weakness of limbs, dry skin, vexation, thirst, cough with little sputum, yellow and small amount of urine, constipation, red tongue with little fur and thready and rapid pulse.

[Main Points of Differentiation] Onset with fever, after abatement of fever appearing weakness of limbs, cough, dry throat, red tongue with little fur.

This type can be observed in acute poliomyelitis, periodic paralysis and acute infective polyneuritis.

[Pathogenesis] Warm-heat invading the lung, causing the lung-heat to impair body fluid and making body fluid fail in spreading resulting in malnutrition of muscles, tendons and vessels.

[Treatment] Clearing away heat, moisturzing dryness and nourishing the lung to produce body fluid.

[Recipe] *Qing Zao Jiu Fei Tang*[254]

In case of excessive heat in the *qifen* with symptoms of high fever, thirst and sweating, take larger amout of *Gypsum Fibrosum*, and add *Flos Lonicerae*, *Rhizoma Anemarrhenae* and *Fructus Forsythiae* to remove pathogenic heat; in case of cough with little phlegm, add *Fructus Trichosanthis*, *Cortex Mori Radicis* and *Folium Eriobotryae* to moisten the lung; in case of abating fever, poor appetite, serious dry mouth and throat due to impairment of lung-*yin* and the stomach-*yin*, use *Yi Wei Tang*[217] plus *Semen Coicis*, *Rhizoma Dioscoreae* and *Fructus Oryzae Germinatus* to reinforce the stomach to produce fluid.

[Nursing Points] Keep the ward air fresh and cool and moist. Take light and sweet food and food of moistening property, and avoid pungent and fried diet.

2. Damp-heat invading the body and failure of *qi* and blood in circulation

[Symptoms] Flaccidity of limbs, tiredness, sometimes complicated with swelling, numbness especially in legs, some with fever, stuffiness in chest and epigastrium, scanty dark urine, difficulty and pain in micturition, yellowish and greasy fur, soft-floating, and rapid pulse

[Main Points of Differentiation] Flaccidity of limbs, stuffiness in epigastrium, dark urine, yellowish and greasy fur.

This type is seen in actue osteomyelitis, acute infective polyneuritis and periodic paralysis.

[Pathogenesis] Dampness-heat invading tendons and muscles in limbs to obstruct the circulation of *qi* and blood causing malnutrition of muscles, tendons and vessels.

[Treatment] Eliminating dampness and heat and easing joint movement.

[Recipe] *Jia Wei Er Miao San*[96]

Caulis Aristolochiae, *Semen Coicis*, *Excrement a Bombycum*, *Fructus Chaenomelis* and *Radix Achyranthis Bidentatae* may be added to promote diuresis and remove obstruction in the collaterals. In case of excessive dampness with symptoms of stuffiness in chest and heavy feeling in limbs with swelling, add *Cortex Magnoliae Officinalis*, *Poria* and *Rhizoma Alismatis* to regulate the flow of *qi* and remove dampness. In summer and autumn, add *Herba Agastachis* and *Herba Eupatorii* to remove dampness with herbs fragrant in flavour. If there is symptoms of stasis such as nunbness of limbs, difficulty of joints in moving, purplish tongue, thready and uneven pulse, add *Semen Persicae*, *Flos Carthami*, *Radix Salviae Miltiorrhizae* and *Radix Paeoniae Rubra* to promote the circulation of blood and remove obstruction in the collaterals; in case of excessive heat to injure *yin* with symptoms of thin physique, hot sensation in legs, vexation, red tongue or absence of fur in the middle of the tongue, thready and rapid pulse, subtract *Rhizoma Atractylodis*, and add *Radix Rehmanniae*, *Plastrum Testudinis* and *Radix Ophiopogonis* to nourish *yin* and clear away heat.

[Nursing Points] Keep the ward clean, and the air fresh, cool, dry and well ventilated. Have light food and avoid pungent, fat and sweet diet, and alcohol which are likely to generate heat and dampness.

3. Deficiency of the spleen and stomach causing food essence fo fail to be transported to the whole body

[Symptoms] Weakness of limbs to become more severe gradually, poor appetite, fullness of abdomen, loose stool, dim complexion and swelling face, short breath, listlessness, pale tongue, thin and whitish fur, thready pulse.

[Main Points of Differentiation] Weakness of limbs to become more severe gradually, poor appetite, loose stool and pale tongue.

This type is common in myasthenia gravis, myodystrophy, progressive myatropgy and infective sequelae of central nervous system with the symptom of flaccidity paralysis.

[Pathogenesis] Deficiency of the spleen and stomach causing the inadequate production of *qi* and blood resulting in malnutrition of muscles, tendons and vessels.

[Treatment] Invigorating the spleen and replenishing *qi* to promote their functions of transporting and transforming food essence.

[Recipe] *Shen Ling Bai Zhu San*[169].

In case of dibility due to long illness and deficiency of *qi* and blood, largen the amount of *Radix Codonopsis Pilosulae*, *Rhizoma Dioscoreae* and *Rhizoma Atractylodis Macro Cephalae*, and add *Radix Astragali seu Hedysari* and *Radix Angelicae Sinensis* to invigorate *qi* and blood; if the patient is fat with the symptom of polyphlegm, adopt *Liu Jun Zi Tang*[45] to reinforce the spleen and resolve phlegm.

[Nursing Points] Have easily digested diet able to replenish *qi* and invigorate the spleen, such as gruel made with hyacinth bean, Chinese yam or *Semen Coicis*.

4. Deficiency of the liver and kidney and myoatrophy

[Symptoms] Slow onset, flaccidity of the lower limbs, soreness of the loins, inability to stand long, sometimes accompanied with blurred vision, losing hair, dry throat, tinnitus, emission, abnormal menstruation (in females), even inability to walk and myoatrophy of the legs if serious; red tongue with little fur, thready and rapid pulse.

[Main Points of Differentiation] Slow onset, flaccid lower limbs, soreness of the loins, tinnitus, red tongue with little fur.

This type is observable in myasthenia gravis, myodystrophy, progressive myatrophy and infective sequelae of central nervous system with the symptoms of flaccidity and paralysis.

[Pathogenesis] Deficiency of the liver and kidney causing their failure in nourishing muscles, bones and channels.

[Treatment] Invigorating the liver and kidney and nourishing *yin* to clear away heat.

[Recipe] *Hu Qian Wan*[151].

This recipe is commonly adopted in practice for flaccidity due to deficiency - *yin* of the liver and kidney accompanied with heat. In case of excessive heat, subtract *Herba Cunomorii* and *Rhizoma zingiberis*; if accompanied with sallow complexion, palpitation, pink tongue, thready and weak pulse, add *Radix Astragali seu Hedysari*, *Radix Codonopsis Pilosulae*, *Radix Angelicae Sinensis* and *Caulis Spatholobi* to enrich *qi* and blood; in case of deficiency of *yin* affecting *yang* due to long illness with symptoms of aversion to cold, impotence, watery urine, pale tongue, deep, thready and weak pulse, subtract *Cortex Phellodendri* and *Rhizoma Anemarrhenae*, and add *Cornu Cervi*, *Fructus Psoraleae*, *Herba Epimedii*, *Radix Morindae officinalis*, *Cortex Cinnamomi* and *Radix Aconiti praeparate* to tonify the kidney and reinforce *yang*.

Besides, the powder made from *Placenta Hominis* and boiled pork marrow or beaf marrow pounded together with rice flour and sugar may be taken by the patient.

[Nursing Points] Take proper exercise and avoid sexual intemperance; Better have a diet able to nourish *yin* and replenish *qi* and refrain from pungent food.

Other treatments such as acupuncture and moxibustion, massage therapy and *qigong* may be adopted in combination, and the patient needs to exercise the limbs moderately which is very important to the recovery, and helps to improve the therapeatic effect.

The prognosis of flaccidity syndrome is related to the course of disease as well as its quality of syndromes, i. e. excess syndrome or deficiency syndrome. The former is chiefly seen in the early stage of some acute cases which have a mild state of illness with a better therapeutic effect, and the patient is easily recovered. Deficiency syndrome and chronic cases display a long course of illness with little effect within a short period, and the patient has difficulty in recovery. The prognosis is unsatisfactory esp. for the patients of old or poor heath.

Summary

Flaccidity syndrome
- Excess syndrome
  - Impairment of body fluid by the lung-heat — Treated by clearing away heat, moistening and nourishing the lung to produce body fluid; recipe: *Qing Zao Jiu Fei Tang*
  - Damp-heat invading the body — Eliminating dampness and heat and keeping the collaterals unobstructed; recipe: *Jia Wei Er Miao San*
- Deficiency syndrome
  - Deficiency of the spleen and stomach — Treated by invigorating the spleen and *qi* to promote transporting and transforming food essence; recipe: *Shen Ling Bai Zhu San*
  - Deficiency of the liver and kidney — Treated by invigorating the liver and kidney and nourishing *yin* to clear away heat; recipe: *Hu Qian Wan*

Discussions

1. What is the definition of flaccidity syndrome?
2. How many types is flaccidity syndrome classified into? What are their respective main points of differentiation, treatments and recipes?
3. How is flaccidity syndrome distinguished from *Bi* syndrome?

39 Fever Due To Internal Injury

General

Fever due to internal injury is caused by deficiency of *qi*, blood and *yin* - essence, and dysfunction of the *zang* and *fu* organs. It is marked by slow onset and long course of illness and the clinical symptom of low fever, and high fever is possible only in a few cases. And in some cases, there is no fever by thermometer, but self - felt fever and dysphoria with feverish sensation in chest, palms and soles.

The differentiating treatments for the disease are referential to neurotic low fever, rheumatic fever, tuberculosis, hyperthyroidism, chronic infectional fever and fever by malignant tumor.

Etiology and Pathogenesis

1. Accumulation of heat in the liver channel   Depressed emotions causes disorder of the liver - *qi* to accumulate and turn into fire resulting in fever; or fury leads to excessive liver - fire resulting in fever. This kind of fever is called "fire caused by the disorders of five emotions", for it is closely related to emotions.

2. Accumulation of blood stasis   Blood stasis due to stagnation of *qi*, tiredness, trauma or bleeding will cause obstruction of the channels and collaterals and the unsmooth circulation of the *qi* and blood resulting in fever.

3. Deficiency of *yin* - essence   Usual deficiency of *yin*, or protracted course of febrile disease, or impairment of *yin* due to long - time diarrhea of misuse or abuse of herbs in warm and dry property will lead to deficiency of *yin* - essence and cause the kidney - fluid to fail to restrain the heart - fire and hyperactivity of *yang* - *qi* resulting in fever.

4. Malnutrition due to blood deficiency   Blood deficiency in the heart and liver due to long illness, or failure of the spleen in blood production or bleeding and excessive loss of blood after delivery or operation will lead to blood deficiency and malnutrition, resulting in fever.

5. Deficiency of *qi* in middle - *jiao*   Overstrain, or improper diet, or lack of nutrition after long illness will cause deficiency of the spleen - *qi* and stomach - *qi* in middle - *jiao* to bring on *yin* - fire resulting in fever which is named "fever due to deficiency of *qi*".

Key Points:

Emotional depression
Blood stasis
Deficiency of *yin* - essence
Deficiency blood and malnutrition
Deficiency of *qi* in middle - *jiao*
} Deficiency of *qi*, blood and *yin* - essence, dysfunction of the *zang* and *fu* organs } - Fever due to internal injury

Diagnosis and Discrimination

Fever due to internal injury is caused by deficiency of *qi*, blood and *yin* - essence, and dysfunction of *zang* - *fu*.

Clinical discrimination should be made between this disease and fever due to exopathogen, for both have the symptom of fever.

Discrimination \ Disease	Fever due to internal injury	Fever due to exopathogenic affection
Etiology	Caused by overstrain, improper diet and emotional disorder	Affected by exopathogen
Onset features	Slow onset, long course, or repeated attack	Acute onset, short course
Fever features	Mainly low fever without aversion to cold, or feeling cold but lessened with quilt, the fever being by fits and starts and appearing irregularly, or only self - felt fever and feverish sensation in the palms and sloes	Mainly high fever, at the early stage with aversion to cold, even if quilt added, the cold - feeling not lessened, fever unable to be relieved unless exopathogens eliminated
Complicated symptoms	Dizziness, listlessness, self - sweating, night sweating, weak pulse	Headache and general pain, nasal obstruction, cough, floating pulse

Selecting Treatment by Differentiating Syndromes

In differentiating syndromes of the disease, etiologies and pathogeneses, and deficiency syndrome and excess syndrome should be distinguished. Stagnation of *qi* and blood stasis belongs to excess syndrome, while deficiency of *qi*, blood and *yin* belongs to deficiency syndrome. According to various conditions, adopt different treatments, such as regulaging *qi* by alleviating mental depression, promoting blood circulation, invigorating *qi*, nourishing the blood and replenishing *yin*. Do not use drugs of pungent flavor which will induce perspiration or drugs bitter in taste and cold in nature for all kinds of fever, for the former will consume body fluid and *qi*, and the latter will impair the spleen-*yang* and make dryness-transformation to impair *yin*, which will make the disease worse.

Common Syndromes:

1. Fever due to stagnation of the liver-*qi*

[Symptoms] Often feeling fever and vexation, the fever condition changing according to the patient's moods, depressed mood, or irritation, fullness in the chest and hypochondrium, being susceptible to sighing, bitter taste, dry mouth, in women, irregular menstruation, abdominal pain or mammary swelling in menstrual period, yellowish fur, and wiry and rapid pulse.

[Main Points of Differentiation] Fever, vexation, the fever condition changing according to the patient's moods, fullness in hypochondrium, bitter taste, wiry and rapid pulse.

This type is common in hyperthyroidism and neurotic low fever.

[Pathogenesis] Emotional depression causing stagnation of the liver-*qi* to turn into fire resulting in fever.

[Treatment] Relieving the depression and purging the liver of pathogenic fire.

[Recipe] *Dan Zhi Xiao Yao San*[52].

In case of dominant heat syndrome, dry mouth and constipation, subtract *Rhizoma Atracthodis Macrocephalae* and *Poria*, and add *Radix Scutellariae* and *Radix Gentianae* to purge the liver of pathogenic fire; in case of pain in hypochondrium, add *Fructus Meliae Toosendan* and *Radix Curcumae* to regulate the flow of *qi* and relieve pain; in case of long-time stagnation of *qi* and pathogenic heat impairing *yin*, or usual deficiency of *yin* complicated with stagnation of the liver-*qi*, use *Zi Shui Qing Gan Yin*[271] to nourish the liver and kidney, sooth the liver and clear away heat; in case of stagnation of *qi* turning into fire with dominant heat syndrome, flushed face, vexation, irritation, dark urine, constipation, deep-red tongue, rapid pulse, adopt *Long Dan Xie Gan Tang*[64] to purge the liver of pathogenic fire.

[Nursing Points] Adjusting emotions to avoid fury; do not eat pungent food.

2. Fever due to blood stasis

[Symptoms] Fever in the afertnoon or at night, dry mouth and throat with no desire for drinking, fixed pain-spot or mass in the trunk or limbs, squamous and dry skin, darkish or sallow complexion, dark purplish tongue or tongue with ecchymosis, and uneven pulse.

[Main points of Defferentiation] Fever in the afternoon or at night, fixed pain-spot or mass in the body, dark purplish tongue.

This type is seen in malignant tumor and rheumatic fever.

[Pathogenesis] Blood stasis obstructing the flow of *qi* and blood resulting in fever.

[Treatment] Promoting blood circulation to remove blood stasis.

[Recipe] *Xue Fu Zhu Yu Tang*[119].

In case of dominant heat syndrome, add *Cortex Moutan Radicis*, *Radix Cynanchi Atrati*, *Radix Salviae Miltiorrhizae* and *Radix et Rhizoma Rhei* to promote blood circulation and clear away heat from blood. In case of marked pain, add *Rhizoma Corydalis* and *Faeces Trogopterorum* to relieve pain by promoting blood circulation.

[Nursing Points] Adjusting emotions; taking food warm in nature; avoiding cold and uncooked food and overstrain.

3. Fever due to deficiency of *yin*

[Symptoms] Fever in the afternoon or at night, feverish sensation in the palms and soles, or hectic fever, vexation, night sweating, insomnia and dreamful sleep, dry mouth and throat, constipation, dark and scant urine, red and dry or crackled tongue with little or without fur, thready and rapid pulse.

[Main Points of Differentiation] Fever in the afternoon or at night, feverish sensation in the palms and soles, night sweat, dreamful sleep, red and dry tongue with little or without fur.

This is observable in neuralfunctional fever, and fever due to tuberculosis and malignant tumor.

[Pathogenesis] Hyperactivity of *yang* due to *yin* deficiency and water failing to control fire resulting in fever.

[Treatment] Nourishing *yin* to clear away heat.

[Recipe] *Qing Gu San*[251].

In case of insomnia, add *Semen ziziphi Spinosae*, *Semen Biotae* and *Caulis Polygoni Multiflori* to nourish heart and tranquilize the mind; in case of severe night sweating, add *Concha Ostreae Calcined*, *Fructus Tritici Levis* and *Radix Oryzae Glutinosae* to strengthen exterior and reduce sweat; in case of severe *yin* deficiency, add *Radix Rehmanniae*, *Radix Scrophulariae* and *Radix Polygoni Multiflori* to strengthen the effect of nourishing *yin*; in case of deficiency of *qi* and *yin* with symptoms of short breath, dizziness and tiredness, add *Radix Codonopsis Pilosulae*, *Radix Glehniae*, *Radix Ophiopogonis* and *Fructus Schisandrae* to supplement *qi* and nourish *yin*.

[Nursing Points] Have sweet food and food apt to produce fluid instead of pungent and fried food and food apt to induce fire; avoid excessive sexual intercourse and overstrain; adjust emotions.

4. Fever due to blood deficiency

[Symptoms] Low fever, dizziness, blurred vision, pale complexion, palpitation, fatigue and weakness, pale lips and nails, pale tongue, thready and weak pulse.

[Main Points of Differentiation] Low fever, dizziness, blurred vision, pale complexion, pale lips and nails.

This type can be observed in malignant tumor, rheumatic fever and neurotic fever.

[Pathogenesis] Deficiency of *yin*-blood failing to control *yang* resulting in fever.

[Treatment] Replenishing *qi* and blood.

[Recipe] *Gui Pi Tang*[95] or *Dang Gui Bu Xue Tang*[115].

[Nursing Points] Have nourishing and light food; avoid pungent food and over-working.

5. Fever due to *qi* deficiency

[Symptoms] Fever often occurring or aggravated after tiredness with various degrees, listlessness, short breath, laziness to talk, dizziness, spontaneous sweat, being apt to catch cold, poor appetite, loose stool, pale tongue with thin and whitish fur, thready and weak pulse.

[Main Points of Differentiation] Fever often occurring or aggravated after tiredness, poor appetite, loose stool, short breath and being lazy to talk.

This type is common in malignant tumor, tuberculosis and fever due to chronic pyelonephritis.

[Pathogenesis] *Qi* deficiency in the spleen and stomach causes *qi* of the middle-*jiao* to descend and deficient fire to generate inside, resulting in fever.

[Treatment] Replenishing *qi* and invigorating the spleen, and relieving fever with drugs of sweet flavor and warm nature.

[Recipe] *Bu Zhong Yi Qi Tang*[140].

In case of seriouse spontaneous sweat, add calcined *Concha Ostreae*, calcined *Os Draconis* and *Fructus Tritici Levis* to strengthen exterior to reduce sweating; if complicated with pathogenic dampness with stuffiness in chest and epigastrium, whitish and greasy fur, add *Poria*, *Rhizoma Atractylodis*, *Herba Agastachis* and *Fructus Amomi* to invigorate the spleen and dry dampness; in case of feeling cold and hot by fits and starts, sweating and aversion to wind, add *Ramulus Cimmamomi* and *Radix Paeoniae Alba* to regulate *Ying* and *Wei*.

[Nursing Points] Do not toil; avoid pungent, fat and sweet food. Have porridge of *Radix Astragali seu Hedysari*, of lotus seed, and of oatmeal to invigorate the spleen and stomach. Besides, there is fever due to *yang* deficiency with the symptoms of fever, aversion to cold, warmless limbs or legs, pale complexion, dizziness, having a liking for lying, soreness in the loins and knees, large and moist tongue or with teeth-pints, whitish and moist fur, deep, thready and weak pulse, or floating, large and weak pulse, use *Jin Gui Shen Qi Wan*[163] to treat it by warming and tonifying the kidney-*yang*. Fever due to *yang* deficiency includes other special type. One is *yang* kept externally by *yin*-excess in the interior and the other displays false heat syndrome but actual cold syndrome, manifested as fever, flushed complexion, no aversion to cold, coldness of limbs, discharge of indigested food, feeble pulse. For emergency case of the former, use *Radix Aconiti Praeparata*, *Rhizoma Zingiberis*, *Radix Glycyrrhizae*, *Radix Ginseng* to recuperate the depleted *yang* and rescue the patient from danger.

Summary

Complicated as its illness condition is and long its course, it is necessary to observe and differentiate it with a careful consideration of the case history, characteristics of fever and accompaning symptoms so that a gradual effect will be achieved.

It is chiefly caused by emotional disorder, improper diet or overstrain with deficiency *qi*, blood and *yin* essence and dysfunction of the *zang* and *fu* as its pathogenesis. It should be discriminated from fever caused by exopathogen, and different methods should be used for different syndromes. However, the different causes are often interrelated or interchangeable or accompanied with one another. For example, fever due to stagnated liver-*qi* may gradually impair *yin* and consume the body fluid, thus convert into fever due to stagnated *qi* and deficient *yin*; *qi* and blood deficiency may interact each other or occur mixedly; *yang* will be affected after long period of fever due to *qi* deficiency, causing fever due to *yang* deficiency. Therefore, differentiation should be carried out in light of the idea of development and interaction so as to have the initiative on treatment. Besides, it is helpful to the treatment and recovery if the patient can keep high spirit, avoid overstrain, and regulate his diet.

Depression	Deficiency of *qi*, blood and *yin*-essence; and dysfunction of the *zang* and *fu*	Fever due to internal injury	Fever due to stagnation of the liver-*qi*	Relieving the depressed liver-*qi* and purging the liver of pathogenic fire; recipe: *Dan Zhi Xiao Yao San*
Stagnation by blood stasis			Fever due to blood stasis	Promoting blood circulation to remove blood stasis; recipe: *Xue Fu Zhu Yu Tang*
Deficiency of *yin*-essence			Fever due to *yin* deficiency	Nourishing *yin* to clear away heat; recipe: *Qing Gu San*
Deficiency of *qi* and blood			Fever due to blood deficiency	Replenishing *qi* and blood; recipe: *Gui Pi Tang*
			Fever due to *qi* deficiency	Replenishing *qi* and invigorating the spleen to relieve fever; recipe *Bu Zhong Yi Qi Tang*
			Fever due to *yang* deficiency	Warming and tonifying the kidney-*yang*; recipe: *Jin Gui Shen Qi Wan*

Discussions

1. How do you distinguish fever due to internal injury from exopathogenic fever?
2. What are the common types of fever due to internal injury? And what are the respective main points of differentiation of each?

40 Consumptive Disease (*Xu Lao*)

General

Consumptive Disease (*Xu Lao*), also called *Xu Sun*, is due to many factors. It is a general term for some chronic consumptive syndromes with deficiency of *zang-fu* organs and insufficiency of *qi* and blood, *yin* and *yang* as the main pathogenesis. Cases belonging to this category are morbid conditions arising from congenital insufficiency and malnutrition after birth, endogenous impairment caused by overstrain, and persistent deficiency, all of which show consumptive syndromes.

Selecting treatment by differentiation of symptoms and signs can be served as a reference to some chronic or consumptive diseases in Western Medicine such as Sheehan's syndrome, Addison's disease, hypothyroidism, aplastic anemia, chronic granulocytic leukemia, etc.

Etiology and Pathogenesis

1. Patients with congenital insufficiency or general asthenia are mostly caused by parents' inadequate essence and blood due to old age and constitutional weakness; by mothers' lack of proper care during pregnancy resulting in deficient development of fetus; or by improper feeding causing infants' malnutrition; or by infants' hereditary defect, etc. Because of general asthenia, it is likely for people to be attacked by pathogenic factors due to overstrain, or to be weak due to disease, and consequently there comes consumptive disease after a long course of lingering morbid condition.

2. Consumptive disease is caused by overanxiety and overstrain impairing the five-*zang* organs. Cases are mostly found in the clinic manifesting impairment of the heart and the spleen due to overanxiety and overstrain, or impairment of the kidney due to early marriage and many births, and overstrain from sexual intemperance.

3. Consumptive disease is the result of the impaired spleen and stomach by irregular food-intake. Intemperance in eating and drinking; habitual preference for a certain kind of food stuff, malnutrition, and excessive alcohol may impair the spleen and the stomach, leading to dysfunction of them in digesting and transmitting food essence, in producing *qi* and blood. If there is a prolonged impairment of the spleen and the stomach, there will certainly be insufficiency of *qi* and blood, resulting in the failure in regulating the function of five *zang*-organs and six *fu*-organs interiorly, and the failure in distributing *qi* and blood in *ying*, *wei* and channels exteriorly, which gradually develops into consumptive disease.

4. Consumptive disease occurs for lack of regulating and nursing after serious dis-

ease or a long course of illness. There usually appears impairment of *zang-qi* due to excessive pathogenic factors after serious disease, or consumption of *yin* and blood due to persistent febrile disease, or impairment of *yang* and vital-*qi* because of prolonged retention of pathogenic cold, or failure in production of fresh blood resulting from internal stagnation of blood stasis, or the failure in nursery after diseases leading to difficult recovery of vital-*qi*. All of the above-mentioned factors may bring about impairment of *qi* and blood, *yin* and *yang*, which gradually develops into consumptive disease in the end.

Key Points:

Deficiency causes illness leading to *Xu Lao*

Deficiency is caused by illness, a long course of which leads to *Xu Lao*

→ Impairment of five *zang*-organs → Deficiency of *qi*, blood, *yin* and *yang* → Consumptive disease

Diagnosis and Discrimination

Consumptive disease is a general term for syndromes of many chronic asthenic diseases.

Careful discrimination should be made among such diseases as consumptive disease, deficiency syndromes and pulmonary tuberculosis that all present asthenic symptoms.

Although consumptive disease is similar to deficiency syndromes manifested by some other diseases in the clinical symptoms, treatment and recipes, there indeed exists difference between the two types of diseases. Consumptive disease is characterized by a series of symptoms of deficiency of essence *qi*, while the deficiency syndromes of other diseases are characterized by the principal symptom shown by these diseases as prominent characteristics. For example, deficiency type of *qi* and blood of vertigo and the type of hypoactivity of the spleen-*yang* of edema are characterized respectively by dizziness and edema as the basic and prominent symptoms. Moreover, consumptive disease usually shows characteristics of a long course and lingering of illness, which is also different from the deficiency syndrome of other diseases.

As to the differentiation of consumptive disease and pulmanary tubuculosis, the latter is an infectious disease caused by invasion of tuberculosis germs, and its diseased region is mainly in the lungs, pathologically marked by excessive heat due to deficiency of *yin*, and clinically manifested by cough, hemoptysis, hectic fever, night sweat, emaciated constitution. While the former is a non-infective disease caused by many factors and the lesion parts are chiefly in five *zang*-organs, pathogenically characterized by consumption of *qi*, blood, *yin* and *yang*, and manifested by various clinical symptoms showing deficiency of *qi*, blood, *yin* and *yang* in five *zang*-organs.

Selecting Treatment by Differentiating Syndromes

The differentiation of consumptive disease can be induced to four types such as deficiency of *qi*, blood, *yin* and *yang*.

Consumptive disease	Deficiency of *qi*	Shortness of breath and listlessness, spontaneous sweat, poor appetite, loose stool, pale tongue and weak pulse	Supplementing *qi*
	Deficiency of blood	Dim complexion, pale lips and tongue, thready and weak pulse	Nourishing blood
	Deficiency of *yin*	Dysphoria with feverish sensation in chest, palms and soles, flushing of zygomatic region, dryness of the mouth and throat, red tongue with little saliva, thready and rapid pulse	Nourishing *yin*
	Deficiency of *yang*	Lassitude with inclination to lie in bed, chilliness and coldness of the extremities, borborygmus and diarrhea, pale and enlarged tongue, weak or deep and slow pulse.	Warming *yang*

In the differentiation, attention should be paid to the mutual influence of different kinds of deficiency caused by different factors; when one *zang*-organ is diseased, other *zang*-organs may get involved; one kind of deficiency may gradually lead to many kinds of deficiency. For instance, disease of the spleen may affect the lung, disease of lungs may involve the kidney, deficiency of *qi* will bring about failure in producing blood, deficiency of blood will result in failure of production of *qi*, the gradual declination of *yang* will follow deficiency of *qi*, insufficiency of *yin* will accompany with deficiency of blood, impairment of *yin* involves *yang*, impairment of *yang* involves *yin* and so on. Therefore in the clinical differentiation treatment should be planned in view of the development and changes of cases.

The treatment of consumptive disease should follow the basic principle of tonifying and invigorating. Based on the different kinds of pathological nature, it is applicable to use recipes respectively for invigorating *qi*, nourishing the blood, nourishing *yin* and warming *yang*, and to select medicines in accordance with the different diseased regions of five *zang*-organs for a better therapeutic effect. Moreover, since *qi* and blood of the human body are originated congenitally, and the reproduction of them lies in the nursing and nourishing postnatally, it is significant to tonify and invigorate the spleen and the kidney in the treatment of consumptive disease.

The types of this disease commonly seen are as follows:

1. Deficiency of *qi*

(1) Deficiency of the lung-qi

[Symptoms] Shortness of breath, spontaneous sweat, a low and weak voice, alternative coldness and hotness, liability to catching cold, pale complexion, pale tongue and weak pulse.

[Main Points of Differentiation] Shortness of breath, spontaneous sweat, liability to catching cold.

[Pathogenesis] Insufficiency of the lung-qi and a failure of superficial-qi to protect the body against diseases resulting in disharmony between *ying* and *wei*.

[Treatment] Invigorating the lung-qi.

[Recipe] *Bu Fei Tang*[143].

The above-mentioned recipe combined with *Mu Li San*[144] is applicable to cases with excessively spontaneous sweating for invigorating qi and consolidating superficial resistance to arrest sweating. In case of deficiency of both qi and yin accompanied with hectic fever, night sweat, add *Carapax Trionycis*, *Cortex Lycii Radicis*, *Radix Gentianae Macrophyllae*, etc. to nourish yin and clear away heat.

[Nursing Points] Protecting from wind and cold, caring for daily life, avoiding uncooked and cold food.

(2) Deficiency of the spleen-qi

[Symptoms] Decreasing in food-intake and uncomfortable feeling of the stomach after eating, lassitude, loose stool, sallow complexion, pale tongue with thin fur and weak pulse.

[Main Points of Differentiation] Poor appetite, loose stool, sallow complexion.

[Pathogenesis] Insufficient source of qi and blood due to dysfunction of the spleen in transportation and transformation and abnormal function of the gastrointestine to transfrom.

[Treatment] Invigorating the spleen and supplementing qi.

[Recipe] *Jia Wei Si Jun Zi Tang*[97].

In case of distending fullness of the stomach, vomiting and eructation, add *Rhizoma Pinelliae*, *Pericarpium Citri Reticulatae* for regulating the function of the stomach to lower the adverse flow of qi. In the case accompanied with indigestion, add *Semen Raphani*, *Massa Fermentata Medicinalis*, *Fructus Hordei Geminatus*, *Endothelium Corneum Gigeriae Galli*, *Fructus Crataegi* to help digest and strengthen the stomach. In case of deficiency of qi involving yang resulting in gradual deficiency of the spleen-yang, manifested by diarrhea with abdominal pain, chillness of hands and feet, add *Cortex Cinnamoni*, baked ginger to warm the middle-*jiao* to dispel cold. In case of deficiency of the spleen-qi chiefly manifested by sinking of qi due to insufficiency of qi in the middle-*jiao*, apply *Bu Zhong Yi Qi Tang*[140] to invigorate qi of the middle-*jiao* and to elevate the spleen *yang*.

[Nursing Points] Preferring light nutritious food, avoiding eating raw and cold food.

Among deficiency types of *qi*, blood, *yin* and *yang*, deficiency of *qi* is mostly seen in the clinic, especially deficiency of the lung – *qi* and the spleen – *qi*, and other deficiency types such as deficiency of the heart – *qi* and the kidney – *qi* are also usually found clinically, the treatment of which may refer to the therapeutic method of deficiency of the heart – *yang* and of the kidney – *yang*.

2. Deficiency of blood

(1) Deficiency of the heart blood

[Symptoms] Severe palpitation, amnesia, insomnia and dreamy sleep, pale complexion, pale tongue, thready or intermittent pulse.

[Main Points of Differentiation] Severe palpitation, pale complexion, intermittent pulse.

[Pathogenesis] Insufficiency of blood circulation for lack of blood nourishment of the heart due to deficiency of the heart blood.

[Treatment] Enriching the blood and calming the mind

[Recipe] *Yang Xin Tang*[185].

In case of palpitation with intermittent pulse, apply *Zhi Gan Cao Tang*[165] to make a recovery of the normal pulse beating, and to arrest palpitation.

[Nursing Points] Preferring tonic food, avoiding intemperance in eating caring for daily life, regulating emotions and avoiding overstrain.

(2) Deficiency of the liver blood

[Symptoms] Dizziness, blurring of vision, hypochondriac pain, numbness of limbs, tense tendons and spasm of muscles, abnormal menstruation or even amenorrhea in women cases, pale complexion, pale tongue, wiry and thready pulse or uneven and thready pulse.

[Main Points of Differentiation] Dizziness, blurring of vision, tense tendons.

[Pathogenesis] Deficiency of the liver blood due to a failure of blood to nourish the liver, and insufficiency of blood failing to nourish tendons and channels.

[Treatment] Enriching the blood and nourishing the liver.

[Recipe] *Si Wu Tang* [79].

Add *Radix Polygoni Multiflori Praeparata*, *Fructus Lycii*, *Caulis Spatholobi* to increase the effect of enriching the liver blood. In case of dizziness and tinnitus, add *Fructus Ligustri Lucidi*, *magnetite*, *Concha Ostreae*, etc. to nourish *yin* and suppress the excessive *yang*. In case of hypochondriac pain, add *Radix Bupleuri*, *Radix Curcumae*, *Rhizoma Cyperi* and *Fructus Meliae Toosendan* to regulate the flow of *qi* so as to remove obstruction in the collaterals.

[Nursing Points] Preferring tonic food, regulating emotions and avoiding overstrain.

In the cases of blood deficiency, the deficiency of the heart blood, the spleen blood and the liver blood are mostly seen. Because deficiency of blood is usually accompanied with the symptoms of deficiency of *qi* to various degrees, in the treatment of this disease, enriching blood should be properly applied with herbs for supplementing *qi* for therapeutic purpose of supplementing *qi* to promote production of the blood.

3. Deficiency of *yin*

(1) Deficiency of the lung – *yin*

[Symptoms] Dry cough, or cough with blood, dry throat, even aphonia, hectic fever and night sweat, flushed complexion, red tongue with little saliva, thready and rapid pulse.

[Main Points of Differnetiation] Dry cough, dry throat, hectic fever and night sweat, red tongue with little saliva.

[Pathogenesis] Deficiency of the lung – *yin* resulting in a failure of nourishing the lung and causing internal production of asthenic fire, followed by impairment of the lung.

[Treatment] Nourishing *yin* and moistening the lung.

[Recipe] *Sha Shen Mai Men Dong Tang*[138].

In case of severe cough, add *Radix Stemonae*, *Flos Farfarae* and *Radix Asteris* for purifying the lung to relieve cough. In case of cough with blood, add *Rhizoma Bletlillae*, *Herba Agrimoniae*, *Fresh Rhizoma Phragmitis* to remove heat from the blood in order to stop bleeding. In case of hectic fever, add *Cortex Lycii Radicis*, *Radix Stellariae*, *Carapax Trionycis* to nourish *yin* and eliminate heat. In case of night sweat, add *Concha Ostreae*, *Fructus Tritici Levis*, *Radix Ephedrae* to consolidate superficial resisitance to stop perspiration.

[Nursing Points] Avoiding pungent and fried food that produces heat to impair *yin*, preferring fruits, vegetable, *Bulbus Lini*, fresh *Lotus Rhizoma* and other things sweet in flavor, cool and moist in nature.

(2) Deficiency of the heart – *yin*

[Symptoms] Palpitation, insomnia, irritability, hectic fever and night sweat, flushed complexion, aphthae, red tongue with little saliva, thready and rapid pulse.

[Main Points of Differentiation] Palpitation, insomnia, hectic fever and night sweat, red tongue with little saliva.

[Pathogenesis] Deficiency of the heart – *yin* giving rise to a failure in nourishing the heart, and the accumulated internal heat due to deficiency of *yin* resulting in insufficiency of the body fluid.

[Treatment] Nourishing *yin* and nourishing the heart.

[Recipe] *Tian Wang Bu Xin Dan*[32].

In case of irritability and restlessness, aphthae, add *Rhizoma Coptidis*, *Caulis Aristolochiae Manshuriensis*, *Lophatherum* to clear away the heart – fire and induce heat to flow downward.

[Nursing Points] Avoiding pungent and fried food that produces heat to impair *yin*, preferring the food good for nourishing *yin* and the heart such as *Fructus Schisandrae*, *Ophiopogon*, etc., decocting them in water and taking as tea.

(3) Deficiency of the spleen - *yin* and the stomach - *yin*

[Symptoms] Dry mouth, poor appetite, dry stool, vomiting, hiccup, flushed complexion, dry tongue with little fur or without any fur, thready and rapid pulse.

[Main Points of Differentiation] Poor appetite, dry mouth, dry stool, and dry tongue with little fur.

[Pathogenesis] Deficiency of the spleen - *yin* and the stomach - *yin* brings about dysfunction of the spleen and the stomach in transport and transformation and results in production of the internal heat with impairment of the body fluid.

[Treatment] Nourishing *yin* and regulating the stomach.

[Recipe] *Yi Wei Tang*[217].

In case of poor appetite, add *Fructus Oryzae Germinatus*, *Fructus Hordei Germinatus*, *Semen Dolichoris* and *Rhizoma Dioscoreae* to tonify the stomach and invigorate the spleen. In case of severely dry lips and mouth, add *Herba Dendrobii* and Pollen to nourish the stomach - *yin*. In case of hiccup, add *Semen Canavaliae*, *Calyx Kaki* and *Caulis Bambusae in Taeniam* to bring down upward adverse flow of *qi* and relieve hiccup.

[Nursing Points] Regulating emotions, avoiding pungent and fried food, preferring food sweet in flavor and moist, and beneficial to nourishing *yin* such as *Rhizoma Polygonati Odorati*, *Herba Dendrobii*, etc., decocting them in water and taking as tea.

(4) Deficiency of the liver - *yin*

[Symptoms] Headache, dizziness, tinnitus, dryness of the eyes and photophoria, blurred vision, vexation and irritability, numbness of the limbs, tense tendons and spasm of muscles, flushed complexion, dry and red tongue with little fur, wiry and thready and rapid pulse.

[Main Points of Differentiations] Dryness of the eyes and photophobria, tense tendons and spasm of muscles, dry and red tongue with little fur.

[Pathogenesis] Deficiency of the liver - *yin* gives rise to excessive fire due to deficiency of *yin*, a failure in nourishing tendons and channles and vessels, and an internal flow of wind of deficiency type.

[Treatment] Nourishing the liver - *yin*.

[Recipe] *Bu Gan Tang*[142].

In case of severe headache, dizziness and tinnitus, or tense tendons and spasm of muscles, add *Concha Heliotidis*, *Flos Chrysanthemi*, and *Ramulus Uncariae cum Uncis* to subdue exuberant *yang* of the liver. In case of dryness of the eyes and photophoria, blurred vision, add *Fructus Ligustri Lucidi*, *Semen Cassiae*, *Fructus Lycii* to nourish the liver and improve visual acuity. In case of vexation and irritability, dark urine and constipation, red tongue and rapid pulse, add *Radix Gentianae*, *Radix Astragali Seu*

Hedysari, *Capejasmine* to remove heat from the liver. In case of costalgia, add *Fructus Meliae Toosendan*, *Radix Curcumae* to relieve the depressed liver - *qi* and regulate the flow of *qi* to alleviate pain.

[Nursing Points] Regulating emotions, avoiding anxiety and anger, prohibiting pungent and fried food, and food of hot and dry nature.

(5) Deficiency of the kidney - *yin*

[Symptoms] Lassitude in the loins, emission, flaccidity of feet, dizziness, tinnitus, even deafness, dry mouth and sore throat, hectic fever and flushing of zygomatic region, red tongue with little saliva, deep and thready pulse.

[Main Points of Differentiation] Lassitude in the loins, emission, hectic fever, dry throat, red tongue with little saliva.

[Pathogenesis] Deficiency of the kidney - *yin* results in production of the interior heat of deficiency type, the kidney's failure in arresting discharge of essence and malnutrition for the brain.

[Treatment] Nourishing and invigorating the kidney - *yin*.

[Recipe] *Zuo Gui Wan*[65].

In case of severe lassitude in the loins and emission, add *Concha Ostreae*, *Fructus Rosae Laevigatae*, *Semen Euryales*, *Stamen Nelumbinis* to consolidate the kidney and arrest spontaneous seminal emission.

[Nursing Points] Caring for daily life, moderating sexual life, avoiding overstrain, prohibiting pungent and fried food, preferring tonic foodstuffs sweet in flavor and moist in nature.

4. Deficiency of *yang*

(1) Deficiency of the heart - *yang*

[Symptoms] Palpitation, spontaneous perspiration, listlessness and inclination to lie in bed, oppressed feeling and pain in the chest, chilliness and cold limbs, pale complexion, pale or dim purplish tongue, thready and weak pulse or deep and slow pulse.

[Main Points of Differentiation] Palpitation, spontaneous perspiration, chilliness and oppressed feeling in the chest.

[Pathgoenesis] Deficiency of the heart - *yang* brings about insufficiency of *yang* - *qi*, which results in the heart to beat feebly, as a result, there appears stagnation of *qi*.

[Treatment] Supplementing *qi* and warming *yang*.

[Recipe] *Zheng Yang Li Lao Tang*[180].

In case of oppressed feeling and pain in the chest, add *Radix Notoginseng*, *Flos Carthami*, *Radix Salviae Miltiorrhizae* and *Radix Curcumae* to remove stagnation by promoting the circulation of the blood, and to regulate *qi* in order to relieve pain.

[Nursing Points] Avoiding wind and cold; prohibiting raw and cold food; regulating emotions.

(2) Deficiency of the spleen - *yang*

[Symptoms] Sallow complexion, poor appetite, loose stool, borborygmus and abdominal pain aggravated with attack of cold and careless eating, chilliness, listlessness and fatigue, shortness of breath, disinclination to talk, pale tongue with whitish fur, feeble and weak pulse.

[Main Points of Differentiation] Poor appetite, loose stool, chilliness and fatigue, pale tongue and feeble pulse.

[Pathogenesis] Deficiency of the spleen - *yang* brings about dysfunction of the spleen in transport and transformation, and cold of the middle - *jiao* due to deficiency of *qi*.

[Treatment] Warming the middle - *jiao* and invigorating the spleen.

[Recipe] *Fu Zi Li Zhong Wan*[146].

In case of cold and pain of the abdomen, persistent loose stool, add *Rhizoma Alpiniae Officinarum*, *Pericarpium Zanthoxyli*, *Semen Myristicae* and *Fructus Psoraleae* to warm the middle - *jiao* and expel cold, and to reinforce the function of intestinal tract so as to arrest diarrhea.

[Nursing Points] Preferring warm food, avoiding raw, cold and greasy food.

(3) Deficiency of the kidney - *yang*

[Symptoms] Aching of the loins and back, seminal emission and impotence, polyuria or incontinence of urine, pale complexion, intolerance to cold and coldness of the limbs, diarrhea with undigested food in the stool, diarrhea before dawn, pale and enlarged tongue with teeth prints, whitish fur, deep and slow pulse.

[Main Points of Differentiation] Aching of the loins and back, seminal emission and impotence, diarrhea before dawn.

[Pathogenesis] Weakness of the kidney - *yang* gives rise to the decline of the vital - portal - fire, thus leading to the excessiveness of severe pathogenic cold.

[Treatment] Warming and tonifying the kidney - *yang* in combination with nourishing essence and blood.

[Recipe] *You Gui Wan*[68].

In case of seminal emission, add *Fructus Rosae Laevigata*, *Oetheca Mantidis*, *Stamen Nelumbinis* or combined with *Jin Suo Gu Jing Wan*[164] to astringe and arrest spontaneous seminal emission. In case of diarrhea before dawn, the main recipe used in combination with *Si Shen Wan*[82] to warm the kidney and arrest diarrhea. If there is syndrome characterized by dyspnea and shortness of breath getting more serious with patient's motion, which suggests failure of the kidney in receiving air, such herbs as *Fructus Psoraleae*, *Fructus Schisandrae* and *Gecko* should be added to tonify the kidney so as to receive air.

[Nursing Points] Working properly, regulating diet, moderating sexual life, avoiding raw and cold food. It is applicable to eat gruel of *Semen Juglandis* or *Placenta Juglandis*.

In most of the cases, deficiency of *yang* develops gradually from deficiency of *qi*. Deficiency of *yang* gives rise to the production of pathogenic cold characterized by more serious symptoms than the symptoms manifested by deficiency of *qi*. As the kidney – *yang* is original *yang* of the human body, a long course of deficiency of the heart – *yang* and the spleen – *yang* usually involves the kidney, presenting syndromes of deficiency of the heart – *yang* and the kidney – *yang* as well as deficiency of the spleen – *yang* and the kidney – *yang*, to which treatment should be applied in careful consideration of both cases.

Summary

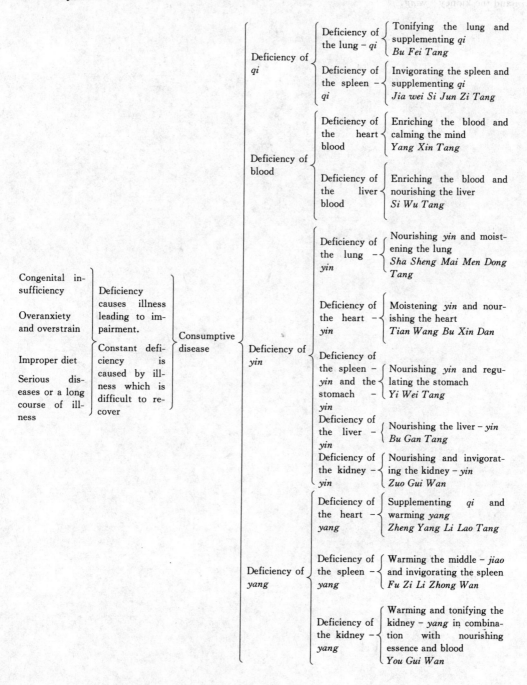

Discussions

1. What are the differences in etiology, diseased regions and clinical manifestations of pulmonary tuberculosis and *Xu Lao*?

2. Retell the main points of differentiation, treatment and recipe respectively of deficiency of the heart blood, deficiency of the liver blood, of the lung - *qi*, of the spleen - *yang* and of both the kidney - *yin* and the kidney - *yang*.

Appendix

1. Indexes of Recipes

[1] Yi Guan Jian: *Radix Adenophorae Strictae, Radix Ophiopogonis, Radix Angelicae Sinensis, Radix Rehmannia, Fructus Lycii, Fructus Meliae Toosendan*

[2] Er Chen Tang: *Rhizoma Pinelliae, Pericarpium Citrl Reticulatae, Poria, Radix Glycyrrhizae Praeparata*

[3] Er Yin Jian: *Radix Rehmanniae, Radix Ophiopogonis, Semen Ziziphispinosae, Radix Glycyrrhizae, Radix Scrophulariae, Poria, Rhizoma Coptidis, Caulis Akebiae, Medulla Junci, Lophatherum*

[4] Er Shen San: *Spora Lygodii, Talcum*

[5] Shi Hui San: *Herba Seu Radix Cirsii Japonici, Herba Cephalanoploris, Cacumen Platycladi, Folium Nelumbinis, Radix Rubiae, Radix Pittospori, Rhizoma Imperatae, Radix et Rhizoma Rhei, Cortex Moutan Radicis, Cortex Trachycarpi*

[6] Shi Zao Tang: *Radix Knoxiae, Flos Genkwa, Radix Euphorbiae Kansui, Fructus Ziziphi Jujubae*

[7] Ding Xiang San: *Flos Syzygii Aromatici, Calyx Kaki, Rhizoma Alpiniae Officinarum, Radix Glycyrrhizae Praeparata*

[8] Qi Wei Du Qi Wan: *Radix Rehmanniae, Fructus Corni, Rhizoma Dioscoreae, Poria, Moutan Radicis, Rhizoma Alismatis, Fructus Schisandrae*

[9] Qi Li San: *Resina Draconis, Moschus, Borneolum Syntheticum, Resina Boswelliae Carterii, Commiphora Myrrha, Flos Carthami, Cinnabaris, Acacia Catechu*

[10] Ren Shen Hu Tao Tang: *Radix Ginseng, Juglandis Regiae, Rhizoma Zingiberis Recens*

[11] Ren Shen Yang Ying Tang: *Radix Ginseng, Radix Glycyrrhizae, Radix Angelicae Sinensis, Radix Paeoniae Alba, Radix Rehmanniae Praeparata, Cortex Cinnamomi, Fructus Ziziphi Jujubae, Radix Astragali Seu Hedysari, Rhizoma Atractylodis Macrocephalae, Poria, Fructus Schisandrae, Radix Polygalae, Exocarpium Citri Grandis, Rhizoma Zingiberis Recens*

[12] Ba Zheng San: *Caulis Akebiae, Semen Plantaginis, Herba Polygoni Avicularis, Herba Dianthi, Talcum, Radix Glycyrrhizae, Radix et Rhizoma Rhei, Radix Pittospori, Medulla Junci*

[13] Ba Zhen Tang: *Radix Ginseng, Rhizoma Atractylodis Macrocephalae, Poria, Radix Glycyrrhizae, Radix Angelicae Sinensis, Radix Paeoniae Alba, Rhizoma Ligustici Chuanxiong, Radix Rehmanniae Praeparata, Rhizoma Zingiberis Re-*

cens, Fructus Ziziphi Jujubae

[14] San Zi Yang Qin Tang: Fructus Parillae, Semen Sinapis Albae, Semen Raphani

[15] San Ren Tang: Semen pruni Armeniacae, Semen Amonicardamoni, Semen Coicis, Cortex Magnoliae Officinalis, Rhizoma Pinelliae, Medulla Tetrapanacis, Talcum, Lophatherum

[16] Da Qi Qi Tang: Pericarpium Citri Reticulatae Viride, Pericarpium Citri Reticulatae, Radix Platycodi, Herba Agastachis, Cortex Cinnamoni, Radix Glycyrrhizae, Rhizoma Sparganii, Rhizoma Zedoariae, Rhizoma Cyperi, Fructus Alpiniae Oxyphylla

[17] Da Bu Yuan Jian: Radix Ginseng, Rhizoma Dioscoreae Praeparata, Radix Rehmanniae Praeparata, Cortex Eucommiae, Fructus Lycii, Radix Angelicae Sinensis, Fructus Corni, Radix Glycyrrhizae Praeparata

[18] Da Bu Yin Wan: Rhizoma Anemarrhenae, Cortex Phellodendri, Radix Rehmanniae Praeparata, Plastrum Testudinis, Porcine Medulla Spinalis

[19] Da Ding Feng Zhu: Radix Paeoniae Alba, Colla Corii Asini, Plastrum Testudinis, Radix Rehmanniae, Frutus Cannabis, Fructus Schisandrae, Concha Ostreae, Radix Ophiopogonis, Radix Glycyrrhizae Praeparata, Gallus Domesticus, Carapax Trionycis

[20] Da Jian Zhong Tang: Pericarpium Zanthoxyli, Rhizoma Zingiberis, Radix Ginseng, Maltose

[21] Da Cheng Qi Tang: Radix et Rhizoma Rhei, Cortex Magnoliae Officinalis, Fructus Aurantii Immaturus, Mirabilitum

[22] Da Qin Jiu Tang: Radix Gentianae Macrophyllae, Radix Angelicae Sinensis, Radix Glycyrrhizae, Rhizoma seu Radix Noto – pterygii, Radix Ledebouriellae, Radix Angelicae Dahuricae, Radix Rehmanniae Praeparata, Poria, Gypsum Fibrosum, Rhizoma Ligustici Chuanxiong, Radix Paeoniae Alba, Radix Angelicae Pubescentis, Radix Scutellariae, Radix Rehmanniae, Rhizoma Atractylodis Macrocephalae, Herba Asari

[23] Chuan Xiong Cha Tiao San: Rhizoma Ligustici Chuanxiong, Herba Schizonepetae, Herba Menthae, Rhizoma seu Radix Noto – pterygii, Herba Asari, Radix Angelicae Dahuricae, Radix Glycyrrhizae, Radix Ledebouriellae

[24] Ji Jiao Li Huang Wan: Radix Stephaniae Tetrandrae, Semen Zanthoxyli, Semen Lepidii seu Descurainiae, Radix et Rhizoma Rhei

[25] Xiao Ban Xia Jia Fu Ling Tang: Rhizoma Pinelliae, Rhizoma Zingiberis Recens, Poria

[26] Xiao Ban Xia Tang: Rhizoma Pinelliae, Rhizoma Zingiberis Recens

[27] Xiao Qing Long Tang: Herba Ephedrae, Ramulus Cinnamomi, Radix Paeoniae Alba, Radix Glycyrrhizae, Rhizoma Zingiberis, Herba Asari, Rhizoma Pinelliae, Fructus Schisandrae

[28] Xiao Jian Zhong Tang: *Ramulus Cinnamomi, Radix Paeoniae Alba, Radix Glycyrrhizae, Rhizoma Zingiberis Recens, Fructus Ziziphi Jujubae, Maltose*

[29] Xiao Cheng Qi Tang: *Radix et Rhizoma Rhei, Cortex Magnoliae Officinalis, Fructus Aurantii Immaturus*

[30] Xiao Chai Hu Tang: *Radix Bupleuri, Radix Scutellariae, Rhizoma Pinelliae, Radix Ginseng, Radix Glycyrrhizae, Rhizoma Zingiberis Recens, Fructus Ziziphi Jujubae*

[31] Xiao Ji Yin Zi: *Radix Rehmanniae, Herba Cephalanoploris, Talcum, Medullar Tetrapanacis, Pollen Typhae Praeparata, Herba Lophatherum, Nodus Nelumbinis Rhizomatis, Radix Angelicae Sinesis, Radix Pittospori, Radix Glycyrrhizae*

[32] Tian Wang Bu Xin Dan: *Radix Ginseng, Radix Scrophulariae, Radix Salviae Miltiorrhizae, Poria, Fructus Schisandrae, Radix Polygalae, Radix Platycodi, Radix Angelicae Sinensis, Radix Asparagi, Radix Ophiopogonis, Semen Biotae, Semen Ziziphi Spinosae, Radix Rehmanniae, Cinnabaris*

[33] Tian Ma Gou Teng Yin: *Rhizoma Gastrodiae, Ramulus Uncariae Cum Uncis, Concha Haliotidis, Radix Cyathulae, Ramulus Loranthi, Cortex Eucommiae, Radix Pittospori, Radix Scutellariae, Herba Leonuri, Cinnabaris et Poriae, Caulis Polysoni Multiflori*

[34] Wu Bi Shan Yao Wan: *Rhizoma Dioscoreae, Herba Cistanchis, Radix Rehmanniae Praeparata, Fructus Corni, Poriacum Ligno Hospite, Semen Cuscutae, Fructus Schisandrae, Halloysitum Rubrum, Radix Morindae Officinalis, Rhizoma Alismatis, Cortex Eucommiae, Radix Achyranthis Bidentatae*

[35] Mu Fang Ji Tang: *Radix Cocculi Trilobi, Gypsum Fibrosum, Ramulus Cinnamomi, Radix Ginseng*

[36] Mu Xiang Shun Qi San: *Radix Aucklandiae, Pericarpium Citri Reticulatae Viride, Pericarpum Citri Reticulatae, Radix Glycyrrhizae, Fructus Aurantii, Cortex Maynoliae Officinalis, Radix Linderae, Rhizoma Cyperi, Rhizoma Atractylodis, Fructus Amomi, Cortex Cinnamomi, Rhizoma Ligustici Chuanxiong*

[37] Zhi Sou San: *Herba Schizonepetae, Radix Platycodi, Radix Glycyrrhizae, Rhizoma cynanchi Vincetoxici, Pericarpium Citri Reticulatae, Radix Stemonaem, Radix Asteris*

[38] Zhong Man Fen Xiao Wan: *Cortex Mangoliae Officinalis, Fructus Aurantii Immaturus, Rhizoma Coptidis, Radix Scutellariae, Rhizoma Anemarrhenae, Rhizoma Pinelliae Pericarpium Citri Reticulatae, Poria, Polyporus Umbellatus, Rhizoma Alismatis, Fructus Amomi, Rhizoma Zingiberis, Rhizoma Curcumae Longae, Radix Ginseng, Rhizoma Atractylodis Macrocephalae, Radix Glycyrrhizae Praeparata*

[39] Wu Ren Wan: *Semen Persicae, Semen pruni Armeniacae, Semen Biotae, Semen Pinus Koraiensis, Semen Pruni, Pericarpium Citri Reticulatae*

[40] Wu Pi San: *Cortex Mori Radicis, Pericarpium Citri Reticulatae, Exocarpium Zingiberis Recens, Pericarpium Arecae, Pericarpium Poria*

[41] Wu Ling San: *Ramulus Cinnamomi, Rhizoma Atractylodis Macrocephalae, Poria, Polyporus Umbellatus, Rhizoma Alismatis*

[42] Wu Ji San: *Radix Angelicae Dahuricae, Pericarpium Citri Reticulatae, Cortex Magnoliae Officinalis, Radix Angelicae Sinensis, Rhizoma Ligustici Chuanxiong, Radix Paeoniae Alba, Poria, Radix Platycodi, Rhizoma Atractylodis, Fructus Aurantii, Rhizoma Pineliae, Herba Ephedrae, Rhizoma Zingiberis, Cortex Cinnamomi, Radix Glycyrrhizae*

[43] Wu Mo Yin Zi: *Radix Linderae, Lignum Aquilariae Resinatum, Semen Arecae, Fructus Aurantii Immaturus, Radix Aucklandiae*

[44] Liu Yi San: *Talcum, Radix Glycyrrhizae*

[45] Liu Jun Zi Tang: *Radix Ginseng, Radix Glycyrrhizae Praeparata, Poria, Rhizoma Atractylodis Macrocephalae, Pericarpium Citri Reticulatae, Rhizoma Pinelliae Praeparata*

[46] Liu Wei Di Huang Wan: *Radix Rehmanniae Praeparata, Rhizoma Dioscoreae, Poria, Cortex Moutan Radicis, Rhizoma Alismatis, Fructus Corni*

[47] Liu Mo Tang: *Lignum Aquilariae Resinatum, Radix Aucklandiae, Semen Arecae, Radix Linderae, Fructus Aurantii Immaturus, Radix et Rhizoma Rhei*

[48] Hua Chong Wan: *Semen Arecae, Fructus Carpesii, Radix Meliae Toosendan, Alumen Exsiccatum, Fructus Quisqualis, Fructus Ulmi Macrocarpae*

[49] Hua Gan Jian: *Pericarpium Citri Peticulatae Viride, Pericarpium Citri Reticulatae, Radix Paeoniae Alba, Cortex Moutan Radicis, Fructus Gardeniae, Rhizoma Alismatis, Bulbus Fritillariae Thunbergii*

[50] Hua Ji Wan: *Rhizoma Sparganii, Rhizoma Zedoariae, Resina Ferulae, Pumex, Rhizoma Cyperi, Realgar, Semen Arecae, Lignum Sappan, Concha Arcae, Faeces Trogopterorum*

[51] Dan Shen Yin: *Radix Salviae Miltiorrhizae, Lignum Santali, Fructus Amomi*

[52] Dan Zhi Xiao Yao San: *Radix Angelicae Sinensis, Radix Paeoniae Alba, Rhizoma Atractylodis Macrocephalae, Radix Bupleuri, Poria, Radix Glycyrrhizae, Rhizoma Zingiberis Praeparata, Herba Menthae, Cortex Moutan Radicis, Radix Pittospori*

[53] Wu Tou Tang: *Radix Aconiti, Herba Ephedrae, Radix Paeonia Alba, Radix Astragali seu Hedysari, Radix Glycyrrhizae*

[54] Wu Tou Chi Shi Zhi Wan: *Pericarpium Zanthoxyli, Rhizoma Aconiti, Radix Aconiti Praeparata, Rhizoma Zingiberis, Halloysitum Rubrum*

[55] Wu Tou Gui Zhi Tang: *Radix Aconiti, Ramulus Cinnamomi, raw Radix Patrniae Albe, Radix Glycyrrhiza preparata, fresh Rhizoma Zingiberis, Fructus Ziziphi Jujubae honey and bee*

[56] Wu Mei Wan: *Fructus Mume, Rhizoma Coptidis, Cortex Phellodendri, Radix Ginseng, Radix Angelicae Sinensis, Radix Aconiti Praeparata, Ramulus Cinnamomi, Pericarpium Zanthoxyli, Rhizoma Zingiberis, Herba Asari*

[57] Shao Fu Zhu Yu Tang: *Fructus Foeniculi, Rhizoma Zingiberis, Rhizoma Corydalis, Lignum Aquilariae Resinatum, Radix Angelicae Sinensis, Rhizoma Ligustici Chuanxiong, Cortex Cinnamomi, Radix Paeoniae Rubra, Pollen Typhae, Faeces Trogopterorum*

[58] Shui Lu Er Xian Dan: *Fructus Rosae Laevigatae, Semen Euryales*

[59] Yu Nu Jian: *Gypsum Fibrosum, Radix Rehmanniae Praeparata, Radix Ophiopogonis, Rhizoma Anemarrhenae, Radix Achyranthis Bidentatae*

[60] Yu Shu Dan: *Bulbus Cremastrae, Semen Euphorbiae Lathyriditis, Radix Knoxiae, Moschus, Realgar, Cinnabaris, Fructus Schisandrae*

[61] Yu Ping Feng San: *Radix Astragali seu Hedysari, Rhizoma Atractylodis Macrocephalae, Radix Ledebouriellae*

[62] Zheng Qi Tian Xiang San: *Radix Linderae, Rhizoma Cyperi, Rhizoma Zingiberis, Fructus Perillae, Pericarpium Citri Reticulatae*

[63] Shi Wei San: *Folium Pyrrosiae, Fructus Malvae Verticillatae, Herba Dianthi, Talcum, Semen Plantaginis*

[64] Long Dan Xie Gan Tang: *Radix Gentianae, Rhizoma Alismatis, Caulis Akebiae, Semen Plantaginis, Radix Angelicae Sinensis, Radix Bupleuri, Radix Rehmannia*

[65] Zuo Gui Wan: *Radix Rehmanniae Praeparata, Rhizoma Dioscoreae, Fructus Corni, Semen Cuscutae, Fructus Lycii, Radix Achyranthis Bidentatae, Colla Cornus Cervi, Colla Plastri Testudinis*

[66] Zuo Gui Yin: *Radix Rehmanniae Praeparata, Fructus Corni, Fructus Lycii, Rhizoma Dioscoreae, Poria, Radix Glycyrrhizae*

[67] Zuo Jin Wan: *Rhizoma Coptidis, Fructus Evodiae*

[68] You Gui Wan: *Radix Rehmanniae Praeparata, Rhizoma Dioscoreae, Fructus Corni, Fructus Lycii, Cortex Eucommiae, Semen Cuscutae, Radix Aconiti Praeparata, Cortex Cinnamomi, Radix Angelicae Sinensis, Colla Cornus Cervi*

[69] You Gui Yin: *Radix Rehmanniae Praeparata, Fructus Corni, Fructus Lycii, Rhizoma Dioscoreae, Cortex Eucommiae, Radix Glycyrrhizae, Radix Aconiti Praeparata, Cortex Cinnamomi*

[70] Ping Wei San: *Rhizoma Atractylodis, Cortex Magnoliae Officinalis, Pericarpium Citri Reticulatae, Radix Glycyrrhizae, Rhizoma Zingiberis Recens, Fructus Ziziphi Jujubae*

[71] Gan Mai Da Zao Tang: *Radix Glycyrrhizae, Fructus Hordei, Fructus Ziziphi Jujubae*

[72] Gan Jiang Ling Zhu Tang: *Radix Glycyrrhizae, Rhizoma Zingiberis, Poria, Rhizoma Atractylodis Macrocephalae*

[73] Gan Sui Ban Xia Tang: *Radix Euphorbiae Kansui, Rhizoma Pinelliae, Radix Paeoniae Alba, Radix Glycyrrhizae*

[74] Gan Lu Xiao Du Dan: *Talcum, Herba Artemisiae Scopariae, Radix Scutellariae, Rhizoma Acori Graminei, Bulbus Fritillariae Cirrhosae, Caulis Akebiae, Herba Agastachis, Rhizoma Belamcandae, Fructus Forsythiae, Herba Menthae, Semen Amomi Cardamomi*

[75] Si Qi Tang: *Folium Perillae, Rhizoma Pinelliae Praeparata, Cortex Magnoliae Officinalis, Poria, Rhizoma Zingiberis Recens, Fructus Ziziphi Jujubae*

[76] Si Miao Wan: *Rhizoma Atractylodis, Cortex Phellodendri, Radix Achyranthis Bidentatae, Semen Coicis*

[77] Si Jun Zi Tang: *Radix Codonopsis Pilosulae, Rhizoma Atractylodis Macrocephalae, Poria, Radix Glycyrrhizae*

[78] Si Wei Hui Yang Yin: *Radix Ginseng, Radix Aconiti Praeparata, Rhizoma Zingiberis Praeparata, Radix Glycyrrhizae Praeparata*

[79] Si Wu Tang: *Radix Angelicae Sinensis, Radix Paeoniae Alba, Rhizoma Ligustici Chuanxiong, Radix Rehmnniae Praeparata*

[80] Si Ni Tang: *Radix Aconiti Praeparata, Rhizoma Zingiberis, Radix Glycyrrhizae Praeparata*

[81] Si Ni San: *Radix Glycyrrhizae Praeparata, Fructus Aurantii Immaturus, Radix Bupleuri, Radix Paeoniae Alba*

[82] Si Shen Wan: *Fructus Psoraleae, Semen Myristicae, Fructus Evodiae, Fructus Schisandrae, Rhizoma Zingiberis Recens, Fructus Ziziphi Jujubae*

[83] Si Hai Shu Yu Wan: *Gecko Pulveratum, Thallus Laminariae, Sargassum, Os Sepiellae seu Sepiae, Thallus Laminariae seu Eckloniae, Pericarpium Citri Reticulatae, Radix Aristolochiae*

[84] Sheng Mai San: *Radix Ginseng, Radix Ophiopogonis, Fructus Schisandrae*

[85] Sheng Tie Luo Yin: *Radix Asparagi, Radix Ophiopogonis, Bulbus Fritillariae Thunbergii, Arisaemacum Bile, Exocarpium Citri Grandis, Radix Polygalae, Rhizoma Acori Graminei, Fructus Forsythiae, Poria, Poriacum Lingo Hospite, Radix Scrophulariae, Ramulus Uncariae Cum Uncis, Radix Salviae Miltiorrhizae, Cinnabaris, Ginder*

[86] Shi Xiao San: *Faeces Trogopterorum, Pollen Typhae*

[87] Dai Di Dang Wan: *Radix et Rhizoma Rhei, Radix Angelicae Sinensis, Radix Rehmanniae, Squama Manitis, Mirabilitum, Semen Persicae, Cortex Cinnamomi*

[88] Bai Tou Weng Tang: *Radix Pulsatillae, Cortex Fraxini, Rhizoma Coptidis, Cortex Phellodendri*

[89] Bai Hu Jia Ren Shen Tang: *Rhizoma Anemarrhenae, Gypsum Fibrosum, Radix Glycyrrhizae, Polished round - grained rice, Radix Ginseng*

[90] Bai Hu Jia Gui Zhi Tang: *Rhizoma Anemarrhenae, Gypsum Fibrosum, Radix Gly-*

cyrrhizae, Polished round - grained rice, Ramulus Cinnamomi

[91] Bai Hu Tang: *Rhizoma Anemarrhenae, Gypsum Fibrosum, Radix Glycyrrhizae, Polish round - grained rice*

[92] Ban Xia Bai Zhu Tian Ma Tang: *Rhizoma Pinelliae, Rhizoma Atractylodis Macrocephalae, Rhizoma Gastrodiae, Pericarpium Citri Reticulatae, Poria, Radix Glycyrrhizae, Rhizoma Zingiberis Recens, Fructus Ziziphi Jujubae*

[93] Ban Xia Hou Pu Tang: *Rhizoma Pinelliae, Cortex Magnoliae Officinalis, Fructus Perillae, Poria, Rhizoma Zingiberis Recens*

[94] Ban Liu Wan: *Rhizoma Pinelliae, Sulfur*

[95] Gui Pi Tang: *Radix Codonopsis Pilosulae, Radix Astragali seu Hedysari, Rhizoma Atractylodis Macrocephalae, Poriacum Ligno Hospite, Semen Ziziphi Spinosae, Arillus Longan, Radix Aucklandiae, Radix Glycyrrhizae Praeparata, Radix Angelicae Sinensis, Radix Polygalae, Rhizoma Zingiberis Recens, Fructus Ziziphi Jujubae*

[96] Jia Wei Er Miao San: *Cortex Phellodendri, Rhizoma Atractylodis, Radix Angelicae Sinensis, Radix Achyranthis Bidentatae, Radix Stephaniae Tetrandrae, Rhizoma Dioscoreae, Plastrum Testudinis*

[97] Jia Wei Si Jun Zi Tang: *Radix Ginseng, Poria, Rhizoma Atractylodis Macrocephalae, Radix Glycyrrhizae Praeparata, Radix Astragali seu Hedysari, Semen Dolichoris Album*

[98] Jia Wei Si Wu Tang: *Radix Paeoniae Alba, Radix Angelicae Sinensis, Radix Rehmannia, Rhizoma Ligustici Chuanxiong, Fructus Viticis, Flos Chrysanthemi, Radix Scutellariae, Radix Glycyrrhizae*

[99] Jia Wei Qing Wei San: *Radix Rehmannia, Cortex Moutan Radicis, Radix Angelicae Sinensis, Rhizoma Coptidis, Fructus Forsythiae, Cornu Rhinoceri, Rhizoma Cimicifugae, Radix Glycyrrhizae*

[100] Jia Jian Cheng Qi Tang: *Radix et Rhizmoa Rhei, Natrii Sulfas Exsiccatus, Fructus Aurantii Immaturus, Chloriteschist Praeparata, Spina Gleditsiae, Pig's bile, Acetum*

[101] Jia Jian Fu Mai Tang: *Radix Glycyrrhizae Praeparata, Radix Rehmanniae, Radix Paeoniae Alba, Radix Ophiopogonis, Colla Corii Asini, Fructus Cannabis*

[102] Jia Jian Wei Rui Tang: *Rhizoma Polygonati Odorati, Caulis Allii Fistulosi, Radix Platycodi, Radix Cynanchi Atrati, Semen Sojae Praeparatum, Herba Menthae, Radix Glycyrrhizae Praeparata, Fructus Ziziphi Jujubae*

[103] Bai He Gu Jin Wan: *Radix Rehmanniae, Radix Rehmanniae Praeparata, Radix Ophiopogonis, Bulbus Fritillariae Thunbergii, Bulbus Lilii, Radix Angelicae Sinensis, Radix Paeoniae Alba Praeparata, Radix Glycyrrhizae, Radix Scrophulariae, Radix Platycodi*

[104] Di Huang Yin Zi: *Radix Rehmanniae, Radix Morindae Officinalis, Fructus*

Corni, Herba Dendrobii, Herba Cistanchis, Fructus Schisandrae, Cortex Cinnamomi, Poria, Radix Ophiopogonis, Radix Aconiti Praeparata, Rhizoma Acori Graminei, Radix Polygalae, Rhizoma Zingiberis Recens, Fructus Ziziphi Jujubae, Herba Menthae

[105] Di Yu San: Radix Sanguisorbae, Radix Rubiae, Radix Scutellariae, Rhizoma Coptidis, Radix Pittospori, Poria

[106] Xiong Zhi Shi Gao Tang: Rhizoma Ligustici Chuanxiong, Radix Angelicae Dahuricae, Gypsum Fibrosum, Flos Chrysanthemi, Rhizoma ligustici, Rhizoma seu Radix Noto-pterygii

[107] Shao Yao Tang: Radix Scutellariae, Radix Paeoniae Alba, Radix Glycyrrhizae Praeparata, Rhizoma Copttdis, Radix et Rhizoma Rhei, Semen Arecae, Radix Angelicae Sinensis, Radix Aucklandiae, Cortex Cinnamomi

[108] Shao Yao Gan Cao Tang: Radix Paeoniae Alba, Radix Glycyrrhizae Praeparata

[109] Zhi Bao Dan: Cinnabaris, Moschus, Benzoinum, Silver et Gold, Cornu Rhinoceri, Calculus Bovis, Succinum, Realgar, Carapax Eretmochelydis, Dryobalanops Aromatica

[110] Jiao Tai Wan: Rhizoma Coptidis, Cortex Cinnamomi

[111] An Gong Niu Huang Wan: Calculus Bovis, Radix Curcumae, Cornu Rhinoceri, Rhizoma Coptidis, Cinnabaris, Borneolum Syntheticum, Margarita, Radix Pittospori, Realgar, Radix Scutellariae, Moschus, Native Gold

[112] An Shen Ding Zhi Wan: Poria, Poriacum Ligno Hospite, Radix Polygalae, Radix Ginseng, Rhizoma Acori Graminiei, Dens Draconis

[113] Dang Gui Liu Huang Tang: Radix Angelicae Sinensis, Radix Rehmanniae, Radix Rehmanniae Praeparata, Rhizoma Coptidis, Radix Scutellariae, Cortex Phellodendri, Radix Astragali seu Hedysari

[114] Dang Gui Long Hui Wan: Radix Angelicae Sinensis, Radix Gentianae, Fructus Gardeniae, Rhizoma Coptidis, Radix Scutellariae, Cortex Phellodendri, Radix et Rhizoma Rhei, Indigo Naturalis, Aloe, Radix Aucklandiae, Moschus

[115] Dang Gui Bu Xue Tang: Radix Astragali seu Hedysari, Radix Angelicae Sinensis

[116] Zhu Ye Shi Gao Tang: Lophatherum, Gypsum Fibrosum, Radix Ophiopogonis, Radix Ginseng, Rhizoma Pinelliae, Rice, Radix Glycyrrhizae Praeparata

[117] Zhu Li Da Tan Wan: Chlorite-schist Praeparata, Lignum Aquilariae Resinatum, Radix et Rhizoma Rhei, Radix Scutellariae, Succus Bambosae, Rhizoma Pinelliae, Exocarpium Citri Grandis, Radix Glycyrrhizae, Poria, Radix Ginseng

[118] Zhu Ru Tang: Caulis Bambusae in Taeniam, Rhizoma Pinelliae, Rhizoma Zingiberis, Radix Glycyrrhizae, Rhizoma Zingiberis Recens, Fructus Ziziphi Jujubae

[119] Xue Fu Zhu Yu Tang: Radix Angelicae Sinensis, Radix Rehmanniae, Semen Persicae, Flos Carthami, Fructus Aurantii, Radix Paeoniae Rubra, Radix Bupleuri, Radix Glycyrrhizae, Radix Platycodi, Rhizoma Ligustici Chuanxiong, Radix

Achyranthis Bidentatae.

[120] Dao Chi San:*Radix Rehmanniae*, *Caulis Akebiae*, *Herba Lophatheri*, *Radix Glycyrrhizae*.

[121] Dao Tan Tang:*Rhizoma Pinelliae*, *Pericarpium Citri Reticulatae Fructus Aurantii Immaturus*, *Poria*, *Radix Glycyrrhizae*, *Rhizoma Arisaematis Praeparatae*.

[122] Fang Ji Huang Qi Tang:*Radix Stephaniae Tetrandrae*, *Rhizoma Atractylodis Macrocephalae*, *Radix Astragali seu Hedysari*, *Radix Glycyrrhizae*, *Rhizoma Zingiberis Recens*, *Fructus Ziziphi Jujubae*.

[123] Fang Feng Tang:*Radix Ledebouriellae*, *Radix Angelicae Sinensis*, *Poria*, *Semen Armeniacae Amarum*, *Radix Scutellariae*, *Radix Gentianae Macrophyllae*, *Radix Puerariae*, *Herba Ephedrae*, *Cortex Cinnamomi*, *Rhizoma Zingiberis Recens*, *Radix Glycyrrhizae*, *Fructus Ziziphi Jujubae*.

[124] Mai Men Dong Tang:*Radix Ophiopogonis*, *Radix Ginseng*, *Rhizoma Pinelliae*, *Radix Glycyrrhizae*, *Semen Oryzae Sativae*, *Fructus Ziziphi Jujubae*.

[125] Mai Wei Di Huang Wan:*Rhizoma Rehmanniae Praeparatae*, *Fructus Corni*, *Rhizoma Dioscoreae*, *Cortex Moutan Radicis*, *Rhizoma Alismatis*, *Poria*, *Radix Ophiopogonis*, *Fructus Schisandrae*.

[126] Cang Zhu Er Chen Tang:*Rhizoma Atractylodis*, *Rhizoma Atractylodis Macrocephalae*, *Poria*, *Pericarpium Citri Reticulatae*, *Radix Glycyrrhizae*, *Rhizoma Pinelliae*.

[127] Su Zi Jiang Qi Tang:*Fructus Perillae*, *Exocarpium Citri Grandis*, *Rhizoma Pinelliae*, *Radix Angelicae Sinensis*, *Radix Peucedani*, *Cortex Magnoliae Officinalis*, *Cortex Cinnamomi*, *Radix Glycyrrhizae*, *Rhizoma Zingiberis Recens*.

[128] Su He Xiang Wan:*Rhizoma Atractylodis Macrocephalae*, *Radix Aucklandiae*, *Cornu Rhinoceri*, *Rhizoma Cyperi*, *Cinnabaris*, *Fructus Chebulae*, *Lignum Santali*, *Benzoinum*, *Lignum Aquilariae Resinatum*, *Moschus*, *Flos Syzygii Aromatici*, *Fructus Piperis Longi*, *Resina Liquidambaris Orientalis*, *Resina Boswelliae Carterii*, *Borneolum Syntheticum*.

[129] Qi Ju Di Huang Wan:*Fructus Lycii*, *Flos Chrysanthemi*, *Rhizoma Rehmanniae Praeparatae*, *Fructus Corni*, *Rhizoma Dioscoreae*, *Rhizoma Alismatis*, *Cortex Moutan Radicis*, *Poria*.

[130] Xing Su San:*Semen Armeniacae Amarum*, *Folium Perillae*, *Exocarpium Citri Grandis*, *Rhizoma Pinelliae*, *Rhizoma Zingiberis Recens*, *Fructus Aurantii*, *Radix Platycodi*, *Radix Peucedani*, *Poria*, *Radix Glycyrrhizae*, *Fructus Ziziphi Jujubae*.

[131] Geng Yi Wan:*Aloe*, *Cinnabaris*.

[132] Miao Xiang San:*Rhizoma Dioscoreae*, *Poria*, *Poria cum Ligno Hospite*, *Radix Polygalae*, *Radix Astragali seu Hedysari*, *Radix Ginseng*, *Radix Platycodi*, *Radix Glycyrrhizae*, *Radix Aucklandiae*, *Cinnabaris*, *Moschus*.

[133] Lian Po Yin: *Cortex Magnoliae Officinalis Praeparatae, Rhizoma Coptidis, Rhizoma Acori Graminei, Rhizoma Pinelliae Praeparatae, Semen Sejae Praeparatum, Fructus Gardeniae, Rhizoma Phragmitis.*

[134] Lian Li Tang: *Radix Ginseng, Rhizoma Atractylodis Macrocephalae, Rhizoma Zingiberis, Radix Glycyrrhizae Preaparata, Rhizoma Coptidis, Poria.*

[135] Wu Zhu Yu Tang: *Fructus Euodiae, Radix Ginseng, Rhizoma Zingiberis Recens, Fructus Ziziphi Jujubae.*

[136] Chen Xiang Jiang Qi San: *Lignum Aquilariae Resinatum, Fructus Amomi, Radix Glycyrrhizae, Rhizoma Cyperi, Fructus Meliae Toosendan, Rhizoma Corydalis.*

[137] Chen Xiang San: *Lignum Aquilariae Resinatum, Folium Pyrrosiae, Talcum, Radix Angelicae Sinensis, Exocarpium Citri Grandis, Radix Paeoniae Alba, Fructus Malvae Verticillatae, Radix Glycyrrhizae, Semen Vaccariae.*

[138] Sha Shen Mai Dong Tang: *Radix Adenophorae Stritae, Radix Ophiopogonis, Rhizoma Polygonati Odorati, Folium Mori, Radix Glycyrrhizae, Radix Trichosanthis, Semen Dolichoris Alba.*

[139] Liang Fu Wan: *Rhizoma Alpiniae Officinarum, Rhizoma Cyperi.*

[140] Bu Zhong Yi Qi Tang: *Radix Ginseng, Radix Astragali seu Hedysari, Rhizoma Atractylodis Macrocephalae, Radix Glycyrrhizae, Radix Angelicae Sinensis, Pericarpium Citri Reticulata, Rhizoma Cimicifugae, Radix Bupleuri.*

[141] Bu Yang Huan Wu Tang: *Radix Angelicae Sinensis, Rhizoma Ligustici Chuanxiong, Radix Astragali seu Hedysari, Semen Persicae, Lumbricus, Radix Paeoniae Rubra, Flos Carthami.*

[142] Bu Gan Tang: *Radix Angelicae Sinensis, Radix Paeoniae Alba, Rhizoma Ligusticum Wallichii, Rhizoma Rehmanniae Praeparatae, Semen Ziziphi Spinosae, Fructus Chaenomelis, Radix Glycyrrhizae Praeparata.*

[143] Bu Fei Tang: *Radix Ginseng, Radix Astragali seu Hedysari, Rhizoma Rehmanniae Praeparatae, Fructus Schisandrae, Radix Asteris, Cortex Mori Radicis.*

[144] Mu Li San: *Concha Ostreae Usta, Radix Astragali seu Hedysari, Radix Ephedrae, Fructus Tritici Levis.*

[145] Shen Tong Zhu Yu Tang: *Radix Gentianae Macrophyllae, Rhizoma Ligustici Chuanxiong, Semen Persicae, Flos Carthami, Radix Glycyrrhizae, Rhizoma seu Radix Notopterygi, Resira Commiphorae Myrrhae, Rhizoma Cyperi, Faeces Trogopterorum, Radix Achyranthis Bidentatae, Lumbricus, Radix Angelicae Sinensis.*

[146] Fu Zi Li Zhong Wan: *Radix Aconiti Praeparate, Radix Ginseng, Rhizoma Atractylodis Macrocephalae, Rhizoma Zingiberis Praeparata, Radix Glycyrrhizae Praeparata.*

[147] Qing E Wan: *Fructus Psoraleae, Cortex Eucommiae, Juglandis Regiae, Bulbus Allii.*

[148] Qing Lin Wan: *Radix et Rhizoma Rhei, fresh Cacumen Biotae, mung bean sprouts, soya bean sprouts, Ramulus Sophorae, Folium Mori, Folium Persicae, Semen Plantaginis, fresh Fructus Foeniculi, Pericarpium Citri Reticulatae, Folium Nelumbinis, Flos Lonicerae, Folium Perillae, Folium Artemisiae Argyi, Rhizoma Pinelliae, Cortex Magnoliae Officinalis, Radix Scutellariae, Rhizoma Cyperi, Fructus Amomi, Radix Glycyrrhizae, Rhizoma Alismatis, Polyporus Umbellatus, milk, ginger juice, pear juice, urine of boy under 12, Wine.*

[149] Ling Gan Wu Wei Jiang Xin Tang: *Poria, Radix Glycyrrhizae, Fructus Schisandrae, Rhizoma Zingiberis, Herba Asari.*

[150] Ling Gui Zhu Gan Tang: *Poria, Ramulus Cinnamomi, Rhizoma Atractylodis Macrocephalae, Radix Glycyrrhizae.*

[151] Hu Qian Wan: *Plastaum Testudinis, Cortex Phellodendri, Rhizoma Anemarrhenae, Rhizoma Rehmanniae Praeparatae, Radix Paeoniae Alba, Herba Cynomorii, Pericarpium Citri Reticulatae, Os Tigris, Rhizoma Zingiberis.*

[152] He Che Da Zao Wan: *Placenta Hominis, Rhizoma Rehmanniae Praeparatae, Cortex Eucommiae, Radix Asparagi, Radix Ophiopogonis, Plastsum Testudinis, Cortex Phellodendri, Radix Achyranthis Bidentatae.*

[153] Xie Xin Tang: *Radix et Rhizoma Rhei, Radix Scutellariae, Rhizoma Coptidis.*

[154] Xie Bai San: *Cortex Mori Radicis, Cortex Lycii Radicis, Radix Glycyrrhizae, Semen Oryzae Sativae.*

[155] Qiang Huo Sheng Shi Tang: *Rhizoma seu Radix Notopterygii, Radix Angelicae Pubescentis, Rhizoma Ligustici Chuanxiong, Fructus Viticis, Radix Glycyrrhizae, Radix Ledebouriellae, Rhizoma Ligustici.*

[156] Ding Zhi Wan: *Radix Codonopsis Pilosulae, Poria cum Ligno Hospite, Rhizoma Acori Graminei, Radix Polygalae, Radix Glycyrrhizae.*

[157] Ding Xian Wan: *Rhizoma Gastrodiae, Bulbus Fritillariae Cirhosae, Arisaemacum Bile, Rhizoma Pinelliae Praeparatae.*

[158] Ding Chuan Tang: *Semen Ginkgo, Herba Ephedrae, Cortex Mori Radicis, Flos Farfarae, Rhizoma Pinelliae, Semen Armeniacae Amarum, Fructus Perillae, Radix Scutellariae, Radix Glycyrrhizae.*

[159] Shi Pi Yin: *Radix Aconiti, Rhizoma Zingiberis, Rhizoma Atractylodis Macrocephalae, Radix Glycyrrhizae, Cortex Magnoliae Officinalis, Radix Aucklandiae, Fructus Tsaoko, Semen Arecae, Fructus Chaenomelis, Rhizoma Zingiberis Recens, Fructus Ziziphi Jujubae, Poria.*

[160] Zhi Bai Di Huang Wan: *Rhizoma Anemarrhenae, Cortex Phellodendri, Rhizoma Rehmanniae Preparatae, Fructus Corni, Rhizoma Dioscoreae, Poria, Cortex Moutan Radicis, Rhizoma Alismatis.*

[161] Jin Shui Liu Jun Jian: *Radix Angelicae Sinensis, Rhizoma Rehmanniae Praeparatae, Pericarpium Citri Reticulatae, Rhizoma Pinelliae, Poria, Radix*

Glycyrrhizae Praeparata, Rhizoma Zingiberis Recens.

[162] Jin Ling Zi San: Fructus Meliae Toosendan, Rhizoma Corydalis.

[163] Jin Gui Shen Qi Wan: Ramulus Cinnamomi, Radix Aconiti Praeparata, Rhizoma Rehmanniae Praeparatae, Fructus Corni, Rhizoma Dioscoreae, Poria, Cortex Moutan Radicis, Rhizoma Alismatis.

[164] Jin Suo Gu Jing Wan: Semen Astragali Complanati, Fructus Tribuli, Semen Euryales, Stamen Nelumbinis, Os Draconis, Concha Ostreae, Semen Nelumbinis.

[165] Zhi Gan Cao Tang: Radix Glycyrrhizae Praeparata, Radix Ginseng, Ramulus Cinnamomi, Rhizoma Zingiberis Recens, Colla Corii Asini, Radix Rehmanniae, Radix Ophiopogonis, Fructus Cannabis, Fructus Ziziphi Jujubae.

[166] Zhu Che Wan: Rhizoma Coptidis, Colla Corii Asini, Radix Angelicae Sinensis, Rhizoma Zingiberis.

[167] Shen Fu Tang: Radix Ginseng, Radix Aconiti Praeparata, Rhizoma Zingiberis Recens, Fructus Ziziphi Jujubae.

[168] Shen Su Yin: Radix Ginseng, Folium Perillae, Radix Puerariae, Radix Peucedani, Rhizoma Pinelliae Praeparatae, Poria, Exocarpium Citri Grandis, Radix Glycyrrhizae, Radix Platycodi, Fructus Aurantii, Radix Aucklandiae, Rhizoma Zingiberis Recens, Fructus Ziziphi Jujubae.

[169] Shen Ling Bai Zhu San: Radix Ginseng, Poria, Rhizoma Atractylodis Macrocephalae, Radix Platycodi, Rhizoma Dioscoreae, Radix Glycyrrhizae, Semen Dolichoris Album, Semen Nelumbinis, Fructus Amomi, Semen Coicis.

[170] Shen Jie San: Radix Ginseng, Gecko.

[171] Chun Ze Tang: Rhizoma Atractylods Macrocephalae, Ramulus Cinnamomi, Polyporus Umbellatus, Rhizoma Alismatis, Poria, Radix Ginseng.

[172] Zhi Shi Dao Zhi Wan: Radix et Rhizoma Rhei, Fructus Aurantii Immaturus, Radix Scutellariae, Rhizoma Coptidis, Massa Fermentata Medicnalis, Rhizoma Atractylodis Macrocephalae, Poria, Rhizoma Alismatis.

[173] Jing Fang Bai Du San: Herba Schizonepetae, Radix Ledebouriellae, Rhizoma seu Radix Notopterygii, Radix Angelicae Pubescentis, Radix Bupleuri, Radix Peucedani, Rhizoma Ligustici Chuanxiong, Fructus Aurantii, Poria, Radix Platycodi, Radix Glycyrrhizae.

[174] Fu Ling Gan Cao Tang: Poria, Ramulus Cinnamomi, Radix Glycyrrhizae Praeparata, Rhizoma Zingiberis Recens.

[175] Yin Chen Wu Ling San: Herba Artemisiae Scopariae, Ramulus Cinnamomi, Poria, Rhizoma Atractylodis Macrocephalae, Rhizoma Alismatis, Polyporus Umbellatus.

[176] Yin Chen Zhu Fu Tang: Herba Artemisiae Scopariae, Rhizoma Atractylodis Macrocephalae, Radix Aconiti, Rhizoma Zingiberis, Cortex Cinnamomi, Radix Glycyrrhizae Praeparata.

[177] Yin Chen Hao Tang: *Herba Artemisiae Capillaris*, *Fructus Gardeniae*, *Radix et Rhizoma Rhei*.

[178] Qian Gen San: *Radix Rubiae*, *Radix Scutellariae*, *Colla Corii Asini*, *Cacumen Biotae*, *Radix Rehmanniae*, *Radix Glycyrrhizae*.

[179] Zhi Mi Fu Ling Wan: *Poria*, *Fructus Aurantii*, *Rhizoma Pinelliae*, *Rhizoma Zingiberis Recens*.

[180] Zheng Yang Li Lao Tang: *Radix Ginseng*, *Radix Astragali seu Hedysari*, *Cortex Cinnamomi*, *Radix Angelicae Sinensis*, *Rhizoma Atractylodis Macrocephalae*, *Radix Glycyrrhizae*, *Pericarpium Citri Reticulata*, *Fructus Schisandrae*, *Rhizoma Zingiberis Recens*, *Fructus Ziziphi Jujubae*.

[181] Qian Zheng San: *Rhizoma Typhonii*, *Bombyx Batryticatus*, *Scorpic*.

[182] Wei Ling Tang: *Rhizoma Atractylodis*, *Cortex Magnoliae Officinalis*, *Pericarpium Citri Reticulatae*, *Radix Glycyrrhizae*, *Rhizoma Zingiberis Recens*, *Fructus Ziziphi Jujubae*, *Ramulus Cinnamomi*, *Rhizoma Atractylodis Macrocephalae*, *Rhizoma Alismatis*, *Poria*, *Polyporus Umbellatus*.

[183] Ji Chuan Jian: *Radix Angelicae Sinensis*, *Radix Achyranthis Bidentatae*, *Herba Cistanchis*, *Rhizoma Alismatis*, *Rhizoma Cimicifugae*, *Fructus Aurantii*.

[184] Ji Sheng Shen Qi Wan: *Radix Rehmanniae*, *Rhizoma Dioscoreae*, *Fructus Corni*, *Cortex Moutan Radicis*, *Poria*, *Rhizoma Alismatis*, *Radix Aconiti Praeparata*, *Ramulus Cinnamomi*, *Radix Achyranthis Bidentatae*, *Semen Plantaginis*.

[185] Yang Xin Tang: *Radix Astragali seu Hydysari*, *Poria*, *Poria cum Ligno Hospite*, *Radix Angelicae Sinensis*, *Rhizoma Ligustici Chuanxiong*, *Radix Glycyrrhizae Preaparata*, *Rhizoma Pinelliae*, *Semen Biotae*, *Radix Polygalae*, *Fructus Schisandrae*, *Radix Ginseng*, *Cortex Cinnamomi*.

[186] Shen Zhu San: *Rhizoma Atractylodis*, *Pericarpium Citri Reticulatae*, *Cortex Magnoliae Officinalis*, *Radix Glycyrrhizae*, *Herba Agastachis*, *Fructus Amomi*.

[187] Shen Xi Dan: *Cornu Rhinoceri*, *Rhizoma Acori Graminei*, *Radix Scutellariae*, *Radix Rehmanniae*, *Flos Lonicerae*, *Faeces Water*, *Fructus Forsythiae*, *Radix Isatidis*, *Semen Sojae Praeparatum*, *Radix Scrophulariae*, *Radix Arnebiae seu Lithospermi*, *Radix Trichosanthis*.

[188] Xiang Fu Xuan Fu Hua Tang: *raw Rhizoma Cyperi*, *Flos Inulae*, *Semen Coicis*, *Rhizoma Pinelliae*, *Exocarpium Citri Grandis*, *Poria*, *Fructus Perillae*.

[189] Xiang Sha Liu Jun Zi Tang: *Radix Aucklandiae*, *Fructus Amomi*, *Pericarpium Citri Reticulatae*, *Rhizoma Pinelliae Praeparatae*, *Radix Codonopsis pilosulae*, *Rhizoma Atractylodis Macrocephalae*, *Poria*, *Radix Glycyrrhizae*.

[190] Fu Yuan Huo Xue Tang: *Radix Bupleuri*, *Radix Trichosanthis*, *Radix Angelicae Sinensis*, *Flos Carthami*, *Radix Glycyrrhizae*, *Squama Manitis*, *Radix et Rhizoma Rhei*, *Semen Persical*.

[191] Shun Qi Dao Tan Tang: *Rhizoma Pinelliae*, *Pericarpium Citri Reticulatae*,

Poria, Radix Glycyrrhizae, Rhizoma Zingiberis Recens, Arisaemacum Bile, Fructus Aurantii Immaturus, Radix Aucklandiae, Rhizoma Cyperi.

[192] Bao Yuan Tang: *Radix Ginseng, Radix Astragali seu Hedysari, Cortex Cinnamomi, Radix Glycyrrhizae, Rhizoma Zingiberis Recens.*

[193] Bao He Wan: *Massa Fermentata Medicinalis, Fructus Crataegi, Poria, Rhizoma Pinelliae, Pericarpium Citri Reticulatae, Fructus Forsythiae, Semen Raphani.*

[194] Du Shen Tang: *Radix Ginseng.*

[195] Du Huo Ji Sheng Tang: *Radix Angelicae Pubescentis, Ramulus Loranthi, Radix Gentianae Macrophyllae, Radix Ledebouriellae, Herba Asari, Radix Angelicae Sinensis, Radix Paeoniae Alba, Rhizoma Ligustici Chuanxiong, Radix Rehmanniae, Cortex Eucommiae, Radix Achyranthis Bidentatae, Radix Ginseng, Poria, Radix Glycyrrhizae, and Cortex Cinnamomi.*

[196] Zhui Chong Wan: *Semen Arecae, Omphalia, Radix Aucklandiae, Cortex Melia, Gleditsia Sinensis Lam, Semen Pharbitidis, and Herba Artemisiae Capillaris.*

[197] Qin Jiu Bie Jia San: *Cortex Lycii Radicis, Radix Bupleuri, Radix Gentianae Macrophyllae, Rhizoma Anemarrhenae, Radix Angelicae Sinensis, Carapax Trionycis, Herba Artemisiae, and Fructus Mume.*

[198] Zhen Ren Yang Zang Tang: *Terminalia chebula Retz., Pericarpium Papaveris, Semen Myristicae, Rhizoma Atractylodis Macrocephalae, Radix Ginseng, Radix Aucklandiae, Cortex Cinnamomi, Radix glycyrrhizae Praeparata, Rhizoma Zingiberis Recens, and Fructus Ziziphi Jujubae.*

[199] Zhen Wu Tang: *Radix Aconiti (praeparata), Rhizoma Atractylodis Macrocephalae, Poria, Radix Paeoniae, and Rhizoma Zingiberis Recens.*

[200] Gui Zhi Tang: *Ramulus Cinnamomi, Radix Paeoniae, Rhizoma Zingiberis Recens, Radix Glycyrrhizae Praeparata, and Fructus Ziziphi Jujubae.*

[201] Gui Zhi Gan Cao Long Gu Mu Li Tang: *Ramulus Cinnamomi, Radix Glycyrrhizae Praeparata, Os Draconis Fossilia Ossis Mastodi, and Concha Ostreae.*

[202] Gui Zhi Jia Fu Zi Tang: *Ramulus Cinnamomi, Radix Paeoniae, Radix Glycyrrhizae Praeparata, Rhizoma Zingiberis Recens, Fructus Ziziphi Jujubae, and Radix Aconiti (praeparata).*

[203] Gui Zhi Shao Yao Zhi Mu Tang: *Ramulus Cinnamomi, Radix Paeoniae, Radix Glycyrrhizae Praeparata, Herba Ephedrae, Rhizoma Atractylodis Macrocephalae, Rhizoma Anemarrhenae, Radix Ledebouriellae, Radix Aconiti (praeparata), and Rhizoma Zingiberis Recens.*

[204] Tao Hong Yin: *Semen Persicae, Flos Carthami, Rhizoma Ligustici Chuanxiong, Radix Angelicae Sinensis, and Radix Clematidis.*

[205] Tao Hua Tang: *Halloysitum Rubrum, Rhizoma Zingiberis, and Oryza Sativa L.*

[206] Tao Ren Hong Hua Jian: *Radix Salviae Miltiorrhizae, Radix Paeoniae Rubra, Semen Persicae, Flos Carthami, Rhizoma Cyperi (praeparata), Rhizoma Cory-*

dalis, *Pericarpium Citri Reticulatae Viride*, *Radix Angelicae Sinensis*, *Rhizoma Ligustici Chuanxiong*, and *Radix Rehmanniae*.

[207] Gua Lou Gui Zhi Tang: *Fructus Trichosanthis*, *Ramulus Cinnamomi*, *Radix Paeoniae*, *Radix glycyrrhizae*, *Rhizoma Zingiberis Recens*, and *Fructus Ziziphi Jujubae*.

[208] Gua Lou Xie Bai Ban Xia Tang: *Fructus Trichosanthis*, *Bulbus Allii Macrostemi*, *White Wine*, and *Rhizoma Pinelliae*.

[209] Gua Lou Xie Bai Bai Jiu Tang: *Fructus Trichosanthis*, *Bulbus Allii Macrostemi*, and *White Wine*.

[210] Gua Lou Xie Bai Gui Zhi Tang: *Fructus Trichosanthis*, *Bulbus Allii Macrostemi*, *Ramulus Cinnamomi*, *Cortex Magnoliae Officinalis*, and *Fructus Aurantii Immaturus*.

[211] Chai Hu Shu Gan San: *Radix Bupleuri*, *Fructus Aurantii*, *Radix Paeoniae*, *Radix Glycyrrhizae*, *Rhizoma Cyperi (praeparata)*, and *Rhizoma Ligustici Chuanxiong*.

[212] Chai Zhi Ban Xia Tang: *Radix Bupleuri*, *Radix Scutellariae*, *Rhizoma Pinelliae*, *Fructus Aurantii*, *Radix Platycodi*, *Semen Armeniacae Amarum*, *Fructus Trichosanthis*, *Pericarpium Citri Reticulatae Viride*, and *Radix Glycyrrhizae*.

[213] Liang Ge San: *Radix et Rhizoma Rhei*, *Natrii Sulphas*, *Radix Glycyrrhiazae*, *Fructus Gardeniae*, *Herba Herba Menthae*, *Radix Scutellariae*, and *Fructus Forsythiae*.

[214] Run Chang Wan: *Radix Angelicae Sinensis*, *Radix Rehmanniae*, *Fructus Cannabis*, *Semen Persicae*, and *Fructus Aurantii*.

[215] Di Tan Tang: *Rhizoma Pinelliae (praeparata)*, *Rhizoma Arisaematis (praeparata)*, *Pericarpium Citri Reticulatae*, *Fructus Aurantii Immaturus*, *Poria*, *Radix Ginseng*, *Rhizoma Acori Graminei*, *Caulis Bambusae in Taeniam*, *Radix Glycyrrhizae*, and *Rhizoma Zingiberis Recens*.

[216] Xiao Ke Fang: *Rhizoma Coptidis Pulveratum*, *Radix Trichosanthis pulveratum*, *Radix Rehmanniae*, *Nodus Nelumbinis Rhizomatis*, *milk*, *Rhizoma Zingiberis Recens*, and *Mel*.

[217] Yi Wei Tang: *Radix Glehniae*, *Radix Ophiopogonis*, *Radix Rehanniae*, *Rhizoma Polygonati*, and *Saccharose*.

[218] Tiao Wei Cheng Qi Tang: *Radix et Rhizoma Rhei*, *Natrii Salphas*, and *Radix Glycyrrhizae Praeparata*.

[219] Tiao Ying Yin: *Rhizoma Zedoariae*, *Rhizoma Ligustici Chuanxiong*, *Radix Angelicae Sinensis*, *Rhizoma Corydalis*, *Radix Paeoniae Rubra*, *Herba Dianthi*, *Radix et Rhizoma Rhei*, *Semen Arecae*, *Pericarpium Citri Reticulatae*, *Pericarpium Arecae*, *Semen Lepidiiseu Descurainiae*, *Poria Rubra*, *Cortex Mori Radicis*, *Herba Asari*, *Cortex Cinnamomi*, *Radix Angelicae Dahuricae*, *Radix Gly-*

cyrrhizae Praeparata, Rhizoma Zingiberis Recens, and Fructus Ziziphi Jujubae.

[220] Mi Jing Wan: Semen Cuscutae, Semen Alliituberosi, Concha Ostreae, Os Draconis Fossilia Ossis Mastodi, Ootheca Mantidis, Poria, Fructus Schisandrae, and Halloysitum Alba.

[221] She Gan Ma Huang Tang: Rhizoma Belamcandae, Herba Ephedrae, Herba Asari, Radix Asteris, Flos Farfarae, Rhizoma Pinelliae, Fructus Schisandrae, Rhizoma Zingiberis Recens, and Fructus Ziziphi Jujubae.

[222] Xiao Yao San: Radix Bupleuri, Rhizoma Atractylodis Macrocephalae, Radix Paeoniae Alba, Radix Angelicae Sinensis, Poria, Radix Paeoniae Alba, Radix Angelicae Sinensis, Poria, Radix Glycyrrhizae Praeparata, Herba Menthae, and Rhizoma Zingiberis.

[223] Tong Qiao Huo Xue Tang: Radix Paeoniae Rubra, Rhizoma Ligustici Chuanxiong, Semen Persicae, Flos Carthami, Moschus, Bulbus Allii Fistulose, Rhizoma Zingiberis Recens, Fructus Ziziphi Jujubae, and Wine.

[224] Tong Yu Jian: Radix Angelicae Sinensis, Fructus Crataegi, Rhizoma Cyperis (praeparata), Flos Carthami, Radix Linderae, Pericarpium Citri Reticulatae Viride, Radix Aucklandiae, and Rhizoma Alismatis.

[225] Sang Bai Pi Tang: Cortex Mori Radicis, Rhizoma Pinelliae, Fructus Perillae, Semen Armeniacae Amarum, Bulbus Fritillariae, Radix Scutellariae, Rhizoma Coptidis, and Fructus Gardeniae.

[226] Sang Xing Tang: Folium Mori, Semen Armeniacae Amarum, Radix Glehniae, Bulbus Fritillariae, Semen Sojae Fermentatum, Fructus Gardeniae, and Pericarpium Pyri.

[227] Sang Ju Yin: Folium Mori, Flos Chrysanthemi, Fructus Forsythiae, Herba Menthae, Radix Platycodi, Semen Armeniacae Amarum, Rhizoma Phragmitis, and Radix Glycyrrhizae.

[228] Sang Piao Xiao San: Ootheca Mantidis, Radix Polygalae, Rhizoma Acori Graminei, Os Draconis Fossilia Ossis Mastodi, Radix Ginseng, Poria, Radix Angelicae Sinensis, and Plastrum Testudinis.

[229] Li Zhong Wan: Radix Ginseng, Rhizoma Atractylodis Macrocephalae, Rhizoma Zingiberis, and Radix Glycyrrhizae.

[230] Huang Tu Tang: Terra Flava Usta, Radix Glycyrrhizae, Radix Rehmanniae, Rhizoma Atractylodis Macrocephalae, Radix Aconiti (praeparata), Colla Corii Asini, and Radix Scutellariae.

[231] Huang Lian E Jiao Tang: Rhizoma Coptidis, Colla Corii Asini, Radix Scutellariae, yolk, and Radix Paeoniae.

[232] Huang Lian Qing Xin Yin: Rhizoma Coptidis, Radix Rehmanniae, Radix Angelicae Sinensis, Radix Glycyrrhizae, Semen Ziziphi Spinosae, Poria, Radix Polygallae, Radix Ginseng, and Semen Nelumbinis.

[233] Huang Lian Wen Dan Tang: *Rhizoma Pinelliae, Pericarpium Citri Reticulatae, Poria, Radix Glycyrrhizae, Fructus Aurantii Immaturus, Caulis Bambusae in Taeniam, Rhizoma Coptidis, and Fructus Ziziphi Jujubae.*

[234] Huang Qi Tang: *Radix Astragali seu Hedysari, Pericarpium Citri Reticulatae, Fructus Cannabis, and Mel.*

[235] Huang Qi Jian Zhong Tang: *Radix Astragali seu Hedysari, Radix Paeoniae Album, Ramulus Cinnamommi, Radix Glycyrrhizae Praeparata, Rhizoma Zingiberis Recens, Fructus Ziziphi Jujubae, and Saccharum Granorum.*

[236] Huang Bing Jiang Fan Wan: *Cortex Magnoliae Officinalis, Rhizoma Atractylodis Lanceae, Pericarpium Citri Reticulatae, Radix Glycyrrhizae, Ferrous Sulfate, and Fructus Ziziphi Jujubae.*

[237] Zhi Zi Chi Tang: *Fructus Gardeniae, and Semen Sojae Fermentatum.*

[238] Kong Xian Dan: *Radix Euphorbiae Kansui, Radix Euphorbiae Pekinensis, and Semen Sinapis Albae.*

[239] Lu Rong Wan: *Cornu Cervi Pantotrichum, Radix Ophiopogonis, Radix Rehmanniae Praeparata, Radix Astragali seu Hedysari, Fructus Schisandrae, Herba Cistanchis, Endothelium Corneum Gigeriae Galli, Fructus Psoraleae, Radix Scrophulariae, Poria, and Cortex Lycii Radicis.*

[240] Ma Zi Ren Wan: *Fructus Cannabis, Radix Paeoniae, Fructus Aurantii Immaturus (praeparata), Radix et Rhizoma Rhei, Cortex Magnoliae Officinalis, and Semen Armeniacae Amarum.*

[241] Ma Xing Shi Gan Tang: *Herba Ephedrae, Semen Armeniacae Amarum, Gypsum Fibrosum, and Radix Glycyrrhizae Praeparata.*

[242] Ma Huang Tang: *Herba Ephedrae, Ramulus Cinnamomi, Semen Armeniacae Amarum, and Radix Glycyrrhizae Praeparata.*

[243] Ma Huang Lian Qiao Chi Xiao Dou Tang: *Herba Ephedrae, Semen Armeniacae Amarum, Cortex Catalpae Ovatae Radicis, Fructus Forsythiae, Semen Phaseoli, Radix Glycyrrhizae, Rhizoma Zingiberis Recens, and Fructus Ziziphi Jujubae.*

[244] Xuan Fu Dai Zhe Tang: *Flos Inulae, Ochra Haematitum, Radix Ginseng, Rhizoma Pinelliae, Radix Glycyrrhizae Praeparata, Rhizoma Zingiberis Recens, and Fructus Ziziphi Jujubae.*

[245] Xuan Fu Hua Tang: *Flos Inulae, and Bulbus Allii Fistulosi.*

[246] Ling Yang Jiao Tang: *Cornu Saigae Tataricae, Plastrum Testudinis, Radix Rehmanniae, Cortex Moutan Radicis, Radix Paeoniae Alba, Radix Bupleuri, Herba Menthae, Periostracum Cicadae, Flos Chrysanthemi, Spica Prunellae, and Concha Haliotidis.*

[247] Ling Yang Gou Teng Tang: *Cornu Saigae Tataricae, Folium Mori, Bulbus Fritillariae, Radix Rehmanniae, Ramulus Uncariae cum Uncis, Flos Chrysanthemi, Radix Paeoniae Alba, Radix Glycyrrhizae, Caulis Bambusae in Taeniam, and*

Poria.

[248] Qing Jin Hua Tan Tang: *Radix Scutellariae, Fructus Gardeniae, Radix Platycodi, Radix Ophiopogonis, Cortex Mori Radicis, Bulbus Fritillariae, Rhizoma Anemarrhenae, Fructus Trichosanthis, Exocarpium Citri Reticulatae, Poria, and Radix Glycyrrhizae.*

[249] Qing Fei Yin: *Poria, Radix Scutellariae, Cortex Mori Radicis, Radix Ophiopogonis, Semen Plantaginis, Fructus Gardeniae, and Caulis Aristolochiae Manshuriensis.*

[250] Qing Wei San: *Radix Angelicae Sinensis, Radix Rehmanniae, Cortex Moutan Radicis, Rhizoma Cimicifugae, and Rhizoma Coptidis.*

[251] Qing Gu San: *Radix Stellariae, Rhizoma Picrorhizae, Radix Gentianae Macrophyllae, Carapax Trionycis, Cortex Lycii Radix Glycyrrhizae.*

[252] Qing Ying Tang: *Cornu Rhinocerotis, Radix Rehmanniae, Radix Scrophulariae, Herba Lophatheri, Radix Ophiopogonis, Radix Salviae Miltiorrhizae, Radix Coptidis, Flos Lonicerae, and Fructus Forsythiae.*

[253] Qing Wen Bai Du Yin: *Gypsum Fibrosum, Radix Rehmanniae, Cornu Rhinocerotis, Radix Coptidis, Fructus Gardeniae, Radix Platycodi, Radix Scutellariae, Bulbus Fritillariae, Radix Paeoniae Rubra, Radix Scrophulariae, Fructus Forsythiae, Radix Glycyrrhizae, Cortex Moutan Radicis, and Herba Lophatheri.*

[254] Qing Zao Jiu Fei Tang: *Folium Mori, Gypsum Fibrosum, Semen Armeniacae Amarum, Radix Glycyrrhizae, Radix Ophiopogonis, Radix Ginseng, Colla Corii Asini, Fructus Cannabis, and Folium Eriobotryae(praeparata).*

[255] Yin Qiao San: *Flos Lonicerae, Fructus Arctii, Herba Menthae, Radix Platycodi, Spica Schizonepetae, Radix Glycyrrhizae, Herba Lophatheri, and Rhizoma Phragmitis.*

[256] Zhu Du Wan: *Rhizoma Atractylodis Macrocephalae, Radix Sophorae Flavescentis, Concha Ostreae, and Gaster Hys Trichis.*

[257] Zhu Ling Tang: *Polyporus, Poria, Rhizoma Alismatis, Colla Corii Asini, and Talcum.*

[258] Ban Long Wan: *Radix Rehmanniae Praeparata, Semen Cuscutae, Fructus Psoraleae, Semen Biotae, Poria, Colla Cornus Cervi, and Cornu Cervi Degelatinatum.*

[259] Ge Gen Tang: *Radix Puerariae, Herba Ephedrae, Ramulus Cinnamomi, Rhizoma Zingiberis Recens, Radix Glycyrrhizae, Radix Paeoniae, and Fructus Ziziphi Jujubae.*

[260] Ge Gen Qin Lian Tang: *Radix Puerariae, Radix Scutellariae, Radix Coptidis, and Radix Glycyrrhizae Praeparata.*

[261] Ting Li Da Zao Xie Fei Tang: *Semen Lepidii seu Descurainiae and Fructus Ziziphi Jujubae.*

[262] Yue Bi Jia Zhu Tang: *Herba Ephedrae, Gypsum Fibrosum, Radix Glycyrrhizae, Fructus Ziziphi Jujubae, Rhizoma Atractylodis Macrocephalae,* and *Rhizoma Zingiberis Recens.*

[263] Yue Bi Jia Ban Xia Tang: *Herba Ephedrae, Gypsum Fibrosum, Rhizoma Zingiberis Recens, Fructus Ziziphi Jujubae, Radix Glycyrrhizae,* and *Rhizoma Pinelliae.*

[264] Yue Ju Wan: *Rhizoma Ligustici Chuanxiong, Rhizoma Atractylodis Lanceae, Rhizoma Cyperi, Fructus Gardeniae (praeparata),* and *Massa Fermentata Medicinalis.*

[265] Jiao Mu Gua Lou Tang: *Semen Zanthoxyli, Semen Trichosanthis, Semen Lepidii seu Descurainiae, Folium Mori, Fructus Perillae, Rhizoma Pinelliae, Poria, Exocarpium Citri Reticulatae, Fructus Tribuli,* and *Rhizoma Zingiberis Recens.*

[266] Xiao Shi Fan Shi San: *Potassium Nitrate* and *Alumen.*

[267] Zi Xue Dan: *Talcum, Gypsum Fibrosum, Calcitum, Magnetitum, Cornu Saigae Tataricae, Radix Aristolochiae, Cornu Rhinocerotis, Lignum Aquilariae Resinatum, Flos Caryophylli, Rhizoma Cimicifugae, Radix Scrophulariae, Radix Glycyrrhizae, Natrii Sulphas, Cinnabaris, Moschus, Aurum,* and *Potassium Nitrate.*

[268] Hei Xi Dan: *Galenite, Sulphur, Fructus Meliae Toosendan, Semen Trigonellae, Radix Aucklandiae, Radix Aconiti Praeparata, Semen Myristicae, Actinolitum, Lignum Aquilariae, Resinatum Fructus Foenicuii, Cortex Cinnamomi,* and *Fructus Psoraleae.*

[269] Tong Xie Yao Fang: *Rhizoma Atractylodis Macrocephalae, Radix Paeoniae Alba, Radix Ledebouriellae,* and *Pericarpium Citrii Reticulatae (praeparata).*

[270] Wen Dan Tang: *Rhizoma Pinelliae, Pericarpium Citrii Reticulatae, Radix Glycyrrhizae, Fructus Aurantii Immaturus, Caulis Bambusae in Taeniam, Rhizoma Zingiberis Recens,* and *Poria.*

[271] Zi Shui Qing Gan Yin: *Radix Rehmanniae, Fructus Corni, Poria, Radix Angelicae Sinensis, Rhizoma Dioscoreae, Cortex Moutan Radicis, Rhizoma Alismatis, Radix Paeoniae Alba, Radix Bupleuri, Fructus Gardeniae,* and *Semen Ziziphi Spinosae.*

[272] Cheng Shi Bi Xie Fen Qing Yin: *Rhizoma Dioscoreae Septemlobae, Semen Plantaginis, Poria, Plumula Nelumbinis, Rhizoma Acori Graminei, Cortex Phellodendri, Radix Salviae Miltiorrhizae,* and *Rhizoma Atractylodis Macrocephalae.*

[273] Xi Jiao Di Huang Tang: *Cornu Rhinocerotis, Radix Rehmanniae, Cortex Moutan Radicis,* and *Radix Paeoniae.*

[274] Xi Jiao San: *Cornu Rhinocerotis, Rhizoma Coptidis, Rhizoma Cimicifugae, Fructus Gardeniae,* and *Herba Artemisiae Capillaris.*

[275] Shu Zao Yin Zi: *Radix Phytolaccae, Rhizoma Alismatis, Semen Phaseoli, Semen Xanthoxyli, Caulis Aristolochiae Manshuriensis, Poria, Pericarpium Arecae, Semen Arecae, Rhizoma Zingeberis Recens, Rhizoma seu Radix Notopterygii, and Radix Gentianae Macrophyllae.*

[276] Hao Qin Qing Dan Tang: *Herba Artemisiae, Caulis Bambusae in Taeniam, Rhizoma Pinelliae, Poria, Radix Scutellariae, Fructus Aurantii, Percarpium Citri Reticulatae, Bi Yu San (Talcum, Radix Glycyrrhizae, and Indigo Naturalis).*

[277] Nuan Gan Jian: *Cortex Cinnamomi, Fructus Foenicuii, Poria, Radix Linderae, Fructus Lycii, Radix Angelicae Sinensis, Lignum Aquilariae, Resinatum and Rhizoma Zingiberis Recens.*

[278] Xin Jia Xiang Ru Yin: *Herba Elscholtziae seu Moslae, Flos Dolichoris, Cortex Magnoliae Officinalis, Flos Lonicerae, and Fructus Forsythiae.*

[279] Jie Yu Dan: *Rhizoma Typhonii, Rhizoma Acori Graminei, Radix Polygalae, Rhizoma Gastrodiae, Scorpio, Rhizoma seu Radix Notopterygii, Rhizoma Arisaematis, Radix Aucklandiae, and Radix Glycyrrhizae.*

[280] Suan Zao Ren Tang: *Semen Ziziphi Spinosae, Rhizoma Anemarrhenae, Rhizoma Ligustici Chuanxiong, Poria, Radix Glycyrrhizae.*

[281] Gao Lin Tang: *Rhizoma Dioscoreae, Semen Euryales, Os Draconis Fossilia Ossis Mastodi, Concha Ostreae, Radix Rehmanniae, Radix Codonopsis Pilosulae, and Radix Paeoniae Alba.*

[282] Ge Xia Zhu Yu Tang: *Faeces Trogopterorum, Radix Angelicae Sinensis, Rhizoma Ligustici Chuanxiong, Semen Persicae, Cortex Moutan Radicis, Radix Paeoniae Rubra, Radix Linderae, Rhizoma Corydalis, Radix Glycyrrhizae, Rhizoma Cyperi(praeparata), Flos Carthami, and Fructus Aurantii.*

[283] Zeng Ye Tang: *Radix Scrophulariae, Radix Ophiopogonis, and Radix Rehmanniae.*

[284] Zeng Ye Cheng Qi Tang: *Radix et Rhizoma Rhei, Natrii Sulphas, Radix Scrophulariae, Radix Ophiopogonis, and Radix Rehmanniae.*

[285] Yi Yi Ren Tang: *Semen Coicis, Rhizoma Ligustici Chuanxion, Radix Angelicae Sinensis, Herba Ephedrae, Ramulus Cinnamomi, Rhizoma seu Radix Notopterygii, Radix Angelicae Pubescentis, Radix Ledebouriellae, Radix Aconii, Rhizoma Atractylodis Lanceae, Radix Glycyrrhizae, and Rhizoma Zingiberis Recens.*

[286] Ju Pi Zhu Ru Tang: *Radix Ginseng, Pericarpium Citri Reticulatae, Caulis Bambusae in Taeniam, Radix Glycyrrhizae, Rhizoma Zingiberis Recens, and Fructus Ziziphi Jujubae.*

[287] Dai Ge San: *Indigo Naturalis and Concha Meretricis seu Cyclinae.*

[288] Huo Xiang Zheng Qi San: *Herba Agastachis, Perillae Frutescens, Radix Angelicae Dahuricae, Radix Platycodi, Rhizoma Atractylodis Macrocephalae, Cortex Magnoliae Officinalis, Rhizoma Pinelliae (praeparata), Pericarpium Arecae,*

Poria, Pericarpium Citri Reticulatae, Radix Glycyrrhizae, and Fructus Ziziphi Jujubae.

[289] Meng Shi Gun Tan Wan: Lapis Chloriti, Lignum Aquilariae Resinatum, Radix et rhizoma Rhei, Radix Scutellariae, and Natrii Sulphas.

[290] Bie Jia Jian Wan: Carapax Trionycis, Rhizoma Belamcandae, Radix Scutellariae, Radix Bupleuri, Armadillidium Vulgare, Rhizoma Zingiberis, Radix et Rhizoma Rhei, Radix Paeoniae, Ramulus Cinnamomi, Semen Lepidii seu Descurainiae, Folium Pyrrosia, Cortex Magnoliae Officinalis, Cortex Moutan Radicis, Herba Dianthi, Radix Campsis, Rhizoma Pinelliae, Radix Ginseng, Eupolyphaga seu Steleophaga, Colla Corii Asini, Nidus Vespae, Allomyrina, and Semen Persicae.

[291] Zhen Gan Xi Feng Tang: Radix Achyranthis Bidentatae, Os Draconis Fossilia Ossis Mastodi, Radix Paeoniae, Radix Asparagi, Fructus Hordei Germinatus, Ochra Haematitum, Concha Ostreae, Radix Scrophulariae, Fructus Meliae Toosendan, Herba Artemisiae Capillaris, Radix Glycyrrhizae, and Plastrum Testudinis.

2. Indexes of Diseases of Western Medicine

A

- acute cholecystitis (411)
- acute enteritis (382)
- acute gastritis (365)(371)
- acute hepatitis (411)
- acute leukemia (434)
- acute lumbar muscle sprain (466)
- acute myelitis (487)
- acute nephritis (447)
- acute pancreatitis (405)
- Addison's disease (500)
- adhesive ileus (405)
- amebic dysentery (388)
- anemia (300)(333)(340)
- anemic insomnia (345)
- angina pectoris (308)
- ankylosing spondylitis (466)
- aplastic anemia (434)(500)
- arrhythmia (300)
- ascariasis (400)
- ascariasis of biliary tract (411)
- ascites due to cirrhosis (428)
- atelectasis (277)
- auditory vertigo (373)

B

- bacillary dysentery (388)
- bronchial asthma (270)(285)
- bronchiectasis (262)(434)
- bronchitis (262)
- bronchopulmonary carcinoma (434)

C

- carcinoma of colon (391)
- carcinoma of stomach (369)(426)(434)
- cardiac edema (447)
- cardiac neurosis (300)(306)
- cardiogenic shock (314)
- cardiomyopathy (306)
- celiac tumor (422)

- cerebral embolism (321)
- cerebral thrombosis (321)
- cerebroma (329)(333)(337)
- cerebrovascular spasm (314)
- cholecystitis (416)
- cholelithiasis (416)
- cholestatic hepatitis (416)
- chronic asthmatic bronchitis (270)(277)
- chronic atrophic gastritis (369)(375)
- chronic bronchitis (285)
- chronic cholecystitis (411)
- chronic constrictive pericarditis (428)
- chronic enteritis (382)
- chronic gastritis (365)(369)
- chronic granulocytic leukemia (500)
- chronic hepatitis (411)
- chronic infectional fever (493)
- chronic nephritis (447)
- chronic nonspecific ulcerative colitis (388)(434)
- chyluria (454)
- cirrhosis (411)(422)
- colitis (405)
- congestive heart-failure (285)(300)
- coronary heart disease (304)(309)
- cor pulmonale (277)

D

- diabetes (471)
- diabetes insipidus (471)
- dietetic constipation (394)

E

- epidemic cerebrospinal meningitis (329)
- epidemic encephalitis B (329)
- epilepsy (361)
- exudative pleurisy (285)

F

- fasciolopsiasis (400)
- fever due to malignant tumor (493)

G

- gastrectasia (379)
- gastritis (368)
- gastroduodenal ulcer (365)
- gastrointestinal dysfunction (285)
- gastrointestinal influenza (372)
- gastrointestinal neurosis (377)(382)(396)(405)(409)
- gastroptosia (365)
- glaucoma (333)
- glomerulonephritis (434)
- gout (482)

H

- habitual constipation (394)
- hemorrhagic shock (314)
- hepatic abscess (411)
- hepatic parasitosis (411)
- hepatosplenomegaly (425)
- hookworm disease(ancylostomiasis) (400)
- hyperosteogeny of lumbar vertebra (466)
- hyperpyretic convulsion (329)
- hypertension (333)(340)
- hypertensive encephalopathy (318)
- hypertensive insomnia (345)
- hyperthyroidism (294)(300)(471)(493)
- hypoglycemic shock (316)
- hypotension (340)
- hypothyroidism (500)
- hysteria (314)(353)
- hysterical gasp (277)

- hysterical syncope　　　　　　(316)

I

- icteric infectious mononucleosis　(416)
- icteric viral hepatitis　　　　(416)
- incomplete pylorochesis　　　(285)
- influenza　　　　　　　　　(333)
- insomnia due to dyspepsia　　(345)
- intercostal neuralgia　　　　(411)
- intestinal obstruction　(407)(422)
- involutional psychosis　　　(356)
- irritable colon　　　　　　　(388)

L

- lacunar cerebral infarction　　(321)
- laryngopharyngitis　　　　　(266)
- leptospirosis　　　　　　　(416)
- lumbar muscle strain　　　　(466)

M

- medicamentous liver lesion　　(416)
- manic-depressive psychosis　(356)
- Ménière's disease　　　　　(340)
- menopausal syndrome　(294)(350)
- myasthenia gravis　　　　　(487)
- myxedema　　　　　　　　(447)

N

- nephrotic syndrome　(447)(428)
- psychogenic vomiting　　　　(371)
- neurosis
  　　(333)(340)(345)(350)(356)(451)
- neurotic low fever　　　　　(493)

O

- occipital neuralgia　　　　　(333)
- osseous arthritis　　　　　　(482)
- oxyuriasis　　　　　　　　(400)

P

- pelvic disease　　　　　　　(466)
- peptic ulcer　　　　　(371)(434)
- periodic paralysis　　　　　(487)
- peripheral facial paralysis　　(321)
- pleurisy　　　　　　　　　(306)
- pneumonia　　　　　(262)(434)
- polyneuritis　　　　　　　(487)
- portal cirrhosis　　　　　　(434)
- postconcussional syndrome　　(333)
- progressive myatrophy　　　(487)
- prolapse of gastric mucosa　　(365)
- prolapse of lumbar intervertebral disc　　　　　　　　　　(466)
- prosopalgia　　　　　　　(333)
- prostatitis　　　　　　　　(454)
- psychogenic reaction　　　　(356)
- psychoneurotic constipation　(394)
- pulmonary emphysema　(270)(277)
- pulmonary encephalopathy　　(314)
- pulmonary tuberculosis
  　　　　　(262)(277)(434)(439)
- pylorochesis　　　　　　　(373)

R

- rectal carcinoma　　　　　(391)
- renal tuberculosis　　　　　(434)
- renal tumor　　　　　　　(434)
- rheumatic arthritis　　　　　(482)
- rheumatic fever　　　(294)(493)
- rheumatism　　　　　　　(466)
- rheumatoid arthritis　　　　(482)

S

- scapulohumeral periarthritis　(482)
- schistosomiasis　　　　　　(388)
- schizophrenia　　　　　　(356)
- senile constipation　　　　　(394)

— 533 —

- senile vertigo (340)
- Sheehan's syndrome (500)
- shock (294)
- silicosis (281)
- subarachnoid hemorrhage (321)

T

- tetany (329)
- thrombocytopenic purpura (434)
- toxic dysentery (390)
- transient cerebral ischemia (321)
- tubercular meningitis (329)
- tubercular peritonitis (428)
- tuberculosis (294)(493)
- tuberculosis of lumbar vertebra (466)
- tumor of lumbar vertebra (466)

U

- upper respiratory tract infection (262)(264)
- urinaemia (380)
- urinary infection (454)
- urinary stone (454)
- urinary tract obstruction (461)
- urinary tuberculosis (454)
- urinary tumor (454)

V

- vascular headache (333)
- vasodepressor syncope (316)
- vegetative nerve functional disturbance (294)
- viral myocarditis (300)(306)